Amazon

1998

Purple
Eagle

The Central Nervous System

The Central

New York • Oxford   OXFORD UNIVERSITY PRESS • 1998

Nervous System

Structure and Function

SECOND EDITION

PER BRODAL

Institute of Basic Medical Sciences

University of Oslo

Oxford University Press

Oxford   New York
Athens   Auckland   Bangkok   Bogota
Bombay   Buenos Aires   Calcutta   Cape Town
Dar es Salaam   Delhi   Florence   Hong Kong
Istanbul   Karachi   Kuala Lumpur   Madras
Madrid   Melbourne   Mexico City   Nairobi
Paris   Singapore   Taipei   Tokyo
Toronto   Warsaw

and associated companies in
Berlin   Ibadan

Published by Oxford University Press, Inc.
198 Madison Avenue, New York, New York 10016

Oxford is a registered trademark of Oxford University Press

Library of Congress Cataloging-in-Publication Data

Brodal, Per.
[Sentralnervesystemet. English]
The central nervous system: structure and function / Per Brodal.—
2nd ed.
p.   cm.
Includes bibliographical references and index.
ISBN 0-19-511741-7
1. Neuroanatomy.   2. Central nervous system—Anatomy.   I. Title.
[DNLM: 1. Central Nervous System—physiology.   2. Central Nervous
System—anatomy & histology.   WL 300 B8645s 1998a]
QM451.B78613   1998
612.8—DC21
DNLM/DLC
for Library of Congress   96-40369
CIP

1 2 3 4 5 6 7 8 9

Printed in the United States of America
on acid-free paper

Preface

This book is intended primarily for use by students of medicine, physical therapy, and psychology, that is, for use in neuroscience or neuroanatomy courses for students who need knowledge of the nervous system as a basis for later clinical study and practice.

This second edition is the result of a major revision incorporating the most important new findings of the last five years. Several chapters have been reorganized to include new material and to make the text easy to follow. Two new chapters deal with development, aging, and plasticity (Chapter 4) and basic properties of sensory receptors (Chapter 6). New illustrations have been added and others have been redrawn to improve their clarity. Altogether the text is somewhat expanded, but hopefully without making the reading more cumbersome. My intentions remain the same as those of my father, Alf Brodal, when he wrote the Norwegian forerunner of this book many years ago: to stimulate understanding rather than memorization of isolated facts, while at the same time fostering a realistic attitude toward our still-limited ability to explain the marvels of the human brain.

The book aims to present the difficult subject of neuroscience so that it can be understood by those approaching it for the first time. Therefore, many details are left out that might be of great interest to the specialist but would merely obscure the essentials for the beginner. Everyday experiences and clinical examples are integrated in the text throughout to help students link the new material with their prior knowledge and future profession. The nervous system, however, is exceedingly complex both structurally and functionally, and much remains to be learned before we can answer many fundamental questions. Thus, while an undergraduate course can provide only partial insights, no one is served by a presentation that avoids controversial issues and areas of ignorance. Indeed, pointing out what we do *not* know is sometimes better than presenting an oversimplified version. For this reason I have also discussed *how* the data were obtained and the limitations inherent in the various methods.

The main challenge—for both the student and the scientist—is to understand how the nervous system solves its multifarious tasks. This requires an integrated approach, drawing on data from all fields of neurobiology, as well as psychology and clinical research. Textbooks sharing this goal nevertheless differ markedly in how they present the material and where they put the emphasis. Perhaps because my own field of research is the wiring patterns of the brain, I strongly feel that knowledge of how the nervous system is built, in particular how the various parts are interconnected to form functional systems, is a prerequisite for proper understanding of data from other fields. A fair knowledge of brain anatomy is especially important for sound interpretations of the symptoms of brain disease. Textbooks of neuroanatomy often overwhelm the reader with details that are not strictly relevant for either functional analysis or clinical thinking. Neither does a strong emphasis on cellular mechanisms at the expense of the properties of neural systems seem the right choice if the aim is to help readers understand how the brain performs its tasks and how the site of a disease process relates to a patient's symptoms. Therefore, neither anatomical nor cellular and molecular details are included in this book if they cannot in some way be related to function. My hope is that the book presents a balance of cellular and neural systems material that is right for students.

In-depth sections and more advanced clinical material are placed in boxes so that they should not disturb reading of the main text. Since the needs of readers differ, however, they are encouraged to read selectively and pick the material they find most relevant and interesting from *their* perspective, regardless of whether it is placed in the main text or in boxes. The frequent subheadings should facilitate such selective reading. Many difficult or complex subjects are preceded with an overview that may suffice for some readers, while other readers will want to read all the text, including the boxes.

During the preparation of the former and the present editions, I have received help from several colleagues, for which I am truly grateful. Jan Bjaalie, Niels Christian Danbolt, Paul Heggelund, Jan Jansen, Harald Kryvi, Kirsten Osen, Ole Petter Ottersen, Eric Rinvik, and Jon Storm-Mathisen have all provided constructive criticism and advice. I also gratefully acknowledge the expert help of Kari Ruud, who prepared the new line-drawings, and of Gunnar Lothe and Carina Ingebrigtsen, who produced the photographic work.

Oslo, Norway   P. B.
April 1997

Contents

A Brief Survey

The essential building block of the nervous system is the *nerve cell*, specialized for rapid conveyance of signals over long distances and in a very precise manner. Together, billions of nerve cells in the brain form complicated and *highly organized networks* for *communication* and information processing.

The nervous system receives a wealth of information from an individual's surroundings and body. From all this information, it extracts the essentials, stores what may be needed later, and emits a command to muscles or glands if an answer is appropriate. Sometimes the answer comes within milliseconds, as a *reflex* or *automatic response*. At other times it may take considerably longer, requiring cooperation among many parts of the brain and involving conscious processes. In any case, the main task of the nervous system is to ensure that the organism *adapts* optimally to the environment.

The nervous system is equipped with *sense organs*, *receptors*, that react to various forms of sensory information or stimuli. Regardless of the mode of stimulation (the form of energy), the receptors "translate" the energy of the stimulus to the language spoken by the nervous system, that is, *nerve impulses*. These are tiny electric discharges rapidly conducted along the nerve processes. In this way signals are conveyed from the receptors to the regions of the nervous system where information processing takes place.

The nervous system can elicit an external response only by acting on *effectors*, which are either muscles or glands. The response is either *movement* or *secretion*. Obviously, muscle contraction can have various expressions, from communication through speech, facial expression, and bodily posture, to walking and running, respiratory movements, and changes of blood pressure. But one should bear in mind that the nervous system can only act on muscles and glands to express its "will." Conversely, if we are to judge the activity going on in the brain of another being, we have only the expressions produced by muscle contraction and secretion to go by.

On an anatomic basis we can divide the nervous system into the *central nervous system* (CNS), consisting of the brain and the spinal cord, and the *peripheral nervous system* (PNS), which connects the central nervous system with the receptors and the effectors. Although without sharp transitions, the PNS and the CNS can be subdivided into parts that are concerned primarily with the regulation of visceral organs and the internal milieu, and parts that are concerned mainly with the more or less conscious adaptation to the external world. The first division is called the *autonomic* or visceral nervous system; the second is usually called *somatic nervous system*. The latter, also called the *cerebrospinal nervous system*, receives information from sense organs capturing events in our surroundings (vision, hearing, receptors in the skin) and controls the activity of voluntary muscles (made up of cross-striated skeletal muscle cells). In contrast, the autonomic nervous system controls the activity of involuntary muscles (smooth muscle and heart muscle cells) and gland cells. The autonomic system may be further subdivided into the *sympathetic system*, mainly concerned with mobilizing the resources of the body when demands are increased (as in emergencies), and the *parasympathetic system*, which is devoted more to the daily maintenance of the body.

The higher an animal is on the scale of evolution, the more complicated is its central nervous system. The tasks carried out by the CNS are correspondingly complex and varied, reaching a maximal development in humans, in whom the brain provides enormous flexibility and adaptability compared with the brains of lower animals. This evolutionary development depends in part on development of the sense organs, in particular those providing information about events taking place at some distance (vision, hearing, and to some extent, smell). By means of these senses, the range of experience is vastly increased, and the animal can adapt in advance to external events. Thus, the animal may predict on the basis of previous experience what is going to happen and alter its behavior accordingly (escape from enemies, search for food or partner, and so on). For more primitive animals the amount and variety of sensory information that has to be integrated to give an appropriate response is limited. The development of new and specialized senses means, of course, that more information reaches the brain. This would be of little use, however, if the brain had not increased its capacity to process information. Thus, what we see in evolution is that the size of the brain increases because many more nerve cells are needed for the greater number of impulse pathways and interconnections. The brain is increasingly differentiated, in the sense that it can handle a wider variety of information and also vary its responses over a much wider range than is the case in lower animals. The more an animal organizes its activities on the basis of previous experience, and the more it is freed from the dominance of immediate sensations, the more complicated are the processes required of the central nervous system.

The higher processes of integration and association—that is, what we call *mental processes*—are first and foremost a function of the *cerebral cortex*. Consequently, this part of the brain shows the most marked relative increase in number of nerve cells as we go from lower to higher vertebrate. In lower mammals (such as the rat) the modest cerebral cortex is mostly engaged in receiving sensory messages or in sending out commands to the muscles. In higher species, especially anthropoid apes and humans, large parts of the cortex are engaged in comparing and integrating the vast amount of immediate information with that stored from previous experiences. Nevertheless, the basic principles underlying the structure and function of this most elaborate part of the brain are the same as for the more primitive parts, and cannot be understood without knowledge of them.

concerned primarily with the regulation of visceral organs and the internal milieu, and parts that are concerned mainly with the more or less conscious adaptation to the external world. The first division is called the *autonomic* or visceral nervous system; the second is usually called *somatic nervous system*. The latter, also called the *cerebrospinal nervous system*, receives information from sense organs capturing events in our surroundings (vision, hearing, receptors in the skin) and controls the activity of voluntary muscles (made up of cross-striated skeletal muscle cells). In contrast, the autonomic nervous system controls the activity of involuntary muscles (smooth muscle and heart muscle cells) and gland cells. The autonomic system may be further subdivided into the *sympathetic system*, mainly concerned with mobilizing the resources of the body when demands are increased (as in emergencies), and the *parasympathetic system*, which is devoted more to the daily maintenance of the body.

The higher an animal is on the scale of evolution, the more complicated is its central nervous system. The tasks carried out by the CNS are correspondingly complex and varied, reaching a maximal development in humans, in whom the brain provides enormous flexibility and adaptability compared with the brains of lower animals. This evolutionary development depends in part on development of the sense organs, in particular those providing information about events taking place at some distance (vision, hearing, and to some extent, smell). By means of these senses, the range of experience is vastly increased, and the animal can adapt in advance to external events. Thus, the animal may predict on the basis of previous experience what is going to happen and alter its behavior accordingly (escape from enemies, search for food or partner, and so on). For more primitive animals the amount and variety of sensory information that has to be integrated to give an appropriate response is limited. The development of new and specialized senses means, of course, that more information reaches the brain. This would be of little use, however, if the brain had not increased its capacity to process information. Thus, what we see in evolution is that the size of the brain increases because many more nerve cells are needed for the greater number of impulse pathways and interconnections. The brain is increasingly differentiated, in the sense that it can handle a wider variety of information and also vary its responses over a much wider range than is the case in lower animals. The more an animal organizes its activities on the basis of previous experience, and the more it is freed from the dominance of immediate sensations, the more complicated are the processes required of the central nervous system.

The higher processes of integration and association—that is, what we call *mental processes*—are first and foremost a function of the *cerebral cortex*. Consequently, this part of the brain shows the most marked relative increase in number of nerve cells as we go from lower to higher vertebrate. In lower mammals (such as the rat) the modest cerebral cortex is mostly engaged in receiving sensory messages or in sending out commands to the muscles. In higher species, especially anthropoid apes and humans, large parts of the cortex are engaged in comparing and integrating the vast amount of immediate information with that stored from previous experiences. Nevertheless, the basic principles underlying the structure and function of this most elaborate part of the brain are the same as for the more primitive parts, and cannot be understood without knowledge of them.

PART I

MAIN FEATURES
OF STRUCTURE
AND FUNCTION

General information about the structure and function of the nervous system forms a necessary basis for treatment of the specific systems described in subsequent parts of this book. Chapter 1 describes the structure of nervous tissue, while Chapter 2 deals with its properties as a basis for understanding communication between nerve cells. Chapter 3 gives an overview of the macroscopic, and to some extent microscopic, structure of the nervous system with brief descriptions of functions. Chapter 4 deals with the development of the nervous system before and after birth with particular reference to how its incredibly complicated and precise patterns of connections may arise. Furthermore, we treat the plasticity of the nervous system in response to normal challenges and to brain damage, and also the effects of aging. Chapter 5 provides some general approaches to neurobiological research and some methods used to obtain the information presented in this book.

CHAPTER 1

CELLULAR ELEMENTS OF NERVOUS TISSUE

The nervous system is built up of nerve cells, *neurons*, and special kinds of supporting cells, *glial cells*. The nerve cells are responsible for the functions that are unique to the nervous system, whereas the glial cells primarily serve the needs of the neurons. Neurons are characterized by their ability to respond to stimuli with an electrical discharge, a *nerve impulse*, and, further, by their fast conduction of the nerve impulse over long distances. In this way, signals can be transmitted in milliseconds from one place to another, either within the central nervous system or between it and other organs of the body. The functions of the glial cells are still not completely known. It is established, however, that they are responsible for isolating neuronal processes and controlling the environment of neurons and that they take part in repair processes. Glial cells also play important roles during the embryological development of the nervous system.

Figure 1.1 *A neuron*. Half-schematic drawing of a neuron (pyramidal cell) from the cerebral cortex. Note the two types of processes emerging from the perikaryon. Small spikes on the dendrites are called spines (spina, plural spinae).

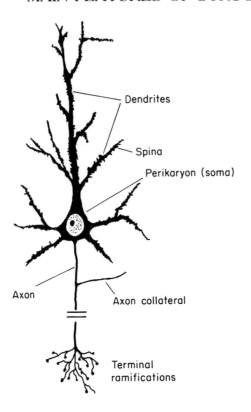

STRUCTURE OF THE NEURON

Neurons Have Long Processes

Like other cells, a neuron has a cell body with a nucleus surrounded by cytoplasm containing various organelles. The cell body is also called the *perikaryon* or *soma*. Long processes extend from the cell body. The number and length of the processes can vary, but they are of two main kinds. There are usually several *dendrites*, whereas there is only one *axon* (Fig. 1.1). The dendrites usually branch and form dendritic "trees" with a large surface to receive signals from other nerve cells. Each neuron has only one axon, which is specially built to conduct the nerve impulse from the cell body to other cells. The axon may have many ramifications, enabling its parent cell to influence many other cells.

To study the elements of nervous tissue, it is necessary to use thin sections that can be examined under the microscope. Different staining methods make it possible to distinguish the whole neuron or parts of it from the surrounding elements (Figs. 1.2 and 1.3). It then becomes evident that the morphology of neurons may vary, with regard to both the size of the perikaryon and the number, length, and branching of the dendrites. The size of the dendritic tree is related to the number of contacts the cell can receive from other nerve cells. Dendrites often have small spikes, *spinae* or *spines*, that are sites of contact from other neurons (Figs. 1.1 and 1.7). The axons also vary, from those that ramify and end close to the perikaryon to those that extend for more than 1 meter. These structural differences are closely connected to functional differences.

Figure 1.2 *Neuronal somata* (cell bodies, perikarya). Photomicrographs of section of the spinal cord stained to show cell bodies (Nissl staining). The stain (thionine) binds primarily to nucleic acids (DNA in the nucleus and RNA in the cytoplasm and nucleolus). The deeply stained clumps in the cytoplasm represent aggregates of rough endoplasmic reticulum (rER), formerly called Nissl granules. Two motor neurons, one large and one small, are shown. Only the proximal parts of the dendrites are stained. Magnification, ×800.

Communication between Nerve Cells Takes Place at Synapses

The terminal branches of an axon have club-shaped enlargements called *boutons* (Figs. 1.1 and 1.4). The term *terminal bouton* is often used when the bouton sits at the end of an axon branch. In other instances the bouton is just a thickening along the course of the axon, with several such *en passage* boutons along one terminal branch. In any case, the bouton is found close to the surface membrane of another cell, usually on the dendrites or the perikaryon. Such a place of close contact between a bouton and another cell is called a synapse. In the peripheral nervous system, synapses are formed between boutons and muscle cells. *The synapse is where information is transmitted from one neuron to another.* This transmission does not occur by direct propagation of the nerve impulse from one cell (neuron) to another, but by liberation of signal molecules that subsequently influence the other cell. Such a signal molecule is called a *neurotransmitter* or, for short, a *transmitter* (the term *transmitter sub-*

Figure 1.3 *Neurons*. Photomicrographs of sections stained with two different methods. To the **right**, only the cell bodies (perikarya) of a group of neurons are stained and visible in the section. The dark region surrounding the group of neurons is made up of myelinated fibers that are also stained. The section to the **left** is from the same cell group, but treated in accordance with the Golgi method so that the dendrites as well as the cell bodies are visualized. Magnification, ×150.

Figure 1.4 *A synapse*. Schematic drawing based on electron micrographs.

stance is also used). The neurotransmitter is (at least partly) located in small vesicles in the bouton called *synaptic vesicles* (Figs. 1.4 and 1.5). How the synapse and the transmitters work is treated later in this chapter. At the moment we will restrict ourselves to the structure of the synapse.

The membrane of the bouton is separated from the membrane of the other nerve cell by a narrow cleft about 20 nm wide (that is, 2/100,000 mm). This *synaptic cleft* cannot be observed in the light microscope. Only when electron microscopy of nervous tissue became feasible in the 1950s could it be demonstrated that neurons are indeed anatomically separate entities. In the electron microscope, one can observe that the membranes facing the synaptic cleft are thickened. This is due to accumulation of specific proteins that are of crucial importance for transmission of the synaptic signal. Many of these protein molecules are receptors for neurotransmitters; others form channels for passage of charged particles, as discussed later. The membrane of the bouton facing the cleft is called the *presynaptic membrane*, and the membrane of the cell that is contacted is called the *postsynaptic membrane*. We also use the terms *pre-* and *postsynaptic neurons*.

Figure 1.5 *Synapses*. Electron micrographs showing boutons (B) in synaptic contacts with dendrites (D), and dendritic spines (Sp). A bundle of unmyelinated axons (A) is seen in the electron micrograph to the **right**. Magnifications, ×20,000 (left) and ×40,000 (right).

Figure 1.6 *Two types of synaptic contacts*. **A**. Numerous club-shaped boutons on a cell body (axosomatic synapses). **B**. An axon follows the dendritic tree closely, and forms numerous boutons with synapses *en passage*.

Synapses formed on the cell soma are called *axosomatic*, while synapses on dendrites are called *axodendritic* (Figs. 1.6 and 1.7). Where dendrites are equipped with spines, one or two synapses are always formed with the head of the spine (Fig. 1.5). We will return to the functional significance of dendritic spines later in this chapter. Boutons may also form a synapse with an axon (usually close to a terminal bouton), and such synapses are called *axoaxonic*. In general, the placement of the synapse tells us something about how strong its particular influence may be. A synapse on the cell soma is usually more powerful than a synapse far out on a dendrite. Every neuron has many thousands of synapses on its surface, and it is the sum of their influences that determines how active the postsynaptic neuron will be at any moment.

Neurons Are Rich in Organelles for Oxidative Metabolism and Protein Synthesis

When seen in a microscopic section, the nucleus of a neuron is characterized by its large size and light staining (that is, the chromatin is extended, indicating that much of the genome is in use). There is also a prominent nucleolus (Figs. 1.2 and 1.8). These features make it easy to distinguish a neuron from other cells (such as glial cells), even in sections in which only the nuclei are clearly stained. In the neuronal cytoplasm there are many mitochondria, an indication of the high metabolic activity of nerve cells. They depend entirely on aerobic adenosine triphosphate (ATP) production and cannot (unlike most other cell types) utilize anaerobic ATP synthesis. Glucose is the substrate for ATP production in the mitochondria of nerve cells, which cannot (unlike muscle cells, for example) use fat.

Neuronal somata also contain conspicuous amounts of *free ribosomes* and *rough endoplasmic reticulum* (rER) for synthesis of proteins. Large clumps of rER are seen light microscopically in the cytoplasm of neurons over a certain size (Fig. 1.2). These were called *tigroid granules* or *Nissl bodies* long before their true nature was known. There are also as a rule several Golgi complexes, which modify proteins before they are exported or inserted in membranes. The large neuronal production of proteins probably reflects their enormous surface membrane containing many protein molecules that must be constantly renewed. Membrane proteins, for ex-

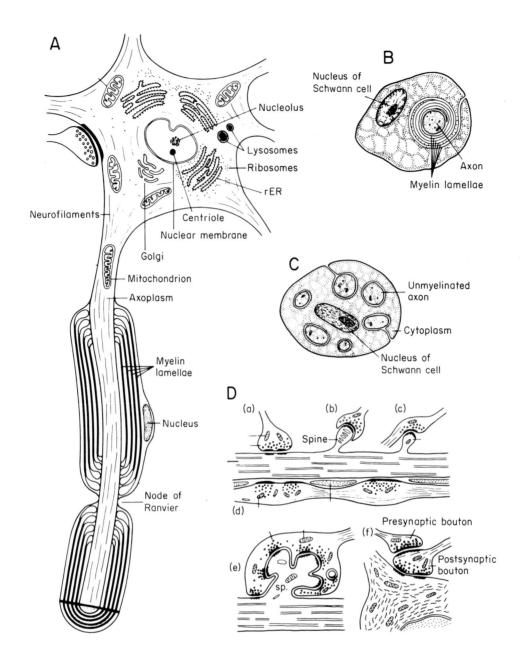

Figure 1.7 *Ultrastructure of the neuron*. Schematic drawings based on electron microscopic observations. **A.** Perikaryon with proximal parts of the dendrites and the axon (myelinated). Various kinds of organelles are shown. The node of Ranvier is where two segments of myelin meets. **B.** Cross section of axon in the process of becoming myelinated. The myelin sheath consists of lamellae formed by the membrane of a glial cell or a Schwann cell. **C.** Unmyelinated axons (in the peripheral nervous system), surrounded by Schwann cell cytoplasm. **D.** Various kinds of synaptic contacts. A bouton may form a synapse directly on (**a**) the shaft of the dendrite, or (**b, c,** and **e**) on a spine, (**d**) the axon may also have several boutons en passage, (**f**) an axoaxonic synapse (a synapse between two boutons).

Figure 1.8 *Ultrastructure of the neuron.* Electron micrograph showing the cell body of a small neuron (**above**) and parts of a larger neuron (**below**). Note the presence of rough endoplasmic reticulum (rER), free ribosomes (r), mitochondria, (m), and Golgi complex (G). Boutons (B) forming axosomatic synapses are also present. N = nucleus, Nu = nucleolus, A = axon, My = myelin. Magnifications, ×9000 (top) and ×15,000 (bottom).

ample, form receptors (binding sites) for neurotransmitters that are constantly being recycled.

Neurons Have a Cytoskeleton That also Serves Transport Functions

The somata and processes of neurons contain thin threads, *neurofibrils*, that can be observed in specially stained microscopic sections (Fig. 1.9). While originally thought to be related to impulse conduction, the neurofibrils are now known to help determine the shape of neurons, as they form the cytoskeleton, and to transport substances in neuronal processes. They also play a role in the growth of the neuron, as when axons grow for long distances in a specific direction.

Electron microscopic and biochemical analyses have shown that the cytoskeleton consists of various kinds of fibrillary proteins, making threads of three main kinds: (1) *actin filaments* (microfilaments) and associated protein molecules (about 5 nm thick), (2) *microtubules* (narrow tubes) and associated proteins (about 20 nm thick), and (3) *intermediary filaments* or *neurofilaments* (about 10 nm thick). *Actin* (microfilaments) is present in the axon, among other places. There it plays an important role during development. When the axon elongates, actin serves to produce movements of the *growth cone* at the tip of the axon (in general, actin is present in cells capable of movement, such as muscle cells). The growth cone continuously sends out thin extensions, like fingers, in various directions. These probably explore the environment for specific molecules that mark the correct direction of growth. In addition, actin is probably important in maintaining the shape of the axon when fully grown.

Microtubules and microtubule-associated proteins (MAPs) are present in all kinds of neuronal processes and are most likely important for their shape. Of special interest is the relation of microtubules to the transport of substances in the axonal cytoplasm (axoplasm). There is a continuous movement of organelles, proteins, and other particles in the axons, both in the direction from the cell body to the terminals of the axon and in the opposite direction. This phenomenon is called *axonal transport*, and is stopped by drugs (such as colchicine) that destroy the microtubules. The need for such axonal transport seems obvious. For example, only the cell soma contains organelles for the synthesis of proteins and for the degradation of particles. Thus, proteins destined for the axonal membrane (such as transmitter receptors) must be transported for long distances. The same is true of enzymes controlling transmitter synthesis and degradation. Furthermore, it is hard to imagine how the nervous system could function without feedback to the cell soma (and the genes in the nucleus) from the synapses and the postsynaptic neuron.

Transport from the cell soma toward the nerve terminal is called *anterograde axonal transport*, and movement toward the cell body is called *retrograde axonal transport*. By *anterograde* transport, substances that are synthesized only in the cell body can be moved to the axon terminals; these include mitochrondria and, as mentioned, various proteins of importance for synaptic transmission. By *retrograde* transport, signal molecules taken up by the axon terminals can reach the cell body and thereby alter its activity (for example, increased or decreased synthesis of transmitters and receptor molecules). Retrograde transport also serves to bring axonal particles that need to be broken down (for example, "worn-out"

More About Axonal Transport and Its Machinery

The injection of radioactively labeled substances taken up by neurons has shown that axonally transported material moves in at least two different phases. One phase is rapid, with particles moving 1 meter or more per day; the other is slow, with movement between 1 and 10 mm per day. As mentioned, microtubules are of particular importance for axonal transport. Each microtubule is composed of smaller building blocks of the protein *tubulin*. The formation of tubes from many tubulin molecules is helped by microtubule-associated proteins. MAPs also anchor the microtubules to the cell membrane and to other parts of the cytoskeleton, such as neurofilaments. Two kinds of MAPs found only in neurons—*MAP2* and *tau*—stiffen the microtubules. Other kinds of MAPs carry out anterograde and retrograde transport and are therefore called the *motors* of axonal transport. These are ATPases (enzymes that split ATP), and the released energy alters their form, thus producing movement. The transported particles, such as vesicles and mitochondria, move along the microtubule by temporarily binding to MAPs sticking out from the microtubule, so that they move almost like the oars of a boat. One microtubule can transport in both directions, depending on the kind of motor to which a particle binds. *Kinesin* is responsible for anterograde movement, *dynein* for retrograde movement. Dynein is a more complex protein than kinesin but both exist in different forms. These differences are probably related to the kinds of particles they transport.

Injections into nervous tissue of substances that are transported axonally and later can be detected in tissue sections are widely used to trace neuronal connections, that is, to reveal the "wiring pattern" of the brain (see Chapter 5).

Figure 1.10 *Peripheral nerve*. Myelinated and unmyelinated axons and the perineurium. Electron micrograph of cross section of the sciatic nerve. Note the large difference in diameter among various myelinated axons (My = myelin, A = axon). The thickness of the myelin sheath increases apace with the increase in axonal diameter. In between the myelinated axons there are numerous unmyelinated ones (UA) and occasional fibroblasts (f). Schwann cells (Schw.) are also associated with unmyelinated axons. The perineurium (Perin.) is formed by several lamellae of flattened cells. Magnification, ×4000.

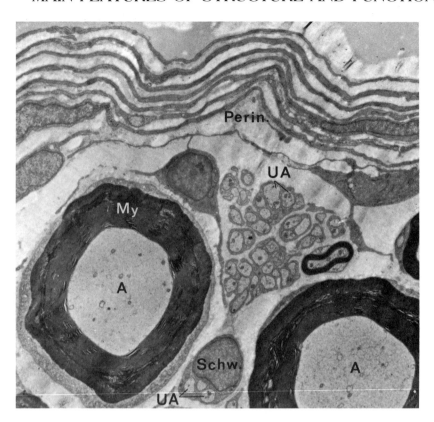

mitochondria) to the cell body, where there are lysosomes containing enzymes necessary for degradation of the particles.

The functional role of the *intermediary filaments* (neurofilaments) is uncertain, although they make up about 10% of axonal proteins. One function might be to maintain the diameter of thick myelinated axons—as an internal scaffolding. Whatever their normal role, it is noteworthy that neurofilaments are altered in several degenerative neurological diseases. In Alzheimer's disease for example, a characteristic feature is disorganized tangles of intermediary filaments in the cerebral cortex (neurofibrillary tangles).

Many Axons Are Isolated to Increase the Speed of Impulse Propagation

The velocity with which the nerve impulse travels depends on the diameter of the axon, among other factors. In addition, how well the axon is insulated is of crucial importance. Many axons have an extra layer of insulation (in addition to the axonal membrane) called a *myelin sheath*. Such axons are therefore called *myelinated*, to distinguish them from those without a myelin sheath, which are called *unmyelinated*.

Many of the tasks performed by the nervous system require very rapid conduction of signals. If unmyelinated axons were to do this, they would have to be extremely thick. Nerves bringing signals to the muscles of the hand, for example, would be impossibly thick, and the brain would also have to be much larger. Insulation is thus a very efficient way of saving

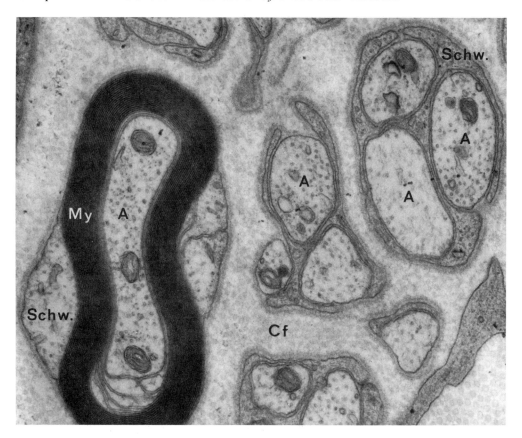

space and expensive building materials. Efficient insulation of axons is in fact a prerequisite for the dramatic development of the nervous system that has taken place in vertebrates as compared with invertebrates.

Oligodendroglia and Schwann Cells Make Myelin

The *myelin sheaths* mentioned above consist mainly of lipids, with smaller amounts of proteins. Together, the material ensheathing the axons is called *myelin*. The myelin sheath forms a cylinder around the axons (Figs. 1.7, 1.10, and 1.11), reducing the loss of current from the axon to the surrounding tissue fluid during impulse conduction. This contributes to the much higher conduction velocity in myelinated axons than in unmyelinated axons (see Chapter 2, *Impulse Conduction in Axons*). The thickest myelinated axons conduct at about 120 m/sec.

Myelin is whitish in color because of its high lipid content. With special methods for staining lipids, the myelin sheaths can be observed in light and electron microscopes (Figs. 1.10, 1.11, and 1.14). In viewing longitudinal sections one can then see that the myelin sheath is interrupted at intervals (Fig. 1.7), forming the *nodes of Ranvier*. With the electron microscope, it can be seen that the axolemma (the axonal membrane) is "naked" at the node; that is, it is exposed to the interstitial fluid. Thus, only at the node of Ranvier can current in the form of ions pass from the axon to the interstitial fluid (and in the opposite direc-

Figure 1.11 *Myelinated and unmyelinated axons*. Detail from Figure 1.10. Note the myelin lamellae (My), formed by Schwann cells (Schw.). The unmyelinated axons (A) are completely surrounded by Schwann cells. Between the axons are numerous collagen fibrils (Cf). Magnification, ×30,000.

tion). This arrangement makes it possible for the nerve impulse to "jump" from node to node, thus increasing the speed of impulse propagation.

Electron microscopically, the myelin sheath has been shown to consist of numerous layers of cell membrane. The layers or *lamellae* are formed when a special kind of glial cell wraps itself around the axon (Fig. 1.7B). During this process, the cytoplasm of the glial cell is squeezed away so that the layers of cell membrane lie closely apposed. The nodes of Ranvier exist because the glial cells forming myelin lie in a row along the axon, each cell making myelin only for a restricted length, or segment, of the axon. In the central nervous system (CNS), myelin is made by *oligodendrocytes* (oligodendroglia), whereas *Schwann cells* are responsible for its manufacture in the peripheral nervous system. The structure of the myelin sheath is nevertheless the same in both places. Oligodendrocytes and Schwann cells are not identical, however. One difference is that a single oligodendrocyte usually sends out processes to produce myelin segments for several axons, whereas each Schwann cell forms a myelin segment for only one axon. The length between two nodes of Ranvier in the peripheral nervous system may be 0.5 mm or more. The myelination of the axons starts prenatally, but many neural pathways in the human are not fully myelinated until two years after birth (see Chapter 4, *Myelination*). The process of myelination is closely related to functional maturation.

The *unmyelinated axons* conduct much more slowly (at less than 1 m/sec) than the myelinated ones. This is so because they are thinner and they lack the extra insulation provided by the myelin sheath. In the central nervous system, unmyelinated axons are often found in closely packed bundles without any glial cells separating them (Fig. 1.5). In the peripheral nervous system, however, unmyelinated axons are always ensheathed in Schwann cells that do not make layers of myelin (Fig. 1.11). Several axons become embedded in the cytoplasm of the Schwann cells by invagination of the Schwann cell membrane. This arrangement probably serves to protect the axon from potentially harmful substances in the interstitial fluid. Such protection is not necessary in the central nervous system, since the composition of the interstitial fluid is governed in other ways.

Demyelinating Diseases Block Impulse Conduction

In *demyelinating diseases* of the nervous system, the myelin sheaths degenerate. The commonest among these diseases is *multiple sclerosis*, which typically manifests in young adults and usually has a long course of progressive degeneration. Its cause is still unknown, but the symptoms are caused by isolated, apparently randomly distributed regions of inflammation and demyelination. In these regions, which are called *plaques*, impulse conduction in the axons is severely slowed or halted. Multiple sclerosis is considered to be an *autoimmune* disease, in which the immune system attacks cells of the body (in this case oligodendroglia). For some reason, the optic nerve is often the first to be affected, resulting in reduced vision. Later symptoms that usually occur in varying proportions are muscle weakness, uncoordination, and sensory disturbances. Typically, the symptoms are episodic and often are characterized by fluctuation in the inflammatory process. Thus periods of marked symptoms (such as paresis of extremities) are followed by periods of partial recovery. The improvement of symptoms is due to partial *remyelination* of the affected regions. As the disease progresses, however, not only the myelin sheaths but also the axons may degenerate, leading to permanent and progressive disability.

Diseases of Peripheral Nerves

Schwann cells do more than produce myelin sheaths. Recent studies suggest that they also influence the thickness of axons, their content of neurofilaments, and axonal transport. For example, a mouse strain with an inherited disease affecting peripheral nerves has a mutation of a gene coding for a specific myelin protein (PMP-22). Most likely, this mutation is responsible for the loss of myelin and subsequent axonal degeneration in such mice.

Diseases involving degeneration of peripheral nerves are called *neuropathies*, and can have various causes in humans. For example, neuropathy is a well-known complication of diabetes, and can also be caused by toxic substances (such as lead). However, a large group of neuropathies are inherited; among them, Charcot-Marie-Tooth disease (peroneal muscle atrophy). In most cases the disease is inherited dominantly. The disease usually starts before the age of 20 and it leads to gradually increasing pareses and sensory loss, starting distally in the legs. The symptoms are caused by loss of myelin and degeneration of axons. Although it is not yet clear whether Charcot-Marie-Tooth disease destroys neurons (axons) or Schwann cells first, the latter possibility is supported by the fact that most patients have a doubling of the PMP-22 gene. The gene is located at the short arm of chromosome 17 in humans.

Peripheral Nerves Are Built for Protection of the Axons

Fresh nervous tissue is rather soft, almost jellylike, having virtually no mechanical strength in itself. Protection of the central nervous system against external mechanical forces is provided by its location within the skull and the vertebral canal and by its "wrapping" in membranes of connective tissue. For peripheral parts of the nervous system, the situation is different. Often located superficially, the peripheral bundles of axons and groups of nerve cells are exposed to various mechanical stresses. They are also subject to considerable stretching by movements of the body. Axons can be stretched only slightly before their impulse conduction suffers, and they may even break. To prevent this, *peripheral nerves contain large amounts of dense connective tissue* with numerous collagen fibers arranged largely longitudinally (Figs. 1.10 and 1.11). The collagen fibers, specialized to resist stretching, protect the axons effectively. The presence of connective tissue in peripheral nerves explains why the nerves become so much thicker where they leave the skull or the vertebral canal.

The connective tissue components of peripheral nerves are arranged in distinctive layers. An external thick layer of mostly longitudinally running collagen fibers is called the *epineurium*. Internal to this layer, the axons are arranged into smaller bundles, fascicles, wrapped in the *perineurium* (Fig. 1.10). The rather sparse collagen fibers and fibroblasts within the fascicles constitute the *endoneurium*. The perineural sheath is special in that it contains several layers of flattened cells. The cells, which in some respects resemble epithelial cells, are connected by various kinds of junctions, suggesting that the perineurium constitutes a barrier preventing certain substances from reaching the interior of the fascicles with the axons. Experimental data indicate that this is indeed the case. It is not surprising that peripheral nervous tissue also needs some extra protective mechanisms to ensure that its environment is kept optimal for conducting impulses.

Projection neuron   Interneuron

Figure 1.12 *Projection neuron and interneuron*. Examples from the brain stem of a monkey, based on sections treated according to the Golgi method.

Projection Neurons and Interneurons

Some neurons influence cells that are far away, and their axon is correspondingly long (more than a meter for the longest). They are called *projection neurons* or Golgi type 1 (Fig. 1.12). Neurons convey signals from the spinal cord to the muscles are examples of projection neurons; others are neurons in the cerebral cortex with axons contacting cells in the brain stem and the spinal cord. The axons of projection neurons as a rule send out branches, *collaterals*, in their course (Figs. 1.12, 2.14, and 20.5). Thus, one projection neuron may send signals to neurons in various other parts of the nervous system.

The other main type of neuron is the *interneuron* or Golgi type 2 (Figs. 1.12 and 20.6), characterized by a short axon that branches extensively in the vicinity of the cell body. Its name implies that an interneuron is intercalated between two other neurons. Even though, strictly speaking, all neurons with axons that do not leave the central nervous system are thus interneurons, the *term is usually restricted to neurons with short axons that do not leave one particular neuronal group.* The interneurons thus mediate communication between neurons within one group. Since interneurons may be *switched* on and off, the possible number of interrelations among the neurons within one group increases dramatically. The number of interneurons is particularly high in the cerebral cortex, and it is the number of interneurons that is so much higher in the human brain than in any other animal. The number of typical projection neurons interconnecting the various parts of the nervous system, and linking the nervous system with the rest of the body, as a rule varies more with the size of the body than with the stage of development.

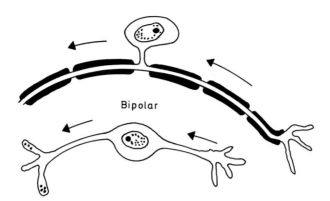

Figure 1.13 *Pseudounipolar and bipolar neurons.*

The distinction between projection neurons and interneurons is not always very clear, however. Many neurons previously regarded as giving off only local branches have been shown by modern methods also to give off long axonal branches to more distant cell groups. Thus, they function both as projection neurons and interneurons. On the other hand, many of the "classical" projection neurons give off collaterals ending within the cell group in which the cell body is located (Fig. 20.5).

Most Neurons Are Multipolar

Neurons described above usually have several processes, and are therefore called *multipolar*. Special kinds of neurons, however, may be different. Thus, neurons conducting sensory signals from the receptors to the central nervous system have only one process that divides close to the cell body. One branch conducts impulses from the receptor toward the cell soma; the other conducts impulses toward and into the central nervous system. Such neurons are called *pseudounipolar* (Fig. 1.13). In accordance with the usual definition, the process conducting toward the cell body should be termed a dendrite. With regard to both structure and function, however, this process must be regarded as an axon. Some neurons have two processes, one conducting toward the perikaryon, the other away from it. Such neurons, present in the retina and some other locations, are called *bipolar*.

Neurons Are Collected in Nuclei and Ganglia

When examining sections from the *central nervous system* under the microscope, one sees that the perikarya of the neurons are not diffusely spread out but are collected in groups. Such a group is called a *nucleus* (Figs. 1.2 and 1.14). Neurons collected in this manner share many connections with other groups and constitute in certain respects a functional unit. In the *peripheral nervous system*, a corresponding collection of perikarya is called a *ganglion*.

Axons from the neurons of one nucleus usually have common targets and therefore run together, forming bundles. Such a bundle of axons con-

Figure 1.14 *Nuclei and tracts*. Photomicrographs showing two nuclei in the brain stem (the hypoglossal nucleus and the dorsal motor nucleus of the vagus) and a tract (the medial lemniscus). In addition, some minor bundles of myelinated fibers can be seen. The sections are stained with thionine to visualize neuronal cell bodies (Nissl staining) and with another method that stains myelin. Magnification, ×75.

necting one nucleus with another is called a *tract* (tractus) (Fig. 1.14). In the peripheral nervous system, a collection of axons is called a *nerve* (nervus).

Schematically, the large tracts of the nervous system are the main routes for nerve impulses—to some extent comparable to highways connecting big cities. In addition, there are numerous smaller pathways often running parallel to the highways, and many smaller bundles of axons leave the big tracts to terminate in nuclei along the course. The number of smaller "footpaths" interconnecting nuclei is enormous, making possible (at least theoretically) the spread of impulses from one nucleus to almost any part of the nervous system. Normally, the spread of impulses is far from random, but rather is highly ordered and patterned. As a rule, the bigger tracts play more significant roles than the smaller ones in the main tasks of the nervous system. Consequently, diseases affecting such tracts usually produce marked symptoms that can be understood only if one has a fair knowledge of the main features of the wiring patterns of the brain.

Nuclei and Tracts Make Up Gray and White Matter

The surfaces made by cutting nervous tissue contain some areas that are whitish and others that have a gray color. The whitish areas consist mainly of myelinated axons, the myelin being responsible for the color. Such regions are called *white matter*. The gray regions, called *gray matter*, contain mainly cell bodies and dendrites (and, of course, axons passing to and from the neurons). The neurons themselves are grayish in color. Owing to this difference in color, one can macroscopically identify the major nuclei (gray) and tracts (white) in brains that have been cut (see, for example, Fig. 3.28). This is dealt with in Chapter 3.

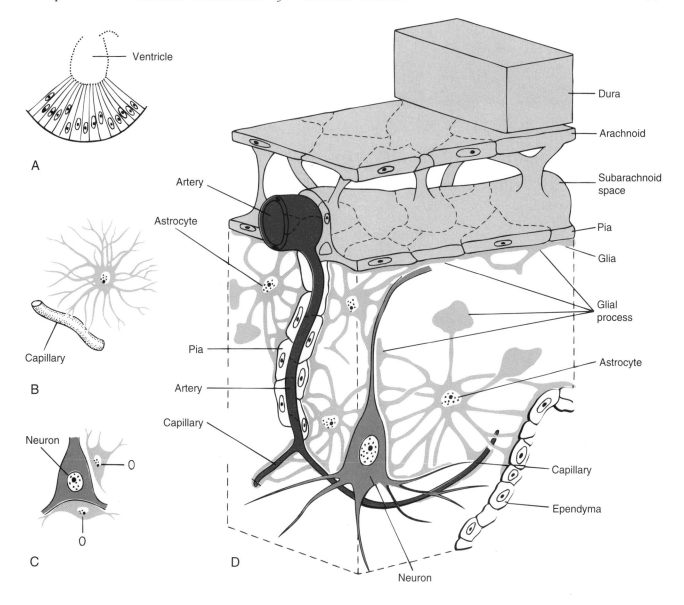

GLIAL CELLS

We have already encountered glial cells briefly. All are equipped with processes, but these are not responsible for the conduction of impulses. The significance of glial cells lies in their crucial role in the functioning of nerve cells. In fact, the number of glial cells is much higher than that of neurons. The name derives from the original, erroneous belief that the glial cells mainly served as "glue," keeping the neurons together.

Most of the tasks today ascribed to glia had been suggested by the turn of the century on the basis of microscopic observations of their structure and relation to other elements of nervous tissue. Nevertheless, only by modern methods has it been possible to study directly the properties and functional roles of glia, and much still remains unknown. The study of glial cells has recently been greatly facilitated by immunocytochemical methods that identify certain cytoplasmic or surface molecules.

Figure 1.15 *Glial cells*. **A:** Ependymal cells lining the wall of the ventricular system. **B:** Astrocyte. **C:** Oligodendrocytes (o) close to the perikaryon of a neuron. **D:** Scheme showing the three-dimensional arrangement of astrocytes and the vessels of the brain. Note that astrocytes are closely related to vessels, ependymal cells, and the innermost part of the cerebral meninges (Pia).

Figure 1.16 *Astrocytes*. Photomicrograph of section from the cerebral cortex treated according to the Golgi method. Magnifications, ×200 and ×400, left to right, respectively.

It is customary to group glial cells in three categories, *astrocytes* (astroglia), *oligodendrocytes* (oligodendroglia), and *microglial cells* (microglia). Each is structurally and functionally different from the others. (Fig. 1.15).

In addition to these three kinds, there are other specialized forms of glial cells. The surface of the cavities inside the central nervous system is lined with a layer of cylindrical cells called *ependyma* (Fig. 1.15 and see Fig. 4.6). There are also special types of glial cells in the retina (Müller cells), the cerebellum (Bergman cells), and the posterior pituitary gland (pituicytes).

Astrocytes Contact Both Capillaries and Neurons

Astrocytes have numerous short or long processes and may be divided on this basis into two kinds: protoplasmic astrocytes and fibrillary astrocytes. The processes extend in all directions (Fig. 1.16). Some contact the surface of capillaries with expanded "feet," and most of the capillary surface is covered by astrocytic processes (Fig. 1.15). The astrocytes are probably of importance for the capillary permeability to certain substances. Other processes contact neuronal surfaces; in this manner, parts not contacted by boutons are mainly covered by glia.

The intimate contact between astrocytes and neurons indicates that they may *exchange substances*, and several examples of this are known. One important function is apparently to *remove or degrade neurotransmitters* released from boutons into the interstitial space. This prevents accumulation of transmitters extracellularly, which would be deleterious to the neurons. Another task appears to be the *regulation of extracellular K^+ ion concentration*. This is important because neuronal excitability is strongly influenced by the extracellular potassium concentration, and prolonged neuronal activity may lead to the accumulation of K^+ extracellularly. Since the extracellular space in the brain is very limited, the potassium concentration could easily reach high values were it not for effective means of removal by glia. Astrocytes are connected by numerous *gap junctions* (nexus), allowing passage of small molecules (such as ions) from cell to cell. This presumably increases the efficiency of K^+ removal, because the astrocytes function as a continuous, large fluid volume. Astrocytes furthermore contribute to the extracellular *pH control* by removing CO_2.

There is also much evidence that glial cells are important during *development* of the nervous system—for example, by providing surfaces and scaffoldings for the axons to follow during outgrowth.

Astrocytes also form a continuous, thin sheet where nervous tissue borders connective tissue. Such a *limiting membrane* (membrana limitans) is found around the big vessels and on the inside of the coverings of the brain and spinal cord (meninges).

Oligodendrocytes Make Myelin Sheaths

Oligodendrocytes have relatively few and short processes (*oligo* = few, little). The cell body is often closely apposed to a neuronal perikaryon (Fig. 1.15), and for this reason oligodendrocytes are also called *satellite cells*. As mentioned above, oligodendrocytes are responsible for myelination of axons in the central nervous system, but their position in relation to nerve cell somata suggests that they also have other tasks. We do not know, for example, whether *all* oligodendrocytes form myelin.

Microglial Cells Are Phagocytes

The third kind of glial cell, *microglia*, were given their name because of their small size (Fig. 1.15). Microglial cells were first described light microscopically in sections treated with heavy metal impregnation methods. Estimates indicate that microglia may constitute 5%–20% of all glial cells, being fairly evenly distributed through all parts of the central nervous system. Although the identification of microglia is not as straightforward as that of the other glial types (for example, they have no distinctive ultrastructural features), immunocytochemical identification of specific membrane proteins has solved several controversial issues. Specifically, microglial cells were originally considered to be of *mesodermal origin*; that is, they had presumably invaded the nervous system during embryonic development. Although this assumption has been debated for a long time, recent immunocytochemical studies support it. Several surface markers (antigens) are common to blood monocytes and microglia, and cells that express such antigens first occur in the central nervous system (of rodents) in late embryonic development. After invading nervous tissue, the cells undergo morphological changes that make them closely resemble microglial cells as identified in the adult. The invasion of the CNS by monocytes may correspond in time to a period of cell death (during development a surplus of neurons is produced, with subsequent elimination of a large number during a restricted period of time). The number of microglial cells is fairly stable after the prenatal invasion. Thus, under *normal conditions* the stock of microglial cells is apparently not supplemented by cells entering the brain from the bone marrow. This has been shown in experimental animals in which the bone marrow was destroyed by intense radiation and then replaced by stem cells from another animal (chimeras). In this way, cells in the central nervous system (or elsewhere) originating from the "new" bone marrow can be identified.

After injury, the number of cells with phagocytic activity (macrophages) increases in the central nervous system. This increase appears to be due primarily to the movement of macrophages from the blood stream and only to a lesser extent to activation of microglial cells.

The Reaction of Nervous Tissue to Injury and Inflammation

Tissue damage leads to an inflammatory reaction, in which the invasion and activation of immunocompetent cells play a central role. The purpose of the invasion is to kill microorganisms, remove debris, and aid reparative processes. However, the inflammatory reaction is different in the central nervous system than in other tissues of the body. Thus, there is often no invasion of neutrophil granulocytes, and the activation of microglia and invading monocytes to macrophages may take several days. Overall, immune reactions are weaker and slower in the central nervous system than elsewhere. This may be explained—at least in part—by the lack of lymphatic drainage from the central nervous system. The immune system, therefore, is not well informed about nervous tissue conditions, in contrast to tissues of most other organs. Normally, only a small number of monocytes and T lymphocytes, entering from the blood stream, patrol the central nervous system. Perhaps these special conditions are necessary to prevent neuronal damage from potent substances liberated from granulocytes and activated macrophages. For example edema—a central component of inflammation—may become harmful and even life-threatening when it occurs in the brain (because of the limited possibilities of expansion within the skull). Nevertheless, immune reactions *do* occur in the brain, sometimes with serious consequences, as in multiple sclerosis.

The main *task of astrocytes after injury* is probably to strengthen their normal function of keeping the extracellular fluid composition constant. Tissue damage—regardless of whether it is caused by bleeding, contusion, or circulatory arrest—increases the flow of ions and transmitters from the neurons to the extracellular fluid. Astrocytes increase their uptake to counteract such disturbances of the neuronal environment. Because the substances taken up are osmotically active, the astrocytes may swell quickly—seconds or minutes after the damage (if the normal uptake capacity is surpassed). This may contribute to brain edema, a dangerous complication of head injuries. In the long term, astrocytes produce a kind of scar tissue at sites where neurons are lost.

In Chapter 4 we discuss the plastic processes of the nervous system that permit functional recovery after injuries (such as stroke).

Microglia and AIDS

Acquired immune deficiency syndrome (AIDS) caused by the HIV-1 virus, also affects the brain. Although the HIV-1 virus does not infect neurons, considerable neuronal death may occur (even without other infections of the central nervous system). This leads to disturbances of voluntary movements, sensation, and mental functions. The virus probably enters the central nervous system via infected T lymphocytes (as mentioned above, a few T lymphocytes and monocytes patrol the nervous system). Microglial cells, after being infected, may secrete toxic substances that kill neurons—perhaps by binding to the so-called NMDA receptor (see the sections on *The NMDA Receptor: A Mediator of Both Learning and Neuronal Damage?* in Chapter 2, and *Ischemic Cell Damage and the Glutamate Hypothesis* in Chapter 4). Thus, microglial cells express at their surface the CD4 antigen that binds HIV-1. Furthermore, human monocytes, macrophages, and microglial cells grown in culture and infected with HIV-1 excrete substances that are toxic to neurons. A protein of the cap of the virus particle (gp120) is neurotoxic in cell culture. It is not clear, however, whether this protein is excreted by microglial cells and directly damages neurons, or whether it induces microglial cells (and other macrophages) to produce other kinds of toxic substances.

CHAPTER 2

FUNCTIONAL PROPERTIES OF NEURONS

BASIS OF EXCITABILITY AND IMPULSE PROPAGATION

Some of the characteristic properties of neurons, such as their *excitability* and their ability to *conduct impulses*, are mentioned in Chapter 1. The term excitability means that the cell can react with a brief electrical discharge, *an action potential*, when sufficiently stimulated. The action potential (the nerve impulse) is conducted along the axon, and is a major element in the communication among nerve cells and between nerve cells and the body. The action potential results from movement of charged particles, *ions*, through the cell membrane. A prerequisite for such a current across the membrane is an electric potential between the inside and the outside of the cell. This is called the *membrane potential* and it results from unequal distribution of positively and negatively charged particles on either side of the membrane.[1]

This chapter will deal with the basis for neuronal excitability and impulse conduction, and for communication between nerve cells at synapses.

Excitability Depends on Ion Channels in the Neuronal Membrane

The normal stimulus for a neuron is the synaptic effect evoked by other neurons acting on it. The signal is conveyed from one neuron to the next by the presynaptic release of a *neurotransmitter*. Thus, the nerve impulse—that is, an electric current—is transformed to a chemical signal. The neurotransmitter binds briefly to receptor molecules in the postsynaptic membrane. Usually, the receptor is closely associated with *ion*

Figure 2.1. *Ion channels*. Schematic representation of a small part of the lipid bilayer of the cell membrane with interspersed ion channels.

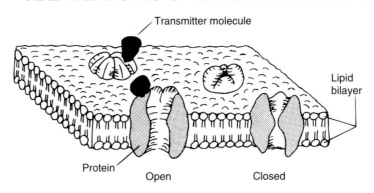

channels in the membrane, and these change their *opening state* when the transmitter binds to the receptor (Figs. 2.1 and 2.2). In this discussion we will restrict our attention first to situations in which the transmitter produces *opening* of ion channels by binding *directly* to them (as we will see later, transmitters can also close channels and act indirectly via intracellular signals). Opening of ion channels produces a brief current carried by ions passing through the membrane. There are many types of ion channels, each *selectively permeable* to one or a few kinds of ions (the most important being Na^+, K^+, Ca^{2+}, and Cl^-). By selectively controlling the opening of ion channels, the transmitters regulate the membrane potential and the excitability of the neuron. By "selectively permeable," we mean that the channel lets certain kinds of ions pass through more easily than others. Some channels are highly selective, allowing the passage of one kind only (such as Ca^{2+} ions), whereas others are less selective and will let through, for example, most cations. Channels that are permeable for anions in general are usually termed *chloride (Cl^-) channels* because Cl^- is the only abundant anion that can pass the membrane. Size and charge of the ion influence its permeability but other—not fully understood—factors are important too. By regulating the channel opening, the transmitter controls the flow of ions through the membrane, and thus regulates the excitability of the neuron.

Figure 2.2. *Ion channels*. Five protein subunits are arranged around a central opening that can admit ions. At the outer side the channel proteins are equipped with receptor sites for neurotransmitter molecules that regulate the opening of the channel. The figure shows the probable appearance of an acetylcholine receptor. Based on Changeux (1993).

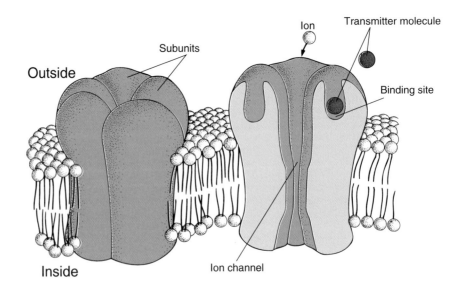

Since ions are charged particles, their passage through channels creates *electric currents*. Thus, *the nerve impulse produces release of the transmitter from the presynaptic bouton; this chemical signal then evokes a brief electric current across the postsynaptic membrane.*

Ion Channels May Be Ligand-Gated or Voltage-Gated

When the opening of a channel is controlled by neurotransmitters (or other chemical substances), the channel is called *transmitter-gated* or *ligand-gated* (the term *transmitter-activated* is also used). Binding of the transmitter to a specific site at the external face of a channel polypeptide may change the form of the polypeptides, thus changing the diameter of the channel (Fig. 2.2). Usually, the channel is open only briefly after binding of a transmitter molecule.

Many channels are not controlled primarily by chemical substances but by the magnitude of the membrane potential, and are therefore called *voltage-gated*. Such channels are, for example, *responsible for the action potential* and thus for the propagation of impulses in the axons. Voltage-gated channels are responsible for the activation of nerves and muscles by external electrical stimulation. Thus, electrical stimulation of a peripheral nerve may produce muscle twitches by activating motor nerve fibers as well as sensations due to activation of sensory nerve fibers.

The *structure of several ligand-gated ion channels* has now been determined. They consist of several polypeptide subunits arranged around a central pore (Fig. 2.2). The subunits span the membrane and extend to the external and internal faces of the membrane. Thus, molecules inside the cell also may influence the opening of the ion channel. We will return to this later (see the section titled *Two Main Kinds of Transmitter Actions: Fast and Slow*). *Voltage-gated channels* resemble ligand-gated ones, consisting of several (probably four) subunits arranged around a central pore. They are members of a related gene family, and subtle differences between the subunits forming the channel probably explain their high selectivity to particular ions (Na^+, K^+, or Ca^{2+}).

Cell Membrane Permeability Is Determined by Ion Channels

Ions cross the cell membrane almost exclusively through specific ion channels since their electrical charges prevent them from passing the lipid bilayer. It follows that the ease with which an ion can pass through the membrane—that is, the *membrane permeability*[2] to that particular kind of ion—depends on how densely the channels are distributed in the membrane and on their degree of opening.

The current of ions through the membrane, however, depends not only on the density and opening of channels. An additional important factor is the *concentration gradient* across the membrane for the ion: the steeper the gradient, the greater the flow of ions will be from high to low concentration (provided that the membrane is not totally impermeable to the ion). Furthermore, since ions are electrically charged particles, the *volt-*

age gradient across the membrane (that is, the membrane potential) will also be of importance. Thus, if the inside of the cell is negative in relation to the outside, positively charged ions, *cations*, on the outside will be exposed to a force attracting them into the cell, while inside cations will be subjected to forces that tend to drive them out. The strength of these attractive and expulsive forces depends on the magnitude of the membrane potential. Thus, the *concentration gradient and the membrane potential together determine the flow of ions through the membrane.*

The Membrane Potential

In a typical nerve cell, the potential across the cell membrane is stable at around 60 mV (millivolt) in the resting state—that is, as long as the cell is not exposed to any stimuli. We therefore use the term *resting potential* in this situation (in different kinds of nerve cells, the resting potential may vary from about 45 mV to about 75 mV). The resting potential is due to a small surplus of negatively charged ions, *anions* inside the cell as compared with the outside, and it has arbitrarily been decided to define the resting potential as negative—for example, −60 mV.

The resting potential is primarily caused by two factors:

1. the cell membrane is *selectively permeable*—that is, some kinds of ion may pass through the membrane with much greater ease than other kinds (in the resting state the membrane is primarily permable to K^+ ions)

2. the *concentration of several ions—among them K^+ ions—differs greatly inside and outside the cell.*

The unequal distribution of ions is established and maintained by energy-requiring "pumps" in the cell membrane that actively transport ions through the membrane against a concentration gradient. Several ions are unequally distributed (Fig. 2.3A). It should be emphasized that the unequal concentrations of ions inside and outside the cell cannot alone explain the membrane potential. Thus, if the membrane were completely impermeable, the result would be electric neutrality as depicted in Figure 2.3A. If the membrane were made permeable to K^+ ions but not to others, however, then K^+ would start to move out of the cell, driven by the concentration gradient. This is, in fact, the situation in the resting state: only K^+ ions can pass through the membrane (the membrane is selectively permeable to K^+). Thus, to explain the membrane potential we can, for the time being, ignore other ions than K^+ (Fig. 2.3B). The concentration gradient will drive K^+ out of the cell because the concentration of K^+ ions is much higher inside than outside the cell. Furthermore, K^+ ions can pass the membrane with relative ease through a particular kind of potassium channel that is open in the resting state. Although the concentration gradient for Na^+ is also large (Fig. 2.3A), there are very few open sodium channels in the resting state. Thus, *at rest only K^+ can pass through the membrane* with some ease, while the membrane is very slightly permeable to, for example, Na^+. This means that *positive charges are lost from the inside of the cell, making the in-*

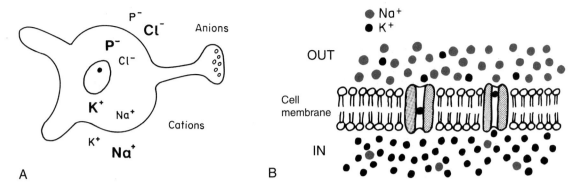

A   B

side negative compared to the outside, and creating a membrane potential.

The membrane potential reaches only a certain value, however, because it will oppose the movement of K$^+$ ions out of the cell. *Two opposite forces are thus at work:* the *concentration gradient* tending to drive K$^+$ out of the cell and the *electrical gradient* (membrane potential) tending to drive K$^+$ into the cell (Fig. 2.4). When the membrane potential is about -75 mV, these two forces are equally strong; that is, the flow of K$^+$ into the cell equals the flow out. This is therefore called the *equilibrium potential for K$^+$*, and its magnitude is determined by the concentration gradient for potassium ions.

The resting potential in most neurons, however, is lower than the equilibrium potential for K$^+$. This is because the cell membrane is *slightly* permeable to Na$^+$ (about $1/50$ th of the permeability to K$^+$). Thus, some positive charges (Na$^+$) pass into the cell, driven by both the concentration gradient and the membrane potential, making the inside of the cell less negative than the equilibrium potential for K$^+$. The membrane potential is thus changed somewhat in the direction of the *equilibrium potential for Na$^+$*, that is, $+55$ mV.

Even though the two opposite currents of K$^+$ and Na$^+$ in the resting state are small, over time they would eliminate the concentration gradients of these ions across the membrane (Fig. 2.3B) were it not for the *sodium—potassium pump.* This pump actively expels Na$^+$ ions from the inside, in exchange for K$^+$ at the same rate that the ions leak through the membrane. Thus, as long as the cell is in the resting state, there is equilibrium between flow of ions into and out of the cell.

Figure 2.3. *Ions of importance for the membrane potential.* **A.** Unequal distribution of some ions. **B.** Unequal distribution of K$^+$ ions is of particular significance for the resting membrane potential, whereas the unequal distribution of Na$^+$ is crucial for the action potential.

Figure 2.4. *Forces acting on the K$^+$ ions.*

Distribution of Anions

For simplicity we have so far dealt with only two of the cations, K^+ and Na^+, because they are the most important ones for the membrane potential and also for the nerve impulse. However, several other kinds of ions are also unequally distributed. Of the *anions*, chloride ions (Cl^-) and negatively charged protein molecules (abbreviated to P^-) make up the bulk (Fig. 2.3A). These are also unequally distributed, so that *chloride is the major extracellular anion, whereas proteins are the major intracellular ones*. The proteins are so big that they cannot pass the membrane—the membrane is impermeable to protein molecules. The membrane is, however, somewhat permeable to Cl^-. The concentration gradient tends to drive chloride into the cell, whereas the membrane potential tends to drive it out, making the net flow of Cl^- small. In fact, the equilibrium poten-

The Sodium–Potassium Pump, the Membrane Potential, and Osmotic Control

The unequal distribution of ions is, as we have seen, of fundamental importance for the membrane potential. How is this unequal distribution produced in the first place, and how is it maintained? This was briefly alluded to above. Again, the selective permeability of the cell membrane is crucial. We may start with a hypothetical situation with only potassium chloride, KCl, inside the cell. This is in the form of K^+ and Cl^- ions. No other ions are present either inside or outside the cell. As mentioned above, the membrane is somewhat permeable to both ions, and they will therefore diffuse slowly out of the cell until the concentrations are equal on both sides of the membrane. Imagine that we now add a large number of negatively charged protein molecules, P^-, to which the cell membrane is impermeable, and an equal number of cations, which in this case are K^+ (cations must follow the anions in order to ensure electrical neutrality). The equilibrium between positive and negative charges inside the cell is thus not disturbed by adding KP. However, the concentration of K^+ becomes higher inside the cell than outside. Thus, some K^+ ions move out of the cell, driven by the concentration gradient, and Cl^- follows, driven by the electric potential (inside negative) that arises when K^+ ions move out. After a while, a new state of equilibrium is reached, at which the electrical gradient produced by the outward flow of K^+ ions equals the concentration gradient for K^+. When this equilibrium is reached, the concentration of K^+ is still higher inside than outside, while the concentration of Cl^- has become highest outside. This situation may appear to be stable. However, because of the protein molecules, which cannot pass through the membrane, the total concentration of ions is higher inside than outside the cell. In this situation, water would flow into the cell by *osmosis* (the water concentration being lower inside than outside the cell). The cell would swell and ultimately disintegrate. This obviously does not happen with the cells in our body. The reason is that, unlike the hypothetical situation described above, the extracellular fluid contains NaCl (as Na^+ and Cl^-), making the total ion concentration equal outside and inside the cell. However, to prevent Na^+ from entering the cell (driven by both concentration and electrical gradients) and thus unsettling the osmotic balance, the cell membrane must have a very low permeability to Na^+. Although this permeability is low, however, it is not zero. Some Na^+ therefore would flow into the cell, and some K^+ would flow out (because the membrane potential would be lowered by cations coming into the cell) were it not for the sodium–potassium pump. In fact, *all cells, not only nerve cells, are dependent on the activity of the sodium–potassium pump to maintain osmotic equilibrium* between the intracellular and extracellular fluid compartments. Unique to nerve cells (and, for example, muscle cells) is that the pumping activity has to be increased in relation to action potentials, since these are produced by an inward current of Na^+ ions and an outward current of K^+ ions. The activity of the pump is increased in pace with increases of the intracellular Na^+ concentration.

A significant part of our energy in the form of ATP is spent on driving the sodium–potassium pump. In the resting state of nerve cells it may constitute approximately one-third, whereas after high-frequency trains of action potentials it may increase to two-thirds of the total energy requirement.

tial for Cl$^-$, -65 mV, is close to the resting potential of most nerve cells. Therefore, no active mechanism for pumping of chloride is needed.

Alteration of the Membrane Potential: Depolarization and Hyperpolarization

As already mentioned, in the resting state the membrane permeability for Na$^+$ is low. If for some reason Na$^+$ channels are opened so that the permeability is increased, Na$^+$ ions will flow into the cell and thereby reduce the magnitude of the membrane potential (that is, change it toward the equilibrium potential of Na$^+$ at $+55$ mV). Such a reduction of the membrane potential is called *depolarization*. The membrane potential is made less negative by depolarization. Correspondingly, one may foresee that when the membrane permeability for K$^+$ is increased, the membrane potential will become more negative than the resting potential. This is called *hyperpolarization*. The same would be achieved by opening channels for chloride ions, enabling negative charges (Cl$^-$) to flow into the cell.

In conclusion, the membrane potential is determined by the relative permeability of the various ions that can pass through the membrane. At rest, the membrane is primarily permeable to K$^+$, and the resting potential is therefore close to the equilibrium potential of K$^+$. As we will see in the following discussion, the action potential is caused by a sudden increase in the Na$^+$ permeability.

The Action Potential

The basis of the action potential is found in the presence of voltage-gated Na$^+$ channels, which are opened by depolarization of the membrane. Depolarization may be induced in several ways; for example, under artificial conditions by direct electrical stimulation. Normally, however, it is caused by the action of neurotransmitters acting on transmitter-gated channels. Thus, depolarization is often started by the opening of transmitter-gated Na$^+$ channels. Opening of the voltage-gated channels requires that the membrane be depolarized to a certain *threshold value*—that is, the threshold for producing an action potential (Fig. 2.5). When voltage-gated channels are opened, the permeability to Na$^+$ is increased beyond what was achieved by the opening of transmitter-gated channels, and Na$^+$ flows into the cell driven by both the concentration gradient and the membrane potential. The membrane is more depolarized, this in turn opens more voltage-gated channels, and so on. Thus, the permeability to Na$^+$ increases in an explosive manner as soon as the membrane is depolarized to the threshold value. Even with all sodium channels fully open, however, the inward current of Na$^+$ ions stops when the membrane is depolarized to $+55$ mV; at that value the inward concentration force is equal to the outward electrical force (the membrane potential). As mentioned above, $+55$ mV is the equilibrium potential of Na$^+$. Figure 2.4 shows how, during an action potential, the membrane potential quickly changes to positive values and then returns almost as rapidly to approximately the resting value.

Figure 2.5. *The action potential.*

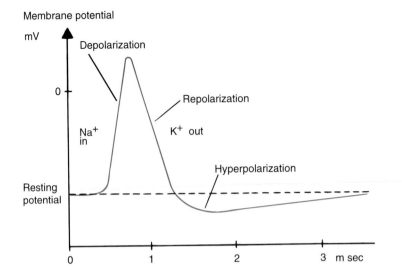

This happens because the membrane again becomes impermeable to Na^+; the *Na^+ channels are closed or inactivated.* Thus at the peak of the action potential and for a short time afterward, no Na^+ can pass through the membrane. In this situation with a positive membrane potential, K^+ is driven out both by the concentration gradient and the membrane potential (electrical force). Since no Na^+ can enter the cell, there is a net outward flow of positive charges, again making the interior of the cell negative. We say that the membrane is repolarized. The speed of repolarization is increased by the presence of voltage-gated K^+ channels, which open when the membrane is sufficiently depolarized. The opening of the voltage-gated K^+ channels is somewhat delayed compared with the Na^+ channels, but whereas the Na^+ channels inactivate after about 1 msec, the K^+ channels stay open for several milliseconds. *In summary, the action potential is caused by a brief inward current of Na^+ ions, followed by an outward current of K^+ ions.* The whole sequence of depolarization—repolarization is generally finished in 1–2 msec. If the threshold is reached, an action potential of a certain magnitude arises, regardless of the strength of the stimulus that produced the depolarization.

One might think that an action potential would cause significant changes in the concentrations of Na^+ and K^+ on the two sides of the membrane. This, however, is not the case. The number of ions actually passing through the membrane during an action potential is extremely small compared with the total number inside the cell and in its immediate surroundings. Even in an axon with a diameter of about 1 μm, with a very small intracellular volume compared to the membrane surface area, only 1 of 3000 K^+ ions moves out during the action potential. In addition, active pumping (the sodium–potassium pump) ensures that Na^+ is moved out and K^+ moved in between each action potential and in periods of rest. Even when the sodium–potassium pump is blocked experimentally, a nerve cell can produce several thousand action potentials before concentration gradients are reduced so much that the cell loses its excitability.

The action potential usually arises in the first part of the axon, *the initial segment*, where the density of voltage-gated Na^+ channels is higher than in the membrane of the dendrites and the cell soma. The current spreads electrotonically (passively) from dendritic and somatic synapses toward the initial segment. If the depolarization is sufficiently strong (reaches threshold), voltage-gated Na^+ and K^+ channels open and thus produce an action potential that is propagated along the axon.

Frequency Coding: How Nerve Cells Can Vary Their Messages

So far we have treated the action potential as a unitary phenomenon. As mentioned, the strength of each action potential of a neuron does not vary—whenever depolarized to the threshold, the cell fires action potentials of constant magnitude. Thus, the action potential is an *all-or-none phenomenon*, and one might think that each neuron would only be able to tell whether or not a stimulus occurs. We know, however, that the individual nerve cell can inform others about the *strength* of the

---

Calcium

Calcium and the Action Potential

A cation other than Na^+, namely Ca^{2+}, may also contribute to the rising phase of the action potential. For Ca^{2+} too the extracellular concentration is much higher than the intracellular one, and there are voltage-gated calcium channels in the membrane.

Cellular influx of calcium can be visualized after intracellular injection of a substance that fluoresces when Ca^{2+} binds to it. During the action potential, calcium enters the cell, partly through Na^+ channels, partly through voltage-gated calcium channels, which have a more prolonged opening-closing phase than the sodium channels. There are also transmitter-gated calcium channels. In most neurons the contribution of Ca^{2+} to the action potential is nevertheless small compared with that of Na^+. In certain other cells such as *heart muscle*, however, calcium is the ion largely responsible for the action potential. Because the calcium channels open and close more slowly than the Na^+ channels, an action potential produced by calcium currents lasts longer than one produced by flow of Na^+.

Another aspect of the functional role of calcium is that the *extracellular calcium concentration influences the membrane excitability*. This is most likely mediated through effects on the Na^+ and K^+ channels. Reducing the calcium concentration in the blood and interstitial fluid—*hypocalcemia*—lowers the threshold for evoking action potentials in neurons and muscle cells, whereas increasing the concentration—*hypercalcemia*—has the opposite effect. A typical symptom of hypocalcemia is muscle spasms due to hyperexcitability of nerves and muscles. Severe hypercalcemia can cause drowsiness, nausea, and anorexia.

Calcium Is an Important Signal Molecule for Nerve Cells

Cellular influx of calcium has other and probably more important effects on most neurons than contributing directly to the action potential. Calcium is an important signal molecule in itself, functioning intracellularly as a *second messenger* and influencing other second messengers like cyclic adenosine monophosphate (cAMP). One well-known effect is that calcium influx into boutons is necessary for *release of neurotransmitters* (corresponding to conditions in secretory cells). We return to this below.

Another important effect calcium may have as a signal molecule is to produce (via intermediaries) changes of *gene expression* and *protein synthesis*. This may be crucial, for example, in relation to long-term changes in neuronal properties underlying learning and memory. Calcium influx can apparently be restricted to only certain parts of the neuronal membrane; for example, on part of a dendrite subjected to particularly strong synaptic influences. This may produce changes in the properties of the synapses only on this part of the neuron, whereas synapses at other sites remain unchanged.

stimulation it receieves—such as the intensity of light or a sound, of something touching the skin, and so forth. It does so by *varying the frequency* of action potentials. To understand this, we need to know that a neuron is more or less continuously influenced by impulses from many other neurons. A sustained synaptic input that is strong enough to depolarize the cell to threshold does not merely produce one action potential but rather several in succession. The stronger the depolarization, the shorter the time required to reach the threshold after each action potential. Consequently, *the firing frequency depends on the strength of depolarization*. The maximal frequency of action potentials in some neurons may be more than 100 sec (1 Hertz), whereas in others it may be much lower.

Many neurons produce *trains of action potentials* in rapid succession and then pause for a while before a new train of impulses arises. Each neuronal type has its characteristic *frequency pattern*, caused by differences in membrane properties and synaptic inputs (see below, *The Refractory Period*). Neurons with high maximal impulse frequency especially tend to discharge in bursts, with trains of impulses interrupted by periods of rest. Such differences in the pattern of impulses may also be of informational value. Thus, the same mean frequency of impulses may carry different information depending on whether the cell fires impulses with a regular interval or in bursts. Some neurons can switch between these two modes of firing impulses.

In conclusion, the code for the information carried by an axon is the frequency and pattern of action potentials since the strength of action potential is always the same.

The Refractory Period

After an action potential, some time must elapse before the neuron can again produce an action potential in response to a stimulus. The cell is said to be in a *refractory state*. This ensures that the cell always gets at least a minimal rest between each action potential and thus puts an upper limit on the frequency with which the cell can fire. The length of the refractory period, and thus the maximal frequency of firing, varies considerably among different kinds of nerve cells.

Two conditions are responsible for the refractory period. One is the above-mentioned *inactivation of the voltage-gated Na^+ channels*, and the other is the fact that *the membrane is hyperpolarized immediately after the action potential* (Fig. 2.5). The inactivation of Na^+ channels means that they cannot be opened, regardless of the strength of the stimulus and the ensuing depolarization. Hyperpolarization occurs because the K^+ channels remain open longer than required just to bring the membrane potential back to resting value. These two different mechanisms can explain why the refractory period consists of two phases. During the first phase, the *absolute refractory period*, the cell cannot be made to discharge however strong the stimulus may be; during the *relative refractory period*, stronger depolarization than normal is needed to produce an action potential.

Impulse Conduction in Axons

We will now consider how the action potential moves along the axon. The ability of the axon to conduct electrical current depends on several conditions, some of which are given by the physical properties of axons, which are very different from, for example, copper wire. In addition, some conditions vary among axons of different kinds. An axon is a poor conductor compared with electrical conductors made of metal. This is so because the axoplasm through which the current has to pass consists of a weak solution of electrolytes (that is, low concentrations of charged particles in water). In addition, the diameter of an axon is small (from less than 1 to 20μm) with a correspondingly enormous *internal resistance* to the current in the axoplasm. Furthermore, the axonal membrane is not a perfect insulator, so that charged particles are lost from the interior of the axon as the current passes along its length. The amount of current being lost is determined by the degree of *membrane resistance* (that is, the resistance offered by the membrane to charged particles trying to pass). Finally, the axonal membrane (like all cell membranes) has an *electrical capacity*; that is, it can store a certain number of charged particles in the same way a battery does. This further contributes to the rapid attenuation of a current that is conducted along an axon—the membrane has to be charged before the current can move on.

From the foregoing it can be concluded that *how well the current is conducted in an axon depends on its internal resistance (its diameter), the membrane resistance (how well insulated it is), and the capacity of the axonal membrane.* If the propagation of the action potential along the axon took place only by passive, electrotonic movement of charged particles, the internal resistance and loss of charges to the exterior would cause the action potential to move only a short distance before it "died out." The solution to this problem is that the *action potential is regenerated as it moves along the axon.* Thus, it is propagated with undiminished strength all the way from the cell body to the terminal boutons. As discussed above, the strength of the action potential—that is, the magnitude of the changes of the membrane potential taking place—is the same regardless of the strength of the stimulus that produced it (as long as the stimulus depolarizes the membrane to threshold). *Increasing the strength of the stimulus increases the frequency of action potentials, whereas the magnitude of each action potential remains constant.*

When the cell membrane close to the site where the axon leaves the cell body is depolarized to threshold, an action potential is produced and is conducted passively a short distance along the axon. From then on, what happens differs somewhat in myelinated and unmyelinated axons. We will consider *unmyelinated axons* first (Fig. 2.6). The action potential is produced by positive charges penetrating to the interior of the axon, which at that point becomes positive relative to more distal parts along its length. Positive charges then start moving in the distal direction (along the electrical gradient that has been set up). Outside the axon, a corresponding current of positive charges moves in the opposite direction, so that an *electrical circuit* is established. Movement of positive charges in

Figure 2.6. *Impulse conduction in unmyelinated axons.*

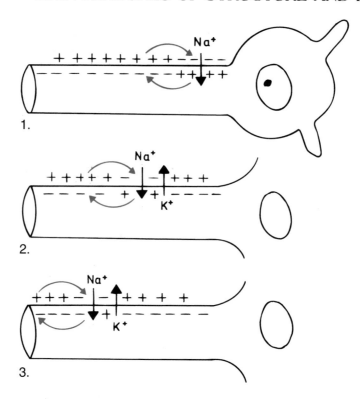

the distal direction inside the axon means that the membrane is depolarized as the charges move along. This depolarization leads to the opening of enough voltage-gated Na^+ and K^+ channels to produce a "new" action potential. In this manner, the action potential moves along the axon at a speed that depends on the speed with which the charged particles (that is, ions) move inside the axon and on the time needed for full opening of the ion channels. The membrane capacity represents a further factor slowing the propagation, because the membrane has to be charged before there can be a net flow of charges through it.

In essence, the *action potential is propagated as a wave of depolarization*, followed closely by a corresponding wave of repolarization. When the membrane has just completed this cycle, it is in the *refractory state* for some milliseconds. This delay prevents the action potential from spreading "backward" toward the perikaryon (antidromic impulse conduction), and ensures that under normal conditions the impulse conduction is unidirectional. If, however, the axon is artificially stimulated (for example, electrically) at some distance from the cell body, the action potential spreads toward both the cell body and the end ramifications (orthodromic impulse conduction). *Antidromic impulse conduction*, however, may occur in branches of peripheral sensory axons upon natural stimulation, and play a role for certain disease symptoms.

In *myelinated axons*, the action potential is also regenerated along the axon (Fig. 2.7). But, in contrast to that in unmyelinated axons, *the action potential is regenerated only at each node of Ranvier*—that is, where the axon membrane lacks covering by the myelin sheath and is in direct contact with the extracellular fluid. As in unmyelinated axons, the action potential arises in the first part of the axon where it

Figure 2.7. *Impulse conduction in myelinated axons.*

emerges from the perikaryon. The current then spreads passively (electrotonically) to the first node of Ranvier. Here, the depolarization of the membrane leads to opening of voltage-gated channels and a "new" action potential. The density of voltage-gated sodium channels is particularly high in the axonal membrane at the node of Ranvier. The current can flow electrotonically as far as the first node of Ranvier (and probably sometimes farther) because the axon is so well insulated by myelin, preventing loss of charges from the interior of the axon. (Myelin increases dramatically the resistance across the membrane and also reduces the membrane capacity.) In addition, the axonal diameter is larger in myelinated than in unmyelinated axons, thus reducing the internal resistance.

In conclusion, in myelinated axons the action potential does not move smoothly and slowly along, as in unmyelinated axons, but instead "jumps" from one node of Ranvier to the next. While the impulse propagation is very rapid between nodes, at each node there is a delay due to the time required for opening of channels and establishment of sufficient flow of current.

Conduction Velocities in Myelinated and Unmyelinated Axons

The main reason myelinated axons conduct so much more rapidly than unmyelinated ones is that the action potential needs to be regenerated only at certain sites. A figure for conduction velocity (expressed in meters per second) in myelinated axons is obtained by multiplying the axonal diameter (in micrometers) by 6. An axon of 20 μm (the maximal diameter) thus conducts at approximately 120 m/sec, whereas the thinnest myelinated axons of about 3 μm conduct at 18 m/sec. In comparison, a typical unmyelinated axon of about 1 μm conducts at less than 1 m/sec.

SYNAPTIC TRANSMISSION

So far, we have discussed the basis of nerve impulses and how they are conducted over long distances. Now we will look into the synaptic transfer of the signal represented by an action potential. We will also examine what leads up to the discharge of an action potential.

Transfer of Signals between Nerve Cells Is Usually Chemically Mediated

We can sum up the signal transfer as follows (Fig. 2.8): First, an action potential reaches the nerve terminal (bouton) and depolarizes it. This *depolarization opens Ca^{2+} channels*, enabling Ca^{2+} to enter the bouton. Increase in intracellular Ca^{2+} concentration is a signal for *release of transmitter* from vesicles by exocytosis. The released transmitter binds briefly to receptors in the postsynaptic membrane. This leads directly or indirectly to alteration of the opening of ion channels and thus to transient changes in membrane permeability to certain ions and alteration of the membrane potential. The potential change arising as a result of such synaptic influence is called a *synaptic potential*. If the synaptic influence depolarizes the postsynaptic cell, the probability that the cell will fire action potentials is increased. This synaptic effect is called an *excitatory synaptic potential*. If the synaptic potential hyperpolarizes the cell, it is called an *inhibitory synaptic potential* because the probability of the cell's firing is diminished.

Transmitters Are Contained in Vesicles and Released in Quanta

We have previously described *synaptic vesicles*, aggregated near the presynaptic membrane of boutons (Fig. 2.8). Although the question is not finally settled, we assume that all transmitters, once they are ready for release, are localized in synaptic vesicles. In addition, "free" transmitter molecules are present in the cytoplasm of the bouton, but most likely these have to be taken up in vesicles before release. The release then takes place by *exocytosis*. The vesicle moves toward the presynaptic membrane and the vesicle membrane fuses with the presynaptic membrane. This also opens the vesicle, and the content of transmitter molecules enters the synaptic cleft. While some vesicles empty their contents, others move toward the presynaptic membrane and get ready for "docking." The synaptic vesicles can therefore be divided into two main groups: those situated close to the membrane that are ready for release when the Ca^{2+} concentration rises around them, and those that must move to the membrane before transmitter release.

For some synapses, in particular those between motor nerve terminals and striated muscle cells (at the neuromuscular junction, see Figure 11.3), there is convincing evidence that the transmitter (acetylcholine) is released in packets, or *quanta*, corresponding to the transmitter content of one vesicle. Calculations from experiments with such synapses indicate that one

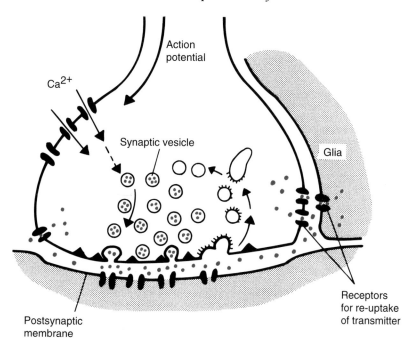

vesicle contains on the average 10,000 acetylcholine molecules. Only a few thousand molecules of each quantum are likely to bind to a receptor before they diffuse away or are removed by other means. Release of one quantum elicits a tiny *excitatory postsynaptic potential (EPSP)—a miniature EPSP*. If stimulation is increased, so that more transmitter is released, the depolarization of the muscle cell membrane increases in steps corresponding to one miniature EPSP. Each bouton probably releases from none to a few quanta for each presynaptic action potential. The situation at the neuromuscular junction is special since each motor axon ramifies into about 50 terminal boutons on one muscle cell (Fig. 11.3). An action potential in the motor axon therefore invades *all* the boutons and leads to release of many quanta. Thus—although each bouton releases only the content of one vesicle—the subsequent depolarization always becomes large enough to reach threshold for an action potential in the muscle cell.

It should be noted that an action potential does not necessarily elicit transmitter release; it merely *increases the probablity of release*. In the central nervous system as well, *each action potential invading a bouton releases the transmitter content of none to a few vesicles*. This differs from the situation in the neuromuscular junction because a single presynaptic action potential would not be able to depolarize a postsynaptic neuron to the threshold. As we shall discuss below, many presynaptic action potentials must coincide to fire a postsynaptic neuron.

Transmitter Release Is Ca^{2+}-Dependent

Depolarization of the presynaptic membrane (by the action potential) is the normal event preceding transmitter release. The transmitter release depends on Ca^{2+} entering the bouton (Fig. 2.8) through voltage-gated calcium channels that are opened by depolarization. The more Ca^{2+} that enters, the more quanta of transmitter are released. Axoaxonic synapses (Fig. 2.10) may regulate the opening of Ca^{2+} channels in the presynaptic membrane. This makes it possible for other neurons to influence the amount of transmitter released. The voltage-gated Ca^{2+} channels must be localized close to the site of exocytosis at the presynaptic membrane; otherwise, there would not be sufficient time for diffusion since it takes only 0.1–0.2 msec from calcium inflow to the occurrence of exocytosis (Figure 2.8 is therefore somewhat misleading).

That vesicles fuse with the postsynaptic membrane during release is supported by electron microscopic observations. Thus, the number of vesicles drops upon long-term stimulation (trains of action potentials), while the number increases after a period of rest. How increased intracellular calcium concentration is coupled to the movement and subsequent fusion of vesicles is not fully understood.

Mechanisms for Vesicle Transport and Fusion

The establishment of contact (and subsequent fusion) between a vesicle and the presynaptic membrane is governed by a set of proteins that most likely is common to all cells. These proteins control not only exocytosis but also other processes involving fusion of membranes (for example in the Golgi apparatus). The fusion requires specific binding of proteins in the presynaptic membrane to receptors (proteins) in the vesicle membrane. By influencing this binding, other molecules can regulate transmitter release—for example, in response to altered use of the synapse.

Some kinds of fusion proteins are specifically degraded by *tetanus toxin* and *botulinum toxin* (produced in certain foods if not treated properly). Both toxins are produced by anaerobic bacteria (that is, they only grow in the absence of oxygen) and produce violent muscle spasms and paralysis, respectively. They evoke opposite effects because they act on different kinds of synapses: the tetanus toxin affects primarily a type of inhibitory synapse, whereas botulinum toxin acts at the neuromuscular junction, preventing release of the excitatory transmitter acetylcholine.

Another group of proteins, the *synapsins*, probably bind vesicles to the cytoskeleton, making them less mobile. The activity of the synapsins can be regulated by specific *protein kinases* (phosphorylating proteins). Phosphorylation of synapsin increases mobility of the vesicles and is most likely another way of controlling the amount of transmitter released by an action potential.

Both the fusion proteins and the synapsins are of special interest since their regulation may be involved in nervous system *plasticity*, which is crucial during development, recovery after brain damage, and learning in general. Thus, plasticity is closely related to changing the functional properties of synapses.

Summation of Stimuli Is Necessary to Evoke an Action Potential

Not every impulse leading to transmitter release at a synapse evokes an action potential in the postsynaptic cell. As already mentioned, the membrane has to be depolarized to a *threshold value* (Fig. 2.9) for an action potential to be evoked. A subthreshold depolarization (excitatory synaptic potential) may nevertheless be of functional significance. Thus, if the synaptic potential is followed by another depolarization before the membrane potential has returned to resting value, the second depolarization is added to the first one so that threshold is reached. This phenomenon is called *summation* (Fig. 2.9A). The summation may be in time, as in the

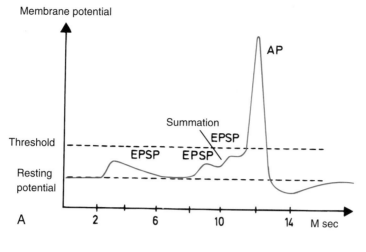

Membrane potential

Threshold

Resting potential

AP

Summation
EPSP
EPSP
EPSP

A   2   6   10   14   M sec

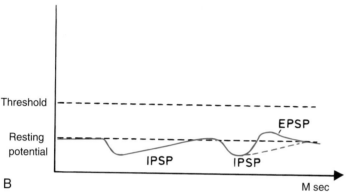

Threshold

Resting potential

EPSP

IPSP   IPSP

B   M sec

Figure 2.9. *Synaptic potentials.* **A.** Diagram showing the time course and polarity of an EPSP. In this example, one EPSP alone does not depolarize the membrane to threshold for eliciting an action potential (AP), but if one or more EPSP follows shortly after the first one, the threshold is reached (summation). **B.** Diagram showing the time course and polarity of an IPSP.

example above, and is then called *temporal summation*, or it may be in space, then called *spatial summation*. In temporal summation, impulses may follow one another in rapid succession in one terminal, whereas in spatial summation, boutons at different places on the cell surface release transmitter and depolarize the cell almost simultaneously.

Summation can be an important mechanism for controlling the activity of nerve cells because the *time course of synaptic potentials is slow* in contrast to the time course of an action potential. The excitatory synaptic potential is caused by simultaneous opening of several types of cation channels (for Na^+ and Ca^{2+} going in, and K^+ going out). Because the cations outside the cell are driven in both by concentration gradients and by the membrane potential, whereas K^+ is driven out only by the concentration gradient, the inward current dominates initially and the membrane is depolarized. This, however, leads to an increased outward current of K^+. Depolarization in itself does not increase the opening of transmitter-gated channels (unlike the case for voltage-gated channels responsible for the action potential). Therefore, the synaptic potential gradually increases and decreases (graded potential). From the site of the synapse, the current spreads passively (electrotonically) along the membrane of the postsynaptic cell, without being regenerated. Thus, because charges (ions) leak through the membrane, the current will gradually become weaker as it moves from the synapse. As already mentioned, the current produced at synaptic sites must reach the initial segment to produce an action potential. If the current is strong enough to depolarize the membrane of the initial segment to threshold, an action potential arises (by opening voltage-gated Na$^+$ channels).

A Neuron Integrates Information from Many Others

We have seen that as a rule many impulses must reach a neuron almost simultaneously to make it fire—that is, to send an action potential through its axon. In other words, *summation* of excitatory synaptic effects is necessary. The stronger the sum of excitatory effects, the shorter the time necessary to depolarize the cell to the threshold for eliciting another action potential. Thus, *the frequency of action potentials, or firing frequency, is an expression of the total synaptic input to a neuron.* Total synaptic input here means the *sum of both excitatory and inhibitory synaptic influences.* Often a neuron is strongly influenced (many synaptic contacts) by one neuronal group as it is weakly influenced by many others. Thus, this particular neuron may be principally involved in signal transmission from one source (a nucleus, a set of receptors, etc.), but the efficiency of transmission may be facilitated or inhibited by many other cell groups.

Consider two *examples* of the integration of different synaptic inputs. The first concerns *motor neurons of the spinal cord.* Such a neuron—sending its axon to innervate hundreds of striated muscle cells in a particular muscle—is synaptically contacted by neurons in many parts of the nervous system. It may receive as many as 50,000 synapses, distributed over its dendrites and cell body. Some synapses inform the cell about sensory stimuli important for the movement produced by the muscle, others about the posture of the body, others about how fast an intended movement should be, and so forth. The sum of all these synaptic inputs—some of them excitatory, others inhibitory—determines the frequency of action potentials sent to the muscle and by that means the force of muscle contraction (each muscle, however, is governed by many such neurons, so that their collective activity determines the behavior of the whole muscle). The other example concerns *neurons in the spinal cord that mediate information about painful stimuli.* While such a neuron receives its strongest synaptic input (most synapses) from sensory organs reacting to painful stimuli, it is also contacted by thousands of synapses from other sources, such as cell groups that are particularly active when the person is anxious. Thus, the final firing frequency of this "pain-transmitting" neuron depends not only on the actual stimuli reaching the receptors but also on the activity within the central nervous system itself. This correlates well with the everyday experience that the pain we feel depends not only on the strength of the peripheral painful stimulus (such as dental drilling) but also on our state of mind. This phenomenon is discussed more fully in Chapter 7.

The Placement of Synapses on the Neuron Influences Their Effectiveness

The efficiency or strength of a certain synaptic input is related not only to the total number of synaptic contacts. The *placement* of a synapse on the neuronal surface is also of importance. Synapses close to the initial segment of the axon have a greater chance of eliciting (or preventing) an action potential than synapses far out on the dendrites. (This finding is related to the loss of current during electrotonic spread of the synaptic potential over long distances.) Thus, a centrally placed synapse may perhaps fire the neuron alone, whereas many peripherally placed synapses will have to cooperate to fire the cell. In this sense, synapses may be more or less *strategically* placed.

Synaptic placement on the neuron is obviously not a matter of chance. Thus, there are several examples of axons coming from different cell groups that end on different parts of the postsynaptic neuron (for example, some end only on proximal dendites, others on distal dendrites or a particular segment of the dendrite).

Many Synapses Are Placed on Spines

Another important point regarding the placement of synapses is that *most excitatory synapses are located on spines* (Figs. 1.1 and 1.5). Most of the neurons in the cerebral cortex conform to this arrangement. Since cortical neurons constitute a major proportion of all neurons in the human brain, suggestions that about 90% of all excitatory synapses are placed on spines may be realistic.

The *functional significance* of this relationship is still under debate. It is not simply a matter of the spines increasing the receiving surface of the neuron since the dendritic membrane between spines may be virtually free of synapses. A spine typically consists of a narrow *neck* and an expanded part called the *spine head* (Fig. 1.7D). Since the microscopic identification of spines in the past century, they have been implicated in *learning and memory*, and recent animal experiments support this hypothesis. For example, the density of spines in the cerebral cortex is higher in rats living in a challenging environment than in those confined to standard laboratory cages (this is more fully discussed in Chapter 4). Electric stimulation of particular axonal populations can produce long-term increases in synaptic efficacy (long-term potentiation, LTP). *LTP* is probably an important mechanism underlying synaptic plasticity, and the induction of LTP appears to be accompanied by changes in the form and number of spines. This effect is observed only among those synapses affected by the increased stimulation. The narrow neck of the spines may ensure that the concentration of signal molecules responsible for LTP induction, such as Ca^{2+}, reach much higher levels in the spine head than in the dendrite. This would facilitate changes in those synapses contacting a particular spine, leaving other synapses unaffected. Spatial restriction of increased Ca^{2+} concentration may also serve a *protective role* since high intracellular Ca^{2+} concentration may damage the neuron (see *Ischemic Cell Damage and the Glutamate Hypothesis* in Chapter 4).

Excitatory Synapses and EPSP

As mentioned above, at a synapse where the transmitter depolarizes the postsynaptic membrane, an EPSP is evoked. If a new EPSP follows before the previous one is finished, summation of depolarizations occurs because more ion channels are open at the same time (Fig. 2.9A). Neurotransmitters producing EPSPs are called *excitatory transmitters*, and we also use the term *excitatory synapses*. One EPSP alone does not as a rule cause sufficient depolarization to give rise to an action potential, but for a short while the cell has increased responsiveness to further excitatory input. Thus repeated stimuli, or an increase in the number of synapses being active, may fire a cell that would not respond with an action potential to a single stimulus.

Neurons Can "Remember" Previous Synaptic Influences

When action potentials reach the nerve terminal at only brief intervals (high firing frequency), the amplitude of the ensuing postsynaptic potentials often increases (the amplitude of the presynaptic action potential remains the same under such conditions). This phenomenon is called *facilitation*. The favored explanation is that some of the Ca^{2+} that enters during one action potential remains in the bouton when the next action potential arrives and again opens calcium channels. Thus the effect of Ca^{2+} on transmitter release is enhanced. Facilitation may last for seconds so that as long as the interval between action potentials is shorter than this, the postsynaptic effect of each action potential may increase by repetitive stimulation. Facilitation appears to be important for the nervous system's capacity for short-term storage of information and for changing responses during learning (plasticity). However, cellular mechanisms other than facilitation are required for more enduring changes in synaptic effects.

A long train of high-frequency stimulation (tetanic stimulation) can render the postsynaptic cell more responsive for minutes to hours. Thus, even hours after the tetanic stimulation, a presynaptic action potential evokes a larger postsynaptic potential. This is called *post-tetanic potentiation*, and like facilitation it is probably explained by increase in transmitter release from the presynaptic bouton. Here the presynaptic terminal "remembers" that it recently received unusually intense stimulation, and alters its behavior accordingly.

Long-term potentiation (LTP) represents an even longer-lasting form of "cellular memory." In this case, changes are most likely occurring both pre- and postsynaptically (not only presynaptically as with facilitation and post-tetanic potentiation). The changes may last very long, probably for years. Such long-term (life-long?) synaptic changes must imply altered neuronal protein synthesis, requiring specific changes of gene expression. *Protein kinases*—enzymes that can alter the opening state of ion channels—are likely candidates in this respect.

The opposite phenomenon to LTP also occurs—that is, a reduction of postsynaptic response after preceding high-frequency stimulation. This is called *long-term depression* (LTD). It also represents a kind of long-term cellular memory, and the mechanisms of induction are similar to those of LTP.

Inhibitory Synapses and Inhibitory Postsynaptic Potential (IPSP)

At many synapses, the transmitter substances released *reduce the probability of the postsynaptic cell responding* with action potentials. One way in which such transmitters work is by *hyperpolarizing* the postsynaptic membrane transiently. Thus, more depolarization is needed to bring the membrane potential to threshold. The potential evoked at such synapses is called an *inhibitory postsynaptic potential* (IPSP). This synaptic potential has a comparatively slow time course and lasts for many milliseconds (Fig. 2.9B). An EPSP occurring during an IPSP will have less probability of evoking an action potential. The postsynaptic cell is therefore inhibited, and we use the terms *inhibitory transmitters* and *inhibitory synapses*.

The mechanism underlying hyperpolarization is usually opening of transmitter-gated K^+ or Cl^- channels. This leads to a flow of K^+ ions out of the cell, with the inside becoming more negative than earlier compared with the outside, or to Cl^- flowing into the cell, with the same effect on the membrane potential. A prerequisite for hyperpolarization to result from opening of K^+ or Cl^- channels is that the membrane potential at the outset is less negative than the equilibrium potentials for K^+ or Cl^-. The equilibrium potential of Cl^- is in fact close to the resting potential in many nerve cells. Nevertheless, even when there is no net flow

Figure 2.10. *Presynaptic inhibition* is mediated by axoaxonic synapses.

of Cl^- into the cell, opening of chloride channels can reduce the effect of simultaneous excitatory transmitters. This is so because Cl^- starts to flow into the cell as soon as the membrane is even slightly depolarized (because this makes the inside less negative) and thus opposes change of the membrane potential. In this manner, the inhibitory transmitter acts to *short-circuit* nearby excitatory synapses.

The kind of inhibition discussed so far acts *postsynaptically*—that is, one neuron reduces the excitability of another neuron. This is the most common kind of inhibition, occurring in all parts of the central nervous system. In addition, however, inhibition may also be exerted *presynaptically*, mediated by axoaxonic synapses (Figs. 1.7D and 2.10). This en-

Axoaxonic Synapses Enable Presynaptic Control of Transmitter Release

In *axoaxonic synapses* (Figs. 1.7D and 2.10), the presynaptic bouton makes synaptic contact with a postsynaptic bouton, which in turn contacts a perikaryon or a dendrite. Release of transmitter from the presynaptic bouton serves to *regulate the amount of transmitter released by the postsynaptic bouton*.

In one type of axoaxonic contact, action potentials in the presynaptic bouton lead to *reduced transmitter release* from the postsynaptic bouton; thus the effect is inhibitory with regard to the neuron contacted by the postsynaptic bouton. A prerequisite for this inhibitory effect to occur, however, is that the presynaptic bouton be depolarized (by an action potential) at the same time as or immediately before an action potential reaches the postsynaptic bouton. This phenomenon is termed *presynaptic inhibition* to distinguish it from the postsynaptic inhibition described above. Two mechanisms may be responsible for presynaptic inhibition. One is the *opening of chloride channels* in the membrane of the postsynaptic bouton, thereby short-circuiting it in the manner described above in connection with postsynaptic inhibition. In such a case, the action potential invading the postsynaptic bouton would elicit less depolarization than normally. Less depolarization means opening of fewer calcium channels, and since the amount of transmitter released is proportional to the influx of Ca^{2+}, less transmitter will be released. Another mechanism for presynaptic inhibition may be *direct influence on calcium channels* by the transmitter released from the presynaptic bouton. Presynaptic inhibition has been found most frequently among fiber systems that transmit sensory information; for example, sensory fibers entering the spinal cord are subject to powerful presynaptic inhibition. Presynaptic inhibition is mediated by the neurotransmitter *glutamic acid decarboxylase (GAD)*, which is also the most common inhibitory transmitter acting postsynaptically (see *Inhibitory Amino Acid Transmitters,* below).

Presynaptic facilitation may be elicited at axoaxonic synapses by transmitters that lead to increased Ca^{2+} influx in the postsynaptic bouton. Increased calcium influx may be caused by closure of K^+ channels by the transmitter. This leads to prolongation of the action potential (the repolarization phase being slower), which enables more Ca^{2+} to enter the postsynaptic bouton.

sures that the excitability of the postsynaptic neuron will remain unaffected while specific synaptic inputs are inhibited. Thus, the neuron may switch from preferentially transmitting one kind of information, to another kind. Such *presynaptic inhibition* plays an important role, for example, in motor control and in transmission of sensory signals.

Why Do We Need Inhibitory Synapses?

Inhibitory synapses are present everywhere in the central nervous system and are of vital importance for its proper functioning. Inhibition is, for example, necessary to *suppress irrelevant sensory information*, thus enabling us to concentrate on certain events and leave others out. Inhibitory synapses also serve to *increase the precision* of sensory information by, for example, enhancing contrast between regions with different light intensity in visual images.

Inhibition is also necessary for another reason—namely, to *dampen or interrupt excitation*, which might otherwise lead to cell damage. As mentioned earlier, ions have to be pumped through the cell membrane in order to maintain osmotic equilibrium. If many neurons fire continuously with high frequency, even maximal pumping may be insufficient in this respect. Increased extracellular potassium concentration depolarizes neurons, thus further increasing the neuronal excitation; this in turn leads to more potassium extracellularly and so on. Epileptic seizures are due to uncontrolled firing of groups of neurons, and drugs reducing the tendency for seizures generally increase the effect of inhibitory transmitters.

Two Main Kinds of Synaptic Effect: Fast and Slow

So far we have considered only fast synaptic effects on the membrane potential, typically lasting only a few milliseconds. If the effects are sufficiently strong, an action potential is elicited. Such synaptic effects are produced by transmitters binding *directly* to ion channels—that is, the external part of the channel protein contains a binding site for the transmitter (Fig. 2.2). In this case we use the terms *ionotropic receptors* and *ionotropic transmitter actions*. Since the binding is direct, the effect on the opening state of the channel is immediate. The effect is also very brief because it ends when the transmitter dissociates from the receptor. In addition, there are mechanisms ensuring rapid removal of the transmitter from the synaptic cleft. The most ubiquitous excitatory and inhibitory transmitters of the central nervous system (glutamate and gamma-aminobutyric acid [GABA], respectively) act in this way. Such transmitters mediate *fast and precise information*, which is obviously of crucial importance for the tasks of the nervous system.

Transmitters may, however, have other kinds of effects as well. Often the transmitter receptor is not an integral part of an ion channel but an independent membrane protein (Fig. 2.11). The transmitter receptor then acts *indirectly* on the ion channel, by way of intracellular signal molecules. It is understandable that such indirect receptors act more slowly

Figure 2.11. *Transmitter receptor with indirect action on ion channels.* Schematic. All indirectly coupled receptors act via G proteins, whereas other elements of the intracellular signal pathway may vary among different receptors. In this example cyclic AMP serves as the second messenger.

than the direct ones (Fig. 2.12) because they initiate a chain of chemical reactions, some of which are enzymatic and slow. It may take seconds to minutes from the binding of an indirectly acting transmitter to its effect on neuronal excitability. On the other hand, the effect may last for seconds or minutes after the transmitter has diffused away. We also apply the term *metabotropic* to such indirectly acting receptors.

Whereas ionotropic transmitters act only on the receptors in the synaptic cleft where the transmitter is released, indirectly acting transmitters may diffuse away from the synaptic cleft and affect other synapses in the vicinity. Thus, *indirect (metabotropic) synaptic effects are less precise than direct (ionotropic) ones, in both time and space.*

G Proteins Mediate Indirect Effects on Ion Channels

All transmitter receptors with indirect actions are coupled to *G proteins*. The G proteins mediate the signal to ion channels via second messengers. The name derives from the ability of G proteins to bind guanosine triphosphate (GTP). So far, more than 1000 receptors acting via G proteins have been described (they are not limited to the nervous system, and their effects may be either stimulatory or inhibitory). They can therefore be regarded as *universal translators—translating many kinds of signals that reach the exterior of a cell into cellular responses.* Two examples are the translation of tasty or odorous chemicals into nerve impulses, and the effects of hormones on cell metabolism. Activation of a receptor coupled to a G protein catalyzes the binding of GTP. This activates the G protein, which in turn initiates a chain of intracellular reactions. The many different kinds of G proteins explain the wide variety of specific effects that can be produced by G protein activation.

Each G protein consists of three subunits: α, β, and γ. The latter two act primarily by binding the α subunit to the cell membrane. When GTP binds to the G protein, the α subunit loosens and can now interact with a target molecule (often an enzyme; see Figure 2.11). Sometimes, however, a G protein can act *directly on ion channels* (without intermediaries) and thus serve as a second messenger itself.

A large group of G proteins exert their effects by activating the enzyme *adenylate cyclase*. This enzyme catalyzes the synthesis of the second messenger *cyclic adenosine monophosphate (cyclic AMP)*, which in turn increases the activity of cyclic AMP-dependent *protein kinases*. The protein kinase then phosphorylates specific channel proteins, thus altering their opening state (Fig. 2.11). Another group of G proteins activate the enzyme *phospholipase* that catalyzes synthesis of two second messengers: *diacylglycerol* (DAG) and *inositol triphosphate* (IP$_3$). IP$_3$ releases Ca^{2+} from the endoplasmic reticulum, while DAG activates a specific protein kinase (C). Several ion channels, among them some potassium and chloride channels, are regulated by the intracellular Ca^{2+} concentration. Here Ca^{2+} acts as a *third messenger*.

Mechanisms of Modulatory Synaptic Effects

A brief train of impulses in axons releasing a transmitter that binds to indirectly acting receptors may keep the membrane depolarized or hyperpolarized for seconds after the train of impulses ends (slow EPSP or IPSP; Fig. 2.12). More intense stimulation may produce depolarization lasting minutes in some neurons. As mentioned, a slow EPSP does not reach the threshold for an action potential but it facilitates the response to fast synaptic actions. Slow EPSPs may be mediated by transmitters closing a kind of *voltage-gated K^+ channel* that is open at the resting membrane potential. This leads to lowered K^+ permeability and reduced flow of K^+ out of the cell, which results in depolarization. Because the membrane potential is shifted toward the threshold, fast depolarization stands a better chance of eliciting an action potential. In addition, the effect on this kind of K^+ channel makes a fast EPSP larger and longer-lasting. This is so because the channel is also acted upon (opened) by the fast transmitter during the repolarization phase of the EPSP (Figs. 2.5 and 2.9). When the modulatory transmitter counteracts the opening of the channel in this phase, the depolarization becomes stronger, and the repolarization phase is prolonged. Thus the fast transmitter, rather than eliciting one, may produce a train of action potentials.

Modulatory synaptic effects may not change the resting membrane potential, if they are confined to channels that are not open at the resting potential. A kind of K^+ receptor—closed at the resting potential—is opened by Ca^{2+} entering the cell during the action potential. This produces a relatively long-lasting hyperpolarization (the refractory period). A modulatory transmitter that reduces the opening of the K^+ channel would shorten the refractory period. As in the example above, a fast excitatory input might produce a train of impulses rather than only one, or the frequency of impulses during a train might be higher than without the modulatory influence.

Slow, long-lasting *hyperpolarizing* synaptic effects (slow IPSP), may be mediated by the indirect opening of K^+ channels. As we discuss below, the inhibitory transmitter GABA can act on receptors with such effect.

Slow Synaptic Effects Modulate the Effect of Fast Ones

Each neuron is influenced by many synapses using different transmitters. Thus, we may safely assume that every neuron receives both fast (direct, ionotropic) and slow (indirect, metabotropic) synaptic inputs. The slow effects *modulate* the effects of the fast ones, and we therefore use the term *modulatory transmitter actions*. A modulatory transmitter (when binding to an indirectly acting receptor) does not by itself evoke action potentials but alters the sensitivity of the neuron to fast, ionotropic transmitter ac-

Figure 2.12. *Fast and slow synaptic actions*. Schematic. A fast EPSP lasts milliseconds and is caused by binding of transmitter molecules directly to channel proteins. A slow EPSP may last seconds or minutes and is due to activation of receptors indirectly coupled to ion channels.

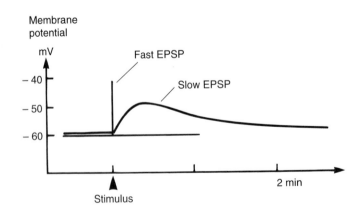

tions. An example may make this clearer: motoneurons in the cord receive fast, excitatory synaptic input from the cerebral cortex. These signals mediate the precise, voluntary control of muscle contraction. In addition, the motoneurons receive slow, modulatory synaptic inputs from cell groups in the brain stem whose activity is related to our degree of motivation for a particular movement. The modulatory input influences the *strength of the response* (frequency of action potentials) to signals from the cerebral cortex—that is, how fast the movement will be. However, the modulatory input cannot initiate movements on its own.

The same type of transmitter may have both fast (direct) and slow, modulatory effects. This depends on whether the postsynaptic membrane presents different kinds of receptors. As we will discuss below, ubiquitous transmitters such as glutamate, GABA, and acetylcholine act on both ionotropic and metabotropic receptors.

Usually, modulatory synaptic effects are mediated by altered opening states of K^+ or Ca^{2+} channels (Fig. 2.11). Thus, the membrane potential and the refractory period can be modulated. The effects are nevertheless varied because there are several kinds of potassium and calcium channels, and each channel may be influenced by several transmitters.

Synaptic Activity May Alter the Metabolism of the Neuron

Synaptic activation, apart from regulating the excitability of neurons, can also influence the metabolic activity of the postsynaptic cell (via intracellular second messengers). This may be related to the growth and development of neurons, which in many cases have been shown to depend on synaptic activity. It probably also relates to plastic changes in neurons

Unusual Synapses: Electrotonic and Dendrodendritic Transmission

Although rare, at some synapses in the central nervous system, the pre- and postsynaptic elements are electrically rather than chemically coupled. Electron microscopically, such electronic synapses differ from chemical synapses in that the synaptic cleft is only 2 nm compared to about 20 nm. The cell contact formed is called a *nexus* or *gap junction*, and consists of *channels that span the synaptic cleft*. Thus, ions (electrical current) can pass directly and quickly from one cell to another with no synaptic delay. In invertebrates and lower vertebrates, electrotonic synapses are formed between neurons mediating short latency responses to stimuli (for example, escape reactions). Electrotonic synapses may also provide electrical coupling between many neurons in a group, so that their activity may be *synchronized*. Chemical synapses may occur close to electrical ones, and serve to uncouple the electrical synapse so that these apparently can be switched on and off. Even a small number of gap junctions between nerve cells—too small to produce efficient electric coupling—may be important by enabling transfer of small signal molecules, such as Ca^{2+}, cyclic AMP, and IP_3. Thus, one neuron may alter the properties of another without ordinary synaptic contact.

Electrical coupling by gap junctions is much more common among glial cells than among neurons, and it occurs regularly among cardiac, smooth-muscle, and epithelial cells.

There are also other unusual types of synapses. *Contacts between dendrites* with all the morphological characteristics of synapses have been observed in several places in the central nervous system. Such *dendrodendritic synapses* are often part of more complex synaptic arrangements. Through dendrodendritic synapses, adjacent neurons can influence each other without being connected with axons. The function of such synapses, however, is not fully understood.

involved in learning and memory. Enduring changes in neurons—at either a molecular or structural level—require *altered gene expression*. We now have much evidence that even synaptic activity lasting for minutes or less may produce altered expression of certain genes that probably encode for transcription factors. The main experimental evidence so far concerns transitory changes of gene expression, however. Furthermore, a causal relationship between the observed changes of gene expression and altered neuronal structure and function has not yet been established.

Long-term (or even permanent) effects may result from changes in synthesis of *receptor proteins* and enzymes involved in *transmitter synthesis*. There may also be changes in the amount and activity of *intracellular second messengers* and *protein kinases* (among other things, regulating ion channels and receptor proteins). If a neuron receives a certain synaptic influence and then liberates more transmitter at its terminals than previously, for example, its effect on other neurons is strengthened. If, however, the density of receptor molecules or ion channels in the neuronal membrane increases because of a synaptic influence, the neuron may react more strongly than before to that synaptic input.

NEUROTRANSMITTERS AND THEIR RECEPTORS

Some general properties of neurotransmitters were outlined earlier in connection with synaptic transmission. We will now explore this topic more fully, and describe the best-known neurotransmitters and their receptors (Table 2.1).

It Is Difficult to Prove That a Substance Functions as a Neurotransmitter

The term *neurotransmitter* or *transmitter* is used to define chemical substances that are released at synapses and transmit a signal from one neuron to another. To prove that a substance present in a neuron actually functions as a neurotransmitter, however, is far from easy. Several complicated anatomic, neurophysiological, and pharmacological techniques are required to demonstrate that the neuron *synthesizes* the transmitter candidate, that it is *stored* in the nerve terminals, that it is *released* by depolarization, that the release is *calcium-dependent*, and that the released substance is directly responsible for the *postsynaptic changes*. There also should be *specific mechanisms for removal* of the substance from the synaptic cleft and its immediate vicinity. For these kinds of studies, we are critically dependent on the availability of specific agonists and antagonists—that is, substances that mimic or prevent the action, respectively, of only the transmitter candidate.

Only a few transmitter candidates have met all of these criteria when tested experimentally. For several others, the probability that they function as transmitters is high, and they are often described as transmitters without reservation. Strictly speaking, however, they should be termed *transmitter candidates* or *putative transmitters*.

TABLE 2.1 The Best-Known Small-Molecular (Classical) Neurotransmitters

Transmitter	Chemical	Receptor Name*, Mechanism, Ion Permeability	Synaptic Actions	Distribution of Receptors in the CNS	Localization of Neurons Synthesizing the Transmitter in the CNS	Localization of Neurons in the PNS
Glutamate	Amino acid	AMPA, direct, Na$^+$ NMDA, direct, Ca^{2+} Indirect (mGluR1–8)	Fast, excitation " " Slow, excitation or inhibition	"Everywhere"	"Everywhere"	
GABA	Amino acid	GABA$_A$, direct, Cl$^-$ GABA$_B$, indirect, K$^+$, Ca^{2+}	Fast, inhibition Slow, inhibition	"Everywhere"	"Everywhere"	Gut, ganglia
Glycine	Amino acid	Direct, Cl$^-$	Fast, inhibition		Spinal cord Brain stem	
Acetylcholine	Quaternary amine	Nicotinic receptors (N), direct, Na$^+$, K$^+$	Fast, excitation	Renshaw cells (spinal cord)	Motoneurons Preganglionic autonomic neurons Basal nucleus	Parasympathetic ganglia
		Muscarinic receptors (m1–5), indirect, K$^+$, Ca^{2+}	Slow, excitation or inhibition	Cerebral cortex (neocortex) Hippocampus and other	Septal nuclei (and neighboring cell groups) Pontine reticular formation (parabrachial region) Basal ganglia	
Norepinephrine	Amine	α receptor, indirect (α_1, α_2)	Slow	Cerebral cortex Spinal cord	Nucleus coeruleus Cell groups in the reticular	Sympathetic ganglia
		β receptor, indirect (β_1, β_2)	Slow	and other	formation	
Dopamine	Amine	D$_1$, indirect D$_2$, indirect (D$_{3–5}$)	Slow	Cerebral cortex (especially frontal lobe) Ventral striatum Basal ganglia and other	Mesencephalon (substantia nigra and nearby cell groups) Hypothalamus	
Serotonin (5 HT)	Amine	5 HT$_{1A}$, indirect, opening K$^+$ 5 HT$_2$, indirect?	Slow, inhibition Slow, excitation	Cerebral cortex Basal ganglia Hippocampus	Raphe nuclei (brain stem)	
		5 HT$_3$, direct, Na$^+$, K$^+$	Fast, excitation	Amygdala Hypothalamus Nucleus solitarius Area postrema		

*There are several subtypes of each receptor.

The table is not complete regarding distribution of neurons and receptors.

As discussed above, the effects of substances released at synapses are multifarious and not limited to excitation or inhibition mediated by direct, fast actions on ion channel permeability. We use the term *modulator* or *neuromodulator* for substances that do not mediate the usual synaptic effects as fast EPSPs and IPSPs. Modulators typically elicit slow, long-lasting changes of neuronal excitability or metabolic changes in the postsynaptic cell.

The Two Main Groups of Chemical Transmitters

The neurotransmitters known today fall into two main chemical groups. One consists of *small molecules*, which with few exceptions (ATP and nitric oxide [NO]) are amino acids or amines (amino acids in which the carboxyl group is removed). The other group consists of larger molecules, namely *peptides* (short proteins consisting of about five to thirty amino acids). In general, the functions of these neuroactive peptides or *neuropeptides* are far less clarified than those of the small-molecular transmitters.

Fast synaptic effects mediated by direct opening or closing of ion channels are produced only by small-molecular transmitters, as far as we know. Some small molecular transmitters produce both fast and *slow, modulatory synaptic effects*, whereas others apparently produce only modulatory effects (Table 2.1). The neuropeptides seem to produce only slow, modulatory effects.

Co-localization of Transmitters

Nerve terminals often contain more than one transmitter; such *co-localization* appears to be the rule rather than an exception. Usually, *a small-molecular, "classical" transmitter is co-localized with one or several neuropeptides*. Therefore, it may be difficult to decide which transmitter is responsible for particular effects. Hypotheses about neural functions and disease symptoms have often been based on the erroneous belief that a particular neuronal group or fiber system uses only one transmitter (the one that was first discovered).

Transmitter Receptors in General

The many transmitters and transmitter candidates (more than fifty, including the neuropeptides) have an even larger variety of receptor types to act on. Several requirements have to be met to conclude that a binding site for a transmitter functions as a receptor. The "final proof" requires that its amino-acid sequence has been determined. After cloning of the protein, one can then find out whether it binds the transmitter (and agonists and antagonists) *and* produces the expected physiological effects.

All the *directly acting, ionotropic, receptors*—being part of ion channel proteins—are similarly built, with several subunits arranged around a central pore (Fig. 2.2). Also the *indirectly acting, metabotropic receptors* share several structural features, although they are quite different from the ionotropic receptors. Thus, the metabotropic receptors usually consist of one large protein mediating its effect via G proteins (Fig. 2.11).

Several receptor types have been identified for each of the best-known transmitters, and each transmitter as a rule acts on both ionotropic and metabotropic receptors, as we have seen. The different receptor types for one transmitter are often differently distributed in the brain. Subtypes of the directly acting GABA receptor (GABA$_A$) and subtypes of the metabotropic glutamate receptor are examples of this. Such differences may explain why drugs mimicking the effect of a transmitter may not have the same effect in all parts of the brain containing the transmitter.

Transmitter receptors are also *localized to the presynaptic membrane* and can by that means regulate transmitter release. We have discussed axoaxonic synapses mediating presynaptic inhibition by acting on receptors in the presynaptic membrane. In addition, the presynaptic membrane can express receptors for the transmitter released by the bouton itself. Here we use the term *autoregulation*. Finally, the bouton may express receptors for transmitters that are released by nearby boutons and reach the receptors by diffusion. This is an important way of regulating transmitter release in the autonomic nervous system.

The transmitter receptors are not static, immutable elements of the nervous system. We have seen that *synaptic plasticity* may be mediated by changes in receptor density and activity. Thus, learning in a wide sense may be accompanied by receptor changes. In animal experiments, for example, stressful psychological experiences leading to altered behavior have been shown to alter the activity of a specific transmitter receptor. Drugs that interfere with transmitter actions often induce changes in the receptor. A drug that blocks the effect of a transmitter on a particular receptor type (antagonists) may indirectly produce increased postsynaptic receptor density. The reverse may happen with drugs mimicking the transmitter (agonist). Probably such *up- or down-regulation of receptors* represents an adaptive response: An abnormally high concentration of the transmitter (or an agonist) is counteracted by reduced receptor activity to maintain normal synaptic transmission. Down-regulation of receptors may explain many of the often dramatic *withdrawal symptoms* occurring when an addict is cut off from a narcotic drug.

Why Are There so Many Different Transmitter Receptors?

One might think that it would suffice to have one kind of receptor mediating excitation and another mediating inhibition. Obviously, this is not so. The fact that almost all receptors known today are coded by separate genes suggests that receptor diversity is important for the organism, rather than an incidental by product of evolution. Presumably, species with a variety of transmitters have an advantage regarding adaptation to their environment. This in turn gives higher survival and reproduction rates. Probably, a variety of receptors enhance the brain's capacity for information processing. It may be especially important that this diversity provides plasticity—that is, the ability of the nervous system to change its performance in response to altered demands. For example, frequent use of a particular GABA synapse might induce the postsynaptic neuron to express a receptor with higher affinity for GABA, thereby changing its response. A large repertoire of receptors also enables a cell group—using one transmitter—to exert differential effects on other cell groups.

Synthesis of Neurotransmitters

The *small-molecular neurotransmitters* are synthesized in the nerve terminals, the synthesis being catalyzed by enzymes transported axonally from the perikaryon. As a rule, the rate of transmitter synthesis is determined by the enzymatic activity. Thus, up- or down-regulation of the enzymatic activity represents one way of changing the properties of nerve cells—for example, with regard to learning. Activation of enzymes often requires that they be phosphorylated, and this may be a result of external stimuli that, via membrane receptors, induce increased intracellular concentration of second messengers (such as Ca^{2+} or cAMP).

Since the organelles necessary for protein synthesis are present only in the perikaryon, the *neuropeptides* have to be synthesized in the perikaryon and subsequently transported to the terminals. Accordingly, substances that block axonal transport, such as colchicine, lead to accumulation of neuropeptides in the perikaryon. Usually, the neuropeptides are produced as larger polypeptides (prepropeptides) that most likely are split into smaller units on their way to the terminals.

How the Action of Neurotransmitters Is Stopped

Synaptic signal transfer is characterized by a precisely timed start and stop, and this is fundamental to many of the functions of the nervous system. We have looked into the mechanisms responsible for precise timing of transmitter release. It is also necessary, however, that the transmitter, once released, be quickly removed from the synaptic cleft. Several different mechanisms are of importance for this task.

An important factor is simple diffusion out of the synaptic cleft. Experimentally, this has been shown to happen very quickly. In addition, *specific uptake mechanisms* actively transport most of the small-molecular transmitters back into the bouton and into glial cells (Fig. 2.8). Several such mechanisms have now been characterized, including those for glutamate, GABA, glycine, and the monoamines. In these cases, the presynaptic membrane and glial membrane contain specific *high-affinity transporters* to bind and transport the transmitter molecules. After entering the bouton, the transmitter may be used again or become enzymatically degraded. The latter is the case for norepinephrine, which is broken down by the enzyme monoamine oxidase. The high-affinity transmitter transporters are also of great interest because their activity can be modified by drugs, thus changing the amount of transmitter available at the synapse. Drugs used to treat serious depression are one example. Furthermore, central nervous system stimulants, such as *cocaine*, act by binding to and inhibiting specific transmitter transporters.

Another mechanism for terminating transmitter action is *extracellular degradation* by specific enzymes. Acetylcholine is broken down by the enzyme *acetylcholinesterase* (AchE), which is present in the synaptic cleft. *Neuropeptides* are also subject to this kind of removal by specific *peptidases*. Overall, however, simple diffusion is probably the most important means of ending the effect of neuropeptides.

Excitatory Amino Acid Transmitters

This group contains the most ubiquitous excitatory transmitter, *glutamate*. Another amino acid with fast excitatory action is *aspartate*. Its role as a neurotransmitter, however, is less clear than that for glutamate. Here we discuss only glutamate.

The dominant effect of *glutamate* in the central nervous system is *fast excitation by direct action on ion channels*. Thus, glutamate is responsible for signal transmission in the majority of the large pathways conveying precise information, such as most sensory and motor tracts and the major connections between various parts of the cerebral cortex.

The synaptic effects of glutamate are nevertheless more complicated than this because glutamate acts on *two main kinds of ionotropic recep-*

tors with quite different properties, as well as on several kinds of *metabotropic receptors*. This action has been studied by using various selective agonists and antagonists and later cloning the receptor proteins. The ionotropic receptors are named after their specific agonists.

The *"classic" type of fast excitation* (fast EPSP) is produced by glutamate binding to so-called amino-methylisoxazole-propionic-acid (*AMPA*) *receptors*. These receptors are integral parts of cation channel proteins. The channels are permeable to Na^+ (and K^+) which is typical of fast excitatory synapses. AMPA receptors most likely mediate the bulk of precise information in the central nervous system—that is, information about *when, where*, and *what*.

The other kind of ionotropic glutamate receptor is the *N*-methyl-D-aspartate (*NMDA*) *receptor*. It has a much slower synaptic action than the AMPA receptor and is engaged in other tasks. The possible relation of the NMDA receptor to *learning and memory* has led to enormous research activity. The ion channel of the *NMDA receptor is much more permeable to Ca^{2+} than to Na^+*. This enables the receptor to exert many effects—besides depolarization—on the postsynaptic cell. As discussed earlier, Ca^{2+} is an important intracellular signal molecule that, among other things, can initiate long-lasting changes in synaptic transmission (LTP). The other important feature of the NMDA receptor is that it is *voltage-dependent*. At the resting membrane potential the channel is blocked by magnesium ions (Mg^{2+}). Depolarization removes the Mg^{2+} ions. Thus, binding of glutamate (or the agonist NMDA) does not open the channel unless the membrane is already depolarized by other synaptic inputs acting on AMPA receptors in the

The NMDA Receptor: A Mediator of Both Learning and Neuronal Damage?

Long-term potentiation, LTP, and its opposite phenomenon with an opposite sign, LTD, were mentioned earlier. In both cases the transmission at an excitatory synapse is changed for a long time when the synapse is active simultaneously with other excitatory synapses in the vicinity (associative LTP and LTD). A sensory input is often of significance to us only in a certain context, and only then should it be remembered. Only a tiny fraction of all the information reaching the brain is retained in memory. Thus, the brain must have mechanisms for detecting and storing coincident stimuli because they often represent the context. The NMDA receptor appears to have just the right properties for such a task because it requires depolarization together with glutamate binding. This occurs when two excitatory inputs of sufficient strength are simultaneously active. However, there are still unanswered questions about the importance of LTP for learning, and the relation between LTP and the NMDA receptor since LTP has been observed in cell groups that lack NMDA receptors.

The NMDA receptor is also one among several candidates for *mediating cell damage upon abnormal excitatory activation*. This happens when nervous tissue receives insufficient oxygen (severely reduced blood pressure, stroke, cerebral bleeding, and so forth). Abnormally intense excitation may also occur during epileptic seizures. Under such circumstances extracellular glutamate concentration rises steeply, and presumably all kinds of glutamate receptors are activated. Activation of NMDA receptors may nevertheless be especially important because it can lead to a dangerous increase of the intracellular Ca^{2+} concentration.

Excitatory amino acid transmitters and the NMDA receptor may also be involved in the cell damage occurring in various *degenerative diseases of the nervous system* (such as amyotrophic lateral sclerosis and Huntington's disease).

vicinity. When it is first opened, the flow of Ca^{2+} lasts longer than an ordinary fast EPSP.

Finally, glutamate acts on indirect, *metabotropic* receptors. So far, eight varieties of such receptors have been identified (mGluR1–8) with somewhat different distributions in the central nervous system. Although all act via G proteins, different G proteins and second messengers are involved. Furthermore, some mGluRs are found presynaptically. Thus, a variety of effects can be produced by metabotropic glutamate receptors, including excitation (depolarization) and inhibition (hyperpolarization).

Studies with immunogold labeling (see Figure 5.4) show that at least one kind of metabotropic glutamate receptor (mGluR1) is located at the periphery of synapses, whereas AMPA receptors occupy the central region. Such segregation might allow the receptors to respond differentially to glutamate: the AMPA receptors could be activated by normal presynaptic stimulation (low frequency of action potentials), whereas mGluRs would be activated only by high-frequency stimulation releasing large amounts of glutamate. If so, this may be related to the observed effects of mGluR activation on *synaptic plasticity* (LTP and LTD).

Inhibitory Amino Acid Transmitters

Gamma-aminobutyric acid (GABA) is the most ubiquitous inhibitory transmitter, being present in nearly all parts of the central nervous system. Perhaps as many as 20% of all synapses are GABAergic. Another inhibitory amino acid transmitter is *glycine*, but its distribution is very restricted compared with that of GABA. We will return to glycine below.

GABA is used as a transmitter mainly by interneurons (projection neurons are most typically glutamatergic). It is synthesized from glutamic acid in one step by the enzyme *glutamic acid decarboxylase* (GAD). Most often, GABA acts by *opening chloride channels*, thus producing a brief hyperpolarizing current (IPSP). The receptor linked with the Cl^- channel is termed $GABA_A$ (there are several subtypes with somewhat different distributions and properties).

In some parts of the central nervous system GABA also binds to $GABA_B$ *receptors* with modulatory actions. By indirectly *opening K^+ channels or blocking Ca^{2+} channels* $GABA_B$ receptors produce long-lasting hyperpolarization (slow IPSP). Like other modulatory receptors, the $GABA_B$ receptor acts via G proteins.

The *$GABA_A$ receptor* is part of an ion channel consisting of several membrane spanning subunits (similar to the acetylcholine receptor shown in Fig. 2.2). This complex has several binding sites besides that for GABA. Thus, *benzodiazepines* and *barbiturates* bind to different sites, although both potentiate the synaptic effect of GABA. The benzodiazepines (for example, diazepam) act by increasing the opening frequency of the Cl^- channels, whereas the barbiturates prolong their opening time. Benzodiazepines are used to reduce anxiety and provide muscle relaxation, and some derivatives are used as hypnotics. The barbiturates have similar effects and were formerly widely used as sedatives and hypnotics (they are now mainly used to induce general anesthesia and to treat epilepsy). Certain *steroid hormones*, among them the female sex hormone progesterone, also bind to GABA$_A$ receptors with actions similar to barbiturates. An anesthetic drug (alphaxalone) was developed on this basis.

Another drug, *baclofen* (Lioresal) binds selectively to the GABA$_B$ receptor and mimics the effect of GABA. It is used to reduce abnormal muscle tension occurring after damage to descending motor pathways (spasticity). The mechanism of action on muscle tension is not clear, however. It was initially assumed that baclofen increases presynaptic inhibition in the spinal cord, but recent data show that this is mediated mainly by GABA$_A$ receptors.

Glycine is used as an inhibitory transmitter by some spinal inhibitory interneurons (Fig. 5.5), and by some brain stem and cerebellar neurons. Like GABA$_A$ receptors, glycine receptors are parts of Cl$^-$ channels, and they produce fast excitatory actions. *Strychnine* blocks glycine receptors (thus blocking inhibition of spinal and brain stem motor neurons), and this explains why strychnine poisoning produces muscle cramps. Likewise, violent muscle spasms are provoked by the *tetanus toxin*, which inhibits synaptic release of glycine.

Acetylcholine

Acetylcholine is a quaternary amine synthesized through the binding of choline to acetyl coenzyme A by the enzyme *choline acetyltransferase* (ChAT). The presence of this enzyme is characteristic of neurons containing acetylcholine, so-called *cholinergic neurons*. Acetylcholine is present in motor neurons in the spinal cord and brain stem—innervating skeletal muscle cells—and in a few other neuronal groups in the central and peripheral nervous system.

Acetylcholine can bind to two kinds of receptors: *nicotinic* and *muscarinic* receptors (nicotine and muscarine being agonists). *The nicotinic receptors produce fast, excitatory synaptic actions, whereas the muscarinic receptors mediate indirect, modulatory effects on neuronal excitability* (Figs. 2.2 and 2.11). *Curare* is an antagonist (blocker) of the nicotinic receptor, whereas *atropine* is an antagonist of muscarinic receptors. The two kinds of receptors are distributed differently, as we will see below. Nicotine, muscarine, and curare are plant alkaloids. Curare has been used as an arrow poison by South American Indians, paralyzing the victim. Muscarine is present in a type of mushroom.

The actions of acetylcholine at the cholinergic synapses between motor neurons and *skeletal muscle cells* are especially well known (Figs. 11.3 and 11.4). There, acetylcholine binds to *nicotinic receptors*, which are part of a channel for cations. Opening of such channels elicits an action potential that spreads out in all directions to reach all parts of the muscle cell membrane. This is the signal that in turn leads to muscle contraction. Using certain toxins (for example, the snake venom α-bungarotoxin) that bind specifically and block the effect of acetylcholine, has helped determine the structure and properties of the nicotinic acetylcholine receptor in great detail (Fig. 2.2). Nicotinic receptors are also present in *autonomic ganglia*.

Although nicotinic receptors are present in several regions, *muscarinic receptors* are dominant in the central nervous system. So far, five subtypes (m1–m5) have been characterized, mediating different and, in part, opposite synaptic effects (all are of the indirect, G protein–coupled type). Thus, one kind closes certain K^+ channels, another opens K^+ channels, a third type reduces Ca^{2+} permeability. In the *cerebral cortex*, which receives many cholinergic nerve terminals, a major effect of acetylcholine is to reduce the permeability of a K^+ channel (by acting on m1 receptors). This makes the neurons more susceptible to other excitatory inputs so that, for example, a neuron will react more easily to a specific sensory stimulus.

Whereas skeletal muscle cells contain only nicotinic receptors, smooth muscle cells are equipped only with muscarinic receptors.

Monoamines (Biogenic Amines)

The *biogenic amines* or *monoamines* constitute a subgroup of the small-molecular transmitters. Neurons using monoamines as transmitters are called *monoaminergic*. The monoamines are synthesized by enzymatic removal of the carboxylic group from an aromatic amino acid. With few exceptions they have only *indirect, modulatory synaptic actions*. Another common feature is that each of the monoamines is used by only a small number of neurons, which, however, have *widely branching axons*. Thus, these few neurons ensure that monoamines can act in most parts of the central nervous system. They can therefore simultaneously modulate the specific information processing in many anatomically separate neuronal groups. This is related to regulation of attention, motivation, and mood. Localization and functions of monoaminergic cell groups are discussed later in this chapter and in Chapters 13, 15, and 17.

Adenosine Triphosphate and Adenosine

There is now convincing evidence that the purine *adenosine triphosphate* (*ATP*) acts as a transmitter in the peripheral nervous system and in certain parts of the central nervous system. At first, ATP was hard to accept as a neurotransmitter, since the molecule is a universal energy supplier present in all cells (for example, to run the sodium–potassium pump and provide energy for muscle contraction). *Purinoreceptors* (ATP receptors) , however, have been identified on many cell types of the body, among them neurons and muscle cells. The purinoreceptors are inhibited by *caffeine* (among other substances). Commonly, ATP is stored in synaptic vesicles together with either acetylcholine or norepinephrine, and is released with them. As a rule, neuronal and smooth muscle ATP receptors appear to be parts of ion channels with *excitatory actions* (there are, however, examples of inhibitory effects of ATP on smooth muscle cells, for example in the longitudinal muscle layer of the large intestine). The channels are most permeable to Ca^{2+}.

Whereas ATP as a transmitter in the autonomic nervous system has been thoroughly studied (see Chapter 17), much less is known about its role in the central nervous system. One effect is presynaptic inhibition of glutamate release at certain sites. ATP is probably also used as transmitter in a subgroup of the sensory neurons conducting impulses from peripheral receptors to the spinal cord (see Chapter 7, *Primary Sensory Fibers and Neurotransmitters*).

The *adenosine* molecule (that is, without phosphorylation) may also function as a transmitter in the spinal cord. Injections of minute amounts of adenosine inhibit neurons transmitting signals about painful stimuli to the brain. Adenosine also appears to be involved—in some yet unknown way—with the analgesic effects of morphine and the morphine-like substances produced in the brain (opioids).

Nitric Oxide

Nitric oxide (NO) is a gas that diffuses freely through biologic membranes. It is also a free radical and as such very reactive and toxic. NO therefore appears *a priori* to be a highly unlikely neurotransmitter candidate, although it is known to act as an intercellular signal molecule in other tissues. Nevertheless, much evidence suggests that NO *has* synaptic messenger functions, especially in the peripheral nervous system. NO differs in important respects from ordinary transmitters since it cannot be stored in vesicles and released by calcium-dependent exocytosis. NO is synthesized from the amino acid arginine by specific enzymes, *NO synthases* (there are several different types). Synthesis of NO in boutons is probably induced by the increase of intracellular Ca^{2+} concentration triggered by a presynaptic action potential. After synthesis, NO diffuses freely in all directions. It is not only delivered into the synaptic cleft but will also enter all cells that are in the vicinity of the bouton. The NO receptor is a water-soluble, cytoplasmatic enzyme, *guanylyl cyclase*, controlling synthesis of cyclic GMP. This is an intracellular messenger with various effects, such as activating protein kinases and acting directly on ion channels.

Various NO synthases are present in neurons in several parts of the central and peripheral nervous system. In the cerebral cortex, they are found in GABAergic neurons, which in addition contain neuropeptides (substance P and somatostatin). In other parts of the brain, NO synthases occur in cholinergic and monoaminergic neurons. We do not know the functions of NO liberated from such neurons, although many effects are possible.

The discovery of NO as a substance of biologic importance was not related to neurons but to *control of vascular musculature*. It produces vasodilatation with resulting increased blood flow, and was named *endothelial derived relaxing factor*. It is produced by endothelial cells after stimulation with (among other substances) acetylcholine. Also, vessels in the central nervous system are strongly affected by NO. Thus, the increased blood flow associated with increased neuronal activity appears to be mediated by NO.

Among the monoamines, *norepinephrine* (noradrenaline), *epinephrine* (adrenaline), and *dopamine* are all synthesized from the amino acid tyrosine and are collectively called *catecholamines*. They are present in distinct cell groups in both the central and peripheral nervous systems. Neurons containing norepinephrine are said to be *noradrenergic*, while those containing dopamine are *dopaminergic* (the same terminology is used for the receptors corresponding to these transmitters). The other monoamines, *serotonin* (5-hydroxytryptamine [5HT]) and *histamine*, are formed from the amino acids tryptophan and histidine, respectively.

The *synaptic effects of the monoamines are complex* because there are several receptor subtypes for each one (Table 2.1). One monoamine transmitter may therefore have different effects on the postsynaptic cell, depending on the repertoire of receptors present. There are two main receptor types, α and β, for *norepinephrine* and *epinephrine*. Their effects are often opposite, and they are also differentially distributed (this is treated in more detail in Chapter 17, *Subgroups of Adrenergic Receptors*). In the cerebral cortex, norepinephrine produces a slow depolarization by binding to β receptors (by indirect, G protein–coupled closure of a K^+ channel). *Dopamine* acts on at least four subgroups of receptors (D_1–D_4) with differential distribution in the central nervous system (see Chapter 13). *Serotonin* acts on several different receptor subtypes ($5HT_1$, $5HT_2$, . . .). Most of these are of the indirect, modulatory type, like the monamine receptors mentioned above. One of the 5HT receptors, however, is directly acting (being part of an ion channel) and belongs to the same protein family as the other ion channel receptors. Serotonin is further discussed in Chapters 7, 11, and 15.

From the above considerations, the monoamines, like other modulatory transmitters, clearly cannot be characterized in simple terms as either excitatory or inhibitory. Furthermore, their widespread distribution suggests that they may influence most of the functions of the nervous system.

Neuropeptides

A large number of neuroactive peptides have so far been identified in the central nervous system, but many of them were first found in the peripheral nervous system and in the gut. Although there is firm evidence of a transmitter function for only a few neuropeptides, many of them have marked effects on physiological processes and behavior if administered locally in the central nervous system. Several of the neuropeptides elicit slow inhibitory or excitatory synaptic potentials when they are administered in minute amounts close to neurons, which would suggest a modulatory transmitter role. This is supported by the identification of several G protein–coupled neuropeptide receptors. Some of the neuropeptides, however, may function more like local hormones than specific neurotransmitters.

It is a characteristic feature that neuropeptides as a rule are co-localized in nerve terminals with small-molecular (classical) transmitters. Whereas small-molecular transmitters are stored in small, electron-lucent vesicles (Figs. 1.4 and 1.5), neuropeptides are found in larger vesicles with an electron-dense center (dense core vesicles; one such is shown in

Examples of Co-localization of Neuropeptides and Small-Molecular Transmitters

Terminals of nerve fibers innervating *salivary glands* contain both *acetylcholine* and the neuropeptide *vasoactive intestinal polypeptide* (VIP). Both substances are released when the nerves are stimulated, but they act on different target cells: Acetylcholine elicits secretion from glandular cells, whereas VIP produces vasodilatation by relaxing smooth muscle cells, thereby increasing blood flow to the organ at the same time as its secretion is increased. Another example concerns *primary sensory neurons* (spinal ganglion cells, Fig. 3.9) mediating information from peripheral sense organs to the spinal cord. Some of these—particularly those related to painful stimuli—probably contain both *glutamate* and the peptides *substance P* (SP) and *calcitonin gene-related peptide* (CGRP). When released with glutamate, these peptides appear to have several actions: they can bind to specific postsynaptic receptors, they can act presynaptically to increase their own release and the release of glutamate, and they can sensitize the postsynaptic glutamate receptors to enhance the effect of glutamate.

Spinal interneurons (Fig 1.7) that receive sensory information exhibit different transmitter combinations. One group of interneurons contains *GABA* and the peptide *enkephalin*. Another group contains both enkephalin and substance P in combination with (most likely) glutamate. Thus, one neuropeptide (enkephalin) may be co-localized with either an inhibitory or an excitatory transmitter with fast synaptic actions. Apparently, spinal interneurons may express a variety of transmitter combinations with correspondingly complex synaptic actions. When we also think of the variety of receptors each neuron expresses, it is easy to understand why unraveling the functional role of a single transmitter can be difficult.

Fig. 1.4). Two or more peptides may also coexist, and there may be more than one small-molecular transmitter together with the peptides. Thus, one neuron may be expected to release several neuroactive substances simultaneously, some with fast synaptic actions, others with long-lasting, modulatory effects. The released substances may also elicit intracellular responses related to growth and development. There is some evidence to suggest, however, that the peptides may not always be released with the classical transmitters. Possibly, the *frequency of action potentials* determines whether peptides are released: It may depend on high-frequency firing or bursts of action potentials. We have already mentioned that some neurons shift from one state of activity with bursting to another with single spikes at regular intervals. Possibly, such altered states are reflected also in the kinds of neurotransmitters released.

Many neuroactive peptides are mentioned in subsequent chapters in relation to various cell groups and neuronal systems.

Modulatory Transmitter Systems

Some neuronal groups are special because they consist of a relatively small number of cells that send axons to large parts of the central nervous system. This happens because the axons ramify extensively. Furthermore, it is characteristic that in most of these groups the neurons contain one of the monoamines. Four monoamines—*norepinephrine, serotonin, dopamine,* and *histamine*—and, in addition, *acetylcholine* appear to be the main transmitters in cell groups with such widely branching axons.

These groups, each containing one of the mentioned transmitters, form more or less distinct entities. For example, neurons containing dopamine form nuclei that are clearly separate from nuclei with neurons containing norepinephrine. Some of these cell groups are treated more specifically in later chapters. Here we will limit ourselves to brief descriptions.

Norepinephrine is primarily localized to neurons forming distributed cell groups in the so-called reticular formation of the brain stem. Many of the neurons form a distinct group in the pons, the *nucleus coeruleus, or the locus coeruleus* (Fig. 15.6).

Dopamine is mostly confined to a large nucleus in the mesencephalon, the *substantia nigra,* and some smaller cell groups in its vicinity (Figs. 13.3 and 13.10).

Serotonin is mostly found in neurons forming a series of nuclei close to the midline in the brain stem, the raphe nuclei (nuclei raphe) (Fig. 15.5).

Acetylcholine is particularly prominent in a few cell groups in the brain stem (the parabrachial nucleus) and in basal parts of the forebrain, among them the *basal nucleus* and the *septal nuclei* (of Meynert; Figs. 4.17, 4.18, and 19.4).

Histamine is found mainly in a small cell group in the hypothalamus, the *tuberomammillary nucleus* (nucleus tuberomammillaris).

Such transmitter-specific cell groups with their widespread axonal ramifications would seem likely to play special functional roles, different from most other neuronal groups with more limited and specific axonal connections. They are, for example, hardly fit to provide precise information about time and space. It seems more likely that they make possible a homogeneous influence on many different parts of the nervous system by exerting general excitatory or inhibitory effects. This probably serves to modulate the excitability of the target neurons, and thus their responsiveness to other inputs carrying specific information. Such assumptions are consistent with the fact that, for example, norepinephrine and acetylcholine both appear to have mostly slow (modulatory) synaptic effects in the central nervous system. Rather diffuse, modulatory synaptic effects are probably of importance in relation to the level of consciousness, different stages of *sleep*, *attention*, *motivation*, and *mood*. Monoamine-containing neuronal groups also appear to influence general changes in the excitability of motor neurons and neurons that carry sensory information.

Nevertheless, it is an oversimplification to regard each transmitter-specific group as a functional entity and to use terms such as "the sero-

Drugs Acting on the Nervous System

Most drugs acting on the nervous system do so by influencing *synaptic transmission*. They may affect the synthesis, release, degradation, or reuptake of transmitters, or the transmitter receptors. There are drugs that have one or more of these actions regarding one or several transmitters.

Most transmitters are present in several parts of the nervous system that are different both anatomically and physiologically. Thus, it should not be surprising that even drugs that apparently influence the actions of only one transmitter nevertheless have multifarious effects. Some of these are desired therapeutic effects, whereas others are disturbing or even dangerous side effects. Development of more specific drugs—for example, drugs acting on only one receptor subtype—may reduce the side effects but will hardly eliminate them. Thus, each receptor type (even one among five different types for a transmitter) is expressed in several functionally different parts of the nervous system. Finally, we should keep in mind that pharmacological manipulation restricted to only one specific set of neurons may lead to changes in remote, interconnected neuronal groups.

We have already mentioned drugs with generalized *sedative effects* (barbiturates, benzodiazepines, and others) that appear to act primarily on GABA receptors. Some of these drugs are particularly effective in reducing anxiety (anxiolytic drugs) but in addition have hypnotic effects. Others have primarily hypnotic effects. Such differences probably reflect specific binding of the drugs to different cell groups that differ with regard to their subtype of GABA receptors (see Chapter 19, *Amygdala, Anxiety, and Neurotransmitters*).

Drugs that are effective in treating *serious mental illness* (psychoses) are characterized generally by prominent effects on dopamine receptors. They tend to act by reducing the postsynaptic sensitivity to the transmitter. Dopamine, however, is present in nuclei and tracts involved in a variety of functions—for example, in motor control and in cognitive processes and emotions. Motor disturbances therefore are commonly seen as a side effect in patients treated with antipsychotic drugs (neuroleptics). Correspondingly, mental disturbances may occur as a side effect in patients with Parkinson's disease treated with dopamine precursors to alleviate their motor symptoms.

Drugs that have proved effective in treating *serious depressive disorders* appear to act largely by inhibiting the reuptake or degradation of monoamine transmitters (particularly norepinephrine and serotonin). Such drugs often alleviate depression but in addition can cause several unwanted side effects (for example, by also blocking cholinergic neurotransmission). Until recently, drugs that inhibit monoamine reuptake nonspecifically (tricyclic antidepressants—TCAs) were mainly used. Now, however, drugs that mainly inhibit serotonin reuptake (selective serotonin reuptake inhibitors—SSRIs) have been developed. They have fewer side effects and lower toxicity than the tricyclic antidepressants.

See also Chapter 13, *Parkinson's Disease*, and Chapter 17, *Drugs with Actions on the Autonomic Nervous System*.

tonin system," "the dopamine system," and so on. First, within each group there are subgroups differing in where they send their axons. Second, the axonal ramifications from each group are not as diffuse as they appeared to be from earlier studies. Thus, in the cerebral cortex, fibers containing serotonin, dopamine, or norepinephrine are largely differentially distributed. Third, not all neurons in the apparently transmitter-specific cell groups contain the same transmitter, and furthermore, in addition to a monoamine transmitter, most neurons also contain one or more neuropeptides. The effects obtained by stimulation of one of these cell groups therefore cannot be ascribed to one transmitter alone. Finally, it should also be recalled that the effects of one transmitter depend on the receptor type present postsynaptically and that there is more than one receptor type for each transmitter.

COUPLING OF NEURONS: PATHWAYS FOR IMPULSES

In addition to the properties of synapses, which determine the transfer of signals among neurons, the function of the nervous system depends on how the various neuronal groups (nuclei) are interconnected (often called the *wiring pattern* of the brain). This determines the pathways that signals may take and the possibilities for cooperation among neuronal groups. Thus, although each neuron is to some extent a functional unit, it is only by proper cooperation that neurons can fulfill their tasks. We will describe here some typical examples of how neurons are interconnected, since such general knowledge is important for understanding the specific examples of connections to be dealt with in later chapters.

Divergence and Convergence Are Fundamental Principles in the Organization of the Nervous System

The simplest example of an impulse pathway is that of the axon of one neuron contacting another neuron that does not receive any other connections (Fig. 2.13A). Such simple arrangements do not exist in the central nervous system, however. Here the connections are frequently arranged so that signals from one neuron are distributed to many others (because the axon sends off collaterals; Fig. 2.13B). In the scheme of Figure 1.13B, it can be seen that all of the neurons that are synaptically contacted by the first one themselves contact several others (in reality, many more than shown here). The end result is that the signal coming from one neuron is transmitted to many others (again, in reality, signals from one group of neurons are transmitted to many other groups). This is an example of the *divergence of connections* that is very common in the nervous system. Thus, information of a particular kind is distributed to many, often functionally diverse, neuronal groups.

Another principle, *convergence of connections*, is shown schematically in Figure 2.13C. In this case, one neuron (*m*) is synaptically con-

Figure 2.13. *Impulse pathways*.
Highly simplified examples.

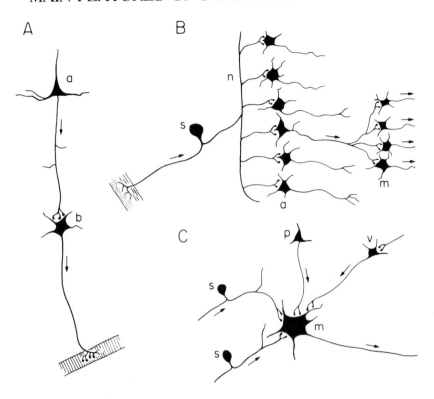

tacted by many other nerve cells (*s*, *p*, and *v*). The sum of excitatory and inhibitory synaptic effects at any given moment determines the activity of the neuron *m*. This neuron is said to represent the *final common path* for the neurons contacting it, since it *integrates* the information from various sources into a unified response. Examples of such a final common path are the motor neurons in the spinal cord, which send their axons to skeletal muscle cells. The frequency at which action potentials are sent to the muscle cell is determined by the sum of all synaptic inputs to the motor neuron.

The signals may not necessarily pass all the way along pathways consisting of several neurons coupled serially (as in Figs. 2.13B and 2.14D). As discussed earlier in this chapter, *summation* of synaptic effects is as a rule necessary for an action potential to be elicited in the postsynaptic neuron. One example is shown in Figure 2.14A. We imagine that an excitatory signal comes from axon *2*. This axon has many boutons that contact the neuron *II*, and together they make the neuron fire an action potential. Axon *2* makes only a few synaptic contacts with neurons *I* and *III* and is on its own unable to make them fire action potentials. If, however, neurons *I* and *III* at the same time receive synaptic inputs from axons *1*, *3*, and *4*, summation may be sufficient to fire the neurons. In this way we may explain why only a few of the many neurons in a nucleus fire action potentials when receiving impulses from an afferent axonal tract. Neurons not eliciting action potentials may nevertheless be depolarized almost to threshold for action potentials and may fire if they receive an additional excitatory input. In such instances, a weak additional excitatory input may elicit a disproportionately large increase in the number of neurons firing.

Many Neurons Are Continuously Active

In the examples mentioned above, the neurons stop firing as soon as excitatory synaptic inputs from other neurons end. In other instances, however, activity in the form of action potentials goes on long after activity has ended in afferent pathways to a nucleus. In fact, most parts of the central nervous system are virtually never totally "silent"—there is always some impulse traffic. In the cerebral cortex, for example, even during sleep there is considerable neuronal activity. *Such neuronal behavior may be partly explained by the membrane properties of many neurons but also by the presence of numerous interneurons.* An example is shown in Figure 2.14C. The axon *n* excites neuron *1*, which in response fires an action potential. At the same time, the interneuron *2* is also excited and fires an action potential, which in turn excites both neurons *1* and *3*. Because of the synaptic delay of a few milliseconds and the time required for impulse conduction in the axons of the interneuron, cell *1* receives excitation in three succeeding waves and may itself fire several action potentials in response. With this kind of arrangement (which in reality would be much more elaborate and complicated than in this example), one impulse (or a brief train of impulses) may set up prolonged impulse activity in a group of neurons.

We mentioned above that the *membrane properties* of neurons may contribute to the activity of neurons in the absence of excitatory synaptic inputs. Such neurons are said to discharge spontaneously and to have *autorhythmicity* or *pacemaker* properties. The frequency and pattern of their firing is nevertheless regulated up or down by afferent synaptic inputs.

Inhibitory Neurons Serve as "Brakes"

In the examples given above, the interneurons were excitatory. Many interneurons, however, are inhibitory. An example is shown in Figure 2.14B. In this case, firing of neuron *1* leads to subsequent inhibition of itself, by way of the inhibitory interneuron *2*. This is called *recurrent inhibition*. In this manner the frequency of action potentials in neuron *1* is prevented from becoming too high. Recurrent inhibition may also ensure that the neuron fires only a few action potentials with high frequency, with a subsequent pause. The typical pattern of activity for this particular neuron is repeated, brief bursts of action potentials. Interneuron *2* is, however, subject to other synaptic influences (although not shown in Fig. 2.14B) that may excite or inhibit it. In this way the recurrent inhibition may be increased or decreased by other neuronal groups; the "brake" may be switched on and off. Recurrent inhibition is found in many places in the nervous system, such as the spinal cord, where it regulates the motor neurons governing the contraction of skeletal muscle.

Signaling by Disinhibition

Inhibition may not only reduce neuronal activity but under certain circumstances may also lead to increased activity. This happens when *in-*

hibitory neurons inhibit other inhibitory neurons, which in turn inhibit excitatory neurons. The result of increased activity of the first inhibitory neuron is reduced inhibitory input to the excitatory neuron, and thus an increased excitatory output from the latter. This phenomenon is called *disinhibition*. If, for example, an inhibitory interneuron has some axonal terminals on an inhibitory neuron and other terminals on an excitatory neuron, it may at the same time excite some neurons and inhibit others. This may be used to switch impulse traffic in the direction required by the situation. Such a mechanism may be of importance in the *spinal cord*, for example, when the central nervous system has to select different combinations of muscles to perform various movements. Disinhibition is also an important mechanism in the *retina* and in the *basal ganglia* (see *Transmitters and Synaptic Actions of Neurons within the Cortex—Basal Ganglia—Cortex Loop: Disinhibition* in Chapter 13).

Interneurons Provide Flexibility of Responses

Figure 2.14D exemplifies another way in which neurons may be interconnected. An action potential in axon *n* activates neuron *1*, which in turn activates neuron *2*, and so on. One might imagine that the same information could have been transferred more economically by the simple connection shown in Figure 2.14E. The intercalated neurons in Figure 2.14D give a delay in impulse propagation, which in itself is a disadvantage. The main point, however, is that the interrupted pathway provides greater flexibility of response from neuron 3 in response to an input in axon n. Neuron *3* is not governed dictatorially by axon *n*, in contrast to the situation in Figure 2.14E, because interneurons *1* and *2* are under the influence of other neurons. Thus the impulse traffic from *n* to neuron *3* may be facilitated or inhibited. Usually, the axons contacting the interneurons (n_1 and n_2) come from nuclei in parts of the central nervous system other than axon *n*. Thus, impulses from very different parts of the nervous system may influence the impulse transmission from *n* to neuron *3*. Identical sensory stimuli, for example, may thus elicit quite different responses, depending on the situation in many, often distant, parts of the nervous system. Such response flexibility is typical of the brains of higher animals, which are characterized by their large number of interneurons.

Nuclei in the Central Nervous System Are Interconnected

Many of the examples given above concern local wiring patterns—that is, connections within groups of neurons. Figure 2.15 gives examples of interconnections among nuclei that are at some distance. Two *parallel pathways* between the two nuclei A and B are shown at the upper left. *One pathway is direct, the other synaptically interrupted* (there are often several pathways of the latter kind). Parallel pathways are common in the central nervous system—for example, for transmission of sensory information. Although their functional significance is not always clear, parallel pathways may be of practical importance after partial brain injury. If,

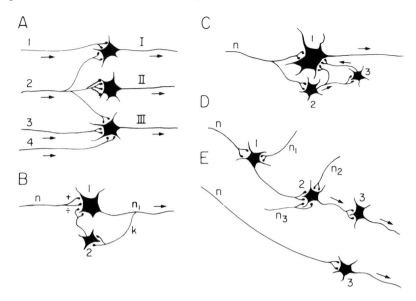

Figure 2.14. *Impulse pathways.* Highly simplified examples.

for example, the direct pathway between *A* and *B* is interrupted, the indirect one may at least partly take over the tasks formerly performed by the direct one (examples of this are discussed in Chapter 4, *Restitution of Function*).

Parallel pathways

Feedback connections

Collaterals

Bilateral connections

Commissural connections

Figure 2.15. *Examples of simple neuronal coupling diagrams.*

Feedback connections between two nuclei represent another common arrangement. When one nucleus sends axons to another, the latter as a rule sends some axons back. In this manner the first nucleus is informed of the outcome of the impulses emitted to the second one. If the influence was too strong, the message back may serve to reduce activity, and vice versa if the influence was too weak. The significance of such feedback connections lies in their ability to *stabilize* the functioning of the nervous system. Thus, many of the symptoms appearing in neurological diseases are due to the failure of stabilizing feedback mechanisms.

Another important general feature is that most nuclei have connections with both sides of the brain: the so-called *bilateral connections* (Fig. 2.15). Some tracts supply both sides with approximately the same number of axons (that is, equal numbers of crossed and uncrossed axons), whereas other tracts are predominantly crossed (contralateral), with only a few axons supplying the same (ipsilateral) side. That there must be extensive cooperation between the two sides of the central nervous system is made even more evident by the vast number of *commissural connections*—that is, direct connections between corresponding parts in the two halves (Fig. 2.14). Such connections occur at all levels of the central nervous system. The most prominent one connects the two halves of the cerebral hemispheres (corpus callosum, Figs. 3.25 and 3.26) and in humans contains probably around 180 million axons.

Cell Populations, Not Individual Cells, Determine What the Nervous System Can Do

For the sake of simplicity, we have considered so far mainly connections between individual nerve cells. This can be justified because the general principles are the same whether the connections are between two neurons or several thousand. It is nevertheless important to realize that the tasks performed by the nervous system do not depend on the function of single cells but on the collective activity of populations of neurons. It is not necessary that all neurons within such a population or group behave correctly; rather, it is a question of a sufficiently high probability for the neurons to send the right signal. If there are many neurons sharing the job, the chance is good that a sufficient number of them at any time will behave correctly. Many of the tasks of the nervous system can still be performed even if the responsible neuronal populations are numerically reduced. Only when the demand on performance is very high may it become apparent that something is wrong. If, however, the number undergoes further reduction, a point may be reached at which obvious functional deficits occur rather abruptly, even though the disease process may have been progressing slowly for years.

NOTES

1. Neither membrane potentials nor action potentials are properties unique to nerve cells. All cells have a membrane potential, although usually of less magnitude than that of neurons. Muscle cells and endocrine gland cells also produce action potentials in relation to contraction and secretion, respectively.

2. To express the membrane permeability of a particular kind of ion more precisely, we use the term *conductance*. The conductance is the inverse of the membrane resistance. In an electrical circuit the current is $I = V/R$, where V is the voltage and R is the resistance (Ohm's law). This may be rewritten by using conductance (g) instead of R, as $I = gV$. Thus, one may obtain quantitative measures of membrane permeability under various conditions. For our purpose, however, it is sufficient to use the less precise termpermeability.

CHAPTER 3

THE DIFFERENT PARTS OF THE NERVOUS SYSTEM

The central nervous system is well protected against external forces as it lies inside the skull and the vertebral canal. In addition to this bony protection, the central nervous system is wrapped in three membranes of connective tissue, with fluid-filled spaces between the membranes. It is, in fact, loosely suspended in a fluid-filled container. Since the specific weight of nervous tissue is only slightly higher than that of water, the brain and spinal cord almost float. This further serves to reduce the impact of external forces on the brain and spinal cord.

The central nervous system can be subdivided anatomically into different parts (Figs. 3.1 and 3.2). The *spinal cord* lies in the vertebral canal, whereas the brain is located in the cranial cavity. The brain is further subdivided into the *brain stem*, which constitutes the upward continuation of the spinal cord, the *cerebellum* ("little brain"), and the *cerebrum* or *cerebral hemispheres*. The cerebellum and cerebrum largely cover the brain stem and constitute the major part of the brain in higher mammals and particularly in humans.

In this chapter we will give an overview of the main features of the anatomy of the central nervous system, with brief mention of the functional significance of the various parts. Structure and function of many of these parts will be treated in more depth in the later chapters dealing with functional systems. It will then be assumed, however, that the reader is familiar with the names and the locations of the major cell groups of

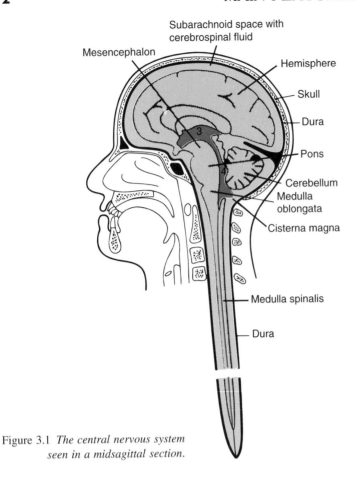

Figure 3.1 *The central nervous system seen in a midsagittal section.*

Figure 3.2 *Magnetic resonance image* (MRI) at a level corresponding to the drawing in Figure 3.1. Most of the structures seen in Figure 3.1 can be identified in this picture. Courtesy of Dr. S. J. Bakke, The National Hospital of Norway, Oslo.

Some Anatomic Terms Used in This Book

The terms *medial*, toward the midline, and *lateral*, away from the midline, are used to describe the relative position of structures in relation to a midsagittal plane of the body. The terms *cranial* or *rostral*, toward the head or nose, and *caudal*, toward the tail, are used to describe the relative position of structures along a longitudinal axis of the body. Thus, for example, nucleus A in the brain stem may lie medial to and rostral to nucleus B, which in turn lies lateral to and caudal to A. The terms *ventral* and *dorsal* are used to describe the relative position of structures in relation to the front (venter = belly) and the back (dorsum) of the body, respectively. *Anterior* (front) and *posterior* (rear) are most often used interchangeably with ventral and dorsal (except for the human forebrain, where anterior means toward the nose and ventral means toward the base of the skull).

the central nervous system. After some comments on the prenatal development of the central nervous system, we start with a description of the spinal cord, since conditions are simplest there.

THE SPINAL CORD

In humans the spinal cord is a 40 to 45 cm-long cylinder of nervous tissue of approximately the same thickness as a little finger. It extends from the lower end of the brain stem (at the level of the upper end of the first

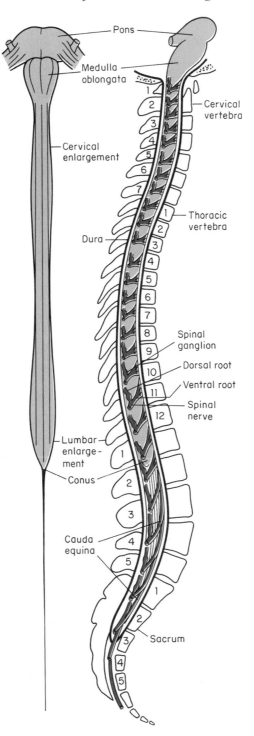

Figure 3.3 *The spinal cord.* To the **left**, the cord from the ventral side. Note the cervical and lumbar enlargements. To the **right**, the cord and the vertebral column from the side, but the right halves of the vertebrae have been removed to expose the vertebral canal with its contents. Below the first–second lumbar vertebrae, the vertebral canal contains only nerve roots (the cauda equina). Note that the roots unite to form the spinal nerves.

cervical vertebra) down the vertebral canal (Figs. 3.1 and 3.3) to the upper margin of the second lumbar vertebra (L_2). Here the cord has a wedge-shaped end called the *medullary conus* (or simply conus). In children the spinal cord extends more caudally, however, and reaches to the third lumbar vertebra in the newborn. This difference between the position of the lower end of the spinal cord in adults and infants is caused by the verte-

Figure 3.4 *Cross section of the spinal cord at a lumbar level.* Note the central H-shaped region of gray matter and the subdivision of the surrounding white matter into funiculi.

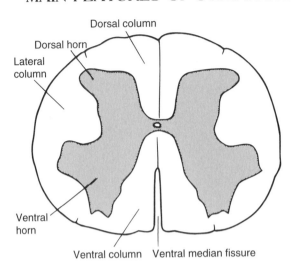

Figure 3.4 *Cross section of the spinal cord at a lumbar level.* Note the central H-shaped region of gray matter and the subdivision of the surrounding white matter into funiculi.

bral column growing more rapidly than the spinal cord. In early embryonic life, the neural tube and the primordium of the vertebral column are equally long (Fig. 3.12).

The spinal cord is somewhat flattened in the anteroposterior direction and is not equally thick along its length. In general, the thickness decreases caudally, but there are two marked intumescences (Fig. 3.3), the *cervical* and *lumbar enlargements* (intumescentia cervicalis et lumbalis). The intumescences supply the extremities with sensory and motor nerves, hence the increased thickness.

In the midline along the anterior aspect of the cord, there is a longitudinal furrow or *fissure* (ventral median fissure, Fig. 3.4). Some of the vessels of the cord enter through this fissure and penetrate deeply into the substance of the cord. At the posterior aspect of the cord there is a corresponding, but more shallow, furrow in the midline (the posterior median sulcus). In addition, on each side there are shallow, longitudinal sulci anteriorly and posteriorly (the anterior and posterior lateral sulci). These laterally placed sulci mark where the spinal nerves connect with the cord.

The color of the spinal cord is whitish because the outer part consists of axons, many of which are myelinated. The consistency of the cord, as of the rest of the central nervous system, is soft and jellylike.

Spinal Nerves Connect the Spinal Cord with the Body

Axons mediating communication between the central nervous system and other parts of the body make up the *peripheral nerves*. The axons (nerve fibers) leave and enter the cord in small bundles called *rootlets* (Fig. 3.5). Several adjacent rootlets unite to a thicker strand, called a *root* or *nerve root*. In this manner, rows of roots are formed along the dorsal and ventral aspects of the cord—the *ventral (anterior) roots* and the *dorsal (posterior) roots*, respectively. Each dorsal root has a swelling, the *spinal ganglion*, which contains the cell bodies of the sensory axons entering the cord through the dorsal root (Figs. 3.3 and 3.5). A dorsal and a ventral root unite to form a *spinal nerve* (nervus spinalis). The spinal ganglion

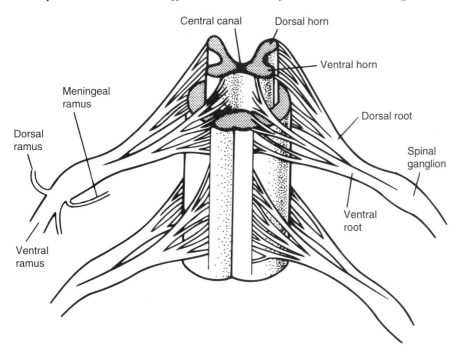

Figure 3.5 *Two segments of the spinal cord* (seen from the ventral aspect). In the upper part, the white matter has been removed. The dorsal and ventral roots emerge from the posterior and anterior lateral sulci, respectively, and unite to form spinal nerves. Note the location of the spinal ganglion at the site where the roots unite.

lies in the *intervertebral foramen* just where the dorsal and ventral roots unite (Fig. 3.6). There is an important functional difference between the ventral and dorsal roots: *The ventral roots consist of efferent (motor) fibers, and the dorsal roots of afferent (sensory) fibers.*

In total, 31 spinal nerves are present on each side, forming symmetrical pairs (Fig. 3.3). They all leave the vertebral canal through the intervertebral foramina on each side. As mentioned, the ventral and dorsal roots unite at the level of the intervertebral foramen to form the spinal nerves. The spinal nerves are numbered (as a general rule) in accordance with the number of verbebrae above the nerve. We therefore have 12 pairs of thoracic nerves, five pairs of lumbar nerves, and five pairs of sacral nerves. In humans, there is only one pair of coccygeal nerves. There are

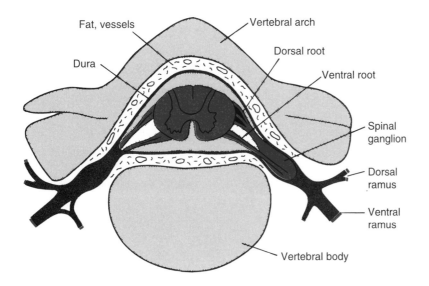

Figure 3.6 *Cross section of the vertebral column* showing the positions of the spinal cord and the spinal nerves. Note the location of the spinal ganglion in the intervertebral foramen. The spinal cord is surrounded by the cerebrospinal fluid contained within the dura. Outside the dura, there is fat and a venous plexus, also serving as soft padding for the cord and the spinal nerves.

seven cervical vertebrae but eight pairs of cervical nerves because the first cervical nerve leaves the vertebral canal above the first cervical vertebra (Fig. 3.3). Therefore, the numbering of the cervical nerves does not follow the general rule given above.

The spinal cord extends caudally only to the level of between the first and the second lumbar vertebrae. Whereas the upper spinal nerves pass approximately horizontally from the cord to the intervertebral foramen, the lower ones have to run obliquely downward in the vertebral canal to reach the corresponding intervertebral foramen, the distance between the site of exit from the cord and the site of exit from the canal increasing steadily (Fig. 3.3). *Below the conus, the vertebral canal contains only spinal nerve roots running longitudinally.* This collection of dorsal and ventral roots is called the *cauda equina* (the horsetail).

The Spinal Cord Is Divided into Segments

The part of the spinal cord giving origin to a pair of spinal nerves is called a *spinal segment*. There are, therefore, as many segments as there are spinal nerves. They are numbered accordingly, the first cervical segment giving origin to the first cervical nerves, and so on. There are no surface markings of the cord to indicate borders between the segments, but the rootlets nevertheless outline them rather precisely (Fig. 3.5).

The cervical enlargement (intumescence) corresponds to the fourth cervical (C_4) segment through the second thoracic (T_2) segment, the lumbar enlargement to the first lumbar (L_1) segment through the second sacral (S_2) segment.

The difference in rostrocaudal level between the spinal segments and the exit from the vertebral canal of the spinal nerves is of practical importance. Thus, identical symptoms may be provoked by a process close to the cord at one level and by one close to the intervertebral foramen at a considerably lower level (as should be clear from the above description; however, this does not concern the nerves in the cervical region).

The Spinal Cord Consists of Gray and White Matter

When cut transversely, the fresh spinal cord can be seen to consist of an outer zone of white matter and a central, H-shaped region of gray matter (Fig. 3.4). The arms of the H, extending dorsally and ventrally, are called the *dorsal horn* (cornu posterius) and *ventral horn* (cornu anterius), respectively. The gray matter extends as a column through the length of the spinal cord (Fig. 3.5). The central canal is seen as a narrow opening in the center of the cord. The central canal ends blindly in the caudal end of the cord, whereas it continues rostrally into the ventricular system of the brain (Fig. 3.1).

The *white matter* of the cord contains axons running longitudinally. Some of these axons convey signals from the cord to higher levels of the central nervous system; others, from higher levels to the cord. Finally, a large proportion of the fibers serve the signal traffic, and hence cooperation, between the segments of the cord. Since the first two groups of axons become successively more numerous in the rostral direction, the proportion of white to gray matter increases from caudal to rostral.

The white matter is divided into *funiculi*, or *columns*, by drawing lines in the transverse plane from the sulci on the surface of the cord to the center (Fig. 3.4). Thus, in each half of the cord, the white matter is divided into a *ventral* or *anterior funiculus*, a *lateral funiculus*, and a *dorsal* or *posterior funiculus*. For the latter, the term *dorsal column* is used most frequently.

The Spinal Gray Matter Contains Three Main Types of Neurons

Among neurons in the gray matter of the spinal cord, there are both morphological and functional differences. Three main types may be identified according to where they send their axons: (1) neurons sending their axons *out of the central nervous system*; (2) neurons sending their axons *to higher levels of the central nervous system* (such as the brain stem); and (3) neurons sending their axons to *other parts of the spinal cord*. We will now consider in some detail each of these three groups.

Efferent Fibers from the Cord Control Muscles and Glands

The cell bodies of the first kind of neuron listed above are located in the ventral horn and at the transition between the dorsal and ventral horns. The *motor neurons* or *motoneurons* have large, multipolar perikarya and are in the ventral horn proper (Figs. 1.2, 3.7, 3.8, 3.10, and 11.2). The dendrites extend for a considerable distance in the gray matter. The axons leave the cord through the ventral root, follow the spinal nerves, and end in *skeletal muscles* (muscles that are controlled voluntarily). The motoneurons are further discussed in Chapter 11.

There is also another group of neurons that sends its axons out of the cord through the ventral root. These supply *smooth muscles* and *glands* with motor signals, and belong to the *autonomic nervous system*. The autonomic system controls the vascular smooth muscles and visceral organs throughout the body. The cell bodies lie in the lateral horn (Fig. 3.8). Most of them form a long, slender column, the *intermediolateral cell column*. This column is present only in the thoracic and upper two lumbar segments of the cord and belongs to the *sympathethic part of the autonomic nervous system*. A corresponding, smaller group of neurons is present in the sacral cord (S_3–S_4) and belongs to the *parasympathetic part of the autonomic nervous system*.

The motor neurons and those in the intermediolateral cell column (and those in the sacral cord) are under synaptic influence from higher levels of the central nervous system.

Figure 3.7 *Three main types of neurons in the spinal cord*. Schematic drawing shows neuronal types classified in accordance with where their axons terminate: (1) *Motoneurons*; α and γ are two different types of motoneuron supplying skeletal muscles. (2) *Sensory neurons*; their axons ascend in the white matter (see also Fig. 3.9). (3) *Interneurons*; their axons are confined to the spinal cord.

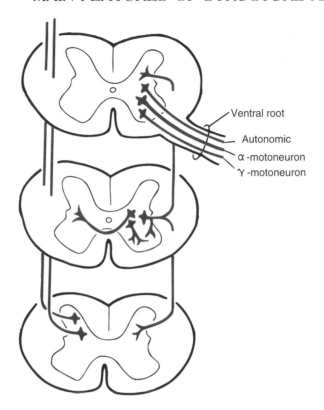

Sensory Neurons in the Cord Are Influenced from the Dorsal Roots and Convey Signals to the Brain

The second main type of spinal neuron mentioned above sends axons to higher levels of the central nervous system. Their perikarya are located mainly in the dorsal horn and in the transition zone between the dorsal and ventral horn (Figs. 3.7 and 3.9). Their job is to inform the brain of the activities of the spinal cord, and especially about what is going on in the body. To fulfill the latter task, the neurons must receive signals from *sense organs—receptors—*in various parts of the body (in the skin, muscles, viscera, and so on). *Sensory*, or *afferent*, nerve fibers conducting impulses from the receptors enter the spinal cord through the dorsal roots and ramify, forming terminal boutons in the gray matter of the cord (Figs. 3.9 and 7.10). The sensory neurons have their perikarya in the *spinal ganglia* and are therefore called *spinal ganglion cells*. These are morphologically special, since they have only one process, which divides shortly after leaving the cell body: One peripheral process connects with the sense organs, and the other extends centrally and enters the spinal cord (Figs. 1.13 and 7.10). In accordance with the usual definition of axons and dendrites, the peripheral process (conducting toward the cell body) should be called a dendrite, whereas the central process is an axon. Both processes are, however, morphologically and functionally axons (for example, by conducting action potentials and by being myelinated).

The dorsal root fibers form synaptic contacts—in part directly, in part indirectly via interneurons—with neurons in the spinal cord, sending their axons to various parts of the brain. Such axons, destined for a common

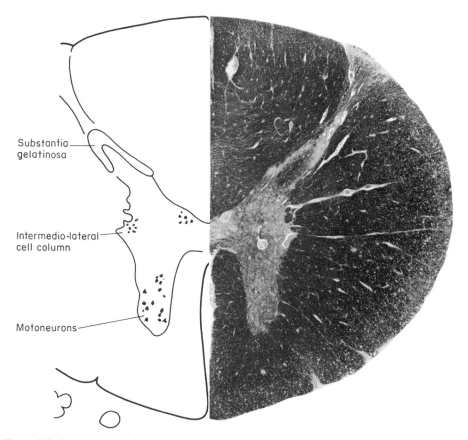

Figure 3.8 *Cross section of the spinal cord at the thoracic level.* Photomicrograph of a section stained so that myelinated axons appear dark. The large motoneurons in the ventral horn have also been stained (Nissl staining) and are just visible (owing to shrinkage, the motoneurons are surrounded by a clear zone).

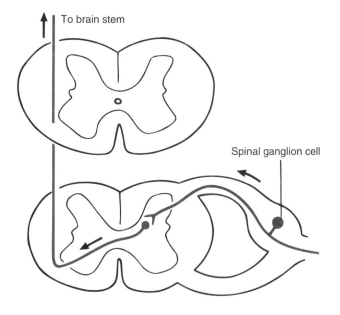

Figure 3.9 *Sensory neuron in the gray substance of the spinal cord.* The neuron, which sends its axon to the brain stem, is synaptically contacted by sensory afferents entering the cord through the dorsal root (pseudounipolar ganglion cell). The presentation is very simplified—in reality, every sensory neuron is contacted by numerous dorsal root afferents.

target in the brain, are grouped together in the spinal white matter, forming *tracts* (tractus). Such tracts are named after the location of the cell bodies and after the target organ. A tract leading from the spinal cord to the cerebellum, for example, is named the *spinocerebellar tract* (tractus spinocerebellaris).

Interneurons Enable Cooperation between Different Cell Groups in the Cord

The axons of the third type of spinal neuron do not leave the spinal cord. Usually, the axons ramify extensively and establish synaptic contacts with many other neurons in the cord, within the segment in which the cell body is located, and in segments above and below (Fig. 3.7). Such neurons are called *spinal interneurons*, to emphasize that they are intercalated between other neurons.[1] Many spinal interneurons are found in an intermediate zone between the dorsal and ventral horns and receive major synaptic inputs from sensory fibers in the dorsal roots. Many of these interneurons establish synaptic contacts with motoneurons in the ventral horn, thus mediating motor responses to sensory stimuli. Most interneurons, however, receive additional strong inputs from other spinal interneurons and from the brain.

As mentioned, spinal interneurons also send collaterals to terminate in segments of the cord other than the one in which their cell body and local ramifications are found. Such collaterals enter the white matter, run there for some distance, and reenter the cord at another segmental level, to ramify and establish synaptic contacts in the gray matter. Axons of this kind in the white matter are called *propriospinal fibers* (that is, fibers "belonging" to the spinal cord itself), to distinguish them from long ascending and descending fibers connecting the cord with the brain. *Propriospinal neurons* is, therefore, another term used for spinal interneurons.[2]

Propriospinal neurons provide opportunities for cooperation among the various spinal segments. In many instances it is necessary for the activity of many segments, each controlling different groups of muscles, to be closely coordinated. Some propriospinal connections are very long, interconnecting segments in the cervical and lumbar parts of the cord that control muscles in the forelimb and hindlimb, respectively. Cooperation between the forelimbs and hindlimbs is necessary, for example, during walking.

The Spinal Gray Matter Can Be Divided into Zones Called Rexed's Laminae

Systematic observations with the microscope of transverse sections of the spinal cord stained to visualize cell bodies show that neurons with different sizes and shapes are also differently distributed (Fig. 3.10). Essentially, neurons with common morphological features are collected into transversely oriented bands or zones. What appear as bands in the transverse plane are, three-dimensionally, longitudinal plates. This laminar pattern is most clear-cut in the dorsal horn, whereas in the ventral horn neu-

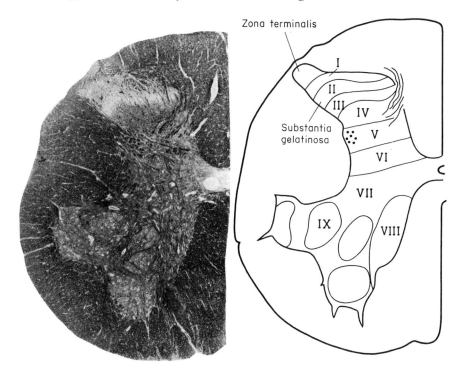

rons are collected into regions forming longitudinal columns rather than plates (Fig. 11.2). Nevertheless, the columns in the ventral horn, as well as the plates in the dorsal horn, are termed *laminae*. This pattern was first described in 1952 by the Swedish neuroanatomist Rexed, and has since proved to be of great help for investigations of the spinal cord. Altogether, Rexed described 10 laminae; laminae 1–6 constitute the dorsal horn, whereas lamina 9 is made up of columns of motoneurons in the ventral horn.

Experimental studies of the connections of the spinal cord and of the functional properties of single spinal neurons have shown that the various laminae differ in these respects. Thus, the laminae may be regarded,

Figure 3.10 *Cross section of the spinal cord at the lumbar level* (lumbar intumescence). Photomicrograph of section stained to show myelin and neuronal cell bodies (perikarya). The drawing shows the borders between Rexed's laminae. Note the groups of motoneurons in the ventral horn (α and γ motoneurons) constituting lamina IX. The zona terminalis (tract of Lissauer) consists primarily of thin dorsal root fibers.

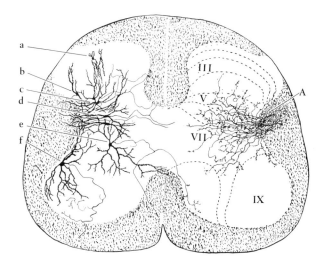

Figure 3.11 *Dendritic arborizations of spinal neurons extend beyond the lamina of their cell bodies.* Composite drawing based on observations in many Golgi-impregnated transverse sections from the spinal cord of the cat. The dendrites extend far, not only in the transverse plane as shown here but also longitudinally. To the right are the terminal ramifications of axons descending to the cord from higher levels of the central nervous system. From Scheibel and Scheibel (1966).

at least to some extent, as the nuclei of the spinal cord. We will return to Rexed's laminae when dealing with the functional organization of the spinal cord in Chapters 7, 11, and 12. It should be emphasized that, even though the laminae of the cord in certain respects are functionally distinct entities, the anatomic identification of a lamina is based solely on the location of the neuronal perikarya. The dendrites of these neurons, however, often extend into neighboring laminae (Fig. 3.11). Therefore, not only axons terminating within a lamina but also those ending in neighboring ones may be expected to influence the spinal neurons within one particular lamina.

The Spinal Nerves Form Plexuses

The dorsal (sensory) and ventral (motor) roots join to form spinal nerves, as described above. Each spinal nerve then divides into several branches just outside the intervertebral foramen (Figs. 3.5 and 3.6). The thickest one, the *ventral ramus* (ramus ventralis), passes ventrally. A thinner branch, the *dorsal ramus* (ramus dorsalis), bends in the dorsal direction. In contrast to the spinal roots, the *ventral and dorsal branches (rami) contain both sensory and motor fibers.* This is caused by mixing of fibers from dorsal and ventral roots as they continue into the spinal nerves.

The dorsal rami innervate muscles and skin on the back, whereas the ventral rami innervate skin and muscles on the ventral aspect of the trunk and neck and, in addition, the extremities. Thus, the ventral rami innervate much larger parts of the body than the dorsal rami, which explains why the ventral ones contain more nerve fibers and are considerably thicker than the dorsal ones. Some of the ventral rami join each other to form plexuses (Fig. 11.1). This will be discussed further in Chapter 11.

Each spinal nerve also sends off a small branch, the *meningeal ramus*, which passes back through the intervertebral foramen to reenter the vertebral canal (Fig. 3.5). These branches supply the meninges of the spinal cord with sensory and autonomic (sympathetic) fibers.

The Spinal Cord Consists of Cooperating Subunits That Are Controlled from the Brain

Each segment of the spinal cord is to some extent a functional unit, since, as we will see in Chapter 7, a pair of spinal nerves relates to a particular "segment" of the body. A spinal segment may be regarded as the "local government" of a part of the body: It receives sensory information from its own district, processes this information, and issues orders through motor nerves to muscles and glands to ensure adequate responses. However, just as local governing bodies in our society must take orders from higher governing bodies (for example, county versus national governments), the spinal segments have only limited independence. Many of the functional tasks of the spinal cord are under strict control and supervision from higher levels of the central nervous system. This control is mediated by fibers from the brain stem and cerebral cortex, which descend in the white matter of the cord and terminate in the gray matter of the spinal segments that are to be influenced. The brain also ensures that the activity of the

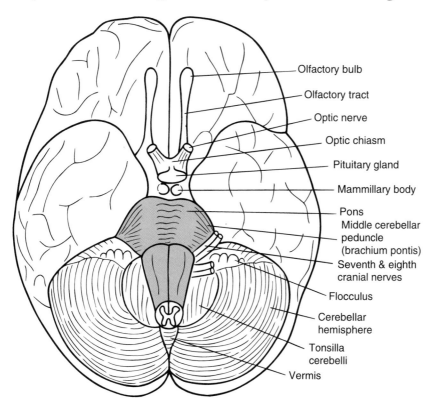

Figure 3.12 *The basal aspect of the brain*. Only some of the cranial nerves are shown.

- Olfactory bulb
- Olfactory tract
- Optic nerve
- Optic chiasm
- Pituitary gland
- Mammillary body
- Pons
- Middle cerebellar peduncle (brachium pontis)
- Seventh & eighth cranial nerves
- Flocculus
- Cerebellar hemisphere
- Tonsilla cerebelli
- Vermis

various spinal segments is coordinated, so that it serves the body as a whole and not only a small part. To be able to carry out this coordination, the brain must continuously receive information about conditions in all the "local districts" of the body and in the spinal segments related to them. This information is mediated by long, ascending fibers in the white matter of the cord terminating in the brain stem. The local cooperation among spinal segments is taken care of by the numerous propriospinal fibers coming from spinal interneurons.

THE BRAIN STEM

The brain stem represents the upward (rostral, cranial) continuation of the spinal cord (Fig. 3.1). It consists of several portions with, in part, clear-cut surface borders between them (Figs. 3.12, 3.13, and 3.14). Whereas the lowermost (caudal) part of the brain stem is structurally similar to the spinal cord, the upper parts are more complicated. The subdivisions of the brain stem are as follows (from caudal to rostral): the *medulla oblongata* (often just called medulla), the *pons* (the bridge), the *mesencephalon* (the midbrain), and the *diencephalon*.

The Brain Stem Contains the Third and Fourth Ventricles

A continuous, fluid-filled cavity varying in diameter stretches through the brain stem (Fig. 3.1). It is the upward continuation of the thin central canal

Figure 3.13 *The brain stem seen from the left side*. The levels of sections shown in several of the following figures are indicated.

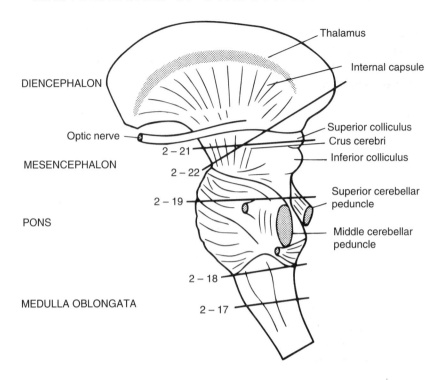

of the spinal cord, and it continues rostrally into the cavities of the cerebrum (Fig. 3.37). Together, these cavities constitute the *ventricular system of the brain and spinal cord*. The cavity in the brain stem has two dilated parts. One, the *fourth ventricle*, is at the level of the medulla and pons, whereas the *third ventricle* is situated in the diencephalon (Fig. 3.36). We will return to the ventricular system later in this chapter.

Figure 3.14 *The cranial nerves*. The brain stem is seen from the ventral side.

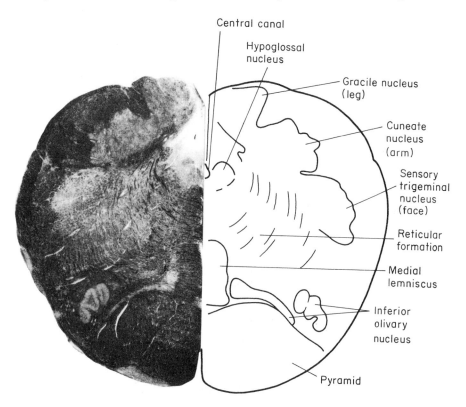

Central canal

Hypoglossal
nucleus

Gracile nucleus
(leg)

Cuneate
nucleus
(arm)

Sensory
trigeminal
nucleus
(face)

Reticular
formation

Medial
lemniscus

Inferior
olivary
nucleus

Pyramid

The Brain Stem Has Similarities to the Spinal Cord: The Cranial Nerves

Examination of the *internal structure of the brain stem* (Figs. 3.15–3.17, 3.19, 3.20, and 3.23) shows that it is more complicated than that of the spinal cord. Even though in both the brain stem and the cord, gray matter is generally located centrally, surrounded by a zone of white matter, the gray matter of the brain stem is subdivided into several regions separated by strands of white matter. The white matter of the brain stem consists of myelinated fibers, as in other parts of the central nervous system. The regions with gray matter contain various nuclei—that is, groups of neurons with common tasks. Many of the nuclei belong to the *cranial nerves*. In total, there are 12 pairs of cranial nerves, which, with the exception of the first, all emerge from the brain stem (Fig. 3.14). They correspond to the spinal nerves but show a more complex and less regular organization. Thus, there is no clear separation of sensory (dorsal) and motor (ventral) roots. The cranial nerves are numbered from rostral to caudal, in accordance with where they emerge on the surface of the brain stem. Figure 3.35 shows the places on the base of the skull where the cranial nerves leave through small holes or fissures.

Many of the cranial nerves contain fibers that conduct impulses out of the brain stem; that is, the fibers are efferent or motor. These fibers

Figure 3.15 *Lower part of the medulla oblongata.* Cross section. See Figure 3.13 for exact level. The **left** half is a photomicrograph of a section with darkly stained myelinated fibers (Woelke method); that is, white matter appears dark and gray matter light.

Figure 3.16 *Upper part of the medulla oblongata*. Cross section. See Figure 3.13 for exact level. Myelin staining as in Figure 3.15.

Figure 3.17 *Upper part of the pons*. Cross section; myelin-stained. See Figure 3.13 for exact level.

belong to neurons with their perikarya in nuclei that are called *motor cranial nerve nuclei*. They correspond to the groups (columns) of neurons in the ventral and lateral horns of the spinal cord. The cranial nerves, like the spinal nerves, also contain sensory, afferent fibers bringing impulses from sense organs. The brain stem cell groups in which these afferent fibers terminate are, accordingly, called *sensory cranial nerve nuclei*. They correspond to the laminae of the spinal dorsal horn. The sensory fibers entering the brain stem have their perikarya in ganglia just outside the brain stem, *cranial nerve ganglia*, corresponding to the spinal ganglia of the spinal nerves. Most cranial nerves are mixed; that is, they contain both motor and sensory fibers, but a few are either purely sensory or purely motor.

The only cranial nerve not emerging from the brain stem is the *first cranial nerve, the olfactory nerve* (nervus olfactorius). This consists of short axons coming from sensory cells in the roof of the nasal cavity, which, immediately after penetrating the base of the skull, terminate in the olfactory bulb (bulbus olfactorius) (Fig. 3.12). The other cranial nerves are briefly mentioned below in connection with a description of the main structural features of the brain stem. More thorough treatment of the cranial nerves and their central connections is found in Chapters 8, 9, 10, and 16.

The Reticular Formation Extends through Central Parts of the Brain Stem

Among the cranial nerve nuclei and other clearly delimited cell groups, there are more diffuse collections of neurons. In microscopic sections stained to visualize the neuronal processes, a networklike pattern is seen. The old anatomists therefore termed these parts—present in the core of most of the brain stem—*the reticular formation* (formatio reticularis, Figs. 3.15–3.17, 3.19, and 15.1). In reality, however, the reticular formation is not one homogeneous structure but rather a conglomerate of cell groups with different connections and functional tasks. Some parts of the reticular formation are, for example, primarily concerned with control of circulation and respiration; other parts are particularly concerned with regulation of sleep and wakefulness. But the collective term, the reticular formation, is still in common use, and it may be practical to retain it to denote parts of the brain stem with certain common anatomic features, without implying that they have common functional tasks. The reticular formation is treated more comprehensively in Chapter 15.

The Medulla Oblongata

Ventrally in the midline, the medulla has a longitudinal sulcus, which is a continuation of the ventral (anterior) median fissure of the cord. The sulcus ends abruptly at the lower end of the pons (Fig. 3.14). The so-called *pyramids* protrude on each side of the longitudinal sulcus. Each pyramid is formed by a thick bundle of axons belonging to the *pyramidal tract*. This important fiber tract conveys signals from the cerebral cortex to the spinal cord (the pyramidal tract is discussed in Chapter 12).

Close to the lower end of the medulla, on the transition to the cord, bundles of fibers can be seen to cross the midline, forming the *pyramidal decussation*. Lateral to the pyramids is an oval protrusion (the olive) formed by a large nucleus, *the inferior olive* (inferior olivary nucleus). This nucleus sends its efferents to the cerebellum (see *Afferents to the Cerebellar Cortex Are of Two Main Kinds*, Chapter 14). Between the olive and the pyramid is a row of small bundles of nerve fibers, which are the rootlets of the *hypoglossal nerve* (the twelfth cranial nerve, nervus hypoglossus). This nerve supplies the striated muscles of the tongue with motor fibers. Lateral to the olive, the rootlets of the *glossopharyngeal* and *vagus nerves* (ninth and tenth cranial nerves, nervus glossopharyngeus and nervus vagus) leave the brain stem. These two nerves supply the pharnyx, the larynx, and most of the viscera with motor and sensory fibers. The *accessory nerve* (eleventh cranial nerve, nervus accessorius) runs cranially along the lateral aspect of the medulla. Most of its fibers come from the upper cervical spinal segments but enter the cranial cavity to leave the skull together with the glossopharyngeal and vagus nerves. The accessory nerve supplies two muscles in the neck with motor fibers.

Figure 3.15 shows a *cross section through the lower part of the medulla*, at a level below the caudal end of the fourth ventricle. The section is stained so that regions with white matter (myelinated fiber tracts) are dark, whereas gray matter (nuclei) appears light. The ventrally located bundle of cross-sectioned fibers is the *pyramidal tract*, forming the pyramid (Fig. 3.16), and containing about 1 million fibers. Dorsal to the pyramid lies a highly convoluted band of gray matter, *the inferior olive*. The *dorsal column nuclei*, the *gracile* and *cuneate* (nucleus gracilis and nucleus cuneatus), are located dorsally in the medulla. The efferent fibers from these nuclei arch ventrally and take up a position close to the midline dorsal to the pyramids, where they form a triangular area of cross-sectioned fibers. This is an important sensory tract, *the medial lemniscus* (lemniscus medialis), leading from neurons in the dorsal column nuclei to nuclei in the diencephalon. The dorsal column nuclei receive afferent fibers that ascend in the dorsal columns (or dorsal funiculi) and convey impulses from receptors (sense organs) in the skin and muscles and around joints. Close to the midline, just ventral to the central canal, lies the *hypoglossal nucleus*, consisting of the perikarya of the motor fibers that form the *hypoglossal nerve*. The efferent fibers of the hypoglossal nucleus pass ventrally and leave the medulla at the lateral edge of the pyramid. Lateral to the motor cranial nerve nuclei are found several sensory cranial nerve nuclei, among them the big *sensory trigeminal nucleus* that receives sensory impulses from the face, carried in the *trigeminal nerve* (the fifth cranial nerve). Note how the nuclei transmitting sensory impulses from the leg, arm, and face are distributed from medial to lateral in the dorsal part of the medulla (Fig. 3.15).

A cross section through the *upper (cranial) part of the medulla oblongata* (Fig. 3.16) shows partly the same fiber tracts and nuclei as the section at a lower level (Fig. 3.15). In addition, we may notice the big *vestibular nuclei* situated dorsally and laterally under the floor of the fourth ventricle (these nuclei also extend cranially into the pons; see Fig. 16.16). They receive sensory impulses from the vestibular apparatus in the inner ear via the *vestibular nerve* (the eighth cranial nerve). One of the main efferent pathways from the vestibular nuclei forms a distinct tract, the *medial longitudinal fasciculus* (fasciculus longitudinalis medialis), close to the midline under the floor of the fourth ventricle (Fig. 3.17). This tract terminates in the motor nuclei of the cranial nerves supplying the eye muscles, thus conveying influences on eye movements from the receptors for equilibrium. Furthermore, Figure 3.16 shows the *motor* and *sensory nuclei of the vagus*, and some of the fibers of the vagus nerve, which pass laterally and ventrally, to leave the medulla lateral to the olive (compare with Fig. 3.14).

The Pons

The pons forms a bulbous protrusion at the ventral aspect of the brain stem, with clear-cut transversely running fiber bundles (Figs. 3.13 and 3.14). It is sharply delimited both caudally and cranially. The transverse fiber bundles are formed by fibers from large cell groups in the pons, the *pontine nuclei* (Fig. 3.17), and terminate in the cerebellum. The fiber bundles join at the lateral aspect of the pons to form the *middle cerebellar peduncle* (brachium pontis) (Figs. 3.13 and 3.17). Several cranial nerves leave the brain stem at the ventral aspect of the pons. At the lower (caudal) edge, just lateral to the midline, a thin nerve emerges on each side. This is the *abducens nerve* (the sixth cranial nerve, nervus abducens) carrying motor fibers to one of the external eye muscles (rotates the eye laterally). Still at the lower edge of the pons, but more laterally, two other cranial nerves leave the brain stem. Most ventrally lies the *facial nerve* (seventh cranial nerve, nervus facialis), bringing motor impulses to the mimetic muscles of the face (it also contains some other kinds of fibers, that are considered in Chapter 16). Closely behind the facial nerve lies the *vestibulocochlear nerve* (the eighth cranial nerve, nervus vestibulo-cochlearis). It carries sensory impulses from the sense organs for equilibrium and hearing in the inner ear. The largest of all the cranial nerves is the *trigeminal nerve* (the fifth cranial nerve, nervus trigeminus). It leaves the brain stem laterally at middle levels of the pons. The largest portion of the nerve consists of sensory fibers from the face, whereas a smaller (medial) portion contains motor fibers destined for the masticatory muscles.

In a *cross section through the pons*, the large *pontine nuclei* can be seen easily (Fig. 3.17). As mentioned, the neurons of the pontine nuclei send their axons to the cerebellum (see *Afferent Connections from the Cerebral Cortex*, Chapter 14). Bordering the pontine nuclei dorsally lies the *medial lemniscus*, which has turned around and moved laterally compared with its location in the medulla (see Figure 3.15). In the lower part of the pons, the nucleus of the abducens nerve, the *abducens nucleus*, is located dorsally and medially, whereas the facial nucleus lies more ventrally and laterally (Fig. 16.18). Figure 16.18 also shows the course taken by the efferent fibers of the abducens and facial nuclei (forming the sixth and seventh cranial nerves, respectively).

Figure 3.17 also shows the *sensory trigeminal nucleus* laterally (this nucleus extends as a slender column through the medulla, pons, and mes-

Third ventricle

Thalamus

Corpus pineale

Superior colliculus

Medial geniculate body

Inferior colliculus

Trochlear nerve

Cerebellar peduncles

Trigeminal nerve

Facial nerve

Vestibulo-cochlear nerve

Dorsal column nuclei (gracile and cuneate tubercles)

Hypoglossal nucleus

Facial colliculus

Figure 3.18 *The brain stem seen from the dorsal aspect.*

encephalon; see also Figs. 3.15–3.17, and 16.2). Medial to the sensory nucleus lies the *motor trigeminal nucleus* (masticatory muscles), but this nucleus is present only in the pons.

The Medulla and Pons Seen from the Dorsal Side

At the dorsal side of the medulla oblongata, at caudal levels, there are two longitudinal protrusions, the *gracile* and *cuneate tubercles* (Fig. 3.18). These are formed by the *dorsal column nuclei*, mentioned above (they are relay stations in pathways for sensory information from the body to the cerebral cortex). The most medial of these nuclei, the *gracile nucleus*, receives impulses from the leg and lower part of the trunk, whereas the laterally situated *cuneate nucleus* receives impulses from the arm and upper part of the trunk. Further laterally, another oblong protrusion (tuberculum cinereum) is formed by the *sensory trigeminal nucleus* (relay station for sensory impulses from the face).

Rostral to the upper end of the dorsal column nuclei, there is a flattened, diamond-shaped area, the *rhomboid fossa* (fossa rhomboides), extending rostrally onto the posterior face of the pons (Fig. 3.18). This constitutes the floor of the fourth ventricle (Fig. 3.37). Laterally and rostrally the rhomboid fossa is delimited by the cerebellar peduncles (these have been cut in Fig. 3.18). Some of the cranial nerve nuclei and some fiber tracts form small protrusions medially at the floor of the fourth ventricle—notably the hypoglossal nucleus and the root fibers of the facial nerve (forming the facial colliculus). (Figure 16.18 shows the peculiar route taken by the facial root fibers.)

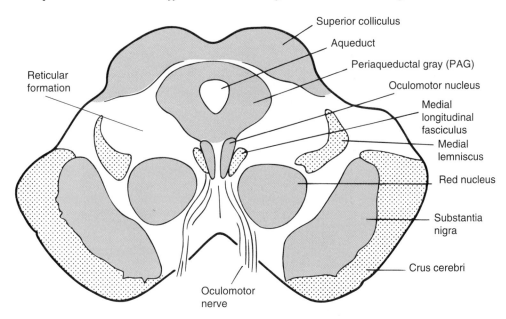

Superior colliculus

Aqueduct

Periaqueductal gray (PAG)

Oculomotor nucleus

Medial longitudinal fasciculus

Medial lemniscus

Red nucleus

Substantia nigra

Crus cerebri

Reticular formation

Oculomotor nerve

The Mesencephalon (Midbrain)

Figure 3.19 *The mesencephalon.* Cross section. The major nuclei are indicated in red and the major tracts in gray. See Figure 3.13 for exact level.

The part of the brain stem rostral to the pons, the mesencephalon, is relatively short (Figs. 3.1, 3.13, and 3.22). Ventrally, an almost half-cylindrical protrusion is present on each side of the midline—the *cerebral peduncle* or the *crus cerebri* (Fig. 3.16).[3] Crus cerebri consists of nerve fibers descending from the cerebral cortex to the brain stem and spinal cord—among these fibers are those of the pyramidal tract. The fibers continue into the pons, where they spread out into several smaller bundles among the pontine nuclei (Fig. 3.17).

In the furrow between the two crura, the *oculomotor nerve* emerges (third cranial nerve, nervus oculomotorius) (Fig. 3.14). As the name implies, the nerve carries motor impulses to muscles that move the eye. The oculomotor nerve innervates four of the six extraocular (striated) muscles and, in addition, two smooth internal muscles that regulate the diameter of the pupil and the curvature of the lens.

At the *dorsal side of the mesencephalon* there is a characteristic formation of four small, rounded protrustions, two on each side of the midline (Fig. 3.18). These are called the *colliculi* (corpora quadrigemina) and consist of, on each side, the *superior colliculus* and the *inferior colliculus*. They contain nuclei that are centers for visual (superior) and auditory (inferior) reflexes. The inferior colliculus is also a relay station in the pathways that bring auditory impulses to awareness.

Below the inferior colliculi there emerges on each side a thin fiber bundle, the *trochlear nerve* (fourth cranial nerve, nervus trochlearis). This is the only cranial nerve that emerges on the dorsal side of the brain stem. It supplies one of the extraocular muscles with motor fibers.

In *cross sections of the mesencephalon* (Figs. 3.19 and 3.20), the crus cerebri can be recognized ventrally, and the superior colliculus dorsally. In the midline just ventral to the colliculi there is a small hole, which is a cross section of the *aqueduct* (aquaeductus cerebri). This a narrow canal

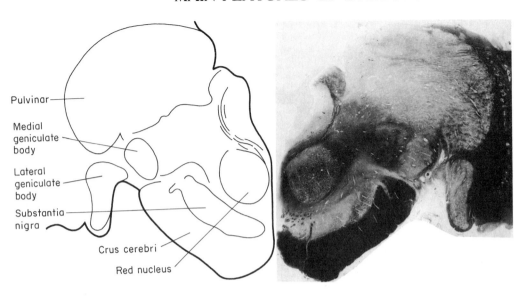

Pulvinar

Medial
geniculate
body

Lateral
geniculate
body

Substantia
nigra

Crus cerebri

Red nucleus

Figure 3.20 *The transition between the mesencephalon and the diencephalon.* Oblique frontal section; myelin staining. See Figure 3.13 for exact plane and level of the section.

interconnecting the third and fourth ventricles (Figs. 3.1, 3.19, and 3.22). Surrounding the aqueduct is a region of gray matter called the *periaqueductal gray substance* (substantia grisea centralis), which is of importance for sensations of pain. Ventral to the periaqueductal gray, close to the midline, we find the *oculomotor nucleus* (or nucleus of the oculomotor nerve). Further ventrally lies the large *red nucleus* (nucleus ruber)—so named because of its slightly reddish color. Just dorsal to the crus and ventral to the red nucleus is the *substantia nigra* (the black substance). The neurons of the substantia nigra contain a dark pigment, making the nucleus clearly visible macroscopically. The red nucleus and the substantia nigra are both of importance for the control of movements.

Figure 3.20 shows how the mesencephalon merges with the diencephalon rostrally without any clear transition.

The Diencephalon Consists of the Thalamus and the Hypothalamus

The diencephalon is not clearly delimited because in early embryonic life it fuses with the primordium of the cerebral hemispheres (Fig. 3.13). The *optic nerve* (the second cranial nerve, nervus opticus) with afferent fibers from the retina ends in the diencephalon.

The largest part of the diencephalon is occupied by the *thalamus*, situated on each side of the third ventricle (Figs. 3.21, 3.26, and 3.30). The thalamus consists of many smaller nuclei and is a *relay station for almost all information transmitted from the lower parts of the central nervous system to the cerebral cortex* (notably most kinds of sensory information). Each thalamus is approximately egg-shaped with a flattened side toward the third ventricle (Figs. 3.21 and 3.22). Lateral to the thalamus lies a thick sheet of white matter, the *internal capsule* (capsula interna). It consists mainly of fibers connecting the cerebral cortex with the brain stem

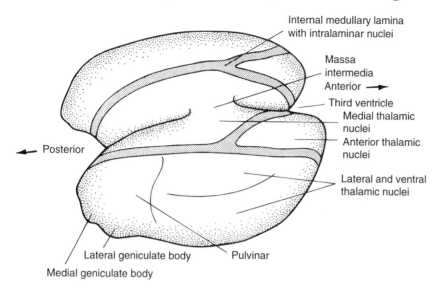

Figure 3.21 *The thalamus*. Drawing of the thalami of both sides, to indicate their three-dimensional form.

and the spinal cord, among them the *pyramidal tract* (Figs. 3.13, 3.23 and 3.26). The crus cerebri is a caudal continuation of many of the fibers of the internal capsule.

In Figure 3.23 (showing a frontal section of the brain), it can be seen that the thalamus is subdivided by narrow bands of white matter forming a Y—*the internal medullary lamina* (lamina medullaris interna) (see also Fig. 3.21). As a result, three major thalamic nuclear subdivisions can be identified, a *medial* (medial thalamic nucleus), a *lateral* (lateral thalamic nucleus), and an *anterior* (anterior thalamic nucleus). On closer (microscopic) inspection, each of these consists of several smaller nuclei that connect to different parts of the cerebral cortex. In addition to the three main nuclei mentioned, the thalamus includes one large nucleus in its posterior part, the *pulvinar* (Figs. 3.20 and 3.21), and two nuclei partly covered by the pulvinar, the *lateral geniculate body* (corpus genicalatum laterale) and the *medial geniculate body* (corpus geniculatum mediale). The latter two nuclei are relay stations for visual and auditory impulses, respectively. Thus, fibers of the *optic nerve* end in the lateral geniculate body.

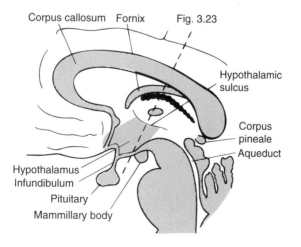

Figure 3.22 *The hypothalamus*. Drawing of midsagittal section showing the upper parts of the brain stem. The hypothalamus is indicated in red.

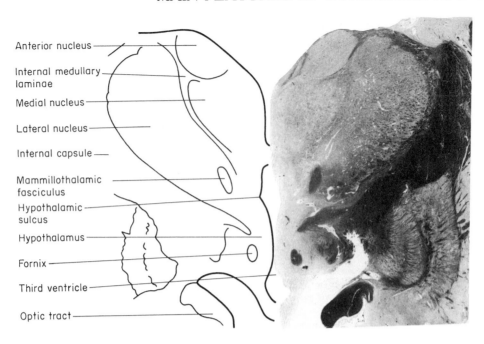

Anterior nucleus

Internal medullary laminae

Medial nucleus

Lateral nucleus

Internal capsule

Mammillothalamic fasciculus

Hypothalamic sulcus

Hypothalamus

Fornix

Third ventricle

Optic tract

Figure 3.23 *The diencephalon.* Frontal section; myelin staining. See Figure 3.22 for exact orientation and level of the section.

The optic nerves from the two eyes unite just underneath the diencephalon and form the *optic chiasm* (chiasma opticum), in which there is a partial crossing of the optic nerve fibers (Figs. 3.12 3.14, and 8.14). In their further course from the optic chiasm to the lateral geniculate body, the fibers form the optic tract (Figs. 3.14 and 3.23).

Anterior and inferior to the thalamus lies the *hypothalamus* (Fig. 3.22), which is particularly involved with *central control of the autonomic nervous system*—that is, with control of the visceral organs and the vessels. The hypothalamus forms the lateral wall of the anterior part of the third ventricle. The border between the thalamus and the hypothalamus is marked by the shallow *hypothalamic sulcus* (Figs. 3.22 and 3.23). The *mammillary body* (corpus mammillare), a special part of the hypothalamus, protrudes downward from its posterior part (Figs. 3.12 and 3.22). The *fornix* is a thick, arching bundle of fibers originating in the cerebral cortex (in the so-called hippocampal region) and terminating in the mammillary bodies (Figs. 3.25 and 19.2). The major efferent pathway of the mammillary body goes to the thalamus, forming a distinct fiber bundle, the *mammillothalamic tract* (fasciculus mammillothalamicus) (Fig. 3.23). In front of the mammillary bodies, the floor of the third ventricle bulges downward like a funnel and forms the stalk of the pituitary gland, the *infundibulum*. The region between the mammillary bodies and the infundibulum is called the *tuber cinereum* (Fig 18.1). It contains cell groups influencing the activity of the pituitary gland.

The *pituitary* (Figs. 3.12 and 3.22) consists of a *posterior lobe*, developed from the central nervous system, and an *anterior lobe*, developed from the epithelium in the roof of the mouth. The anterior lobe, secreting several hormones that control important bodily functions, is itself under the control of the hypothalamus. This is discussed further in Chapter 18.

Epithalamus, the Pineal Body, and Melatonin

The diencephalon also includes a small area called the *epithalamus*, located posteriorly in the roof of the third ventricle. In addition to a small nucleus, the *habenula* (Fig. 3.20), the epithalamus contains the *pineal body* or *gland* (corpus pineale) (Figs. 3.22 and 3.30). This peculiar structure lies in the midline (unpaired), and is formed by an evagination of the roof of the third ventricle. It contains glandular cells, *pinealocytes*, which produce the hormone *melatonin*. Since there are no efferent nerve fibers leaving the pineal body, it is regarded as a purely endocrine gland. The only known afferent nerve fibers arise in the upper cervical sympathetic ganglion (postganglionic fibers). The secretion of melatonin is influenced by the ambient light; *increased light (longer days) inhibits secretion*. In humans, as in experimental animals, the level of melatonin varies with the light-darkness cycle, with the highest level occurring at night. The influence of light is mediated via a tortuous route: signals from the retina reach an area in the hypothalamus called the *suprachiasmatic nucleus* (SCN) by a direct pathway; neurons there forward signal directly or indirectly to the preganglionic sympathetic neurons in the upper thoracic cord, their axons reach the upper cervical ganglion via the sympathetic trunk (Figs. 17.5 and 17.6).

Melatonin can influence several physiological parameters, espcecially those that show a cyclic variation. Its normal role in humans is not clear, however, because most of what we know comes from experiments on rodents. It can inhibit the secretion of gonadotropic hormones from the pituitary (the opposite effect has also been described, however, and the effect may depend on the time of the day it is given). Melatonin also influences sleep, attention, body temperature, and cortisol blood level (see Chapter 18, *The Hypothalamus and Circadian Rhythms*). Intake of melatonin in humans alters the phase of such rhythms, probably by setting the "circadian clock" in the SCN of the hypothalamus. Melatonin is now widely though controversially used to alleviate the unpleasant psychological and physiological effects of *jet lag*. It has also been used to normalize sleep–wake patterns in blind people. (Melatonin is not the only factor governing circadian rhythms, however.) A number of beneficial effects of melatonin that have been reported, such as preventing cancer, and counteracting the process of aging, lack convincing documentation.

The pineal body accumulates *calcified concretions* even before the age of 20. These are visible on X-ray films. Since it is normally located strictly in the midline, lateral displacement of the pineal body may signify a unilateral expansive intracranial process, such as a tumor or hemorrhage.

The *habenula* (Fig. 3.20) is situated just underneath the pineal body (one on each side). This small nucleus (composed of several subnuclei) receives afferents from the *hypothalamus* and the *septal nuclei*, among other sources. Its main efferents go to *nuclei in the mesencephalon*. The functional role of the habenula is not known, but the pathway from the hypothalamus via habenula to the mesencephalon may be engaged in the bodily expressions of strong emotions (for example, rage, fear).

THE CEREBRUM

The cerebrum has an ovoid shape and fills most of the cranial cavity. Whereas its convexity—that is, its upper and lateral surfaces—are evenly curved, the basal surface is uneven. In the center of the basal surface, the brain stem emerges (Figs. 3.12 and 3.25). The cerebrum is almost completely divided in two by a vertical slit, the *longitudinal cerebral fissure* (fissura longitudinalis cerebralis), so that it consists of two approximate half-spheres or *cerebral hemispheres*. Each of the cerebral hemispheres contains a central cavity, the *lateral ventricle* (Figs. 3.26 and 3.36). The lateral ventricles are continuous with the third ventricle through a small

Figure 3.24 *The right cerebral hemisphere seen from the lateral aspect.*

opening, the *interventricular foramen* (Fig. 3.37). The lateral ventricles are surrounded by masses of white matter with some embedded nuclei. The surface of the hemisphere is covered everywhere by a 3 to 5 mm-thick layer of gray substance, the *cerebral cortex* (cortex cerebri). The structure, connections, and functions of the cerebral cortex are covered most completely in Chapter 20, but some main features are briefly described here because knowledge of them is necessary for the chapters dealing with sensory and motor systems.

The neurons of the cerebral cortex receive impulses from lower parts of the central nervous system, most of which are relayed through the *thalamus*. In addition, there are numerous *association fibers*—that is, fibers interconnecting neurons in various parts of the cerebral cortex of one hemisphere. Finally, a vast number of *commissural fibers* interconnects neurons in the two hemispheres. Most of the commissural fibers are collected into a thick plate of white matter, the *corpus callosum*, which joins the two hemispheres across the midline (Fig. 3.25). The fibers in the corpus callosum enable impulses to travel from one hemisphere to the other and thus ensure that the right and left hemispheres can cooperate (see Chapter 20, *The Function of the Commissural Connections*). A few commissural fibers pass in the *anterior commissure* (commissura anterior) (Fig. 3.25).

The Surface of the Hemisphere Is Highly Convoluted and Forms Gyri and Sulci

During embryonic development, the cerebral hemispheres fold as they grow in size (Fig. 3.38). This leads to a great increase in their surface area and thus in the amount of cortex relative to their volume (only about

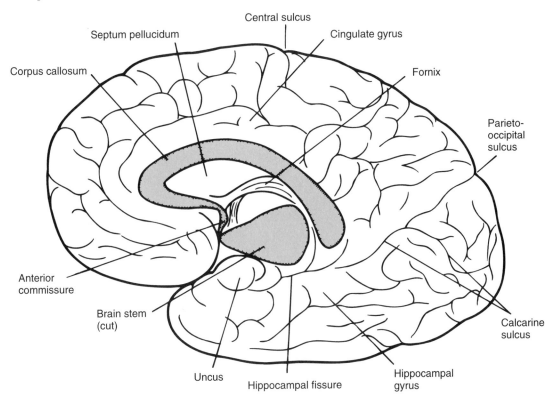

Central sulcus

Septum pellucidum   Cingulate gyrus

Corpus callosum   Fornix

                                                    Parieto-
                                                    occipital
                                                    sulcus

Anterior
commissure

Brain stem
(cut)
                                                    Calcarine
                                                    sulcus

Uncus   Hippocampal fissure   Hippocampal
                                       gyrus

a third of the total cortical surface is exposed). The furrowed, walnut-like appearance of the cerebral hemispheres of man and some higher mammals is highly characteristic (Figs. 3.24 and 3.25). The folding of the hemisphere produces deep *fissures* and more shallow *sulci*. Between the sulci, the surface of the cortex forms rounded *gyri*. Apart from the fissure that divides the two hemispheres along the midline, the longitudinal cerebral fissure, the largest fissure in each hemisphere is the *lateral cerebral sulcus* (fissure) or the *Sylvian fissure* (Fig. 3.24). This fissure follows a course upward and backward, and extends deep into the hemisphere (Fig. 3.26). The small gyri in the bottom of the lateral sulcus form the *insula* (the island) (Figs. 3.26, 3.27, and 3.28, 3.29). More sulci and gyri will be mentioned when dealing with the lobes of the cerebrum.

The pattern of the fissures and the larger sulci in the human brain is fairly constant. Nevertheless, variations are great enough to make it impossible to know exactly where a certain sulcus is located only from landmarks on the outside of the skull. The smaller sulci and gyri are subject to considerable individual variation.

The Hemisphere Can Be Divided into Four Lobes

With more or less sharply defined borders (formed by fissures and sulci), one can distinguish four lobes of the cerebral hemispheres. They are named in accordance with the bone of the skull under which they are located. The *frontal lobe* (lobus frontalis) (Fig. 3.24) lies in the anterior cranial fossa above the orbit. The frontal lobe is separated from the *parietal*

Figure 3.25 *The right cerebral hemisphere seen from the medial aspect.* The brain stem has been removed.

Figure 3.26 *The cerebral hemispheres and the brain stem.* Oblique frontal section. Compare with Figure 3.27.

Figure 3.27 *Magnetic resonance image* (MRI) with plane of sectioning corresponding to that in Figure 3.26. Almost all of the structures that can be identified in a section of a fixed brain can be recognized in the MRI. Courtesy of Dr. S. J. Bakke, The National Hospital of Norway.

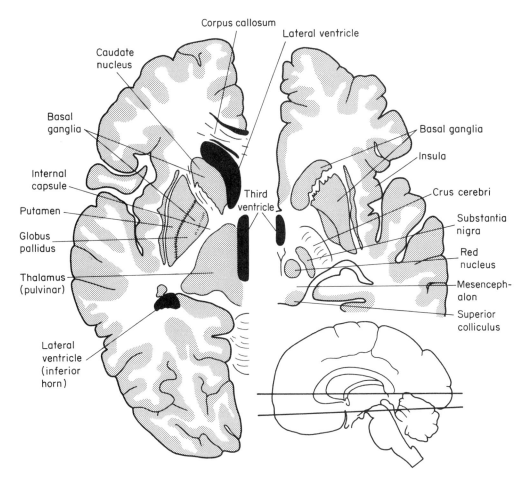

Figure 3.28 *The internal structure of the cerebral hemispheres.*
Drawings of two horizontal sections at slightly different levels,
the right section lowest. Compare with Figure 3.29.

Figure 3.29 *Magnetic resonance image* (MRI). Same direction and level of sectioning as in the left half of Figure 3.28. Courtesy of Dr. S. J. Bakke, The National Hospital of Norway, Oslo.

lobe (lobus parietalis) by the *central sulcus*, which extends from the medial edge of the hemisphere laterally to the lateral sulcus. Below the lateral sulcus lies the *temporal lobe* (lobus temporalis). Neither the parietal nor the temporal lobe has any clearly defined border posteriorly toward the occipital lobe. The occipital lobe lies above the cerebellum, which is located in the posterior cranial fossa (Fig. 3.1). On the medial aspect of the hemisphere, the border between the parietal and the occipital lobe is marked by the parieto-occipital sulcus (sulcus parieto-occipitalis) (Fig. 3.25).

Anatomically and functionally, the cerebral cortex can be divided into different regions, which do not, however, coincide with the different lobes. Here only a few points will be mentioned. The gyrus in front of the central sulcus, the *precentral gyrus* (gyrus precentralis) (Fig. 3.24), coincides fairly closely with the *motor cortex* (MI), which is of special significance for the execution of voluntary movements. If this gyrus is destroyed in one hemisphere, pareses ensue in the opposite side of the body. Many of the fibers in the pyramidal tract come from the precentral gyrus, and, as mentioned above, most of these fibers cross the midline on their way to the spinal cord. The *postcentral gyrus*, situated just posterior to the central sulcus, is the major receiving region for sensory impulses from the skin, musculoskeletal system, and the viscera. This region is called the *somatosensory cortex* (SI). The tracts that conduct impulses from the sense organs to the cortex are also crossed. Thus, destruction of the postcentral gyrus on one side leads to reduced sensibility (for example, of the skin) on the opposite side of the body. We have previously mentioned the medial lemniscus, which is part of the pathways from the sense organs to the postcentral gyrus. The fibers of the medial lemniscus terminate in the lateral thalamic nucleus (Fig. 3.23), and the neurons in this nucleus send their axons to the postcentral gyrus.

The *visual cortex*—that is, the main cortical region receiving information from the eyes—is located in the occipital lobe around a deep sulcus (fissure), the *calcarine sulcus* (sulcus calcarinus) (Fig. 3.25). The impulses start in the retina and are conducted in the optic nerve and the optic tract to the thalamus (the lateral geniculate body) (Figs. 3.20 and 3.21) and from there to the visual cortex (Fig. 8.14). The visual cortex can be distinguished from the surrounding parts of the cortex in sections perpendicular to the surface: It contains a thin whitish stripe running parallel to the surface (caused by a large number of myelinated fibers). Because of the stripe, this part of the cortex was named the striate area by the early anatomists (see also Fig. 8.18).

The *auditory cortex*—that is, the cortical region receiving impulses from the cochlea in the inner ear—is located in the temporal lobe (in the superior temporal gyrus) (Figs. 3.24 and 9.10). The pathway for auditory impulses is synaptically interrupted in the thalamus (the medial geniculate body) (Figs. 3.20 and 3.21).

The *olfactory cortex* is a small region on the medial aspect of the hemisphere near the tip of the temporal lobe. It is part of the so-called uncus (Figs. 3.25 and 10.2) and extends somewhat onto the adjoining hippocampal gyrus. The olfactory cortex receives fibers from the *olfactory bulb* (bulbus olfactorius) through the *olfactory tract* (tractus olfactorius)

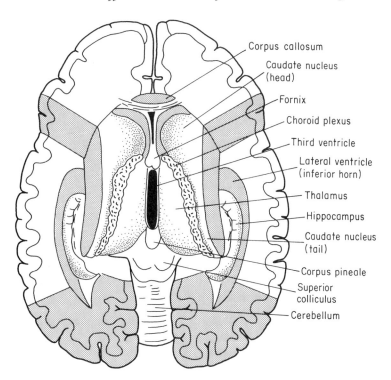

Corpus callosum

Caudate nucleus (head)

Fornix

Choroid plexus

Third ventricle

Lateral ventricle (inferior horn)

Thalamus

Hippocampus

Caudate nucleus (tail)

Corpus pineale

Superior colliculus

Cerebellum

Figure 3.30 *The internal structure of the cerebral hemispheres.* Parts of the hemispheres are removed to open the lateral ventricles. In the anterior part, the caudate nucleus can be seen to form the bottom and lateral wall of the ventricle. In the temporal horn of the ventricle, the hippocampus forms the medial wall.

(Fig. 3.12). The *hippocampal gyrus* and adjoining cortical regions are of particular interest with regard to learning and memory (this is treated further in Chapter 19). The cortex of the hippocampal gyrus extends into the *hippocampal sulcus* (fissure), forming a longitudinal elevation, the *hippocampus* (Figs. 3.26, 3.30, and 19.2). The hippocampus belongs to the phylogenetically oldest parts of the cerebral cortex and has a simpler structure than the newer parts.

The Cerebral Cortex Consists of Six Cell Layers

When the cerebral cortex is examined in a microscopic section cut perpendicular to the surface, it can be seen that the neuronal cell bodies (perikarya) are not randomly distributed (Figs. 20.1 and 20.2). They are arranged into *layers* or *laminae* parallel to the surface. Each layer is characterized by a certain shape, size, and packing density of the perikarya (compare with the Rexed's laminae of the spinal cord). The layers are numbered from the surface inward to the white matter. *Lamina 1* is cell-poor and consists largely of dendrites from neurons with perikarya in deeper layers and of axons with boutons making synapses on the dendrites. *Layers* or *laminae 2 and 4* are made up of predominantly small, rounded cells and are therefore also called the external and internal granular layer, respectively. These two layers have in common that they largely have a receiving function: Many of the afferent fibers to the cerebral cortex terminate and form synapses in layers 2 and 4. Fibers conveying sensory information from lower levels of the central nervous system end predominantly in layer 4, and consequently this layer is particularly well developed in the sensory cortical regions mentioned above. *Layers* or *lam-*

inae 3 and 5 contain cells that are larger than those in layers 2 and 4, and the cell bodies tend to be of pyramidal shape, hence the name *pyramidal cells*. Many of the pyramidal cells in layer 5 send their axons to the brain stem and spinal cord, where they influence motor neurons. Layer 5 is therefore especially well developed in the motor cortex in the precentral gyrus. The pyramidal neurons in lamina 3 send their axons primarily to other parts of the cerebral cortex, either in the same hemisphere (association fibers) or to cortex in the hemisphere of the other side (commissural fibers). The perikarya of *layer 6* are smaller and more spindle-shaped than those in lamina 5. Many of the neurons send their axons to the thalamus, enabling the cerebral cortex to influence the impulse traffic from the thalamus to the cortex (feedback connections).

There are also numerous *interneurons* in the cerebral cortex, providing opportunity for cooperation between the various layers (interneurons with "vertically" oriented axons) and between neurons in different parts of one layer (interneurons with "horizontally" oriented axons). The layers are obviously not independent units.

The Cerebral Cortex Can Be Divided into Many Areas on a Cytoarchitectonic Basis

We have mentioned above that some layers may be particularly well developed in certain regions of the cortex—for example, layer 4 in the sensory receiving areas and layer 5 in the motor cortex. There are many more differences when all layers all over the cortex are systematically compared. Such *cytoarchitectonic* differences (that is, differences in perikaryal size, shape, and packing density) form the basis of a parcellation of the cerebral cortex of each hemisphere into approximately *50 cortical areas* (areae). Maps of the cerebral cortex showing the positions of the various areas were published by several investigators around the turn of the century and are still in use. The most widely used map was published by the German anatomist Brodmann (Fig. 20.3). Such cytoarchitectonically defined areas have later been shown, in many cases, to differ also with regard to connections and functional properties. The numbering of the cortical areas may appear illogical. For example, the motor cortex in the precentral gyrus corresponds to area 4 of Brodmann. This borders posteriorly on area 3 but on area 6 anteriorly. Area 3 borders on area 1, which borders on area 2, and so on (Fig. 20.3). It is not necessary, however, to learn the position of more than a few of the cortical areas, and these will be dealt with in connection with the various functional systems in Parts II–VI.

The Basal Ganglia

The interior of the hemispheres contains regions with a gray substance. Largest among these are the so-called basal ganglia[4] which perform important tasks related to the control of movements. Other nuclear groups (the amygdala, the septal nuclei, and the basal nucleus) are discussed in Chapter 19, and the basal ganglia are discussed in Chapter 13. Here we will mention only a few main points with regard to the anatomy of the basal ganglia.

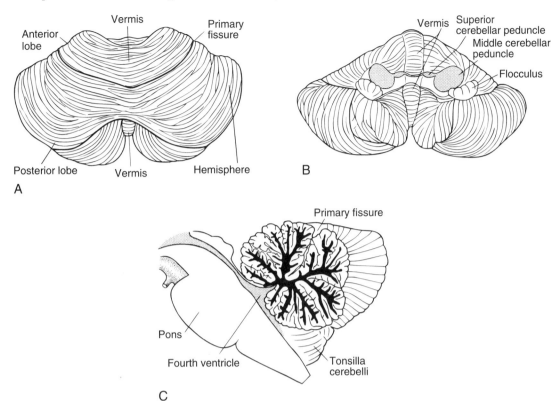

Vermis
Anterior lobe
Primary fissure
Posterior lobe   Vermis   Hemisphere

A

Vermis   Superior cerebellar peduncle
Middle cerebellar peduncle
Flocculus

B

Primary fissure
Pons
Fourth ventricle   Tonsilla cerebelli

C

Fig. 3.31 *The cerebellum.* **A**. Seen from the rostral–posterior aspect. **B**. Seen from the ventral aspect (the side facing the brain stem). **C.** Midsagittal section showing the cerebellar cortex as a thin layer with white matter underneath (indicated in black in the drawing).

The basal ganglia receive massive *afferent connections from the cerebral cortex and acts, by way of their efferent fibers, primarily back on motor regions of the cortex.* Sections through the hemispheres show that the basal ganglia consist of two main parts (Figs. 3.26 and 3.28). In a horizontal section (Fig. 3.28) one large part lies lateral to the internal capsule, and a smaller medial to the internal capsule and anterior to the thalamus. The largest part is called the *lentiform nucleus* (nucleus lentiformis) because of its shape. It consists of two closely apposed parts: The lateral or external part is called the *putamen*, and the medial or internal part is called the *globus pallidus.* The part of the basal ganglia situated medial to the internal capsule is called the *caudate nucleus* (nucleus caudatus). The name describes its form—a large part of the nucleus is indeed formed like a long, curved tail (Figs. 3.30 and 13.1). The caudate nucleus consists of an anterior bulky part, the *caput* (head), and a progressively thinner *cauda* (tail). The cauda extends first backward and then down and forward into the temporal lobe, located in the wall of the lateral ventricle. Figure 3.38 shows how this peculiar form can be explained on the basis of the embryonic development of the cerebral hemispheres.

THE CEREBELLUM

The cerebellum (the "little brain") is first and foremost of importance for the execution of movements; like the basal ganglia, it belongs to the motor system. The cerebellum is located in the posterior cranial fossa, dorsal to the brain stem (Figs. 3.1 and 3.31). It is connected with the brain stem anteriorly by way of three stalks of white matter on each side: *the inferior, middle, and superior cerebellar peduncles* (Figs. 3.13 and 3.15). In general, the inferior cerebellar peduncle or *restiform body* (corpus restiforme) contains fibers carrying impulses from the spinal cord to the cerebellum, whereas the middle cerebellar peduncle or the *brachium pontis* conveys information from the cerebral cortex. The superior cerebellar peduncle or the *brachium conjunctivum* contains most of the fibers conveying impulses out of the cerebellum—that is, the cerebellar efferent fibers.

Like the cerebrum, the cerebellum is covered by a layer of gray substance, the *cerebellar cortex* (cortex cerebellaris), with underlying white matter. Enclosed in the white matter are regions of gray matter, the *central (deep) cerebellar nuclei* (Fig. 13.12). From the neurons in these nuclei come the majority of efferent fibers conveying information from the cerebellum to other parts of the central nervous system.

The cerebellar surface is extensively folded, forming numerous narrow sheets or *folia* that are predominantly oriented transversely (Fig. 3.31). The fissures and sulci between the folia are partly very deep; the deepest among them divide the cerebellum into *lobes* (this is treated further in Chapter 14). In addition, the cerebellum can be subdivided macroscopically on another basis. In the posterior part of the cerebellum a narrow middle region is situated deeper than the much larger lateral parts (Fig. 3.33B). This middle part of the cerebellum is called the *vermis* (worm) and is present also in the anterior part of the cerebellum, although not as clearly distinguished from the lateral parts as posteriorly. The lateral parts are called the *cerebellar hemispheres*. A small bulbous part on each is connected medially with a thin stalk to the vermis. This part is called the *flocculus* (Fig. 3.31B) and lies close to the middle cerebellar peduncle, just posterior to the seventh and eighth cranial nerves. A midsagittal section through the cerebellum (Fig. 3.31C) shows clearly the deep sulci and fissures. The white substance forms a treelike structure and is called the *arbor vitae* (the tree of life—perhaps not very fitting, since the cerebellum is not necessary for life). The fourth ventricle, extending into the cerebellum like the apex of a tent, is also evident in the midsagittal section.

THE COVERINGS OF THE BRAIN

The central nervous system is enclosed in three connective tissue membranes, the *meninges*. The innermost one is the vascular *pia mater* (usually just called *pia*). It follows the surface of the brain and spinal cord closely, and extends into all sulci and depressions of the surface (Figs. 3.32 and 3.33). Thin vessels pass from the pia into the substance of the brain and supply the external parts, such as the cerebral cortex, with blood (the deeper parts of the brain are supplied by vessels entering the brain at its basal surface). The next membrane, the *arachnoid*, does not follow the uneven surface of the brain but extends across depressions, fissures, and sulci. Between the pia and the arachnoid exists a narrow space, the *subarachnoid space*, which is filled with cerebrospinal fluid (Figs. 3.1,

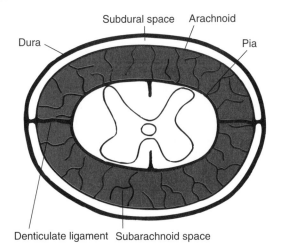

Subdural space   Arachnoid

Dura   Pia

Denticulate ligament   Subarachnoid space

Figure 3.32 *The meninges and sub-arachnoidal space of the spinal cord.*

3.32, and 3.33). Numerous thin threads of connective tissue connect the pia with the arachnoid, thus spanning the subarachnoid space. The depth of the subarachnoid space varies from place to place because the arachnoid, as mentioned, does not follow the surface of the brain. Where it crosses larger depressions, the subarachnoid space is considerably widened, forming so-called *cisterns* filled with cerebrospinal fluid. Several cisterns are found around the brain stem, but the largest one, the *cisterna magna* or cerebellomedullary cistern, is located posterior to the medulla below the cerebellum (Figs. 3.1 and 3.2). The cerebrospinal fluid enters the cisterna magna from the fourth ventricle (Figs. 3.1 and 3.37).

The subarachnoid space is continuous around the whole central nervous system. Substances released into the subarachnoid space at one place are therefore quickly spread out. A *subarachnoid hemorrhage*, for example, most often caused by rupture of a vessel at the base of the brain, quickly leads to all of the cerebrospinal fluid being mixed with blood. Thus, a sample of cerebrospinal fluid taken from the dural sac at lumbar levels will be bloody.

Figure 3.33 *The meninges, the subarachnoidal space, and the superior sagittal sinus.* Schematic drawing of a frontal section through the head, with the skull and the brain. See also Figure 1.15.

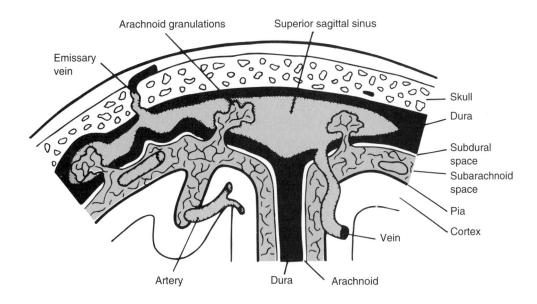

Arachnoid granulations   Superior sagittal sinus

Emissary vein

Skull

Dura

Subdural space

Subarachnoid space

Pia

Cortex

Vein

Artery   Dura   Arachnoid

Figure 3.34 *Folds of the dura and the venous sinuses*. The folds serve to minimize movements of the brain and also contain venous sinuses (red).

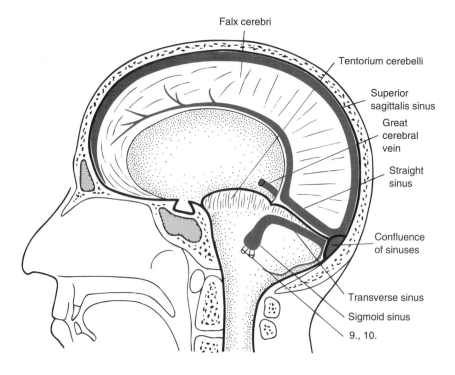

Falx cerebri

Tentorium cerebelli

Superior sagittalis sinus

Great cerebral vein

Straight sinus

Confluence of sinuses

Transverse sinus

Sigmoid sinus

9., 10.

The outermost membrane, the *dura mater* (usually just called the *dura*), is thick and strong because it consists of dense connective tissue (Figs. 3.1, 3.32, and 3.33). The dura covers closely the inside of the skull and constitutes also the periosteum. The arachnoid follows the inside of the dura closely so that there is only a very narrow space between these two meninges, the *subdural space* (Figs. 3.32 and 3.33). The dura extends down into the vertebral canal to enclose the spinal cord. It extends further down than the cord, however, forming a sac around the roots of the lower spinal nerves (the cauda equina). This *dural sac* extends down to the level of the second sacral vertebra. Thus below the level of the first–second lumbar vertebra (the lower end of the cord), the dural sac contains only spinal nerve roots and cerebrospinal fluid (Figs. 3.1 and 3.3). This is a safe place to enter the subarachnoid space with a needle (lumbar puncture) to take samples of the cerebrospinal fluid, since there is no danger of harming the cord.

In a few places *the dura forms strong infoldings*, serving to restrict the movements of the brain within the skull. Large movements can stretch and damage vessels and nerves connecting the brain with the skull (one of the possible effects of head injuries). From the midline, the *falx cerebri* extends down between the two hemispheres (Fig. 3.34). Posteriorly, the falx divides into two parts that extend laterally over the superior face of the cerebellum and attach to the temporal pyramid (Fig. 3.35). These two folds meet in the midline and form the *cerebellar tentorium*. In the anterior part of the tentorium, there is an elongated opening for the brain stem. If the pressure in the skull above the tentorium increases (due to bleeding, a tumor, or brain edema), part of the temporal lobe may be pressed down or *herniate* between the tentorium and the brain stem, harming the brain stem temporarily or permanently.

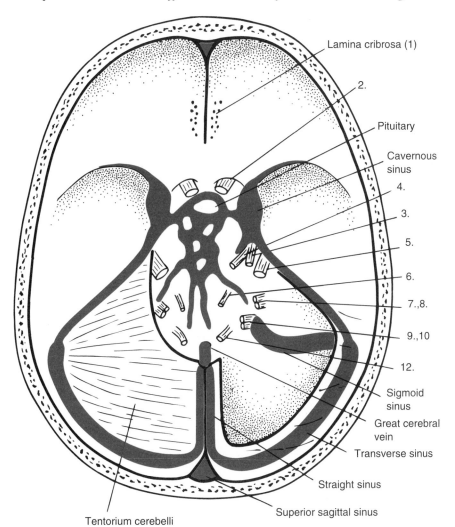

Figure 3.35 *The tentorium cerebelli and the large venous sinuses at the base of the skull.* At the right side, the tentorium is partly removed. The cranial nerves and their sites of exit from the skull are also shown.

Lamina cribrosa (1)

2.

Pituitary

Cavernous sinus

4.

3.

5.

6.

7.,8.

9.,10

12.

Sigmoid sinus

Great cerebral vein

Transverse sinus

Straight sinus

Superior sagittal sinus

Tentorium cerebelli

The Meninges and Stiffness of the Neck

Infection of the meninges, *meningitis*, typically produces *stiffness of the neck*. Every attempt to bend the neck or the back forward evokes an immediate reflexive muscular resistance. When the doctor tries to lift the patient's head off the pillow, the neck is kept straight. The infection causes inflammation of the meninges, which also extends onto the vessels and the nerve roots in the subarachnoid space. Forward bending (flexion) of the vertebral column elongates the spinal canal, as mentioned above, and that stretches the meninges, the vessels, and the nerve roots. Most likely, this accounts for the intense pain associated with any effort to flex the back or neck (similar to the pain felt by stretching an inflamed area of the skin or a joint capsule). Straining or coughing also causes pain in patients with meningitis. *Irritation of the meninges* can be caused by other means than infections by bacteria and viruses, however. One strong irritant is, for example, *blood in the subarachnoid space*. Thus, stiffness of the neck is by itself only a sign of meningeal irritation and does not indicate a specific cause.

Meningeal irritation is usually accompanied by a strong *headache*. This is seen most dramatically with subarachnoid hemorrhage, in which an intense headache starts abruptly the moment the bleeding starts and blood flows into the subarachnoid space. In such instances the cause is usually spontaneous rupture of an *aneurysm* (a sac-like dilatation) on one of the arteries at the base of the skull (Fig. 3.41).

Lateral ventricle

Third ventricle

Lateral ventricle (anterior horn)

Lateral ventricle (central part)

Lateral ventricle (posterior horn)

Interventricular foramen

Third ventricle

Lateral ventricle (inferior horn)

Aqueduct

Fourth ventricle

Figure 3.36 *The ventricular system of the brain.*

The spinal cord is anchored to the meninges partly by the spinal nerves and partly by two thin bands, the *denticulate ligaments* (Fig. 3.32), extending laterally from the cord to the arachnoid and dura (this is not a continuous ligament but one that forms 21 lateral extensions from the cord to the dura). The spinal cord nevertheless moves considerably up and down in the dural sac with movements of the vertebral column (the length of the vertebral canal varies by almost 10 cm from maximal flexion, when it is longest, to maximal extension).

THE CEREBRAL VENTRICLES AND THE CEREBROSPINAL FLUID

We have mentioned the ventricular system several times in connection with treatment of the various parts of the brain. Here we will consider the ventricular system as a whole, along with the cerebrospinal fluid.

The Location and Form of the Ventricles

The thin central canal of the cord continues upward into the brain stem. There the canal widens to form the *fourth ventricle* at the posterior aspect of the medulla and pons (Figs. 3.1, 3.36, and 3.37). The floor of the fourth ventricle is formed by the diamond-shaped *rhomboid fossa* (Fig. 3.18). The lateral walls of the ventricle are formed by the cerebellar peduncles. The ventricle has a tentlike form with the apex projecting into the cerebellum and two lateral evaginations (recessus lateralis).

The *third ventricle* is a thin slitlike room between the two thalami (Figs. 3.30, 3.36, and 3.37). During embryonic development, the primordia of the hemispheres become closely apposed to the diencephalon (Fig. 3.13). The loose masses of connective tissue between the hemispheres form an approximately horizontal plate that constitues the roof of the third ventricle. The choroid plexus is attached to the inside of the roof (Fig. 3.37).

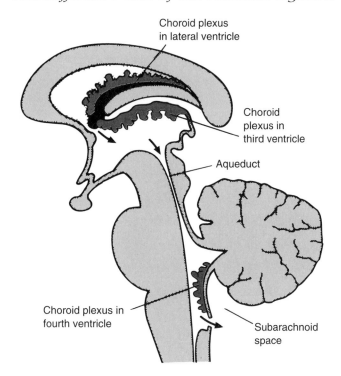

Choroid plexus
in lateral ventricle

Choroid
plexus in
third ventricle

Aqueduct

Choroid plexus in
fourth ventricle

Subarachnoid
space

Figure 3.37 *The ventricular system and the choroid plexus.* The flow of the cerebrospinal fluid is indicated with **arrows** in the drawing. All ventricles contain choroid plexus.

The two *lateral ventricles* represent the first and second ventricles, but these terms are not used. From a central part in the parietal lobe, the lateral ventricles have processes called *horns* into the three other lobes: an *anterior (frontal) horn*, a *posterior (occipital) horn*, and an *inferior (temporal) horn* extending downward and anteriorly into the temporal lobe (Figs. 3.30 and 3.36). The anterior horn is the largest and is bordered medially by the septum pellucidum[5] (Fig. 3.37), whereas the head of the caudate nucleus bulges into it from the lateral side. The central part of the ventricle lies just above the thalamus (Fig. 3.30). The inferior horn starts at the transition between the central part and the posterior horn and follows the temporal lobe almost to its tip. Medially in the inferior horn there is an elongated elevation, the *hippocampus* (Fig. 3.30), formed by invagination of the ventriclar wall from the medial side by the hippocampal fissure (Figs. 3.25 and 3.26).

The form of the lateral ventricles can be understood on the basis of the embryonic development of the cerebrum (Fig. 3.38). Both the lateral ventricles and the nervous tissue in its walls (such as the caudate nucleus and the hippocampus) eventually obtain a curved shape.

The Cerebrospinal Fluid Is Produced by Vascular Plexuses in the Ventricles

All of the ventricles are filled with a clear, watery fluid, the *cerebrospinal fluid* (CSF). Most of the fluid is produced by vascular tufts, the *choroid plexus*.[6] This is present in all four ventricles (Fig. 3.37), but the largest amount is found in the lateral ventricles. The plexuses are formed in early embryonic life by invaginations of the innermost meninx (the pia mater) at sites where the wall of the neural tube is very thin (Figs. 3.39 and 4.10).

Figure 3.38 *Development of the cerebral hemispheres and the lateral ventricles*. The characteristic arched shape of the ventricles can be explained by the manner in which the hemispheres fold during their growth in embryonic life. The caudate nucleus, located in the wall of the lateral ventricle, is indicated in red. All structures in the wall of the ventricles attain the curved shape. The figure also shows the development of gyri and sulci. Compare the pattern in the newborn and in the adult (Fig. 3.24). Based on Hamilton, Boyd, and Mossman (1972).

An elaborate structure of thin, branching protrusions or villi arises here (Fig. 3.40). The choroid plexuses are attached to the wall of the ventricles with a thin stalk (tela choroidea). The surface of the villi is covered by simple cuboid epithelium (which is continuous with the ependyma covering the inside of the ventricles). The epithelial cells have microvilli that increase their surface in contact with the CSF. The interior of the villi is composed of loose connective tissue with numerous capillaries of the fenestrated type, which are rather leaky. Therefore the hydrostatic pressure inside the capillaries produces a net flow of water with solutes (and a fair amount of proteins) into the interstitial space of the villi. This protein-rich fluid cannot leave the villi directly, however, since the epithelial cells covering the villi are attached to each other with tight junctions. The transport of water through the epithelium appears to be caused by active transport of sodium. Thus, the pumping of sodium produces an osmotic gradient so that water diffuses from the interior of the villi into the ventricles. Other ions, such as chloride and bicarbonate, follow the water passively.

The epithelium of the choroid plexus represents a barrier between the blood and the CSF, the *blood–CSF barrier*. Thus, many substances that

Figure 3.39 *Embryonic development of the choroid plexus*. Schematic drawing of a frontal section through the cerebral hemispheres at an early stage, showing how the choroid plexus is formed by invaginations of the pia into the ventricles.

Figure 3.40 *The structure of the choroid plexus, exemplified by one villus.* **Arrows** indicate the flow of fluid from the capillaries to the ventricles.

Cuboidal epithelium

Capillary

Tela choroidea

can leave the capillaries of the choroid plexus cannot enter the CSF. This is obviously important, because neurons are extremely sensitive to changes in the composition of their environment. We will later describe a similar barrier between the blood in the brain capillaries and the brain interstitium.

Composition and Function of the Cerebrospinal Fluid

The concentration of sodium, potassium, and several other ions is about the same in the CSF as in the blood (there are, however, some minor differences). The concentration of glucose is about two-thirds that in the blood. A major difference concerns proteins: There is normally very little protein in the CSF (less than 0.5% of the plasma protein concentration).

Water and soluble substances are freely exchangeable between the CSF and the interstitial fluid of the nervous tissue because the ependyma is freely permeable to water and even small protein molecules. It is, therefore, not surprising that many of the neurotransmitters, peptides, and other neuroactive substances can be found in the CSF. Some substances, notably hormones synthesized in the anterior pituitary, are apparently actively secreted into the CSF and thus reach it not only by passive diffusion. The functional role of the various neurotransmitters and peptides present in the CSF is not yet known.

We mention at the beginning of this chapter that, because the brain almost floats in it, the CSF has important *protective functions*. This buoyancy reduces the weight of the brain to about 50 g, which means less traction on vessels and nerves connected to the central nervous system. Furthermore, the effect of blows to the head on the brain is dampened be-cause water has to be pressed aside before the brain hits its hard sur-roundings (the skull).

Another possible functional role of the CSF can be deduced from the fact, mentioned above, that water and solutes can pass freely between it and the extracellular fluid (interstitium) of the nervous tissue. This means that the accumulation of substances in the nervous tissue (such as potas-sium ions during prolonged periods of intense neuronal activity) may be minimized by diffusion into the CSF. In general, it appears likely that *the CSF contributes to the maintenance of a constant composition of the neu-ronal environment.* This is important for the excitability of the neurons, among other functions. Altogether, however, glial cells are probably much more important than the CSF in this respect. Determining the presence and concentration of various neuroactive substances in the CSF is never-theless of great interest, because it represents an indirect way of examin-ing the extracellular fluid of the brain, which is very difficult to examine directly. Owing to the free permeability of the ependymal layer, the con-centration of a substance in the CSF presumably corresponds closely to its concentration in the extracellular fluid of the nervous tissue—that is, in the immediate vicinity of the neurons.

Circulation and Drainage of the Cerebrospinal Fluid

About one-half liter of CSF is produced each day, yet the total volume of fluid in the ventricles and the subarachnoid space is approximately 130 ml (approximately 20 ml is in the ventricles). Thus, the total amount is renewed several times a day. This means that effective means of drainage must exist.

The fluid produced in the lateral ventricles flows into the third ven-tricle through the *interventricular foramen* (of Monro) (Fig. 3.37). From there the fluid flows through the narrow *cerebral aqueduct* to the fourth ventricle. More fluid is added by the choroid plexuses in the third and fourth ventricles. The fluid leaves the ventricular system and enters the subarachnoid space (more specifically the cisterna magna) through *three openings in the roof of the fourth ventricle*—one in the midline posteri-orly (the foramen of Magendie) and two laterally (the lateral recesses or foramina of Luschka) (Figs. 3.1 and 3.37). The fluid then spreads out over the entire surface of the brain and spinal cord. From the base of the brain, there is an upward stream along the lateral aspects of the hemispheres to-ward the midline. Here, most of the CSF *empties into venous sinuses*. This happens by way of small evaginations of the arachnoid (arachnoid villi) into the venous sinuses. Several villi together form macroscopically visible protrusions called *arachnoid granulations*, which are particularly prominent along the superior sagittal sinus (Fig. 3.33). The passage of fluid from the subarachnoid space to the venous sinuses is probably caused by a difference in hydrostatic pressure—the pressure being higher in the subarachnoid space (about 15 cm H_2O) than in the sinuses (7–8 cm H_2O). Some of the CSF is drained via other routes, such as lymphatic vessels in cranial and spinal nerves.

Diseases Affecting the Ventricles and the Cerebrospinal Fluid

Because the central nervous system and the CSF are located in a closed container with rigid walls, the pressure inside the container increases if, for some reason, the amount of substance inside it increases. The intracranial pressure is the same for the nervous tissue and the CSF, but it can be measured most conveniently in the latter. For each heartbeat, for example, the pressure inside the cerebral ventricles increases slightly because more blood is pumped into the brain. Correspondingly, the pressure increases on coughing and straining because the drainage of venous blood from the cranial cavity and the vertebral canal is reduced. *Regardless of cause, any intracranial expansive process leads to increased intracranial pressure.* When the pressure increases, the blood pressure has to be increased to maintain cerebral blood flow. Thus, abnormally elevated blood pressure, usually combined with slowing of the heart rate, is one of the signs of severely increased intracranial pressure. However, if the increase is above a certain level, the cerebral blood flow is reduced, and the functioning of the brain suffers (with signs of confusion and eventually loss of consciousness). This happens, for example, in patients with *brain edema.* This is a dangerous complication of acute brain damage caused by, for example, head injuries. The edema is caused by extravasation of fluid from the brain capillaries. Similarly, an intracranial hemorrhage, which may arise from vessels inside or outside the brain substance, can also cause a dangerous increase of the intracranial pressure. If the expansion process is located in the posterior fossa (below the tentorium cerebelli), the tonsilla cerebelli (Fig. 3.31C) may be dislocated downward into the foramen magnum and thus compress the medulla (tonsillar herniation). If the expansive process is located above the tentorium cerebelli (in the middle or anterior fossa), the uncus of the temporal lobe (Fig. 3.25) can be dislocated downward beneath the edge of the tentorium and compress the brain stem at the level of the mesencephalon (Fig. 3.26). Both forms of herniation may lead to serious brain damage or death.

If the amount of CSF is increased in the ventricles, the pressure usually increases as well. A condition with an increased amount of cerebrospinal fluid is called *hydrocephalus.* Most often, this is caused by obstruction of the drainage of the CSF—for example, by closure of the aqueduct (inflammation, tumor, bleeding) or the outlets from the fourth ventricles. If this happens in an adult, in whom the sutures of the skull have grown firmly together, the intracranial pressure increases markedly, with dramatic symptoms. If, however, the condition arises in early childhood before the sutures are closed, the size of the head grows abnormally, with the skull yielding to the increased intracranial pressure. This may continue for some time with surprisingly few signs of cerebral dysfunction, but the development of the brain will eventually suffer, with results such as mental retardation. Hydrocephalus in children may be treated by shunting the CSF directly into a big vein outside the skull. A thin tube is inserted through a small hole in the skull into the lateral ventricle and is then directed under the skin, usually to where the internal jugular and the subclavian veins meet. In this manner, damage to the brain may be prevented.

Examination of the CSF can provide valuable information about neurological diseases. A sample of the fluid is usually withdrawn with a thin needle from the subarachnoid space in the dural sac—that is, below the level of the second lumbar vertebra. This way there is no risk of damaging the spinal cord (Figs. 3.1 and 3.3). When the tip of the needle is in the subarachnoid space, the intracranial pressure can also be determined. Examination of the fluid, in part under the microscope, can give information about possible bleeding into the subarachnoid space and about infections and inflammations of the brain itself (encephalitis) or the meninges (meningitis). In the latter case there are numerous leukocytes in the CSF. The concentration of proteins, normally very low, may increase in certain diseases (for example, in multiple sclerosis, in which the proteins are antibodies against components of the nervous tissue).

The shape and size of the ventricles can now be determined noninvasively in living subjects by use of computer tomography (CT) and magnetic resonance imaging (MRI) (Figs. 3.2, 3.27, and 3.29). Atrophy of the nervous tissue of the brain—for example, the atrophy of the cerebral cortex occurring in dementia—leads to dilatation of the ventricles, whereas expansive, space-occupying processes like hemorrhages and tumors may distort and compress the ventricles.

THE BLOOD SUPPLY OF THE CENTRAL NERVOUS SYSTEM

Of all cell types in the body, neurons are the most sensitive to interruption of their supply of oxygen (anoxia). Only a few minutes' stop in the blood flow may cause neuronal death. The oxygen consumption of the brain is high even at rest. Therefore, the blood supply of the central nervous system is ample, and the brain receives about 15% of the cardiac output at rest. Regulatory mechanisms ensure that the brain gets what it needs—if necessary, at the expense of all other organs. The arteries of the brain lie within the cranial cavity and are mostly devoid of anastomoses (connections) with arteries outside the skull. Therefore, other arteries cannot take over if the intracranial ones are narrowed or occluded.

The Blood–Brain Barrier Prevents Many Substances from Entering the Brain

In most organs of our body, small-molecular substances pass the capillary wall with relative ease, and their concentration is therefore similar in the blood plasma and in the interstitial fluid. The composition of the interstitial (extracellular) fluid of the brain differs, however, from that in most other organs. The *blood–brain barrier* (we have previously mentioned a similar barrier between the blood and the CSF) is due to special, selective properties of the brain capillaries. Many small molecules cannot pass the capillary wall at all, whereas others pass with greater ease than in other organs. *Thus, there is not only a barrier intercalated between the blood and the brain but also specific transport mechanisms for certain substances that the brain needs.*

The barrier properties of the brain capillaries appear to result mainly from very extensive tight junctions between the endothelial cells. Substances therefore have to pass through the plasma membrane of the capillaries to enter the brain interstitium.[7] Water-soluble substances are thus effectively prevented from passing (except via specific uptake-mechanisms), whereas lipid-soluble substances can pass the plasma membrane with ease. This is of consequence for whether a drug may gain access to the brain; only lipid-soluble drugs can as a rule reach therapeutic concentrations in the brain. Certain drugs—such as barbiturates used for induction of anesthesia—are highly lipid-soluble and act rapidly. Other drugs, such as penicillin, have low lipid solubility and pass the blood–brain barrier only with difficulty. In serious infections of the central nervous system, penicillin (or another drug with low lipid solubility) may be injected directly into the CSF, usually in the cisterna magna (Fig. 3.1). The drug then easily enters the brain tissue because there is no barrier between the CSF and the brain interstitial fluid.

Glucose is an example of a substance with high water solubility that nevertheless reaches high concentrations in the brain (this is necessary because the neurons depend almost solely on glucose as a source of energy). The reason is that the plasma membrane of the brain endothelial cells is equipped with carrier proteins that transport glucose actively. Similar active mechanisms exist for other water-soluble substances that the brain needs.

There is evidence that the special barrier properties of the brain capillaries depend upon influence from surrounding *astrocytes.* As mentioned earlier, all brain capillaries are surrounded by astrocyte processes (Fig. 1.15D), and these probably induce the special morphological and functional features of the brain capillaries. In several different, unrelated *diseases of the brain, the blood—brain barrier becomes less effective.* At the ultrastructural level the capillaries are changed, with loss of tight junctions as a prominent feature, and at the same time there are changes of the astrocytes.

The blood–brain barrier appears first and foremost to have protective functions. Many foreign substances that would be harmful to the neurons are kept out. Also, neuroactive substances in the bloodstream, such as neurotransmitters and peptides (produced in the peripheral nervous tissue, endocrine organs, and the gut) are prevented from reaching the brain. For example, fluctuations of the plasma level of norepinephrine or serotonin are not accompanied by similar fluctuations in the brain, which would have disturbed its normal functioning.

It is also likely that the endothelial cells of the brain actively pump several ions that are present in different concentrations in the blood plasma and in the extracellular fluid of the brain (Na^+, K^+, Ca^{2+}, and others). Even more than other cells, neurons depend on precise control of the concentrations of such ions for their normal functioning (for example, their excitability is increased by an increase of the extracellular potassium concentration).

Some Parts of the Brain Lack a Blood–Brain Barrier

In a few small regions adjoining the ventricles, the capillaries are fenestrated and hence let substances from the blood pass through easily. At such places neurons are exposed to substances of the blood that do not enter other parts of the brain. These regions are called the *circumventricular organs.* Among these, the *area postrema* is found in the lower end of the fourth ventricle, whereas the *subfornical organ* lies in the roof of the third ventricle just underneath the fornix close to the interventricular foramen. Both the area postrema and the subfornical organ contain many neurons that send their axons to other parts of the central nervous system and can thus mediate various specific influences on the nervous system. Neurons in the area postrema are involved in the vomiting reflex when this is elicited by toxic substances of the blood. Neurons in the subfornical organ monitor the salt concentration of the blood. They send signals to the hypothalamus that can initiate responses necessary to maintain the fluid balance of the body. The subfornical organ (and other parts of the circumventricular organs) are probably also targets of substances in the blood that induce fever and other symptoms of infections.

The *median eminence* (eminentia mediana) in the hypothalamus (Fig. 18.5C) also lacks a blood–brain barrier. This region does not contain neuronal cell bodies but receives nerve fibers from other parts of the hypothalamus. Hormones released from nerve terminals in the median eminence are transported by the blood stream to the anterior pituitary. (This is treated in more depth in Chapter 18.)

The two endocrine glands that are parts of or developed from the brain, the *posterior pituitary* and the *pineal body*, also lack a blood–brain barrier. As with the median eminence, this is related to their release of hormones directly into the bloodstream.

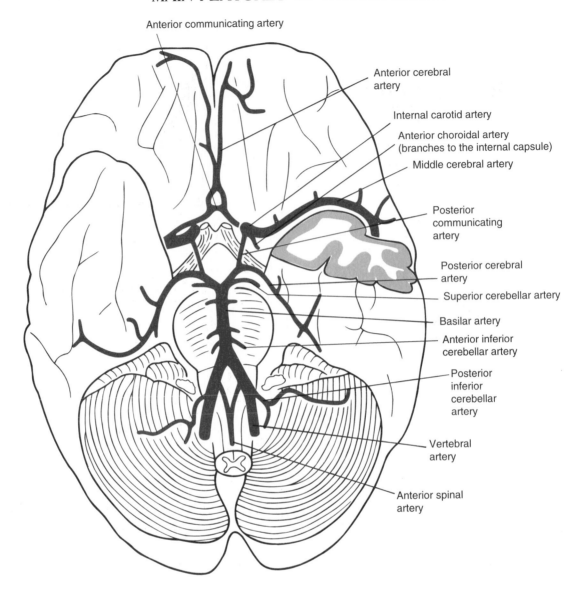

Anterior communicating artery

Anterior cerebral artery

Internal carotid artery

Anterior choroidal artery (branches to the internal capsule)

Middle cerebral artery

Posterior communicating artery

Posterior cerebral artery

Superior cerebellar artery

Basilar artery

Anterior inferior cerebellar artery

Posterior inferior cerebellar artery

Vertebral artery

Anterior spinal artery

Figure 3.41 *The main arteries of the brain*. Note anastomoses between branches of the internal carotid artery and the vertebral artery and between the two anterior cerebral arteries. These anastomoses form an arterial circuit at the base of the brain.

The Brain Receives Arterial Blood from the Internal Carotid and the Vertebral Arteries

Broadly speaking, the internal carotid artery supplies most of the cerebral hemispheres, whereas the vertebral artery supplies the brain stem and the cerebellum.

The *internal carotid artery* (arteria carotis interna) enters the cranial cavity through a canal at the base of the skull (the carotid canal in the temporal bone) and then divides into three branches (Fig. 3.41). The *ophthalmic artery* passes to the orbit through the optic canal and thus does not supply the brain itself (although, strictly speaking, the retina is part of the central nervous system). The *anterior cerebral artery* runs forward over the optic nerve and along the medial aspect of the hemispheres. Its branches reach only a short distance onto the convexity of the hemispheres (Fig. 3.43). The *middle cerebral artery* is the largest branch. It curves laterally into the lateral cerebral fissure and follows this backward and up-

Figure 3.42 *The course of the middle cerebral artery.* In the depth of the lateral fissure, it gives off branches to the internal capsule and the basal ganglia.

Middle cerebral
artery

ward (Figs. 3.42 and 3.43). On its way, numerous branches are given off that supply most of the cerebral cortex on the convexity of the hemispheres, notably the motor and somatosensory cortical areas, except for their most medial parts (with neuronal groups concerned with the motor and sensory functions of the legs; see Figs. 12.4 and 12.8), which are supplied by the anterior cerebral artery. The deep parts of the cerebrum, such as the *basal ganglia* and the *internal capsule*, are supplied by their own branches from the middle cerebral artery (Fig. 3.42) and by a separate branch of the internal carotid artery, the *anterior choroid artery* (Fig. 3.41).

The *vertebral artery* (Fig. 3.41) enters the posterior fossa after ascending through the transverse foramina of the cervical vertebrae. When passing from the atlas through the foramen magnum, the artery is highly convoluted, enabling it to follow the large movements in the upper cervical joints without being overstretched or compressed. Nevertheless, by extreme movements—particularly in elderly people with sclerotic arteries—the vertebral artery may be temporarily occluded. This may lead to loss of consciousness due to lack of blood supply to the brain stem. Backward bending of the head combined with rotation is particularly apt to compress the vertebral artery. The vertebral arteries of the two sides unite at the lower level of the pons to form the *basilar artery* (Fig. 3.41). The vertebral arteries and the basilar artery send off numerous branches to supply the medulla oblongata, the pons, the mesencephalon, and the cerebellum. One of these, the *posterior inferior cerebellar artery* (PICA), supplies the lateral part of the medulla and parts of the cerebellar hemispheres, whereas the *anterior inferior cerebellar artery* supplies lateral parts of the pons and parts of the cerebellum (see Chapter 16, *Brain Stem Infarc-*

Figure 3.43 *The parts of the brain supplied with blood from the main arterial branches*

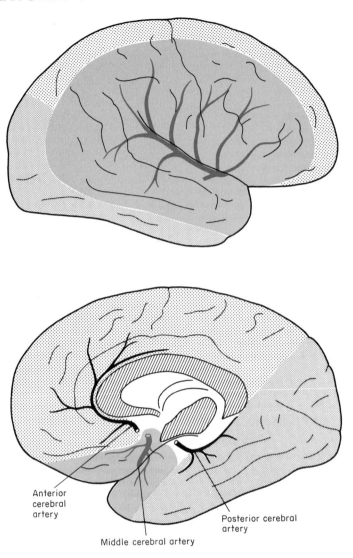

Anterior cerebral artery

Middle cerebral artery

Posterior cerebral artery

tions Can Produce Symptoms from Several Cranial Nerves and Long Tracts).

At the upper end of the pons, the basilar artery divides into its two end branches, the *posterior cerebral arteries*. These curve posteriorly around the mesencephalon and continue at the medial side of the hemisphere to the occipital lobe (Figs. 3.41 and 3.43). The posterior cerebral artery supplies large parts of the occipital lobe, notably the *visual cortex*, and the inferior aspect of the temporal lobe.

It should be noted that the symptoms produced by occlusion of one arterial branch are variable because of individual differences in the size and exact distribution of the various arterial branches. Thus, if one artery is small, another supplying a neighboring territory is usually large. The two inferior cerebellar arteries are examples of this phenomenon. Even the two vertebral arteries often differ markedly in size in one person, explaining why symptoms caused by occlusion of the artery may vary from minimal to life-threatening.

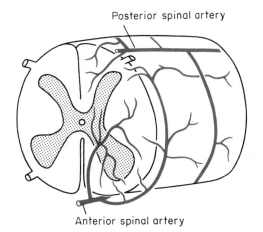

Posterior spinal artery

Anterior spinal artery

Figure 3.44 *The arterial supply of the spinal cord.*

There Are Communications between the Vertebral and Carotid Arteries and between the Arteries of the Two Sides

At the base of the brain there is a connection on each side between the middle and the posterior cerebral arteries, the *posterior communicating artery* (arteria communicans posterior) (Fig. 3.41). This means that if one of the two main arterial trunks (the internal carotid or the vertebral artery) is narrowed or even occluded, the other may to some extent compensate for the loss (as long as the communicating artery is open). There is also a corresponding communicating artery between the two anterior cerebral arteries (Fig. 3.41). In this manner a circle of anastomosing arteries is formed at the base of the skull, the *circle of Willis*, which may be of great clinical significance. It may explain, for example, how some people may have a totally occluded internal carotid artery on one side without any neurological signs.

The Spinal Cord Receives Arteries at Many Levels

In general, the arteries of the cord are arranged with one artery running in the midline anteriorly, the *anterior spinal artery*, and one on each side running along the rows of posterior roots, *the posterior spinal arteries* (Fig. 3.44). All three arteries begin cranially as branches of the vertebral arteries but receive contributions from small arteries entering the vertebral canal along with the spinal nerves.

The *venous blood* is collected in a venous plexus at the surface of the cord. This plexus empties into another, larger plexus at the surface of the dura, the *epidural plexus* (Fig. 3.6). From there the blood is emptied into veins outside the vertebral canal.

The Venous Blood Is Collected in Sinuses and Leaves the Skull in the Internal Jugular Vein

The cerebral veins can be divided into *deep* and *superficial types*. The latter partly accompany the arteries on the surface of the brain. All of the veins empty into large venous sinuses that are formed by folds of the dura (Figs. 3.34 and 3.35). At the base of the skull there are several sinuses, among them the *cavernous sinus* lateral to the pituitary gland. Blood from the pituitary (among other structures) flows into the cavernous sinus, and continues posteriorly in the *inferior petrous sinus* to the internal jugular vein. By threading a thin catheter cranially from the femoral vein, the petrous sinus can be reached. This permits examination of venous blood draining the pituitary in patients with symptoms suggesting a hormone-producing pituitary tumor.

The superficial veins at the dorsal parts of the hemispheres run upward and medially and empty into the large *superior sagittal sinus* in the upper margin of the falx cerebri. Where the falx cerebri meets the tentorium cerebelli, the superior sagittal sinus divides into two parts, the *transverse sinuses*, so named because they follow a transverse course laterally along where the tentorium is attached to the occipital bone. The *sigmoid sinus*—forming the direct continuation of the transverse sinus—empties into the *internal jugular vein* at the jugular foramen. The internal jugular vein leaves the skull and continues downward into the neck.

Most of the blood in the deep cerebral veins collects into the *great cerebral vein* of Galen (vena cerebri magna) (Fig. 3.35). This comes out from the inferior side of the posterior end of the corpus callosum and empties into the *straight sinus* (sinus rectus) in the midline of the tentorium. The sinus rectus drains into the superior sagittal sinus at the confluence region, from which the transverse sinus originates (Fig. 3.35).

Unlike the arteries, the cerebral veins have numerous anastomoses. At some locations there are also *emissary veins* that form connections between intracranial and extracranial veins (Fig. 3.33). Veins draining into the sinuses from the subarachnoid space—for example, along the superior sagittal sinus—are called *bridging veins* (Fig. 3.33). They constitute some of the few attachments that exist between the convexity of the hemispheres and the skull. Head injuries that lead to sudden displacement of the brain inside the skull may cause bridging veins to tear, with venous bleeding as a result. This results in a *chronic subdural hematoma*, which expands very slowly (due to an osmotic effect of the decomposing blood of the hematoma). The name implies that the blood collects between the dura and the arachnoid, in the subdural space. The blood remains localized, in contrast to what happens when the bleeding occurs in the subarachnoid space. The symptoms arising from a subdural hematoma may be due to pressure on the underlying parts of the brain (for example, paresis if the hematoma overlies the motor cortex), or they may be due to increased intracranial pressure with more nonspecific symptoms, such as headache and confusion.

NOTES

1. Strictly speaking, most neurons in the central nervous system are interneurons according to this definition—including, for example, spinal neurons with axons ascending to the brain. In practice the term interneurons is nevertheless restricted to neurons with an axon ramifying in the vicinity of the cell body, thus synaptically coupling neurons within one nucleus.

2. It was formerly believed that propriospinal neurons—that is, spinal neurons with axons entering the white matter but not leaving the spinal cord—and interneurons represented two distinct cell groups. Recent studies have shown, however, that spinal interneurons have local (intrasegmental) branches as well as collaterals destined for other segments (intersegmental).

3. The *pedunculus cerebri*, strictly speaking, includes both the crus cerebri and parts of the mesencephalon dorsal to the crus except the colliculi (connectively termed the *tectum*). The region between the crus cerebri and the tectum is called the tegmentum and includes the periaqueductal gray, the red nucleus, and the substantia nigra. Previously, however, the crus cerebri and pedunculus cerebri were both applied to the ventralmost, fiber-rich part.

4. The name basal ganglia is unfortunate and has been retained from a time when all collections of neurons were called ganglia, regardless of whether they were located inside or outside the central nervous system. Today we use the term ganglion only for collections of neurons *outside* the central nervous system, as discussed in Chapter 1.

5. Between the septum pellucidum of the two sides there is a thin slit that has nothing to do with the ventricles. The slit was originally continuous with the room between the two hemispheres, but has been closed by the corpus callosum growing across the two hemispheres. Downward, the slit is closed by the fornices lying close together.

6. Approximately 70% of the CSF is produced by the choroid plexus while the rest is formed most likely by secretion from the ependyma. Early observations in experimental animals suggested that the choroid plexus cannot be solely responsible for CSF production. Thus, removal of the choroid plexus did not prevent the development of the hydrocephalus after the drainage of CSF was blocked.

7. In the capillary walls of most other organs, there are slits—as a result of less extensive tight junctions between the endothelial cells—where water can flow.

CHAPTER 4

DEVELOPMENT, AGING, AND PLASTICITY OF THE NERVOUS SYSTEM

The fully developed nervous system consists of incredibly complex networks of connections. There are billions of neurons in the human brain, and each one is probably, on average, connected with several thousand others. The number of possible combinations of synaptic contacts is therefore astronomic. Indeed, a section of nervous tissue stained to reveal all neuronal processes may appear as a chaotic jungle. Nevertheless, we have ample evidence that this is very far from the case: Strict order exists everywhere, and the mutual connections between neuronal groups are far from random. Improved methods have made it increasingly clear that precise order prevails even in parts of the nervous system formerly believed to possess only crude localization. Individual nuclei, formerly regarded as structural and functional units, have also been shown to consist of subdivisions differing as to connections and other characteristics. Even within the individual neuron, afferent axons from different sources may terminate on different parts of the dendritic tree. This leads to a number of questions. For example, how do the thousands of individual cell groups find their highly specific positions in the brain? How do the complicated and precisely organized networks arise during development of the individual? What roles do genetic and environmental factors play in the final structure and performance of the brain? Such questions are dealt with in this chapter. In addition, we will discuss the changes taking place in the *aging* brain and their consequences for function. *Plasticity* of the nervous system—that is, its ability to adapt structurally and functionally to altered demands—is mentioned several times below, particularly with reference to *restitution of function after damage to the central nervous system*, such as that caused by a stroke.

DEVELOPMENT OF THE NERVOUS SYSTEM

How neurons assemble into nuclei and how the nuclei are interconnected is largely *genetically determined*. The outer shape of the brain, the position of thousands of neuronal groups (nuclei), and the main neural connections are established prenatally: *our genes contain the "recipe" for the building of the nervous system in considerable detail.* Thus, for the most part, each individual neuron possesses the instructions that determine its final size, the shape of its dendritic tree, and the types of neurotransmitters it uses. This can be verified with neurons grown in culture. Nevertheless, the normal development of a neuron also depends on *influences from other cells in its vicinity* and *proper use of the neurons and their interconnections*. Thus, the development and mature performance of the nervous system depends on interactions of genetic and environmental factors. As mentioned above, the nervous system is *plastic*; that is, its structure and performance may change in response to altered external requirements. The fact that we can learn and memorize tells us that, in some way or another, the nervous system is modifiable. Considering the crucial role of synaptic transmission for all information processing in the brain, it seems *a priori* very likely that modifications take place at the synaptic level, as we will discuss in more detail below.

A Brief Survey of Phases in the Development of the Nervous System

Growth of certain parts of the cellular layer covering the dorsal aspect of the embryo initiates the development of the nervous system. Diffusible substances produced by the underlying tissue induce growth of the cells. This phase of *induction* is an example of how the cells and tissues interact during development. Then follows a more prolonged period where the primitive neurons and glial precursors divide mitotically. This is called the phase of *cell proliferation*. The number of divisions is genetically determined.

To get from the site of proliferation to their final position in the nervous system, the primitive neurons have to *migrate*. After reaching their final location, they start to aggregate into groups, representing the future nuclei. For most neurons *differentiation* starts with the outgrowth of processes after migration. By differentiation, we mean the development of structural and functional features that makes cells different from each other. Very early in differentiation the dendritic tree starts to develop. Fully grown, this pattern is often highly characteristic. While the neuronal processes are developing, the neuronal membranes undergo changes, and the neurotransmitters and other specific synaptic properties of the neurons begin to be expressed.

The next step in the development of the nervous system is the *outgrowth of axons* and *establishment of specific synaptic connections*. During this phase the axons must find their way and recognize the neurons with which they are going to establish synaptic contact. Several factors play a role in this process. Neurons can be equipped with specific recognition molecules, the target region can produce a diffusible substance that "attracts" the axons, and the time of birth of a neuron may determine the synaptic contacts to be established.

Many more neurons are formed during the proliferation phase than the number present in the mature nervous system. In fact, many neurons are eliminated at the time their axons are establishing synaptic contacts. This is called the *phase of selective cell death*, and has been observed in many parts of the nervous system. Usually, about half of the neurons are eliminated during this phase, although there are large regional differences.

The elimination of axon collaterals takes place in some systems at a later stage than selective cell death. This phenomenon, which perhaps may be compared with the pruning of a tree so that only the most viable branches remain, has been most intensively studied with regard to the innervation of skeletal muscles.

As already mentioned, *neuronal activity* is necessary for the proper development of axonal ramifications and for the formation of synapses. During this process, certain connections survive and possibly expand, whereas others are eliminated. There is evidence, however, that impulse activity is not enough for proper development in the central nervous system. The pattern of impulses has to be natural, which probably means that it must contain *meaningful information*, to be of consequence for synapse formation.

Most of the points mentioned in this brief survey are dealt with in more depth in the section that follows.

The Central Nervous System Develops as a Long Tube

A few days after fertilization of the egg, differentiation of the cells of the embryo to the main kinds of tissue has started. From being a round lump of cells, the embryo is transformed into an elongated disc after a week. The disc is covered on the upper or dorsal side and along the edges by primitive epithelium, the *ectoderm*, whereas the under or ventral side is covered by an epithelium—the *endoderm*—which later forms the intestinal tract and its glands. In the third week (after 18 days) the development of the nervous system starts with the formation of a thickening, the *neural plate*, in the prospective cranial end of the disc (Figs. 4.1 and 4.2). The thickening is due to growth of the ectodermal cells so that they form a tall, simple columnar *neuroepithelium*. Formation of the neural plate is induced by diffusible substances from the underlying mesodermal cells.

Figure 4.1 *The neural plate and closure of the neural groove.* Drawing of a 22-day-old human embryo, approximately 1 mm long. The central nervous system is shown in red. Based on Hamilton, Boyd, and Mossman (1972).

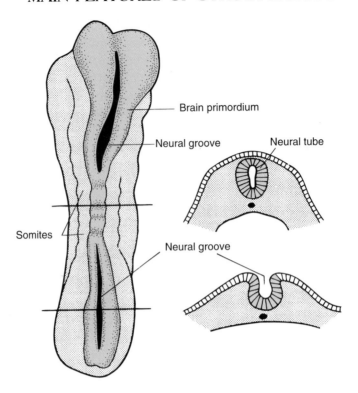

The differentiation of ectodermal cells to neuroepithelium proceeds in a cranial-to-caudal direction. A longitudinal infolding of the ectoderm occurs by the end of the third week (Figs. 4.1 and 4.2). This *neural groove* is subsequently closed in the fourth week; the closing starts in the mid-

Figure 4.2 *The formation of the neural tube and the neural crest.* Schematic cross sections through embryos at different stages of development. The formation of the neural tube is induced by substances diffusing from the underlying mesoderm (black). The neural crest gives origin to spinal ganglion cells and autonomic ganglion cells (and some other cell types). The figure shows how neural crest cells migrate into the body to form ganglia.

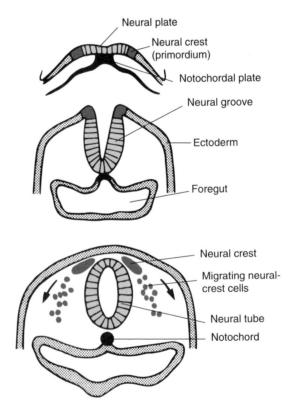

dle part and forms *the neural tube*. This is soon covered by the ectoderm
dorsally. The wall of the tube is formed by primitive neuroepithelial cells,
which proliferate enormously and develop into neurons and glial cells
(Fig. 4.6). The lateral edge of the neural plate forms a distinct cell group,
which later forms a longitudinal column on each side of the neural tube
called the *neural crest* (Fig. 4.2). The neural crest produces the neurons
of the peripheral nervous system, among them spinal ganglion cells and
autonomic ganglion cells. The neural crest also produces Schwann cells
and satellite cells (a kind of glia) in the ganglia.

The Neural Crest Produces More Than Neurons and Glia

Experiments with labeling of neural crest cells before they migrate (Fig. 4.2), show that some differentiate into non-nervous
structures. These include the *smooth muscles of the eye* (intrinsic eye muscles) and most likely *pia* and the *arachnoid* (the
dura mater is believed to originate from the mesoderm). The *dermis and subcutis of the face*, and the *cartilaginous skeleton of the visceral arches* also are formed by migrated neural crest cells. Finally, neural crest cells produce endocrine cells
of the *adrenal medulla*, *melanocytes* of the skin, and parts of the *septum* dividing the pulmonal artery and the aorta.

Early Development of the Cranial End of the Neural Tube

Whereas the caudal end of the neural tube—which develops into the spinal
cord—retains its simple tubular form, the expanded cranial end undergoes marked changes. This happens because different parts grow at different rates, and because the tube bends, forming *flexures* (Fig. 4.3). In
the fourth week three swellings or *primary vesicles* take shape (Figs. 4.3
and 4.4). The cavities inside the primary vesicles are continuous and develop into the ventricular system of the brain (Fig. 3.36). The most cranial vesicle is called *the prosencephalon* (forebrain), the middle one *the*

Figure 4.3 *Early stages of brain development*. To the **right**, a drawing of a
28-day-old human embryo, approximately 3.5 mm long. The **left** drawings
show the cranial part of the neural tube
(the brain primordium) isolated and
magnified compared with the drawing
of the embryo. The flexures of the
neural tube are shown by **arrows**. The
lower left is cut through (seen from the
dorsal aspect) to show the primary
vesicles and the ventricular space.
Based on Hamilton, Boyd, and Mossman (1972)

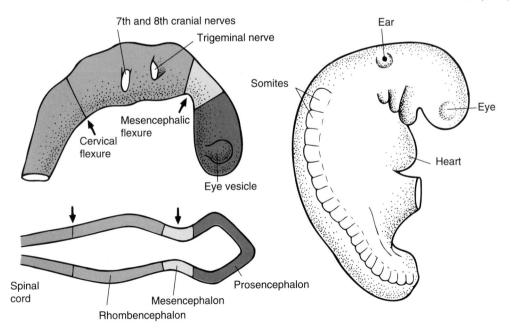

Figure 4.4 *The different divisions of the brain primordium.* Schematic drawing of the cranial part of the neural tube (straightened out and cut open horizontally). **A.** Approximately the same stage as in Figure 4.3; **B.** The same stage as in Figure 4.13A. Note the development of the hemispheres (the telencephalon) that gradually covers the diencephalon.

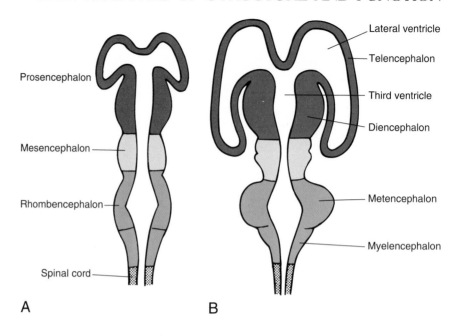

Figure 4.5 *Early development of the brain.* To the **left**, a drawing of a 36-day-old human embryo, approximately 11 mm long. To the **right**, the cranial part of the neural tube at the same stage. Based on Hamilton, Boyd, and Mossman (1972).

mesencephalon (the midbrain), and the caudal-most one *the rhombencephalon* (hindbrain). A ventrally directed bend—*the cervical flexure*—arises at the junction between the rhombencephalon and the spinal cord (Fig. 4.3). Later, a *mesencephalic flexure* arises between the rhombencephalon and the mesencephalon. A dorsally directed bend—*the pontine flexure*—later divides the rhombencephalon into two parts (Fig. 4.5).

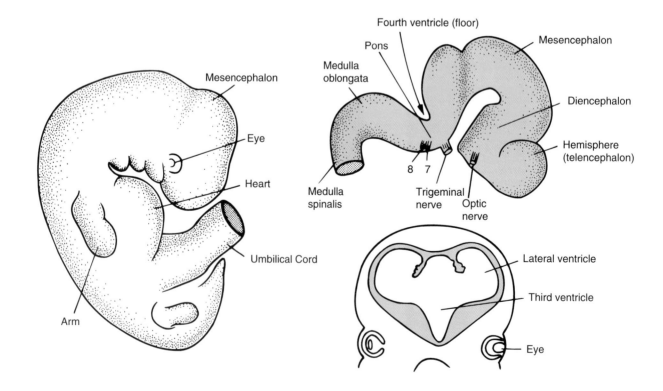

Early in the fourth week, the ventral aspect of the prospective brain exhibits shallow, transverse grooves. These are external signs of *segmentation* of the cranial end of the neural tube, and each segment is called a *neuromere*. The segmentation is most obvious in the rhombencephalon, and the term *rhombomere* is used in this region. Although their external signs disappear by the sixth week, the neuromeres are important because they represent the first segregation of neurons that later differentiate into the various nuclei of the brain stem. Thus, several cranial nerves and their nuclei are first laid down according to a segmental pattern—like the spinal nerves—although later development makes the cranial nerve pattern less regular.

The *mesencephalon* changes little during further development, in contrast to the two other primary vesicles. *The prosencephalon* develops into *the diencephalon* and *the cerebral hemispheres*, whereas *the rhombencephalon* differentiates into *the medulla oblongata, the pons*, and *the cerebellum* (Figs. 4.4 and 4.5). The rostral end of the prosencephalon produces two more vesicles (one on each side), called *the telencephalon*,

Neuromeres and Homeotic Genes

We mentioned above that the rostral part of the neural tube shows transient, external signs of segmentation (neuromeres). Although this phenomenon was observed in the nineteenth century, modern cell biological methods were necessary for closer study of their role in the development of the nervous system. Neuromeres are most convincingly shown in the rhombencephalon, where they are called *rhombomeres*. It is assumed that the mesencephalon consists of two neuromeres, whereas the prosencephalon probably consists of six. It is not known, however, whether the latter really correspond to those of the hindbrain, or whether they represent a later regionalization.

Each rhombomere represents a unit of neurons that do not mix with neurons of other rhombomeres during subsequent development. This specification takes place just when the rhombomere boundaries arise. It is believed that the rhombomeres arise when adjoining groups of neurons begin to express different surface markers. The neurons of one rhombomere are, among other things, specified regarding their future peripheral target (the neurons of the neural crest in the head region are also specified before they start to migrate peripherally). The motor trigeminal nucleus, for example, is formed in the rhombomeres r2 and r3, whereas the motor facial nucleus develops in r4 and r5. The motor and sensory cranial nerve axons already have a specified target when they start growing out from the neural tube (Fig. 4.8). Thus, when a rhombomere is transplanted to another place in the chicken embryonic brain, it develops as if it were still in its original place and not corresponding to its new location. Such specification must be caused by the switching on of certain genes—which start to express themselves by production of mRNA—while perhaps other genes are switched off. Recently, many genes have been identified that are expressed in a pattern corresponding to neuromeric boundaries. Most of these are genes controlling the expression of other genes during specific phases of development. Such *homeotic genes* (hox genes) all contain a piece of DNA (a so-called homeobox) that can bind to specific sites on other genes and thus regulate their expression. Homeotic genes not only control regional development of the nervous system but also act in pattern formation in other parts of the body (in mice about 30 homeotic genes have been identified). When a certain one is switched on, this probably initiates a cascade of changes in the expression of other genes. These provide various gene products that give the neuronal groups their identity, for example regarding location and connections.

Neuromeric borders—identified with genetic markers—are more reliable indicators of future borders between anatomically and functionally different areas than borders between brain vesicles. For example, the cerebellum—traditionally regarded as arising only from the metencephalon—is in addition formed by neurons in the adjoining part of the mesencephalon. The rostral border of neurons forming the cerebellum coincides with a border for the expression of a certain gene (engrailed 2).

Figure 4.6 *Differentiation of the neuroepithelium*. **Left**. Drawing of a section through the wall of the neural tube at an early stage (cf. Fig. 4.7A). **Right**. **Arrows** show how the neuroepithelial cells move while they differentiate into different cell types.

which later forms the cerebral cortex and basal ganglia (Figs. 4.4, 4.5, and 4.13). In addition, *the olfactory bulbs* (Figs. 3.12 and 10.2) are formed as evaginations from the ventral aspect of the telencephalon. The remaining caudal part of the prosencephalon forms *the diencephalon*, which includes the thalamus and hypothalamus. At an early stage (Fig. 4.3), cuplike evaginations—*the eye vesicles*—are formed from the prosencephalon (the part later to become the diencephalon). The eye vesicles develop into the *retina* and *the optic nerve*. The rhombencephalon develops two parts: *the myelencephalon* forming the medulla oblongata, and *the metencephalon* forming the pons and most of the cerebellum (the cerebellum also develops from the mesencephalon, as discussed below).

Early Phases in the Development of the Neuroepithelium

Initially, the wall of the neural tube consists of only one layer of cylindrical neuroepithelial cells (Figs. 4.1 and 4.2), bounded externally by basal membranes (the external limiting membrane, covered by the pia) and internally towards the cavity (by the internal limiting membrane). Intense *proliferation* of neuroepithelial cells soon leads to several layers of nuclei. The epithelium does not become truly stratified, however, since all cells retain a thin process reaching the internal limiting membrane (pseudostratified, Figs. 4.6 and 4.7). The outermost cells move towards the cavity of the neural tube (the future ventricles and central canal). The innermost layer—bordering the cavity—is called *the ventricular zone*. There the cells divide mitotically (Figs. 4.6 and 4.7). The future neurons—*the neuroblasts*—afterwards migrate outwards to form *the mantle zone* that

A   B

Figure 4.7 *Differentiation of the prosencephalic neuroepithelium to the cerebral cortex.* **A**. Photomicrograph of a cross section through the neural tube (prosencephalic part) at an early stage (chicken embryo, corresponding to early 4th week gestation in humans). Note mitotic activity in the ventricular zone.

B. Photomicrograph of a section through the telencephalon (rat) at a much later stage than in A, corresponding approximately to the 4th–5th month in human development. The ventricular zone is densely packed with neuroblasts that will migrate towards the cortical plate. In the further development the cortical plate develops into the adult six-layered cortex.

later becomes the gray matter. A layer without neurons—*the marginal zone*—is formed external to the mantle zone and becomes the white matter. The neurons of the mantle zone send axons into the marginal zone. These axons loop back to the mantle zone, however, to synapse on neurons there (these are the first association connections to arise). Other axons leave the neural tube as motor fibers growing peripherally to contact muscle cells and glands (Fig. 4.8). After neuroblast production ends, various types of glial cells are produced by mitosis of neuropepithelial cells that remain in the ventricular zone. The last to be produced are *the ependymal cells*. These retain their internal position and cover the ventricular face of the neural tube (Fig. 4.6). The cavity is filled with *cerebrospinal fluid* produced by tufts invaginated from the wall into the cavity. These tufts (the future choroid plexus) are covered by ependymal cells (Figs. 3.39, 3.40, and 4.13).

The simple layering of the neural tube, with the mantle zone (gray matter) inside and the marginal zone (white matter) outside, is retained with minor changes in the spinal cord (compare Figs. 3.4 and 4.9). In the cranial part of the neural tube (the future brain), however, major alterations in the mutual positions of gray and white matter occur. In the developing cerebellar and cerebral cortices, for example, neurons migrate from the mantle zone through the marginal zone and form a layered sheet of gray matter externally, just under the pia (Fig. 4.7).

Figure 4.8 *Outgrowth of cranial nerves from the rhombencephalon.* Photomicrograph of a horizontal section through a chicken embryo at about the same stage as in Figure 4.3. Thin bundles of axons leave the marginal zone and penetrate the connective tissue surrounding the brain primordium.

Ventricle

Ventricular zone

Mantle zone

Marginal zone

Cranial nerve (roots)

Further Development of the Spinal Cord and the Brain Stem

Figure 4.9 *Early development of the spinal cord.* **A**. Photomicrograph of a cross section of a chicken embryo (corresponding approximately to a 6-week human embryo, cf. Fig. 4.5). **B**. Drawing based on a photomicrograph of the human spinal cord at about 7 weeks gestation.

In the fourth week, the proliferation of neuroblasts in the mantle zone produces a large ventral thickening and a smaller dorsal one on each side of the neural tube. These thickenings are called *the basal plates* and *the alar plates*, respectively (Figs. 4.9, 4.10, and 4.11). The border between them is marked by a shallow furrow, *the sulcus limitans.* This remains visible in the lower part of the brain stem in the adult (Fig. 3.16), while it disappears early in the spinal cord. The basal plate contains neuroblasts that later become *motor neurons*, whereas many alar plate neuroblasts be-

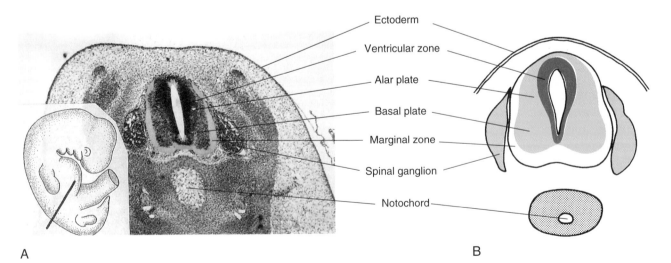

Ectoderm

Ventricular zone

Alar plate

Basal plate

Marginal zone

Spinal ganglion

Notochord

A   B

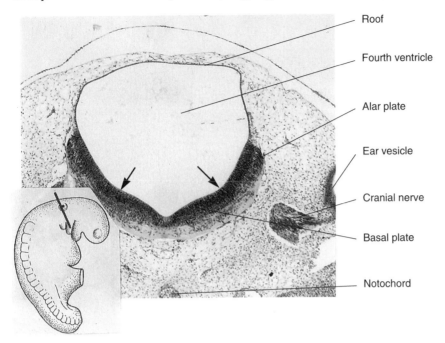

Roof

Fourth ventricle

Alar plate

Ear vesicle

Cranial nerve

Basal plate

Notochord

Figure 4.10 *The rhombencephalon.* Early stage of development, approximately as in Figure 4.3. Photomicrograph of a cross section of a chicken embryo (the inset shows a human embryo at a corresponding stage of development). Note the thin rhombencephalic roof attached to the edge of the alar plate.

come *sensory neurons*. This corresponds to the functional division between the ventral and dorsal horns of the cord. In the adult brain stem, *the sulcus limitans marks the border between the motor and the sensory cranial nerve nuclei* (Fig. 4.11). In the open part of the rhombencephalon—later to become parts of the medulla and the pons—the motor nuclei lie medially and the sensory nuclei laterally (Figs. 16.2 and 16.3). This is caused by lateral bending—away from each other—of the alar plates so that the roof of the rhombencephalon becomes only a thin membrane (Figs. 4.10 and 4.11). At a later stage, *the cerebellum* develops from the margins of the alar plates.

At an early stage, several neuronal groups in the brain stem move away from their "birthplace" in the alar or basal plates. In the *pons*, neuroblasts migrate from the alar plate in a ventral direction and form the pontine nuclei (Figs. 3.17 and 14.7). Similarly, in the medulla the *inferior olive* (another nucleus projecting to the cerebellum, Figs. 3.16 and 16.5) is formed by neuroblasts migrating ventrally from the alar plate. Another example is *motor cranial nerve nuclei* innervating visceral (branchial) arch muscles (Fig. 4.11). These neurons move in a ventral direction during early development after they have started to send out axons. The course of the root fibers in the brain stem therefore shows the path followed by the migrating neurons (Figs. 16.4B and 16.18).

Until the 8th–9th week the cord extends the full length of the spinal canal of the embryo. After that, however, the vertebral column and the coverings of the cord grow more rapidly than the spinal cord itself, producing a gradually increasing length difference (Fig. 4.12). This explains the *oblique course of the spinal nerves* in the vertebral canal before they leave through the intervertebral foramina. The lower end of the cord is at the level of the third lumbar vertebra at birth, in contrast to the first lumbar vertebra in adults. The dural sac, containing spinal nerve roots (the cauda equina), continues down to the second sacral vertebra (Fig. 3.3).

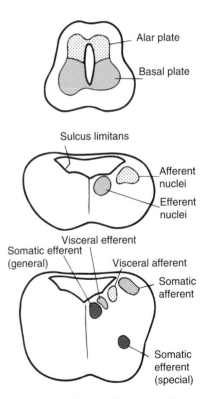

Alar plate

Basal plate

Sulcus limitans

Afferent nuclei

Efferent nuclei

Visceral efferent

Somatic efferent (general)

Visceral afferent

Somatic afferent

Somatic efferent (special)

Figure 4.11 *The development of the cranial nerve nuclei.* Schematic. Three stages are shown to explain the mutual positions of the nuclei. After their formation the special somatic efferent nuclei move ventrolaterally. See also Figures 16.2 and 16.3.

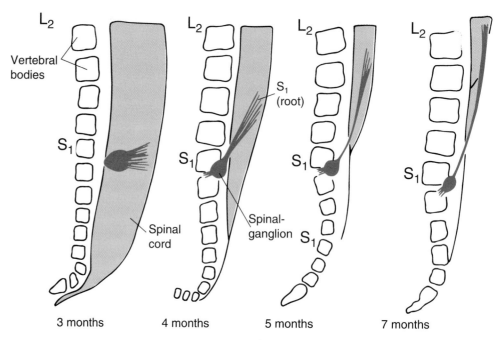

Figure 4.12 *The relationship between the lengths of the spinal cord and the vertebral column.* Based on Hamilton, Boyd, and Mossman (1972).

Cranial Nerves and Visceral Arches

The cranial nerves 5, 7, 9, and *10* (trigeminal, facial, glossopharyngeal, and vagal, Fig. 3.14) innervate structures developed from *visceral arches* (or branchial arches). In fish the two upper visceral arches are parts of the viscerocranium surrounding the oral cavity. They are not equipped with gills, in contrast to the lower (3–6) arches that are true respiratory organs. In mammals, none of the visceral arches have respiratory functions. Parts of them are used for new tasks, whereas other parts have regressed. There are no signs of gill development at any stage of human embryogenesis. The term *branchial arch* (from Greek *brankhion* = gill) is therefore not quite appropriate.

A *visceral arch* consists of a skeletal part (cartilage, later replaced by bone in some arches), muscles, skin, mucous membranes, and a nerve of its own. As mentioned, the skeletal part is formed by neural crest cells. In human embryos some visceral arches appear as ventral bulges in the head and cervical region (Figs. 4.3 and 4.5). The *first visceral arch*—producing the upper and lower jaw with attached masticatory muscles, and the hammer and the anvil of the middle ear—is innervated by the *fifth cranial nerve* (the trigeminal). The *second visceral arch*—forming, among other things, the upper part of the hyoid bone, the stirrup of the middle ear, and the facial muscles—is innervated by the *seventh cranial nerve* (the facial). The *third visceral arch*—forming most of the hyoid bone and the posterior part of the tongue—is innervated by the *ninth cranial nerve* (the glossopharyngeal). The *fourth, fifth,* and *sixth visceral arches* form the cartilaginous skeleton of the larynx and the muscles of the larynx and the pharynx. These structures are innervated for the most part by the *tenth cranial nerve* (the vagus).

The cranial nerves 3, 4, 6, and *12* (the oculomotor, trochlear, abducens, and hypoglossal, Fig. 3.14) innervate structures that most likely develope from segmentally arranged somites (somites are paired cubical masses giving rise to muscles, the axial skeleton, and the dermis of the skin) . These nerves are homologous to spinal ventral roots. As for the *eleventh cranial nerve* (the accessory), it is not settled whether the two muscles it innervates (the sternocleidomastoid and trapezius) develop from somites or from visceral arches. The latter hypothesis is supported by the fact that the accessory nerve root fibers, coming from the upper cervical segments, exit the cord more dorsally than the spinal ventral roots (corresponding to the level where visceral arch nerves leave the brain stem; Figs. 16.1 and 16.7).

Further Development of the Diencephalon

The diencephalon represents the caudal part of the original prosencephalic vesicle (Figs. 4.4 and 4.5). The *lateral wall* in this part becomes thicker at an early stage and develops into the *thalamus*. The *floor plate* forms the *hypothalamus* and the *pituitary* (Figs. 3.22, 3.23 and 18.1). The latter are formed as an evagination of the floor plate. The furrow (sulcus hypothalamicus, Fig. 3.22) marking the border between the thalamus and the hypothalamus might be a continuation of the sulcus limitans (Fig. 4.11). The thin *roof plate* of the diencephalon forms by invagination the *choroid plexus of the third ventricle* (Fig. 3.37). Furthermore, the roof plate produces the *pineal body* by evagination (Figs. 3.22 and 3.30). The *eye vesicle* occurs at an earlier stage (before the further differentiation of the prosencephalon, Fig. 4.3) but retains connection with the diencephalon by the future optic nerve (Fig. 4.5).

Further Development of the Telencephalon

In the fifth week, development of the cerebral hemispheres starts in one vesicle on each side of the prosencephalon (Figs. 4.4 and 4.5). These are called the *telencephalic (cerebral) vesicles*. Their cavities form the lateral ventricles, which initially have wide openings to the third ventricle (interventricular foramen, Fig. 4.13). The mantle zone of the basal part of the telencephalic vesicle thickens rapidly to form the *corpus striatum* of the basal ganglia (Fig. 4.13A). The thinner overlying part, called the *pallium*, becomes the cerebral cortex. The pallium grows dorsally, rostrally, and caudally in relation to the diencephalon (Fig. 4.4). The caudal and ventral parts of the hemispheres later fuse with the diencephalon (Fig. 4.13B).

The *basal ganglia* primordium is later divided into two parts—the *lateral and medial corpus striatum*—by descending axons from the cerebral cortex. These descending axons form the *internal capsule* (Fig. 4.13B). As development proceeds, the caudate nucleus and the thalamus come to lie medial to the internal capsule whereas the lentiform nucleus (the putamen and the globus pallidus) lies laterally (Figs. 3.26 and 13.1).

In the medial wall of the pallium, just above the attachment of the choroid plexus, a thickening arises that bulges into the lateral ventricle (Fig. 4.13A). This is the beginning of the *hippocampus*, which is separated from the rest of the pallium by the *hippocampal sulcus*. As the hemispheres grow, their shape changes so that the temporal lobe comes to lie ventrally (Fig. 3.38). This produces the characteristic curved shape of the lateral ventricles and the structures in their wall, such as the hippocampus and the caudate nucleus (see also Figs. 3.30 and 19.2). The hippocampus thus moves from the position in Figure 4.13A to that in Figure 4.13B.

The *choroid plexus* of the lateral ventricles is formed by invagination of the thin part of the pallium (together with the pia) close to the dorsal aspect of the diencephalon (Figs. 3.39 and 4.13B).

Development of the Cerebral Cortex

At first, the telencephalic vesicle consists of only one layer of neuroepithelial cells. These proliferate, however, producing rapid growth of the

Figure 4.13 *Development of the telencephalon.* **A**. Early stage, in which the telencephalon is still separated from the diencephalon. Descending fibers have started their growth from the pallium (primordium of the cerebral cortex) to the brain stem and the spinal cord. **B**. The telencephalon is now attached to the diencephalon laterally. The medial and lateral striatum have been separated by the internal capsule. Note also that the hippocampus has changed its position, due to the growth of the hemispheres (cf. Fig. 3.38). Based on Hamilton, Boyd, and Mossman (1972).

prospective cerebral hemisphere (Fig. 4.7). At a later stage we can differentiate a ventricular zone, mantle zone, and marginal zone, just as in other parts of the neural tube. At the beginning of the 8th week, neuroblasts from the mantle zone migrate into the marginal zone and start establishing the cerebral cortex. The differentiation from the *cortical plate* (Fig. 4.7B) to the six-layered cortex (Figs. 20.1 and 20.2) is not finished until birth, and is accomplished by waves of cells migrating toward the cortical surface. The deepest cortical layers are established first; thus, neurons destined for superficial layers have to pass through the deep layers. Neuroepithelial cells in the ventricular zone that have ceased dividing are termed *postmitotic*. The migration of postmitotic neurons toward the cortex is guided by *radially oriented glial cells*, with processes extending from the ependyma to the pia (Fig. 4.6). When postmitotic neurons start migrating toward their final destination in the cortex, their future cell type is probably already specified. The exact time a neuron becomes postmitotic—its date of birth—appears to decide which *cortical layer* it will join. It is not quite clear, however, how far the specification goes regarding the

Myelination

Myelination of axons starts in the fourth month of gestation and is completed 2–3 years after birth. Although many axons in the central nervous system remain unmyelinated, the process of myelination is clearly related to functional maturation of neuronal interconnections. Full functional capacity cannot be expected before myelination is completed. As for the individual neuron, myelination starts at the soma and proceeds distally. Different tracts are myelinated at different times. Overall, *tracts concerned with basic tasks, necessary for life, are the first to be myelinated* (such as sucking, swallowing, retraction from harmful stimuli, emptying of bowel and bladder, and so forth). Such connections are also phylogenetically the oldest.

In the *spinal cord*, myelination starts in the cervical region and proceeds in the caudal direction. First to be myelinated are the *propriospinal fibers* (interconnecting various spinal segments). *Ventral root* motor fibers are myelinated earlier than the *dorsal root* sensory fibers. Myelination of *ascending spinal tracts* starts in the 6th fetal month, and tracts descending from the brain stem follow shortly after (reticulospinal and vestibulospinal tracts). These tracts need to be functioning at birth. In contrast, the *pyramidal tract*—controlling the most precise voluntary movements—is fully myelinated about 2 years after birth. Connections from the cerebral cortex to the cerebellum (Fig. 14.7) are myelinated at the same time as the pyramidal tract, which seems logical since these connections are important for coordination of voluntary movements.

Myelination of the *cranial nerves* starts in the 6th fetal month, except for the optic nerve (which is a central tract and not a peripheral nerve). Myelination starts shortly before birth in the optic nerve.

In the *cerebral cortex* myelination begins shortly before birth, first in motor and sensory areas. The association areas are mainly myelinated during the first 4 months after birth, although myelination continues for some time after that period. The last regions to become fully meylinated are the association areas in the frontal lobe (prefrontal cortex).

Malformations of the Nervous System

Malformations of the nervous system—as in other organs of the body—may be caused by genes or environmental factors (or by both). External agents, such as viruses and drugs, are most likely to cause serious malformations or maldevelopment if they act in the period of maximal differentiation—that is, from the 3rd to 8th week of gestation (most organs are formed during the embryonic period from 4th to 8th week). Harmful influences before this stage usually lead to early death of the embryo.

Among the most common malformations is *defective closure of the neural tube*, which may be caused by various genetic and environmental factors. Normally, the closure is completed by the end of the 4th week. Lack of closure may affect the whole length of the neural tube but is most often restricted to either the cranial or the caudal end. When the neural tube does not develop normally, neither do overlying structures such as the skull, parts of the vertebral column, and the skin. Their normal development depends on induction by diffusible substances from the nervous tissue. With defective closure of the cranial end, the brain does not develop and the remainder of the neural plate degenerates. This condition is termed *anencephaly*. Such fetuses may sometimes live until birth but always die shortly after. A defective closure of the spinal cord (most often in the lumbosacral part), is termed *spina bifida* because the vertebral arch and soft tissue dorsal to the cord do not develop normally. This condition may vary in severity. In the most serious cases the vertebral arches, muscles, and skin are absent and there is herniation of the coverings of the cord containing degenerated nervous tissue (meningomyelocele). Less severe cases may involve herniation of the coverings but intact spinal cord, whereas the least affected have only partial lack of the vertebral arch (spina bifida occulta). In the more serious cases the cord does not develop normally, leading to pareses and sensory disturbances of the legs. When the nervous supply is deficient, the muscles do not develop to their normal size and strength.

Reduced drainage of the cerebrospinal fluid caused by, for example, abnormal narrowing or obliteration of the cerebral aqueduct (Fig. 3.37) leads to *hydrocephalus*. If untreated, this will cause death or seriously impair brain development.

Disturbances in periods with neuronal migration may cause defective development, for example of the cerebral cortex, and are sometimes the cause of mental retardation, epilepsy, and other symptoms in infants and children.

cortical area in which the cell is to end. The mature cytoarchitectonic characteristics of an area appear to be influenced mainly by its thalamic afferents: if a piece of visual cortex is transplanted to the somatosensory cortex, the transplanted tissue acquires the cytoarchitectonic features typical of the somatosensory cortex.

How Are Specific Neuronal Connections Established?

We know several mechanisms that can aid axons in selecting their target, but we cannot fully explain the amazing connectional specificity observed in the mature nervous system. Progress is rapid in this field, however, due to the use of techniques for identifying specific markers and growth-promoting molecules, and for making genetic manipulations that alter the establishment of connections. Video recording of growing axons (after labeling with fluorescent substances) affords unique opportunities for direct observations of development.

Trial and error are unimportant for the establishment of specific connections. True enough, the distribution of axonal branches is often more diffuse initially than after maturation, but this is so only within a well-defined target region. Indeed, the growth is often surprisingly goal-directed, with few or no aberrations. Knowing the complexity of the mature nervous system, one might think that most of the human genome has to be devoted to specification of neuronal connections. This, of course, is not the case. We should bear in mind that the whole embryo is only a few millimeters to a couple of centimeters during the stages of most intense axonal outgrowths. Thus, the distances that axons have to grow to reach their targets are usually very short. Furthermore, the topography of the nervous system at these early stages is also much simpler than later, since not all nuclear groups develop simultaneously. Our present knowledge strongly suggests that *combined actions of several different mechanisms— each of them simple—can explain how the specificity of the nervous system arises.*

Genetically programmed time of neuronal birth and axonal outgrowth can explain the development of specific connections in many cases (Fig. 4.14). If, at the time of axonal outgrowth from one neuronal group, only certain neurons are present in the direction of axonal growth, the axons will hit their correct target without specific recognition molecules. In addition, programming of neurons for maximal synapse formation during a limited period ensures that synapses are established upon arrival of the proper axons. The period during which neurons readily produce synapses is usually time-limited. Axons encountering a particular neuronal group at a later stage cannot establish synapses and therefore either retract or grow past to other targets.

Timing of neuronal birth and maturation cannot explain all aspects of specificity, however. For example, what decides the *direction of axonal outgrowths*? For some neurons, such as pyramidal cells in the cerebral cortex (Fig. 1.1), the initial growth direction is genetically determined. After that, however, the direction must be determined by signals in the environment of the axons. Thus, cortical pyramidal cells are occasionally

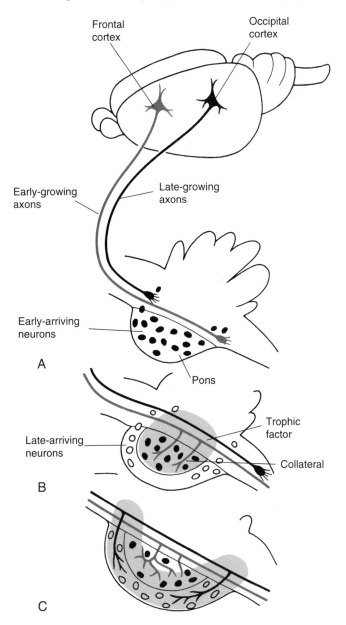

Frontal
cortex

Occipital
cortex

Early-growing
axons

Late-growing
axons

Early-arriving
neurons

A

Pons

Late-arriving
neurons

Trophic
factor

Collateral

B

C

Figure 4.14 *Development of topo-graphically organized connections.* Example from the corticopontine projection (cf. Fig. 14. 7). **A.** Because the axons from the frontal lobe start growing earlier than axons from the occipital lobe, they have reached further down in the brain stem. At this stage neurons migrate into the ventral pons to form the pontine nuclei. **B.** At a later stage the early-arriving pontine neurons produce a trophic substance that attracts collaterals from the descending axons. However, only the axons from the frontal lobe are sufficiently mature to emit collaterals at this stage (two days elapse from the axons arrive in the pons until they can form collaterals). Immature neurons continue to invade the ventral pons and form a shell around the early-arriving neurons. **C.** Late-arriving pontine neurons are now sufficiently mature to produce the trophic factor, whereas the early-arriving ones have stopped their production. At this later stage only the axons from the occipital lobe can emit collaterals. Thus, axons from different parts of the cerebral cortex end in different parts of the pontine nuclei, forming the orderly topographic arrangement seen in the adult (see Fig. 14.8). In this example, the topographic arrangement can be explained by genetically programmed differences in the time of birth for neurons in various parts of the cerebral cortex and the pontine nuclei. Other mechanisms may operate as well. Based on experimental studies in the rat by Leergaard, Lakke, and Bjaalie (1995).

"inverted" with their apical dendrite pointing toward the white matter instead of towards the cortical surface. In such cases, the axons start growing toward the pial surface but soon turn around and grow towards the white matter, as do normal pyramidal cells (Fig. 20.5). In other instances the target organ produces growth promoting substances—*chemotrophic factors*—that diffuse in the tissue. Axons then grow in the direction of increasing concentration of the chemotrophic factor. This factor binds to specific receptors, so that only axons expressing the receptor are influenced. This may explain why some experiments show that axons from a neuronal group grow toward their correct target even if this neuronal group has been transplanted to a new place before axonal outgrowth.

In other instances specific molecules are apparently expressed by neurons or glia along the route—functioning as "*signposts.*" When the first axons—*the pioneers*—have reached their target, the rest of the axons can get there simply by following the pioneers. (The pioneers may have a relatively simple job because, as mentioned above, the distances they grow are very short and the "landscape" is simple.) Axons with a common target can express at their surface *neuronal cell adhesion molecules* (N-CAMs) that make them sticky. Those axons expressing a particular kind of N-CAM are then kept together whereas others are repelled or inhibited in their growth. In this way axons with common targets form bundles or *fascicles*, and the phenomenon is termed *fasciculation*. The well-defined tracts of the nervous system arise in this way.

Examples of Axonal Growth Guided by Chemotrophic Gradients and Local Cues

One example, inverted pyramidal cells, was mentioned above. Another example concerns the development of descending connections from the cerebral cortex, that is, the outgrowth of axons from cortical projection neurons. Many such axons reach the spinal cord and in addition emit collaterals to nuclei in the brain stem. Initially, the axons grow towards the cord without sending out collaterals. After a certain interval or waiting time, however, collaterals grow out and innervate the pontine nuclei (Figs. 4.14 and 4.13). The collaterals to the pontine nuclei arise just when the pontine neurons have reached a certain stage of maturation (postmitotic age). Most likely, the pontine neurons at this stage produce a chemotrophic factor which "attracts" growing axons. Such a mechanism, depending upon diffusion, can only operate over short distances. Thus, it is less likely that chemotrophic factors produced in the spinal cord are responsible for the goal-directed growth of corticospinal axons.

When the distance to the target is too long for chemotrophic factors alone to guide axonal growth, we assume that there are *local cues* (specific molecules) along the route. One example illustrating the importance of such local clues is the *growth of axons from the retina through the optic chiasm*. Figure 8.14 shows how the axons from various parts of the retina are arranged as they pass through the optic chiasm in the adult. Axons from the nasal retina cross to the other side, whereas axons from the temporal retina pass ipsilaterally, that is, without crossing. In the adult crossing and ipsilateral axons are segregated as they approach the optic chiasm. During the first outgrowth, however, axons from the nasal and temporal parts of the retina are mixed. Nevertheless, they take the correct path when they reach the region of the chiasm, even when this requires that some have to bend 90° and that axons have to cross each other. Interaction between axons from the two eyes is not necessary either. Thus, if one eye primordia is removed before the axons have reached the optic chiasm, the axons from the remaining eye still find their correct way through. Neither can chemotrophic factors from the target organ of the axons (a thalamic nucleus) play a decisive role because this nucleus is not yet established at the time the axons grow through the optic chiasm. Therefore, *local clues in the region of the optic chiasm must guide the axons—at least during the first pioneering phase*. The nature of these clues has not yet been established. In the next few weeks—when thousands of axons follow the pioneers through the chiasm—cell adhesion molecules and fasciculation are important. It should be taken into consideration that the environment in the region of the chiasm is quite different at the time the first pioneer axons arrive than later. The pioneers presumably meet primitive glial cells and neuroepithelial cells belonging to the diencephalic floor plate, while at a later stage they encounter only more mature glial cells and other axons of their own kind.

Another example of the importance of local cues for axonal pathfinding is the *development of skeletal muscle nerve supply by spinal motoneurons*. Even after removal of the primordial muscle, the axons that would normally supply it still find their way to the site of the (removed) muscle.

Establishment of Topographic Maps

When axons arrive at their target nucleus, they usually do not establish synapses at random among the neurons but rather in a specific part of the nucleus. Thus, the incoming axons together form a *topographic map* so that, for example, different body parts (Figs. 7.14 and 7.22) or parts of the visual field (Fig. 8.19) are represented by spatially separate neurons. Most connections exhibit some degree of topographic organization; this is not restricted to systems conveying sensory information and motor commands. Some topographic maps are simple, while others may appear highly complex. How such topographic relationships develop is not fully understood, but genetic programing of neuronal time of birth is one important mechanism. (Time of birth also decides the scheduling of axonal outgrowth and the ability to form and receive synapses, as discussed above.) Figure 4.14 illustrates how topographic maps in the pontine nuclei may arise. In the adult, axons from the cerebral cortex end in a precise topographic pattern in the pontine nuclei. Functionally different parts of the cerebral cortex connect with different parts of the nuclei (Fig. 14.8). This pattern appears to arise because axons from different parts of the cortex start growing at different times, and because subgroups of pontine neurons are born at different times.

Although the basic pattern of topography is genetically determined, proper use of the system is necessary to obtain maximal precision of spatial arrangements. This concerns, for example, maps of the visual field and of the body surface in primary sensory regions of the cerebral cortex. We return to this below when considering the effects of the environment on development of the nervous system.

Growth Cones and Their Interactions with N-CAMs and Other Molecules

Much remains to be learned about the exact roles during development of the many chemotrophic factors, molecules functioning as signposts, recognition molecules, and N-CAMs. In the establishment of specific connections, most of the relevant molecules act on the axonal *growth cone*. The growth cone is an expanded part of the tip of a growing axon (Fig. 4.14). It continuously sends out small extensions or *filopodia*, as if exploring its immediate surroundings. Filopodia encountering the proper molecules in the tissue are stabilized and this decides the direction of further growth, while other filopodia retract. The stabilization is related to an increased number of *actin* molecules in the filopodia and of *microtubules* in the axon. Several nerve cell adhesion molecules influence the growth of the axon when they are present near the growth cone. These N-CAM molecules can be expressed at the surface of both the growth cone and the nearby cells. Binding of the N-CAM molecules to each other causes stickiness. In other instances, N-CAMs bind to specific receptors in the growth cone membrane and thus activate intracellular second messengers (by influx of Ca^{2+} ions). N-CAMS are proteins related to the immunoglobulins. There are also *extracellular* molecules with actions on the growth cone, such as *laminin*, which is bound to the basal lamina. Laminin binds to receptors in the growth cone membrane. At some places laminin is expressed transiently along the path of growing axons in the periphery, guiding the growth toward the target organ. Although the action of laminin is not by itself specific, its time-specific expression ensures that only axons present at the proper time will grow. This is another example of the importance of timing—in this case of axonal outgrowth—during development.

Further Elaboration and Refinement of Neuronal Connections

As mentioned, the terminal area of a group of axons is often more extensive initially than after maturation. Thus, many collaterals are eliminated during further development. Sometimes this is caused simply by the death of many neurons during certain phases of development (we return to this phenomenon below). Here we are concerned with the *elimination of some axonal branches*, which may be likened to the *pruning* of a tree. Usually, such elimination may be expected to *increase the spatial precision of connections*. In other instances, neurons initially send axon collaterals to two (or more) distant nuclei but only one collateral survives while the other(s) disappears during further development. This is exemplified by the development of *descending connections from the visual cortex*. Initially, the axons grow down to the spinal cord, sending off collaterals to the pontine nuclei (among other areas) on their way (Fig. 4.14). After the pontine collaterals are established, those to the cord are eliminated (in adult animals there are no connections from the visual cortex to the cord). We do not know how this happens; perhaps chemotrophic factors from the cord or medulla "trick" the axons to grow beyond their real targets. We may furthermore assume that once in the cord, the axons are not able to establish synapses—perhaps due to lack of specific recognition molecules or simply because the spinal neurons are not receptive then. A similar example concerns *descending axons from the forelimb region of the motor cortex* (of rodents). Initially, such axons reach both the cervical and the lumbar parts of the cord (innervating the forelimb and the hindlimb, respectively). Collaterals enter the spinal gray matter only in the cervical region, however, and the branch to the lumbar cord disappears without having established synapses.

Another example concerns development of the *spinal network controlling locomotion*. This network is laid down long before such movement is of any use. In human fetuses, rhythmic movements of the extremities (although incoordinate) have been observed as early as 10 weeks after fertilization. At first, the spinal network initiates movements without any sensory information or commands from higher levels of the central nervous system. Gradually the coordination improves to complete locomotor patterns, and this continues after birth. This improvement is probably due to several factors: altered electric properties of the neurons, expression of novel transmitters and receptors, and development of the connections among the network neurons. These alterations depend on the development of descending connections from the brain stem (especially such that contain serotonin might be important). Maturation of the locomotor function starts with the forelimb and proceeds caudally to the hindlimb, in parallel with the growth of descending axons.

Programed Cell Death and Competition among Neurons for Trophic Factors

As already mentioned, many more neurons are formed during the proliferation phase than are found in the mature nervous system. Cell death usually coincides in time with the period during which the neurons establish synaptic contacts. For the most intensively studied neuronal groups—such as spinal motoneurons and retinal ganglion cells—the amount of elimination depends on target size. If the target (for example, striated muscle cells) is experimentally expanded, more motoneurons survive; whereas reducing the target size increases elimination. This can be explained by the neurons needing a sufficient supply of a growth-promoting substance (trophic factor) to survive. This trophic factor is produced by the target cells in a limited amount; that is, there is not enough to keep *all* neurons alive. The neurons innervating the target *compete* for the trophic factor and only the winners survive. Since only a limited number of synapses can be formed on each neuron, the axons arriving first have an advantage. The trophic factor is taken up at the synaptic sites by the axonal boutons and transported retrogradely to the cell body.

The elimination of surplus neurons appears to take place rapidly—perhaps during a few days in some systems. Overall, this kind of cell death is believed to *ensure optimal numerical relationships between, for example, motoneurons and muscle cells*. It may also serve to *eliminate incorrect synaptic connections*.

Programmed cell death is not uniform throughout the nervous system. In the primordial cerebral cortex probably about 90% of the neurons die, whereas few spinal interneurons die. About 50% of motoneurons die, and a similar rate has been found in a type of retinal interneurons (amacrine cells). We do not know the reasons for such differences. The number of cells that die is not *always* related to the size of the target. Thus, many open questions remain concerning the phenomenon of programed cell death.

Apoptosis and Genetic Death Program

Cell death as a normal developmental process is termed *apoptosis* (in contrast to *necrosis*, which means cell death caused by abnormal, nonphysi-

Nerve Growth Factors

A substance that stimulates axonal growth in the peripheral nervous system was discovered around 1950 by the Italian Nobel Prize winner Rita Levi-Montalcini. This substance—nerve growth factor (NGF)—is a protein produced by the cells of the target organ. Antibodies against NGF inhibit the growth of axons from autonomic ganglion cells and sensory cells derived from the neural crest. In cell cultures, axons grow into an area containing NGF and retract from areas without it. NGF binds to specific membrane receptors and is transported retrogradely to the cell body, inducing structural and functional alterations there.

The discovery of NGF raised expectations of finding many more specific neuronal growth factors. Four substances that are closely related to NGF have been identified; with NGF, they form the *neurotrophin family*. These are *brain-derived neurotrophic factor (BDNF)*—which probably plays a role similar to that of NGF in certain types of central neurons—and *neurotrophin NT-3, NT-4*, and *NT-5*. In addition, other growth factors act also on cell types outside the CNS. Among these are several *fibroblast growth factors (FGFs)*, which increase survival of several kinds of neurons.

It has become evident—after the first surge of enthusiasm—that the growth factors are less specific than researchers believed initially. Their actions are not restricted to specific neuronal populations, and each kind of neuron is influenced by several growth factors. They not only act by retrograde transport but can be transported anterogradely and also secreted from glial cells to act locally.

Nerve growth factors are now being intensely investigated concerning *possible beneficial effects after brain damage*. Thus, administration of growth factors at the site of injured neurons might help them survive. In animal experiments injection of NGF into the ventricular system prevented delayed cell death in the hippocampus after a period without blood supply. The role of growth factors in *degenerative diseases* of the nervous system has also attracted interest. One theory proposes that the senile plaques in the brain of Alzheimer patients down-regulate fibroblast growth factor (FGF) in their environment, thus causing neuronal death. In Parkinson's disease and Huntington's disease (Chapter 13) as well, the level of FGF is apparently reduced. The connection—if any—between such changes and the disease process is not known, however.

Prolonged *stress* can cause neuronal death in experimental animals. This may be mediated by decreased production of growth factors (BDNF in particular). Alterations of growth factors have also been observed in patients with severe depression, and both antidepressive drugs and electroconvulsive therapy have been reported to increase expression of BDNF (among other effects).

ological influences). Apoptosis is characterized by the breakdown of DNA to smaller fragments and the subsequent dissolution of the cell. What triggers this process? When autonomic ganglion cells die without nerve growth factor (NGF), does it happen because the cell needs NGF for vital metabolic processes or because NGF inactivates genes that trigger apoptosis? There is much evidence in favor of the latter explanation, that is, the existence of a *genetic death program* in each cell. Thus, genes necessary for apoptosis have been identified in invertebrates: Mutation of certain genes prevents apoptosis that would have occurred at a certain stage of development. The evidence is less direct in vertebrates, but apoptosis due to lack of NGF can be prevented by inhibiting synthesis of mRNA or proteins. This strongly suggests that gene expression is necessary for apoptosis.

The Role Played by the Environment in Development of the Nervous System

We have so far considered developmental events governed largely or only by genetic factors. The main morphologic features of the nervous system—such as its macroscopic form and the positions of major nuclei and tracts—are established well before birth. In a sense this represents the *hard wiring* of the brain. We know, however, that nervous development is far from finished by birth. The weight of the human brain triples during the first year of life (from 300 to 900 grams). After that the weight increases more slowly to reach almost adult values around the age of ten (1400 grams for men and 1250 for women). We know that this weight gain is not caused by the production of new neurons but rather by the growth of existing neurons, the myelination of axons, and the proliferation of glial cells. The growth mainly involves expansion of the dendritic trees and formation of axon collaterals with boutons. The spreading of dendritic arbors is especially marked in the human cerebral cortex during the first two years of life (Fig. 4.15). There is good evidence that increased dendritic ramifications relate to an increased number of synapses. Myelination of cortico-cortical connections takes place during the same period, and is a sign of functional maturation. Increased conduction velocity would be expected to enhance both the precision and the capacity of the neural networks; that is, their potential for information processing increases.

How much of the postnatal growth of the nervous system—in particular the establishment of billions of new synapses—depends on interaction of the brain with the environment? Though we have no final answer to this question, it is clear that the brain's postnatal growth is largely genetically determined. Yet, the final functional status of the various neural systems and networks depends in large measure on their proper use during a certain period. For example, about one third of all synapses in the cerebral cortex may depend on proper use of the functional system in which they participate. While activity is necessary for the normal development of the nervous system, this does not concern the establishment of connections from one cell group to another, but rather the final number of synapses, their precise distribution, and postsynaptic effects.

Striate area

Parietal association cortex

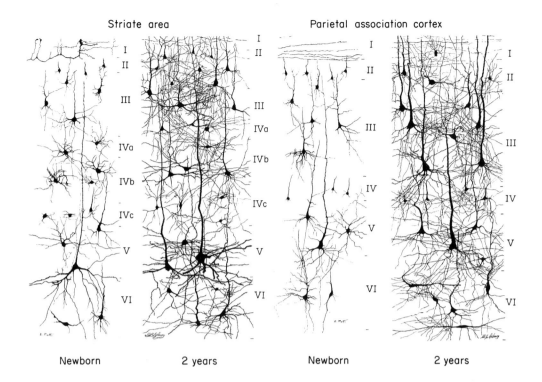

Newborn   2 years   Newborn   2 years

Examples of Environmental Influences on Brain Development

Wild animals have larger brains than tame animals of the same species. The responsible influence must occur quite early, because animals born in the wild and later tamed have the same brain size as wild animals. The difference is not genetic, however, since individuals of the first generation born in captivity have smaller brains than their wild relatives. It is plausible that this phenomenon is related to differences in the amount of *learning*: life in the wild requires a much broader repertoire of adaptive behaviors than life in the cage or the bin. Experiments point in the same direction: dendritic arborizations were found to be more extensive in the cerebral cortex of rats raised in a simulated natural environment with ample space and access to toys than in rats raised in standard laboratory cages.

Another example concerns the *development of connections from the retina to the visual cortex*. At first, neurons in the visual cortex are influenced with equal strength from each eye. Soon after birth, however, neurons in the cortex segregate into groups with a dominant input from one eye and a weaker input from the other. This phenomenon is called *eye dominance*. When all impulse traffic from the retina is blocked in kittens, eye dominance does not develop—that is, each neuron continues to respond equally well to signals from either eye. Artificial electric stimulation of the optic nerve can nevertheless induce eye dominance even though the animal is blind, but only if the signals from the two eyes arrive with a minute time difference (corresponding to what occurs under natural conditions with light falling on the two retinas). With natural use of the system during development, axon terminals conveying signals from the two eyes *compete* for the available synaptic sites on each neuron.

Figure 4.15 *Development of the human cerebral cortex postnatally.* Drawings based on Golgi sections from the visual cortex showing the increase in dendritic arborizations from birth and until the age of 2 years. The increase in dendritic arborization is most likely related to the increase in the number of synapses per neuron. From Conel (1939).

That nerve impulses are not by themselves sufficient for normal development is also supported by the following experiment. In *goldfish exposed only to diffuse light* (devoid of information) at the time retinal axons form synapses in the optic tectum, the normal ordered map of the visual environment is not formed. Both of these examples from the visual system show that *in order to induce the normal synaptic pattern and connectivity, nerve impulses must convey meaningful information—that is, information that helps the animal to adapt to its environment.*

The previous examples of brain size in wild and tame animals, and of environmental effects on dendritic arborizations, strongly suggest that formation of new synapses is closely linked with *learning*. Results from experiments on the motor system support this conclusion: Among young adult rats doing different motor tasks, some developed more synapses per neuron in the cerebellar cortex than others. The decisive factor was not the amount of motor activity, but whether the activity implied learning of new motor behaviors. Other experiments show that learning of specific skills can be accompanied by synaptic changes in cortical areas involved in the task. For example, as monkeys gradually improved their performance in distinguishing tones of different frequencies, the part of the auditory cortex representing the particular frequencies increased in size.

Elimination of Synapses at Puberty

In the primate visual cortex there is an intense proliferation of synapses during infancy, and a surprisingly large elimination of them at puberty. Whereas the number of neurons is only slightly reduced at puberty, the number of synapses per neuron decreases by more than 40%. Presumably, synaptic elimination takes place in other parts of the cortex as well. After puberty the synaptic density in the visual cortex remains fairly constant for a long period. We do not know the cause or functional implications of this synaptic elimination, though it is probably related to sex hormones.

Critical Periods

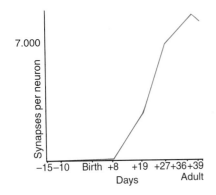

Figure 4.16 *Increase in number of synapses postnatally.* Synapses per neuron increase dramatically shortly after birth in the cat. Note that the steep rise in synapse number starts at the time the kittens open their eyes. Based on Cragg (1972).

The ability of the mature brain to process sensory information depends critically on the system being used during a specific period of time in early postnatal development (this has been most thoroughly studied in the visual system, and we shall discuss several examples below). Furthermore, we know that *extra stimulation later cannot fully compensate for the lack of use of a system during the normal period of most rapid development.* The same holds for development of numerous skills. The term *critical period* is applied to the development of a particular function of the nervous system and refers to the period when that sub-system is maximally plastic—that is, its capacity for structural and functional adaptations is maximal. Critical periods occur at different times and vary in duration for different systems and behaviors. Most likely, they start with a *genetically determined proliferation of synapses in a particular neuronal network*. For example, the increase of synapses per neuron from birth to adulthood in the cat visual cortex is shown in Figure 4.16. The largest increase starts at the time the kittens open their eyes at about 8 days, and ends after about 1 month. Further experiments showed that *part of this* increase takes place only if the visual system is used. In one group of kittens the eyelids were sutured in the first postnatal week, whereas in another group the optic nerves were cut. Both groups had about 30% fewer synapses per neuron in the visual cortex than controls. It is worth noting that the effect was the same regardless of whether the visual cortex was completely cut off from afferent signals from the retina, or only lacked a meaningful sensory input (with sutured eyelids, action potentials still travel in the optic nerve).

The phase of synaptic proliferation has limited duration and *probably must coincide with meaningful use of the system* to ensure optimal development. For example, infant monkeys prevented from using their vision until the age of 3–6 months needed several months afterwards to learn to distinguish a circle from a square. A normal infant monkey learns this simple task in a few days.

It should be emphasized that although the period of intense synaptic proliferation is brief and well-defined, the critical period for functional development is usually much longer and need not have a clearcut endpoint. In humans the critical period for vision, for example, probably lasts several years although the development is most rapid during the first year. Various aspects of vision have different critical periods, and at the cellular level neurons in different layers of the visual cortex develop their characteristic properties at different times.

Compared with other phases of development, a critical period is characterized by both increased *plasticity* and increased *vulnerability* of the nervous structures involved. These factors are mutually dependent—one cannot have the one without the other. Thus, lack of proper stimulation, lack of opportunites for practice, or exposure to harmful influences would have more serious effects during critical periods than at other times.

The cellular mechanisms underlying the enhanced plasticity during critical periods are not fully understood. We know, however, that monamines play an important role. Thus, in the cerebral cortex a sufficient

Examples of Critical Periods in Humans

Infants born with opaque lenses in their eyes (cataracts) can develop normal vision provided the lens is removed at a very early stage. The longer the time before operation, the smaller the chances are that the child will attain normal vision. Persons attaining their sight after puberty (for example, by removal of an opaque lens) have grave difficulties using their sight. The "new" sense may cause trouble rather than being the expected blessing. Some choose to return to a life as blind persons. A boy operated at the age of eight illustrates this problem. Several months of patient training were needed before he could recognize objects by sight (objects he was familiar with from the use of other senses). The surgeon who treated the boy concluded afterwards: "To give back his sight to a congenitally blind patient is more the work of an educationalist than of a surgeon" (cited by Zeki, 1993). The main reason for the problems encountered by this boy (and others in his situation) is most likely that he had not established the cortical networks needed for integrating visual information with other sensory modalities. Thus, his brain was not capable of using the wealth of information provided by his eyes. This is related to synaptic adaptations in various parts of the cerebral cortex (see Chapter 20, *The Parietal Lobe and the Development of the Ability to Integrate Somatosensory and Visual Information*). On the other hand, if the visual system has been used normally during the critical period in infancy and early childhood, even many years of temporary blindness have no serious effects on visual capacities.

level of these transmitters must be present at the time of synaptic proliferation. Monoaminergic fibers are the first to grow into the cerebral cortex during development, perhaps to prepare the ground for the critical period. Through their modulatory actions, monoamines may ensure the necessary responsiveness of neurons to new synapses. After the critical period, levels of monoamines decrease.

THE NERVOUS SYSTEM AND AGING

It is a common notion that we loose a large number of neurons as we grow older. This notion is based partly on the fact that the brain is on average 8% lighter at 80 than at 25. Reduced mental capacities in old people are often explained simply by referring to neuronal death (as we know, lost neurons are not replaced). It is not clear, however, how much of the weight loss is actually caused by cell death, because at the same time neurons become smaller, and their water content is probably reduced (as in other tissues during aging). Especially after 80 years, the cell bodies shrink and the dendritic trees become less ramified in the cerebral cortex. A correlation between brain weight and mental capacities has not been established in healthy human beings, and the loss of brain weight in some patients with dementia is not greater than that which occurs in normal aging. Therefore, a diffusely distributed neuronal loss cannot alone explain intellectual decline in normal aging or Alzheimer's disease.

From a theoretical viewpoint, a diffuse neuronal loss would not necessarily cause marked reductions in the performance of the nervous system. As discussed earlier, large populations of neurons share responsibility for most specific tasks, especially higher mental functions such as abstract thinking, language, and memory. These are the products of distributed networks connecting neuronal groups in many parts of the cerebral cortex and other brain regions. A diffusely distributed reduction of neurons in these networks might not cause functional deficits, or the deficits might appear only with maximal demands on performance. Microscopic findings of moderate neuronal loss cannot readily be correlated with altered behavior or reduced mental functions. Another factor should also be kept in mind: The nervous system remains plastic throughout life, although this capacity diminishes with advancing age. Thus, even in old age the brain can to some extent compensate for a moderate neuronal loss.

It has become clear in recent years that *alterations of brain structures with advancing age are not uniformly distributed but rather are concentrated in specific parts of the brain.* To understand how the aging brain differs from the young one, this is more important than the overall number of neurons dying. Psychological tests show that not all capacities of the brain are significantly reduced by normal aging. In many elderly people the only clear reduction may be of memory for recent events, and speed in solving certain mental tasks. Furthermore, the *individual differences* among elderly people are large, even regarding memory. Investigations of aged rats, monkeys, and humans with standard tests for recent memory reveal that a relatively large minority does as well as young controls, although most show some decline. An investigation of more than

1600 persons with a simple memory test (repeat a list of 20 words just presented), showed that the performance of the oldest group (88 years) overlapped that of the youngest (25 years) by 50%. Thus, even memory is not as strongly correlated with age as is often assumed.

Human Brain Weights

One large study comparing average brain weights at 80 and 25 years of age found for men 1300 and 1400 g respectively, and 1150 and 1250 g for women. Various values of average adult brain weight are found in the literature, however. Usually, such studies are based on brains of adults between the ages of 20 and 40 years. Variations may be explained, at least in part, by different fixation methods and storage time. More interesting than average weight is the *range of variation* among normal individuals. An investigation of brains from 200 persons 17–40 years of age reported variations from 1120 to 1780 g in men and from 1070 to 1550 g in women.

Loss of Peripheral Sensory Cells with Age

For everyday problems of the elderly, changes in the central nervous system may be less important than *loss of sensory cells and neurons of the peripheral sensory organs*. This concerns sight and hearing in particular, but joint sense and sense of equilibrium also deteriorate with advancing age. Transmission of sensory signals at lower levels of the central nervous system is *serial*—that is, the different links in the chain are coupled one after another (see Fig. 7.14). If one link is broken, all transmission stops, and the brain cannot compensate for the loss of sensory information. This contrasts with the high degree of parallel processing taking place at higher levels, particularly in the cerebral cortex.

Dizziness and Loss of Vestibular Receptors

Studies of eye movements in persons over the age 75 show that their *vestibulo-ocular reflex* (VOR) is less accurate than in younger persons. This reflex ensures that the gaze is kept fixed at one point in the environment when the head rotates (to keep the retinal image stable). Furthermore, *optokinetic eye movements* become more sluggish in old age. Such eye movements are elicited when the environment moves—for example when looking out of a car—so that the gaze is kept fixed (see Chapter 16, *Classification of Eye Movements*). Suppression of the VOR, which is necessary when the head rotates in the same direction as the visual scene, is also impaired in many elderly persons. All these changes may cause difficulties with vision and orientation while moving, especially if the movement is rapid. This may be an important factor in the dizziness that bothers many elderly people. At the cellular level, a major cause of impaired equilibrium and eye movements may be loss of sensory cells in the vestibular apparatus. A 40% loss has been reported at 75 years of age.

Biologic Basis of Memory Impairment in the Elderly

Many structural changes in the brain have been regarded as typical of aging. These include a moderate reduction of average *brain weight* mentioned above, the *enlargement of ventricles* (indicative of tissue atrophy), the appearance of *degenerative patches*, and the shrinkage of the neuronal cell bodies that primarily occurs in very old people. *Dendritic trees* and *synaptic numbers* are reduced in certain parts of the cerebral cortex. Reduced blood flow of the whole brain or certain regions has been found in several studies. Several other changes, particularly in neurotransmitters and their receptors, have been reported. The question is, however, *whether any of these changes are directly related to impairments of brain functions and behavior?* Right now we have few decisive answers but there is no lack of hypotheses.

The best data link age-dependent memory-loss to changes in specific areas of the brain. Studies of aged rats indicate that their memory impairments are due to anatomical and physiological changes in the *hippocampal region*. The hippocampus and surrounding parts of the temporal lobe are necessary for the storing and retrieval of events, faces, names, and so forth (see Chapter 19, *The Hippocampal Formation: Learning and Memory*). The changes occurring in the hippocampus are quite specific, and affect only certain kinds of neurons and synapses. Some changes are presumably caused by compensatory mechanisms. For example, one kind of neuron receives fewer synapses, but each synaptic bouton releases more transmitters. Long-term potentiation (LTP) is more difficult to produce and does not last as long in aged rats as in young ones. The memory impairment in aged monkeys has the same characteristics as in young monkeys after removal of the medial temporal lobe. *Thus, it seems likely that age-dependent loss of recent memory is caused primarily by specific changes in the hippocampus and surrounding parts of the medial temporal lobe.*

Reduced levels of different neurotransmitters with age, including acetylcholine, dopamine, and norepinephrine, have been reported but the data are inconclusive. The connection between changes of transmitters with age and functional impairments is not obvious. For instance, compensations may take place in the brain, reducing functional deficits. We should also keep in mind that synaptic transmission depends on pre and postsynaptic receptors as well as on the transmitter itself.

Dementia

Dementia can be defined as an *acquired, global impairment of intellect, reason, and personality, but without impairment of consciousness* (Lishman). It is uncommon before the age of 60 but occurs with increasing frequency, especially after 75. One third of people above 85 years may exhibit signs of dementia, although with varying severity (such estimates are uncertain). Dementia can have different causes, but *most cases include extensive damage to neurons and connections of the cerebral cortex.* Repeated brain infarctions destroying large volumes of tissue, intoxications (alcohol, solvents, and carbon monoxide), large tumors, or infections (for example, HIV) can cause dementia. Most cases, however, are caused by degenerative diseases leading to progressive neuronal loss. Most people in the latter group have *Alzheimer's disease* (AD). This disease was described just after the turn of the century as a distinct kind of dementia, that characteristically developed before the age of 60 (presenile dementia). Around 1970 it was realized, however, that most cases of dementia beginning after age 60 also are of the Alzheimer kind. Despite all the research since then "*... at present, no one theory explains adequately the host of complex biochemical and pathological facets of the disease*" (Smith et al., 1995).

Alzheimer's Disease

The disease manifests itself by *gradual decline of mental functions*. Impaired *recent memory* is an early sign: The person forgets appointments and names, repeats questions, and may appear confused and helpless. There is typically a loss of interest and initiative, and a neglect of daily activities. Initial symptoms are usually vague and hard to distinguish from normal aging. It has been discussed whether Alzheimer's disease (AD) is just an exaggerated form of normal aging, but there is now little doubt that it represents a distinct disease entity, both clinically and pathologically.

Microscopically, AD is characterized by *senile plaques* and *neurofibrillary tangles*. The latter consist of thickened, intraneuronal fibrils. The senile plaques are patchy, degenerative changes with extracellular deposits of *amyloid* and other proteins, in which *amyloid β-protein* (Aβ) is a major component. The plaques also contain many abnormal axon terminals. Aβ is formed from a large membrane protein called *amyloid precursor protein* (APP). We do not know the function of APP, but it is present normally in most neurons and is transported anterogradely in the axons to the terminals. Aβ is normally secreted from neurons, and we do not know why it precipitates in AD. The *neurofibrillary tangles* consist of a specific kind of filaments (paired helical filaments, PHF). A major component of PHF is an abnormal kind of the microtubule-associated protein *tau*. The protein lacks its normal ability to attach to microtubules, however, and this may explain why they aggregate as abnormal filaments.

Electron microscopic observations show that there is a marked *loss of synapses* in AD. Most notable are losses in the layers 2 and 3 (Fig. 20.1) of the cerebral cortex that send out and receive association connections. Thus, the pathologic changes are more severe in the *association areas of the frontal and temporal lobes* than in the primary sensory and motor areas. It appears that severity of dementia shows a closer correlation with the degree of synaptic loss than with the density of senile plaques and neurofibrillary tangles.

Some years ago it was found that Alzheimer patients have a severe neuronal loss in a diffusely distributed cell group at the base of the cerebral hemispheres, called the *basal nucleus* (of Meynert, Figs. 4.17 and 19.4). Many neurons in this nucleus are *cholinergic* (Fig. 4.18) and send their axons to the cerebral cortex (see Chapter 19, *Cholinergic Neurons Projecting to the Cerebral Cortex*). Loss of neurons in the basal nucleus may therefore explain why Alzheimer patients have severely reduced amounts of acetylcholine in the cortex. Acetylcholine raises the excitability and improves the signal–noise ratio of cortical neurons, enhancing their ability to handle information rapidly and accurately. Many neurons in the basal nucleus increase their firing rate when the animal is rewarded for doing a task, and other data also suggest that basal nucleus activity is related to *motivation*. Furthermore, experiments with selective destruction of the nucleus suggest that it is important for attending to visual stimuli and for aspects of learning and problem solving. From such data, the mental impairments in AD were tentatively explained as due to lack of acetylcholine and the resulting lowered excitability of cortical neurons. The *memory impairment* might be explained by *lack of cholinergic input to the hippocampus and nearby cortical regions*.

The relationship between the loss of basal nucleus neurons and the pathological changes in the cerebral cortex is not clear, however. Not all aspects of the functional impairment in AD can be induced by destruction of the basal nucleus in experimental animals, and there has been no clear-cut improvement in patients given drugs that increase acetylcholine in the brain. Also, transmitters other than acetylcholine are affected by AD.

Depleting the cerebral cortex of *acetylcholine, norepinephrine*, or *serotonin* (rats), triggers a rapid rise of APP synthesis. Such transmitter depletion can be produced by destroying the basal nucleus (Fig. 4.17), the raphe nuclei, or the locus coeruleus (Figs. 15.5 and 15.6) but the effect is due to loss of their synaptic actions—not the cell death alone. Thus, injecting the basal nucleus with a drug that temporarily prevents transmitter release increases cortical APP synthesis only while the drug acts. These findings suggest, first, that APP synthesis is normally controlled by synaptic actions and, second, that precipitation of amyloid *might* be caused by loss of transmitter actions.

Patients with AD are quite similar with regard to brain pathology and clinical manifestations but they differ in terms of causal factors. Genetics appears to play a variable role but may be especially important in patients with an early debut of symptoms (before 60 years). Many in the latter group inherit the disease dominantly. In a subgroup of patients, a *mutation of the gene coding for APP* might suffice to cause the disease. This gene sits on chromosome 21. Another group of patients with familial occurrence of the disease have in common a mutation on chromosome 14. The gene product in this case is is not known, however. Another candidate is the gene coding for one *apolipoprotein (ApoE4)*. This gene is on chromosome 19. Normally, the apolipoproteins come in three genetically different kinds, but only the ApoE4 variety is associated with AD. Thus, persons with the ApoE4 gene run a much higher risk of AD than persons with genes for another variety of apolipoprotein. Two to three percent of the population are homozygotes for ApoE4, and their AD risk is five to fifteen times higher than in the rest of the population. The normal task of apolipoproteins is to transport cholesterol in the blood. ApoE4, however, also binds to amyloid β-protein and is present in senile plaques and neurofibrillary tangles. Therefore, it may be instrumental in the precipitation of amyloid.

Figure 4.17 *The basal nucleus* (of Meynert). Frontal section through the left hemisphere (monkey). The cholinergic neurons of the basal nucleus are indicated with red dots. The basal nucleus is continuous anteriorly with the septal nuclei and other cholinergic cell groups of the forebrain. Redrawn from Richardson and DeLong (1988).

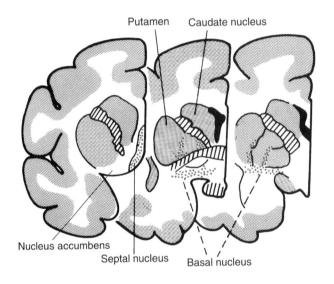

Figure 4.18 *Cholinergic neurons of the basal nucleus*. Photomicrograph of a section treated to demonstrate immunocytochemically the enzyme choline acetyltransferase. The enzyme is necessary for the synthesis of acetylcholine. Magnification, ×300. Courtesy of Dr. J.-E. Aas, Department of Anatomy, University of Oslo.

RESTITUTION OF FUNCTION

The nervous system retains its plasticity throughout life, and this property is a prerequisite for recovery of function after damage after injury or disease. Yet what changes do occur in the brain when a patient recovers functions after a stroke? Are the mechanisms operating in normal development also responsible for plasticity after brain damage? These are questions we will discuss in the rest of this chapter.

Restitution Can Be Divided into Two Phases

After a person has a stroke, there is usually a first phase of rapid improvement lasting from days to weeks, followed by a second phase of

---

Ischemic Cell Damage and the Glutamate Hypothesis

Abolished or reduced blood supply to an organ is called *ischemia*. Even a few minutes of severe brain ischemia may cause massive neuronal death but, surprisingly, the neurons often do not die until several hours after the ischemic episode. This is so because the lack of oxygen (hypoxia) and glucose triggers a cascade of events, in which each step takes some time, but resulting eventually in neuronal death.

Glutamate and *glutamate receptors* are under particularly strong suspicion as the main villains of this drama. According to the *glutamate hypothesis* of ischemic brain damage, the sequence of events after a temporary stop of blood flow is probably as follows:

1. the loss of energy supply rapidly *reduces the activity of the Na^+–K^+ pump*, leading to (among other things);
2. *increased extracellular K^+ concentration* that depolarizes the neurons so they fire bursts of action potentials;
3. steadily worsening *imbalances of ion concentrations* across the cell membrane make the neuron incapable of firing action potentials (electrically silent);
4. at the same time the *extracellular glutamate concentration rises* steeply (perhaps because the ionic imbalances reverse the pumping of glutamate by high affinity transporters) leading to
5. enormous *activation of glutamate receptors*, among them NMDA receptors; this in turn is believed to induce
6. *cell damage*, probably because of an uncontrolled rise in *intracellular Ca^{2+} concentration*. This may harm the cell in various ways, for example by activating enzymes that degrade proteins and nucleic acids. This in turn destroys other vital enzymes.

That NMDA receptors are involved in ischemic cell death is indirectly supported by animal experiments involving NMDA-receptor blockers. If such drugs are given even a few hours after an ischemic episode, they reduce or prevent the cell damage. Also, blockers of AMPA receptors give protection against ischemic cell death in such experiments.

The glutamate hypothesis cannot readily explain all aspects of ischemic cell death, however. For example, after *global ischemia* (shutting down the blood supply to the whole brain, as can occur in cardiac arrest), the *cell death is not diffusely distributed*. Especially vulnerable are the neurons in the CA1 field of the hippocampus (Fig. 19.7). Regional differences in glutamate release or glutamate receptors are probably not the reason. More likely explanations concern differences among regions regarding the presence and regulation of *neurotrophic factors*.

The delay between an ischemic episode and irreversible cell damage gives hope for finding drugs that prevent or reduce the brain damage, and this is now an active field of research. In clinical situations, *focal ischemia* due to occlusion of a brain artery by thrombosis or embolus is more common than global ischemia. In such cases we can hope to reduce the size of the brain infarct by keeping neurons in the peripheral zone of the ischemic region alive until the circulation improves. Improvement may occur spontaneously or by using fibrinolytic drugs that dissolve the vascular obstruction.

slower progress lasting from months to years. After acute damage to neural tissue, secondary changes occur in the tissue surrounding the damaged area, such as *disturbed local circulation* and *tissue swelling (edema)*. This occurs, for example, after the crushing of neural tissue and bleeding caused by head injuries, and after vascular occlusion caused by thrombosis or an embolus. Thus, neurons outside the damaged region may also become temporarily or permanently nonfunctional. If the edema subsides quickly and the circulation improves in the zone around the permanently damaged tissue, many neurons will regain their normal activity (compare with the transient weakness and loss of cutaneous sensation produced by pressure on a peripheral nerve). This is probably why there is often a marked improvement of the patient's condition during the first weeks after the accident. For example, an arm that was totally paralyzed the day after a stroke may in a few weeks be only slightly weaker and more clumsy than before the stroke.

Animal experiments have shown observable plastic changes shortly after an injury (hours, days). Thus, *there is probably no sharp distinction between the rapid and the slow phases of recovery*—the nervous system starts its adaptation to the new circumstances immediately.

Mechanisms Underlying Recovery of Function

We know that *dead neurons are not replaced*, and that *cut axons do not regenerate in the central nervous system* (the latter in contrast to the peripheral nervous system). Therefore, the improvement in function after damage to the central nervous system cannot be due to a directly reparative process. Rather, we must assume that recovery is due to changes among the remaining, undamaged elements. That is, neural circuitries *reorganize* to adapt to a novel situation. We will discuss two kinds of adaptation below, both of which may be regarded as *learning processes*.

In one type of adaptation, called *substitution*, intact neuronal groups take over and substitute for the damaged parts. The neuronal groups responsible for the substitution normally carry out tasks similar to those of the damaged ones. Thus, after a stroke destroys cell groups responsible for intitating certain kinds of movements, cells responsible for other kinds of movements may to some extent take over. For example, other cortical areas may partially substitute for functions lost when a lesion destroys the primary motor cortex (Fig. 12.7), and neuronal groups normally controlling only one side of the body may expand their activity to concern also the other side as well. Substitution, however, can seldom restore a system to its premorbid function. After all, a specialist has been replaced by an amateur, who in addition still has to take care of his former duties!

The other kind of adaptation—called *compensation*—implies that remaining structures change their normal activity so that disturbing symptoms produced by the injury are diminished. This is relevant when the brain damage not only leads to loss of functions, such as muscular weakness or sensory loss, but also produces disturbing phenomena such as involuntary movements. For example, unilateral destruction of the vestibular apparatus in the inner ear initially causes severe dizziness and

Examples of Substitution from Animal Experiments

Clinical recovery after brain damage may be likened to a long-term learning process, involving strengthening of specific synaptic connections by repeated use. As we shall see, however, some redirecting of impulse traffic can occur even immediately after the damage.

When the arm region of the motor cortex (Fig. 12.7) in monkeys doing specific wrist movements is cooled, the movements immediately become slower and weaker. This is expected since the cooling inactivates many pyramidal tract neurons (see Fig. 12.2). Activity in the somatosensory cortex (Fig. 7.21) increases simultaneously, however, as if this region were prepared to take over immediately. If the somatosensory cortex is then also cooled, the monkey becomes paralytic and is unable to do the movements at all. Cooling of the somatosensory cortex alone has almost no effect on the movements, and is not accompanied by increased activity in the motor cortex. These data suggest that the *impulse traffic can be switched very rapidly from one path to another, so that command signals for movements are redirected to the somatosensory* cortex. If the motor cortex were permanently inactivated, we might expect that the new impulse route would gradually become strengthened.

Other experiments suggest, first, that strengthening of connections takes place during recovery and, secondly, that this strengthening is paralleled with the establishment of new synapses. After the first link of the disynaptic pathway from the cerebellum to the motor cortex is severed in monkeys (Fig. 14.7), voluntary movements become jerky and uncoordinated. In two to three weeks, however, most symptoms disappear, and movements are carried out almost as before. Thus, considerable restitution has occurred despite permanent damage to the connections. If the somatosensory cortex is then destroyed, however, the original symptoms recur with full strength. After this second operation, recovery takes much longer and is incomplete. Obviously, during the first phase of recovery, the somatosensory cortex substituted the cerebellum regarding information to the motor cortex. This information is presumably carried by the numerous association connections from the somatosensory to the motor cortex. This assumption is supported by the observation that the motor cortex had increased synaptic density after recovery. These experiments thus suggest that new synapses can be established in the adult after brain damage, even in a neuronal group far removed from the site of injury.

Collateral Sprouting Can Aid Restitution

Neurons that have lost their afferents may be supplied with new ones from normal axons in the vicinity. This is called *collateral sprouting*. In experiments where some afferent axons to a neuronal group are cut (deafferentation), the axons degenerate and their boutons are removed by phagocytic activity of glial cells. In a relatively short time, however, the vacant synaptic sites may be filled with new boutons. This probably occurs because a trophic substance becomes available from the neurons that have lost their afferents. The trophic substance stimulates nearby normal axons to send out sprouts. Collateral sprouting would mainly be of local importance in restoring neuronal activity. There is no evidence that it can restore connections between more distant cell groups. Nor do all systems seem to exhibit collateral sprouting.

It should be emphasized that collateral sprouting *cannot restore the original pattern of innervation* since the neurons responsible for that pattern are gone. Thus, there will always be a loss of specificity of connections compared with the normal situation. Restitution of function seen after brain damage is usually characterized by a loss of precision; for example, the force of movements may be well restored, whereas the ability to carry out delicate movements may never return.

Collateral sprouting may not always be functionally beneficial. For example, after a stroke that damages the motor pathways descending from the cerebral cortex, the vacant synaptic sites on motor neurons in the cord may be filled by axon collaterals from sensory neurons. This would not help to improve the voluntary control of the muscles but might rather contribute to the hyperreactivity of the muscles to sensory stimuli that is characteristic of such cases (spasticity).

disturbances of posture and eye movements. This is due to a mismatch between the vestibular information reaching the brain from the two sides of the body. The symptoms usually subside quickly, because the vestibular system on the intact side compensates by altering its sensitivity and information handling. In this case the sense of equilibrium is not regained but disturbing symptoms are at least reduced. This example of adaptation to vestibular damage also illustrates *substitution*, however. The postural adjustments necessary for the upright position are gradually improved because vestibular information is substituted by visual information. When denied the use of vision (as in the dark), the person becomes very unsteady or completely helpless. In conclusion, neither substitution nor compensation can be expected to provide full restoration of functions after damage to the nervous system.

Studies of Recovery after a Stroke in Humans

Many stroke patients have muscular weakness (pareses) in the opposite side of the body as a dominating symptom. This is called *hemiplegia* (hemi = half; plegia, from Greek plegé = stroke). The symptoms are caused by destruction (due to occlusion of an artery or a bleeding) of motor pathways from the cerebral cortex to the brain stem and the cord (see Fig. 12.2). Usually, the injury occurs in the internal capsule where the descending fibers from the cerebral cortex are collected (Figs. 12.5 and 12.9; see also Fig. 3.42 for arteries supplying the internal capsule). When such injuries cause hemiplegia, we use the term *capsular hemiplegia*. Because patients with this clinical condition are so common, and because the site of their injury is usually well localized, they have been the subjects for many studies of restitution. Some examples elucidating mechanisms behind restitution in humans are presented below.

Regional cerebral blood flow is closely linked with neuronal activity. Thus, when we find altered blood flow in a specific part of the brain after a stroke, it is taken as evidence of altered activity caused by the stroke. One group of *patients with capsular hemiplegia* were tested 3 months after the stroke. They were then completely or substantially recovered; for example, they could all perform opposition movements with the fingers. The test was to touch the thumb sequentially with the fingers, in a rhythm determined by a metronome. In *normal control persons* this task evokes increased blood flow primarily in the *opposite motor cortex*. This fits with the fact that the pyramidal tract—necessary for precise finger movements—is crossed (Fig. 12.5). The patients differed from the controls by showing increased activity in *motor cortical areas on the same side* as the affected hand. In addition, there was increased activity in cortical areas that are not normally activated in this kind of simple, routine movements (parts of the insula, posterior parietal cortex, and the cingulate gyrus). In controls, these areas show increased activity with problem-solving tasks requiring extra attention. The regions have in common that they send association connections to the premotor area (PMA, Fig. 12.7) and by this route can influence voluntary movements. These findings suggest that *functional recovery after hemiplegia is related to (1) the patients learning to use motor areas on the same side as the pareses, and (2) their using larger parts of the cerebral cortex for control of simple finger movements than before the damage.* In some patients, movements of the fingers of the paretic hand were accompanied by movements (involuntarily) of the unaffected hand. This also suggests that the undamaged hemisphere now participates in the control of muscles of the paretic side. The involvement of larger parts of the cerebral cortex may explain why simple, previously effortless movements require much more attention and mental energy than before the stroke.

A peculiar experiment of nature sheds light on what happens during restitution. Two patients with purely motor symptoms who were in clear

Can We Help Restitution?

Why do severed axons regenerate in the peripheral nervous system but not in the CNS? This question, puzzling neuroscientists for a century, has recently been answered at least partly. Under certain conditions, even axons in the CNS can regenerate. If they can make contact with a piece of peripheral nerve containing Schwann cells, central axons will grow into the nerve. Several centimeters of axonal growth have been shown in such experiments. Normally, however, central axons are prevented from growing by *specific, myelin-associated proteins* produced by oligodendroglial cells. These substances cause immediate collapse of the growth cone when an axon starts to grow. *Antibodies* against these myelin-associated proteins enable central axons to grow. Such antibodies have been given to rats after damage to the cord that interrupts the pyramidal tract (among other fiber tracts). Although considerable growth was achieved (up to one centimeter), we do not know whether this approach can help achieve functional restitution in humans with transverse lesions of the cord. For example, axons encounter special problems when trying to cross the damaged region.

Another question is whether we can rescue neurons after brain damage or stimulate plastic changes necessary for restitution. Various neurotrophic factors (NGF, BDNF, and others) are under preclinical trials for such purposes. Although such substances can improve survival of neurons *in vitro* and *in vivo*, their application in the central nervous system meets difficulties. Since they are proteins, the substances do not pass the blood–brain barrier readily, and even if delivered directly into the cerebrospinal fluid, their tissue penetration is restricted. Also, long-term supply of proteins to the brain may have uncontrollable actions and perhaps dangerous side effects. Therefore, the hope is to develop drugs that can stimulate the synthesis of specific neurotrophic factors in the brain itself.

Can We Replace Lost Neurons by Transplantation?

Because early embryonic neurons still can send out axons, the possibility of replacing lost neurons in the adult brain is being investigated by transplanting neuroblasts from an embryo into the host brain (the embryo must be so young that the neuroblasts have not yet sent out axons). Besides numerous animal experiments, this approach has been tried in a limited number of patients with Parkinson's disease (see Chapter 13, *Parkinson's Disease*) with promising results. Animal experiments do show convincingly that neuroblasts can survive and send out axons after transplantation to an adult brain. If transplanted to a site where the adult neurons have been destroyed, the axons may even reach the normal targets of the destroyed neurons. Functional restoration has also been demonstrated in some studies. Embryonic neuroblasts are obviously not affected by the myelin-associated factors that normally inhibit axonal growth in the mature central nervous system.

Many problems complicate the transplantations of embryonic tissue, however. One is the ethical issue of using brains of early abortions for therapy. Others are technical, such as the necessity for growth over long distances in the human brain (as compared with the rat) and survival of a sufficient number of neuroblasts. The chances of success are best with restoring diffusely organized, fairly short connections, whereas with precisely organized, long-ranging connections in the human brain, chances are remote.

recovery from capsular hemiplegia, suffered a second stroke in the other hemisphere. As expected, their previously normal side now became paretic but so did the recovered side. This phenomenon is difficult to explain if not by assuming that the restitution had involved the use of motor pathways from the normal hemisphere to ipsilateral muscles.

Restitution Is a Learning Process

Regardless of whether long-term restitution is caused by other neuronal groups taking over a function or by collateral sprouting (or both), there is good reason to believe that the improvement is a result of a *learning process*, subject to the same rules that underlie learning in an intact nervous system. All learning is likely to involve changes in the properties of existing synapses, formation of new ones, and removal of inappropriate ones. Such use-dependent plasticity continues throughout life, and is the nervous system's means of adapting to new and changing conditions—in the body itself and in the environment. The process is bound to take time and is probably slower in a brain deprived of many neurons. We know, from own experience and from cognitive psychology, the importance of *motivation* and *focused, selective attention* for effective learning. An ex-

Restitution after Damage in Early Childhood

Often restitution is more complete after damage that occurs during development than in the mature brain. This is not always the case, however. We have discussed that during early critical periods of development the brain is not only more plastic but also more vulnerable than later. Examples from development of the visual system illustrated this point. Early damage of the cerebellum in rats was found to produce more severe defects in motor function than similar damage inflicted at a later stage. That restitution is often more complete after early damage, is probably only partly due to the properties of the individual neurons, which may be more apt to send out new collaterals and remove others. Another factor could be as important. In the young brain various regions, particularly of the cerebral cortex, are not yet fully engaged in the tasks for which they are destined. Therefore they may be used more easily for other purposes if necessary. Thus, the right hemisphere of the brain may partly take over the processing of *language* if the left hemisphere (which normally does this) is damaged at an early age.

Even in the immature brain of an infant, connections that are already established are apparently not replaced if damaged. Thus, if the left motor cortex (sending fibers to the right spinal cord) is removed in monkeys shortly after birth, the remaining right motor cortex is not able to supply the denervated right half of the spinal cord with axons. Behaviorally, these monkeys never learn (with their right hand) the kinds of movements that are dependent on direct connections from the cerebral cortex to the cord. This is because these connections are already established at birth in monkeys. Reports of apparent reestablishment of long fiber tracts after early injury are probably based on experiments in which the injury was inflicted *before* the axons from the relevant cell groups had reached their targets. In such instances, the outgrowing axons may also innervate other cell groups than they normally do. This may be due to a lack of normal competition among outgrowing fiber tracts. In humans, direct connections from the cerebral cortex to the cord are established at the 7th gestational month. In children with *inborn hemiplegia* due to damage occurring before this fetal period (often in connection with premature birth) the pyramidal tract innervates abnormal sites. For example, individual pyramidal tract axons from the undamaged hemisphere can branch to innervate motoneurons on both sides of the cord. This is clinically expressed by the children doing *mirror movements*, that is, voluntary movements with one hand are always accompanied by the same movement with the other hand. Normally, the fibers innervating motoneurons for hand movements are purely crossed.

ample of the importance of focused attention concerns infants and children with a *squint* (strabismus). Because the retinal images are different in the two eyes, the child attends to signals from one eye only to avoid contradictory information (double vision). Some children solve the conflict by constantly using one eye and ignoring information from the other, whereas other children use the two eyes interchangeably. It turns out that those always using the same eye eventually get severely reduced vision in the eye that is not used. Those using their eyes interchangeably, however, retain normal vision in both eyes. It should be noted that the actual images reaching the cortex from the two eyes—even with a squint—are almost identical. The crucial factor is whether the information receives attention or not. In anesthetized animals cells in the visual cortex can change their properties after exposure to light stimuli if these are coupled with stimulation of cell groups that are normally active during focused attention. *Thus, the learning effect appears to require that two kinds of synaptic input converge at a neuron—one kind providing specific information, the other "telling" the neuron that this is relevant information that should be stored.* As discussed earlier, the release of monoamines is probably a factor in such plastic changes.

CHAPTER 5

HOW ARE THE STRUCTURE AND FUNCTION OF THE NERVOUS SYSTEM STUDIED?

Many approaches have been used to study the structure and function of the nervous system, from straightforward observations of its macroscopic appearance to determination of the function of single neuronal molecules. Recent years have witnessed a tremendous development of methods, so that problems can be approached today that formerly were a matter of speculation only. The number of neuroscientists has also increased almost exponentially, and they are engaged in problems ranging from molecular genetics to behavior. The mass of knowledge in the field of neurobiology has increased accordingly, and, more importantly, the understanding of how our brains work has improved considerably. Nevertheless, the steadily expanding amount of information has made it more difficult than before for each scientist to have a comprehensive knowledge of more than his or her own field. The rapid advancement of user-friendly computer systems for accessing the voluminous literature may help in this respect.

Traditionally, methods used for neurobiological research were grouped into those dealing with structure (neuroanatomy) and those aiming at disclosing the function of the structures (neurophysiology, neuropsychology). The borders, however, are far from sharp, and it is typical of modern neuroscience that anatomic, physiological, biochemical, pharmacological, psychological, and other methods are combined. Furthermore, the introduction of modern computer-based imaging techniques has opened exciting possibilities for studying the relation between structure and function in the living human brain. The number of methods used in modern neuroscience is so large that only a few will be mentioned here. More and more of the methods originally developed in cell biology and immunology are being applied to the nervous system, and we now realize that neurons are not so different from other cells as was once assumed.

Here we will discuss a selection of methods that form the basis of most of what is presented in this book. The emphasis will be on methods that show the "wiring pattern" of the brain, and those that reveal the relationship between structure and function. Although knowledge of structure alone does not tell us how the brain operates or how its various parts function, such knowledge is nevertheless a prerequisite for sound interpretations of findings obtained with other methods.

SOME GENERAL FEATURES OF NEUROBIOLOGICAL RESEARCH

Animal Experiments Have Been Crucial for Progress

Only a minor part of our present knowledge of the nervous system is based on observations in man; most has been obtained in experimental animals. In humans we are usually limited to comparison of symptoms caused by naturally occurring diseases with the findings made at postmortem examination of the brain. Two cases are seldom identical, and the structural derangement of the brain is often too extensive to enable unequivocal conclusions. In animals, on the other hand, the experimental conditions can be controlled, and the experiments may be repeated, to reach reliable conclusions. The properties of the elements of neural tissue can be examined directly—for example, the activity of single neurons can be correlated with the behavior of the animal. Parts of the nervous system can also be studied in isolation—for example, by using tissue slices that can be kept viable in vitro for hours. This enables recordings and experimental manipulations to be done, with subsequent structural analysis of the tissue. Studies in invertebrates with a simple nervous system have made it possible to discover fundamental mechanisms underlying synaptic function and the functioning of simple neuronal networks.

When addressing questions about functions specific to the most highly developed nervous systems, however, experiments must be performed in higher mammals, such as cats and monkeys, with a well-developed cerebral cortex. Even from such experiments, inferences about the human nervous system must be drawn with great caution. Thus, even though the nervous systems in all higher mammals show striking similarities with regard to their basic principles of organization, there are important differences in the relative development of the various parts. Such anatomic differences indicate that there are functional differences as well. Thus, results based on the study of humans, as in clinical neurology, psychiatry, and psychology, must have the final word when it comes to functions of the human brain. But because clinicians seldom can experiment, they must often build their conclusions on observations made in experimental animals and then decide whether findings from patients or normal volunteers can be explained on such a basis. If this is not possible, the clinical findings may raise new problems that require studies in experimental animals to be solved. Basically, however, the methods used to study the human brain are the same as those used in the study of experimental animals.

Experiments on animals are often criticized from an *ethical* point of view. The question of whether such experiments are acceptable, however, cannot be entirely separated from the broader question of whether mankind has the right to determine the lives of animals by using them for food, by taking over their territories, and so forth. With regard to using animals for scientific purposes, one has to realize that a better understanding of man as a thinking, feeling, and acting being requires, among other things, further animal experiments. Even though cell cultures and computer models may replace some, in the foreseeable future we will still need animal experiments. Computer-based models of the neuronal interactions taking place in the cerebral cortex, for example, usually require further animal experiments to test their tenability. Improved knowledge and understanding of the human brain is, however, also mandatory if we want to improve the prospects for treatment of the many diseases affecting the nervous system. Until today, these diseases—most often leading to severe suffering and disability—have only occasionally been amenable to effective treatment. Modern neurobiological research nevertheless gives hope, and many promising results have appeared in the last few years. Again, this would not have been possible without animal experiments.

Yet there are obviously limits to what can be defended ethically, even when the purpose is to alleviate human suffering. Strict rules have been made by the governmental authorities and the scientific community itself to ensure that only properly trained persons perform animal experiments and that the experiments are conducted so that discomfort and pain are reduced to a minimum. Most international neuroscience journals require that the experiments they publish have been conducted in accordance with such rules.

There Are Sources of Error in All Methods

Even though we will not treat systematically the sources of error inherent in the various methods to be discussed in this book, it should be realized that all methods have their limitations. One source of error when doing animal experiments is to draw premature conclusions about conditions in humans. In general, all experiments aim at isolating structures and processes so that they can be observed more clearly. However necessary this may be, it also means that many phenomena are only studied out of their natural context. Conclusions with regard to how the parts function in conjunction with all of the others must therefore be speculative.

Purely anatomic methods also have their sources of error and have led to many erroneous conclusions in the past about connections between neuronal groups. Such errors in turn may lead to misinterpretations of physiological and psychological data. The study of man also entails sources of error—for example, of a psychological nature. Thus, the answers and information given by a patient or a volunteer are not always reliable; the patient may, for example, want to please the doctor and answer accordingly.

Scientific "Truths" Must Be Revised from Time to Time

That our methods have sources of error and that our interpretations of data are not always tenable are witnessed by the fact that our concepts of the nervous system must be revised regularly. Reinterpretations of old data and changing concepts are often made necessary by the introduction of new methods. As in all areas of science, conclusions based on the available data should not be regarded as final truths but as more or less probable and preliminary interpretations. Natural science is basically concerned with posing questions to nature. How understandable and unequivocal the answers are depends on the precision of our questions and how relevant they are to the problem we are studying—stupid questions receive stupid answers. It is furthermore fundamental to science—although not always easy for the individual scientist to live up to—that conclusions and interpretations be made without any bias and solely on the strength of the facts and the arguments. It should be irrelevant whether the scientist is a young student or a Nobel laureate.

METHODS

Comparative Studies

Comparison of functional specialization and the development of particular parts of the nervous system in different species has given us much insight, and is still a useful and robust method in neuroscience. When a part of the brain is particularly well developed in a species with certain behavioral characteristics and only slightly developed in other species lacking these characteristics, conclusions about the correlation between structure and function can be drawn with some confidence. Such comparative studies have now been extended from purely anatomic ones down to the molecular level.

Dissection and Microscopic Examination Laid the Foundation for Knowledge of the Structure of the Nervous System

Our first knowledge of the structure of the nervous system and its subdivision into different parts was gained by simple macroscopic observation and dissection. The names of the major subdivisions as we use them to-

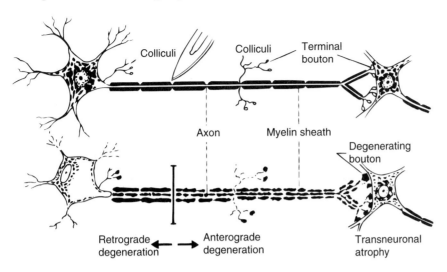

Figure 5.1 *Transection of an axon in the central nervous system.* The distal part of the axon disintegrates and is finally removed. The perikaryon exhibits a characteristic, chromatolytic reaction.

day stem from such investigations with simple and primitive methods, made before there was any knowledge of the construction of the nervous tissue. A better understanding of the building elements of the nervous system and their interconnections was first made possible with the invention of the light microscope in the middle of the nineteenth century. Thus, tissue that was fixed, cut in thin sections, and stained to differentiate among structural elements could be examined. By the turn of the century, the main features of the microscopic structure and many of the interconnections of the major cell groups were known. This was partly achieved with staining methods that predominantly stain cell bodies, *Nissl staining*, which was used for *cytoarchitectonic* characterization of the gray substance, such as dividing the cerebral cortex in different areas and the brain stem in numerous separate nuclei (Figs. 1.3, 1.14, and 20.2). Partly, methods visualizing primarily the *myelin sheaths* (Figs. 3.15–3.17, and 3.23) enabled the early anatomists to follow the course of the major fiber tracts. Methods that visualized neurons by impregnating them with the salts of heavy metals (of silver and gold) made it possible to study also the dendrites and axonal ramifications. The *Golgi method* (introduced by the Italian anatomist Camillo Golgi) was particularly powerful in this respect and is widely used even today. With the Golgi method, only a small percentage of all neurons within a region are impregnated, which provides a clearer view of the neuronal processes (Figs. 1.3 and 20.5). In young animals, before the fiber tracts are myelinated, axons can be followed for considerable distances after Golgi impregnation. It was then possible to formulate basic rules with regard to how neurons are interconnected and communicate. The great Spanish neuroanatomist Ramón y Cajal expressed particularly clearly, on the basis of his own careful observations, that neuronal impulse traffic is one-way and that the synapse is the site of communication betweeen nerve cells.

To study connections between neuronal groups that are far apart, observations in normal material are not sufficient. Experimental methods were developed on the basis of the fact that when an axon is cut, characteristic structural changes occur in the perikaryon and in the parts of the axon distal to the cut (Fig. 5.1). The perikaryon first swells and thereafter shrinks and disappears, undergoing *retrograde degeneration*. By making restricted experimental lesions and looking in the microscope for signs of retrograde degeneration, the main features of the central nervous system's connections were clarified. The axonal changes distal to the cut are called *anterograde degeneration*. The first method that visualized axons undergoing anterograde degeneration was the *Marchi method*, which stains degenerational products of myelin. By destroying the perikarya of a nucleus, it was possible to follow the course and, to some extent, the termination of their axons. Since, however, many axons are unmyelinated, either along their full course or just before they end, the Marchi method cannot visualize all fiber tracts or even for the myelinated ones, their exact sites of termination.

If a neuronal group is destroyed, the target neurons on which they form synapses sometimes also show signs of degeneration. The neurons may shrink and eventually disappear by this *transneuronal degeneration*, which may give valuable information about connectivity. For example, connections from the retina to the thalamus were described in detail on the basis of this method. The transneuronal degeneration is presumably caused by the lack of a trophic substance normally delivered by the presynaptic neuron to the postsynaptic one, but lack of activity also appears to play a role.

In the 1950s, methods were developed that enabled vastly improved precision in the determination of neuronal connectivity. These methods were based on the impregnation of degenerating axons by silver salts, the *silver impregnation methods* (the Nauta method and the Fink and Heimer method have been used most widely). With such methods the axons can in some cases be followed even to their boutons. In about 20 years these methods brought a wealth of new information and improved considerably our understanding of how the nervous system is organized.

By the end of the past century, when neurohistological techniques provided new insight into the internal structure of the nervous system, physiological studies based on the *electrical nature of the nerve impulse* were also in rapid progress. Increasingly sensitive methods were developed to record the activity of nerve cells and to stimulate well-defined parts of the nervous system. From initially being able to record only the activity of large neuronal assemblies, it became possible to record the activity of single neurons.

Modern Methods for Tracing Neuronal Connections

Another great leap forward in the investigation of neuronal connections was made at the end of the 1960s with the introduction of methods using *axonal transport* of tracer substances. In contrast to degeneration methods, they take advantage of the normal processes of the cells and avoid damaging the neurons under study. This eliminates several of the sources of error of the degeneration methods. In addition, the axonal transport methods are more sensitive than the degeneration methods, and in a short time many "new" connections were described. Our concepts of how neurons are interconnected had to be partly revised on the basis of these new findings.

Axonal transport is directed both *anterogradely* and *retrogradely*, as described in Chapter 1. The first method to be utilized was *anterograde transport of radioactively labeled amino acids.* Amino acids are normally taken up by the perikarya and used for protein synthesis. Many of these proteins are transported anterogradely to the boutons. After injection of (most often) tritium-labeled leucine or proline, the transported material can be visualized in tissue sections by autoradiography. This method can also be used for electron microscopy and then enables definite conclusions about synaptic relations. For *retrograde transport* especially, the enzyme *horseradish peroxidase* (HRP) has been widely used, either alone (free HRP) or conjugated to another molecule (wheat germ agglutinin [WGA]) that is taken up more readily by the nerve cells than free HRP. A small amount (for example, $0.1\,\mu$l) of a solution of the tracer is injected and is then taken up by the nerve terminals in the injected area and transported retrogradely to the cell bodies (Figs. 5.2 and 12.3). HRP is, however, also transported anterogradely after perikaryal uptake. Thus, the method can also be used to demonstrate the terminal sites of specific neu-

Figure 5.2 *Retrograde and anterograde axonal transport.* A cat received injections of HRP–WGA in the cerebellum and in the cerebral cortex (0.2 μl in each). The extension of the tracer at the injection site is seen in the sections by the black reaction product obtained after incubation of the sections with tetramethylbenzidine (TMB). The tracer is transported retrogradely from the cerebellum to the pontine nuclei in the brain stem. The retrogradely labeled cells are black in the section from the pontine nuclei shown below. From the injection site in the cerebral cortex, the tracer is transported anterogradely to the pontine nuclei. The terminal ramifications and the boutons of the axons are seen as black dust in the section of the pontine nuclei. Magnifications, $\times 8$ (upper photomicrographs) and $\times 150$.

ronal groups. HRP can be visualized in tissue sections by utilizing its peroxidase activity to form a colored reaction product from a colorless substrate (diaminobenzidine, tetramethylbenzidine, and others). The uptake of HRP takes place by endocytosis, and the enzyme is subsequently internalized in lysosomelike bodies.

Several other substances are also used for axonal transport; some of these are transported only anterogradely, others only retrogradely. Substances that have no enzyme activity to help their visualization may be demonstrated by immunocytochemical techniques using antibodies raised against the transported molecule. This is the case for the plant lectin *Phaseolus vulgaris leukoagglutinin* (PHAL), which is only transported anterogradely. This lectin has the advantage of an extremely small and well circumscribed injection site, yet the transport is good and the labeled terminal fibers are shown in very fine detail in the sections.

Small-molecular, fluorescent substances that are subject to axonal transport have proved very valuable for tracing neuronal connections. Their advantage is that several tracers that fluoresce at different wavelengths of ultraviolet light can be injected in the same animal. This makes it possible to decide, for example, whether a cell group sends axonal collaterals to more than one target. In such double-labeling experiments, two fluorescent tracers are injected (each in a different place) and the region of interest is examined under the fluorescence microscope to look for perikarya that fluoresce under both wavelengths. Axonal transport of fluorescent tracers can also be combined with immunocytochemical methods to show the transmitter candidates of the labeled neurons.

It is also possible to label a transmitter molecule radioactively, and then inject it into the tissue. Only neurons that use this particular transmitter have specific uptake mechanisms for it. After uptake, the transmitter is transported anterogradely and can be subsequently localized in the tissue by autoradiography. Thus connections of transmitter-specific neuronal populations can be determined.

Neuronal connections can also be traced by *electrophysiological methods*. A cell group or nucleus is stimulated electrically, and the subsequent change of neuronal activity in other regions—caused by synaptic influence from the stimulated cell group—is recorded (orthodromic stimulation). By measuring the time from the stimulus to the response, it is usually possible to determine whether connections between two cell groups are monosynaptic or polysynaptic. Stimulation of axons within a fiber tract or their terminal ramifications can be used to determine the location of their parent cell bodies. In this instance the action potentials set up in the axons travel retrogradely toward the cell body (antidromic stimulation).

Electron Microscopic Examination of Nervous Tissue

Toward the end of the 1950s, electron microscopic techniques made it possible to characterize the structure of the subcellular elements of nerve cells in detail (Figs. 1.5, 1.8, 1.10, and 1.11). Of particular importance was the demonstration of the fine structure of the synapse, which enabled correlations to be made with physiological, biochemical, and pharmacological data pertaining to synaptic processes. Electron microscopy also made it possible to describe the various types of filaments involved in axonal tranpsort. Another example is the clarification of the structure of myelin.

Because boutons undergoing degenerative changes after destruction of the perikaryon show characteristic alterations in the electron microscope, the synaptic relations of specific sets of afferents to a nucleus could be determined. Moreover, some axonally transported tracer substances can be identified in the electron microscope. Likewise, the exact subcellular localization of tissue antigens (transmitters, transmitter-related enzymes, and other substances of functional interest) can be identified by electron microscopy after immunocytochemical treatment.

Determination of Neuronal Content of Neurotransmitters and Distribution of Receptors

To understand the functions of a nerve cell, it is necessary to know the transmitters it uses. With biochemical methods, the content of transmitters in parts of the brain and in subcellular fractions can be determined. To obtain further knowledge, however, it is also necessary to link the transmitters to specific neurons with known connections and physiological properties.

The first possibilities of studying the anatomy of neurons with known transmitters arose in the 1960s, when it was discovered that monamine-containing neurons can be made fluorescent by a special treatment with formaldehyde. This marked the beginning of intense investigations, with other methods as well, of characterizing neurons with regard to connections and at the same time with regard to their transmitters. It became evident that neurons with a certain transmitter may not be restricted to cytoarchitectonically homogeneous nuclei and, vice versa, that neurons within one cytoarchitectonically defined nucleus may use different transmitters.

The introduction of immunological methods, such as *immunocytochemistry*, to localize substances in nervous tissue has been of particular importance during recent years. By purifying a potentially interesting substance present in nervous tissue, antibodies may be raised against it (either polyclonal antibodies raised in animals, or monoclonal antibodies produced in cell cultures). The antibodies bind to their antigens at the site where they are exposed in the tissue sections, and the antibodies can be visualized subsequently with the use of secondary antibodies. The secondary antibodies may be labeled with a fluorescent molecule, or they may be identified in other ways. Such methods have been widely used to demonstrate the localization of enzymes that are critical for synthesis or degradation of certain transmitters, such as tyrosine hydroxylase, which is necessary for the synthesis of dopamine and norepinephrine (Fig. 13.11), choline acetyltransferase (ChAT) for synthesis of actylcholine (Fig. 4.18), and GAD for GABA. Even transmitter molecules that are themselves too small to serve as antigens can be specifically identified in tissue sections with immunocytochemical methods when conjugated to

Figure 5.3 *Immunocytochemical demonstration of neurotransmitters.* An antibody binding to a GABA-protein complex in the section. The darkly stained perikarya, showing GABA-like immunoreactivity, are interneurons in a brain stem nucleus (monkey). The darkly stained fibers are partly dendrites, partly axons and boutons.

tissue proteins with glutaraldehyde. This is the case for GABA (Fig. 5.3), glutamate, and glycine. Immunocytochemical methods can also be applied to ultrastructural analysis, in order to determine the transmitter accumulated at specific synapses and also whether the transmitter is localized to certain organelles, such as presynaptic vesicles. Figures 5.4 and 5.5 show examples of demonstrating glycine in the spinal cord and GABA in the cerebellum, using secondary antibodies that are labeled with small gold particles (immuno-gold method). Since the gold particles are electron-dense, they appear as black dots in the electron micrographs. Such methods can also be used quantitatively in studies of relations between transmitters and different functional states and to determine whether diseases are related to alterations in specific transmitters.

Combination of axonal transport methods and immunocytochemical procedures makes it possible to determine both the connections as well as the transmitter candidates and other neuroactive substances of specific neuronal groups.

Figure 5.4 *Electron microscopic, immunocytochemical demonstration of neurotransmitters.* The small black dots represent gold particles bound in the tissue where GABA is present. The gold particles are conjugated to an antibody directed against a GABA-protein complex. The gold particles are concentrated over a particular kind of bouton (b), whereas dendrites (d) and part of a perikaryon (Gr) are not labeled. Another kind of bouton (Mf) is also unlabeled and most likely contains a neurotransmitter other than GABA. Rat cerebellum. Courtesy of Dr. O. P. Ottersen, Department of Anatomy, University of Oslo.

Gly 31

Even though the determination of the transmitter candidates present in a neuron is of great importance, it is not always possible to know whether the substance has been synthesized in the cell or whether it has merely been taken up. Furthermore, the concentration of transmitter in parts of a neuron may be so low that it cannot be reliably detected with immunocytochemical methods. The use of *in situ hybridization techniques* helps to overcome this kind of problem. By these methods, it is not the neuroactive peptides or enzymes related to transmitter metabolism that are demonstrated but the presence of the corresponding mRNA.

Immunocytochemical techniques are also used to study the distribution of molecules other than those assumed to function as transmitters, such as proteins and peptides that may play specific roles during development of the nervous system and molecules that may serve as markers to differentiate types of glial cells.

Techniques of molecular biology have also been instrumental in the localization and characterization of *receptors* and *ion channel proteins*. Receptors, for example, can be localized by binding to specific agonists or antagonists that are radioactively labeled, and their distribution can then be correlated with what is known of connections and distribution of transmitters for the cell groups under study. Specific binding of ligands to receptors also makes it possible to purify the receptor molecules of subsequent determination of their amino acid sequence. It is also possible to study changes in the receptor density after experimental manipulations. Receptor studies can also be carried out postmortally on the human brain—for example, to ascertain whether certain neurological and psy-

Figure 5.5 *Electron microscopic, immunocytochemical demonstration of neurotransmitters*. Experimental procedures corresponding to those in Figure 3.4, except that the antibody gold particle conjugate binds to a glycine protein complex in the tissue. M is part of a spinal motoneuron; B is a labeled bouton forming an axosomatic synapse; and b is an unlabeled bouton. A labeled and an unlabeled axon (Ax) are also seen. Glycine is an inhibitory neurotransmitter. The bar represents 1μm. Courtesy of Dr. O. P. Ottersen.

chiatric diseases are associated with alterations of specific transmitters and their receptors.

Lesion and Stimulation Experiments Are Used to Determine the Functions of Cell Groups

A fundamental approach to the study of the function of specific parts of the nervous system is to make circumscribed *lesions* and to observe the functional disturbances that ensue. Such a lesion may constitute interruption of fiber tracts, destruction of neurons within a nucleus, or removal of large parts, such as a whole lobe of the cerebral hemisphere. It is also possible to *cool* circumscribed regions reversibly, so that neurons are "silenced" only temporarily. Corresponding reversible effects can be obtained with the use of *local anesthetics*. To study the functional and behavioral changes, highly sophisticated test methods may be necessary. Also, control experiments with lesions of other parts are usually crucial.

Examples of lesion experiments in animals and observations in *humans with brain damage* are mentioned throughout in this book. The interpretation of the association between the normal function of the structures and the symptoms that ensue after lesions is often far from straightforward, however. For example, a lesion may destroy not only a certain group of neurons but also fibers passing through the area. The symptoms may in such cases be caused by dysfunction of neuronal groups distant from the lesion. The interpretation is generally least problematic when lesions are confined to large, well-delimited tracts, whereas symptoms after lesions of the cerebral cortex may be much more difficult to interpret. A fundamental problem remains, however, in all such experiments: To what extent can normal function of a part of the brain be deduced from the deficits and disturbances resulting from its removal? In many instances the symptoms occurring are for the most part a consequence of dysfunction and compensations of cell groups not damaged by the lesion.

Electrical stimulation of tracts and specific cell groups can be used to study their function, assuming that the physiological and behavioral effects are closely related to their normal function. One example is electrical stimulation of the motor cortex in the precentral gyrus, which elicits more or less isolated muscle contractions in the opposite side of the body. This example also illustrates the limitations of such methods: The experiments tell us that the motor cortex is of importance for the start of movements but tell us very little about how the complicated pattern of activity in many muscles, which is so characteristic of our voluntary movements, comes about. The difficulties of interpretation become much greater, however, when regions with multifarious connections with other parts of the brain are stimulated (this may be particularly obvious for stimulation experiments of the so-called limbic system; see Chapter 19, *Behavioral Effects after Damage or Stimulation of the Amygdala*).

Since stimulation experiments often have to be performed on anesthetized animals, this further limits the conclusions about normal function. Many cell groups are much less excitable during general anesthesia. This problem can be overcome to some extent by the use of *chronically implanted electrodes*, which enable stimulation to be carried out in conscious animals. Such electrodes are inserted in the brain under general anesthesia and are fixed to the skull to remain in place (the electrodes cause no pain because the nervous tissue is devoid of nociceptors). The behavioral effects of stimulation of specific parts can then be observed repeatedly. After the experiments, the exact location of the electrode can be verified histologically. Such experiments also entail problems of interpretation. After all, the evoked activity is artificial, and one usually cannot know whether identical patterns of activity occur naturally.

With the use of *autoradiography*, it is possible to map the metabolic activity of various brain regions in relation to specific stimuli or behaviors. Radioactively labeled *2-deoxyglucose* is given intravenously and is taken up by the neurons. Unlike glucose, however, deoxyglucose is not metabolized by the neurons and therefore accumulates. The neuronal uptake of glucose is closely related to the level of activity. After autoradiography of tissue sections, neuronal groups with high levels of deoxyglucose can be identified. These have most likely been particularly active just before the death of the animal and are therefore presumably related to whatever specific activities were going on at that time.

Recording of Single-Cell Activity

Microelectrodes, with tips less than 1 μm thick, can be used to record the activity of single neurons and their processes (single units) intracellularly. Among other things, this has made it possible to study in detail the electrical events at the synapses and how they are influenced by various experimental manipulations. The effects of different concentrations of ions intra- and extracellularly have been studied, as have the synaptic effects of various transmitter candidates and drugs. Thin implanted extracellular electrodes can be used to record the activity of single neurons in relation to specific stimuli or behavioral tasks. This method has, for example, provided new insight into functional specializations within various areas of the cerebral cortex.

The *voltage clamp* technique, which permits manipulation of the membrane potential, has been instrumental to our understanding of the properties of synapses and the basic mechanisms underlying their operations. Likewise, great progress has been made with the *patch clamp* technique, making possible measurements of ion currents limited to even single ion channels. The study of the properties of ion channels and membrane receptors is today highly interdisciplinary.

By combining anatomic and physiological techniques, it has been possible to determine the functional properties of structurally defined cell types. After intracellular recording has been made from a neuronal cell body or its axon, it can be filled with a tracer substance, such as HRP, through the same pipette. Afterwards, the neuron with all its processes can be visualized in sections. This has been done, for example, for several neuronal types in the dorsal horn of the spinal cord. Thus, the types of sensory receptors acting on the neuron can be identified before filling the neuron. In general, such techniques have provided important contributions to the correlation of structure and function in the nervous system.

The Living Human Brain Can Be Studied with Computer-Based Imaging Techniques

New techniques for computer-based image analysis of the living human brain have revolutionized the possibilities for localizing disease processes in the brain and for studying normal structure and function. In this chapter we have discussed some problems one encounters when trying to deduce the normal function of a brain structure from the symptoms occurring after the structure is damaged. Modern *neuroimaging techniques* permit the visualization of brain regions activated in conjunction with specific behaviors and mental operations. This is especially valuable for speech, solving abstract problems, and other functions that can only be studied in humans. Such functional studies are usually based on the observation that there is a *relationship between the blood flow through a brain region and the neuronal electrical activity*. The *regional cerebral blood flow* (rCBF) can now be measured with different techniques. A limitation of the rCBF is that it takes from a few hundred milliseconds to several seconds from an increase in neuronal activity to the blood flow increase. It furthermore takes some time—often around 60 sec—to make a reliable measurement, so that the method provides only an average for this period.

The mechanisms responsible for the coupling of neuronal activity to blood flow are not fully known, although animal experiments suggest that NO is at least partly responsible. Theoretically, NO should be well suited: It is produced in many neurons upon synaptic activation, it diffuses freely, and it causes vasodilation.

The first of the imaging techniques that enabled us to identify smaller parts of the living brain is CT. This method makes it possible to see X-ray pictures of thin slices through the brain. The plane of sectioning may be chosen by the examiner. CT affords much more precise visualization of brain structures than conventional X-ray examination, which includes all tissue between the X-ray tube and the film. It also provides good visualization of the ventricular system, which previously could be visualized only by replacing the CSF with air and then making an X-ray examination.

CT can also visualize the distribution of a radioactive substance in the living brain. This method is based on the use of isotopes that emit positrons. Positrons fuse immediately with electrons, producing two gamma rays going in opposite directions. This permits the identification of their origin in the brain with the aid of a powerful computer. This method, called *positron emission tomography* (PET), produces images that show the distribution of an inhaled or injected radioactively labeled substance at a given time. By labeling substances of biological interest, one can determine their distribution in the body. The *flow of blood* through specific parts of the brain, for example, can be correlated with certain stimuli or specific sensory, motor or mental activities. In such cases, radioactively labeled water is injected into the bloodstream. Also, the regional *metabolism* can be examined after injection of radioactively labeled deoxyglucose. Substances known to bind specifically to certain *receptor* types can also be labeled radioactively and injected. Thus, the normal distribution of such receptors can be determined, and possible changes in neurological and psychiatric diseases.

When PET is used to study the relationship between specific mental activities and regional cerebral blood flow, a *subtraction technique* has to be used. Thus, the blood flow measured before the test situation is subtracted from the blood flow during the activity (reading a text, doing a series of finger movements, identifying colors, imagining a familiar landscape, finding verbs to go with nouns, and so forth). There are many problems with the interpretation of such studies, however. One problem is variations among PET studies regarding what is used as the subtraction situation. Another complicating factor is that variations among subjects (regarding emotional status, attention, and so forth) may produce differences in cortical activity patterns even if the test situations are identical. Even with a simple task, such as deciding the orientation of an object, the subject will also covertly analyze other aspects of the object (name, what it is used for, and so forth). Thus, the activity pattern occurring in the test situation may not be related to the test alone.

A further technical development is represented by MRI. This technique is based not on X-rays but on signals emitted by protons when they are placed in a magnetic field. Depending on the proton concentration in different tissue components, the pictures may show clearly, for example, the contrast between gray and white matter (Figs. 3.2, 3.27, 3.29, 13.2, an 19.6). The bone of the skull gives very little or no signal and is seen as black in the pictures. With this technique, the brain can be visualized in slices with a resolution not far from that of a corresponding section through a fixed brain. Areas with changes in the tissue—for example, infarction, bleeding, or tumor—can be identified. Apart from the diagnostic advantages, the MRI technique also improves the correlation of the functional disturbances with the actual damage of the brain. MRI can also be used to study dynamic processes in the brain.

Functional MRI can visualize dynamic changes in the brain. This is because magnetic properties of hemoglobin depend on whether it is oxygenated or not, and small differences in blood oxyhemoglobin concentration can be detected with MRI. For unknown reasons, the oxygen uptake of nerve cells does not increase simultaneously with increased activity. Thus, it appears that neurons work anaerobically during a brief period of increased activity, despite a sufficient oxygen supply. The glucose uptake increases, however, and so does the blood flow. When the blood flow increases without increased oxygen uptake, more oxygen remains in the blood after passing the capillaries—that is, the arteriovenous O_2 difference is reduced. This change can be detected by MRI, and in this way the regions of increased or reduced blood flow can be visualized. An advantage compared with PET is that the picture of blood flow changes can be compared with the precise MRI picture of the same person's brain. This permits localization of blood flow changes to anatomic structures with a spatial resolution down to less than 2 mm.

A drawback of blood flow measurement as an indicator of neuronal activity, as mentioned above, is its low time resolution compared with the time scale for signal transmission in the brain. In this respect, recording the electrical activity of the brain is superior. This is usually done by placing many electrodes on the head, and is called *electroencephalography* (EEG), (see Chapter 15, *EEG*). A drawback with EEG is its low spatial resolution; that is, only a crude correlation is possible between electrical activity and its origin in the brain. A more recent technique, *magnetic encephalography* (MEG), records the magnetic fields produced by the electric activity of the brain. The spatial resolution is much better than with EEG—at best down to a few mm. (For both methods, however, the spatial resolution becomes poorer the deeper in the brain the source of activity is located.) A further advantage with the MEG technique is that it can be combined with MRI. This enables precise localization of the brain areas participating in a task, at the same time as the temporal aspects are analyzed (such as the sequence in which various cell groups are activated).

Methods of stimulating the brain in healthy volunteers are now available. Electric stimulation through the skull (transcranial) requires such high intensity that it is painful, and is therefore of limited use. However, a brief magnetic pulse applied outside the skull—*magnetic brain stimulation*—can activate cerebral cortical neurons without evoking pain. The magnetic field passes the skull and produces an electric current in the brain. It is primarily the superficial parts of the cerebral cortex that appear to be activated. The method has been mainly used to study connections from the motor cortex to spinal motoneurons in humans, both in healthy persons and in patients with neurological diseases, such as multiple sclerosis and stroke.

For the study of human brain function, the methods described above require cooperation between many specialists (physicists, chemists, neurophysiologists, neuroanatomists, neurologists, psychologists, computer experts, and statisticians). Furthermore, the equipment is very costly. Only a small number of centers around the world can therefore be expected to have the necessary competence. Conflicting data from different research groups, for example regarding brain activation during speech or the sensation of pain, betray the difficulties inherent in such studies. Although these methods are truly impressive and represent a great stride forward for neuroscience, they still give very crude pictures of what is really going on in the brain and how it handles mental operations. Sound interpretation requires continuous correlation of imaging data with clinical and neuropathological observations in patients with lesions of the brain, animal experiments, and psychological research.

PART II

SENSORY SYSTEMS

The first chapter in this part covers basic features common to all sensory receptors (sense organs). Such knowledge will make the reading of the following chapters easier. Chapter 7 deals with the *somatosensory system*, which is primarily concerned with sensory information from the *skin, joints, and muscles*; Chapter 8 with the *optic system* (vision); Chapter 9 with the *auditory system* (hearing); and Chapter 10 with the *olfactory* and the *gustatory systems* (smell and taste). For practical reasons, the sense of *equilibrium* is discussed in Chapter 16 (The Cranial Nerves), and sensory information from the *internal organs* (viscera) is dealt with in Chapter 17 (Peripheral Parts of the Autonomic Nervous System).

We use the term *system* to indicate that each of these senses is mediated—at least in part—in different regions of the nervous system. In neurobiology a *system usually means a set of interconnected neuronal groups that share a particular task, or several closely related tasks*. Sensory systems are designed to capture, transmit, and process information about events in the body and in the environment, such as light hitting the eye or the fullness of the bladder. We also use the term *system* for parts of the nervous system dealing with tasks other than sensory ones. The motor system, for example, initiates appropriate movements and maintains bodily postures.

The term *system* is being used rather loosely here: we do not imply that each system can be understood independently of the rest of the nervous system. Furthermore, it is often arbitrary as to which system a particular neuronal group is said to belong. Thus, usually a cell group is used in the operations of several systems. Especially at higher levels of the brain, information from various systems converge. Cortical cell groups, for example, may be devoted to both sensory processing and motor preparation. *Convergence of information* from several sensory systems seems necessary for us to perceive that the different kinds of information actually concern the same phenomenon, whether it is in our own body or in the environment. How do we know, for example, that the round object with a rough surface we hold in the hand is the same as the orange we see with our eyes?

Sometimes the term *system* is misused, so that it confuses rather than clarifies; this happens when we lump together in one system structures about which we know too little, or cell groups that have such widespread connections that they do not belong to a particular system. The wish to simplify a complex reality—and the nervous system *is* complicated—can sometimes become too strong.

CHAPTER 6

SENSORY RECEPTORS IN GENERAL

Sensory impulses from nearly all parts of the body are transmitted to the central nervous system, bringing information about conditions in the various tissues and organs and in our surroundings. The structures where sensory impulses originate are called *sense organs* or *receptors*. The receptors are formed either by the terminal branches of an axon (the skin, joints, muscles, internal organs) or by specialized sensory cells (the retina, taste buds, inner ear) that transmit the message to nerve terminals (Fig. 6.1). Note that we are using the word *receptor* differently here than in earlier chapters where we applied it to molecules with specific binding properties.

Sensory Units and Their Receptive Fields

Regardless of the structure of the receptor, a *sensory neuron* transmits the signal to the central nervous system. We also use the term *sensory unit* for *a sensory neuron with all its ramifications in the periphery and in the central nervous system* (Fig. 6.1). Such *primary* sensory neurons have their perikarya in ganglia close to the cord or the brain stem (similar neurons are found in the retina). The *receptive field* of the sensory neuron is the part of the body or the environment from which it samples information. The receptive field of a cutaneous sensory unit is a spot on the skin (see Fig. 7.10). For a sensory neuron in the retina, the receptive field is a part of the visual field (sending light to a particular spot on the retina). We can determine the receptive field of a sensory unit by recording with a thin electrode the action potentials produced in an axon or a cell body, and then systematically explore where it can be activated.

We will come back to the terms *sensory unit* and *receptive field* and exemplify them in the following chapters. It is important to note, how-

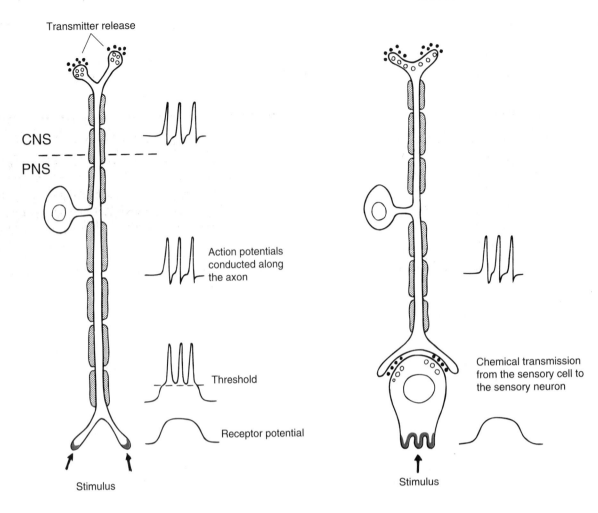

Figure 6.1 *Two main kinds of sensory receptors.* **Left**. The most common kind, found in most parts of the body. The receptor properties are found at the terminal ramifications of a sensory axon belonging to a pseudounipolar ganglion cell. **Right**. The kind found in the sense organs for taste, equilibrium and hearing. The receptor properties are located on a sensory cell that transmits the signal to a ganglion cell. In both kinds a stimulus produces a graded receptor potential. In the ganglion cell to the left an action potential results if the graded potential reaches the threshold. The sensory cell to the right does not produce an action potential but releases a chemical substance that depolarizes the terminals of the ganglion cell. In the CNS the signal is transmitted chemically to central sensory neurons.

ever, that they can be applied to sensory neurons at any level of the pathways leading from the receptors to the cerebral cortex. A neuron in the visual cortex, for example, reacts to light coming from only one particular part of the visual field, which represents the receptive field of the neuron (Fig. 8.8). At the cortical level the receptive field depends on convergence from several sensory units at lower levels (retina, thalamus). Thus, receptive fields are usually larger for cortical sensory units than for those closer to the sense organ.

Transduction: The Translation of Stimuli to Action Potentials

The task of the receptors is to respond to stimuli of various kinds. Regardless of the nature of the stimulus, the receptor "translates" the stimulus to the language spoken by the nervous system—that is, electrical impulses in the form of action potentials. We saw in Chapter 1 how summation of many synaptic inputs evokes an action potential (depolarization to threshold) that is propagated along the axon. In receptors, the *action potential arises close to the terminal branches of the sensory neuron.* This is true regardless of whether the stimulus acts directly on the terminal branches (as in the skin, Fig. 7.1) or indirectly via receptor cells (as in the retinal and the inner ear, Figs. 8.4 and 9.5). The stimulus alters the permeability of the receptor membrane, usually by opening Na^+ channels and thus depolarizing the receptor. The effect of the stimulus on ion channel openings is graded (like a synaptic potential, Fig. 2.9). This graded change in the membrane potential is called a *receptor potential.* The receptor potential arising in the terminal branches spreads electrotonically in the proximal direction (toward the CNS, Fig. 6.1) to the site where an action potential is formed (provided the receptor potential is strong enough). The process is similar to synaptic activation of a neuron since the action potential usually arises where the axon leaves the cell body. In sensory cells the stimulus leads to graded release of a chemical substance (transmitter) that depolarizes the terminals of the sensory cell (Fig. 6.1, right).

The mechanism behind "translation" or *transduction* of a stimulus to a receptor potential is not fully understood. Depolarization of receptors that are sensitive to particular chemical substances is most likely triggered by binding of the chemical to the membrane; either directly to channel proteins or to G protein–coupled receptors. The latter can then alter the opening state of ion channels via intracellular second messengers (such as cyclic adenosine monophosphate or guanosine monophosphate—cyclic AMP or GMP). For receptors sensitive to *mechanical* forces, movements of the cell membrane (stretching or shortening) induce the permeability changes. Since the membrane is fluid, we assume that the mechanical force is transmitted to membrane-receptor proteins via the rigid cytoskeleton (or similar structures outside the nerve terminal). Altering the shape of the protein alters its properties as well. For example, when light hits the photoreceptors in the retina, the photopigment is changed and this, in turn, leads to breakdown of cyclic GMP. Since cyclic GMP keeps Na^+ channels open, this leads to closure of Na^+ channels. Thus, the photoreceptors are hyperpolarized by light.

Receptor Properties

Most receptors are built to respond only or preferably to one kind of stimulus energy (mechanical, chemical, thermal, etc.). The kind of stimulus to which the receptor responds most easily—that is, with the lowest threshold—is called the *adequate stimulus* for the receptor. We also say that the receptor is specific for this type of stimuli, whether it is mechanical, chemical, electromagnetic (light), or thermal (warmth, cold). As we shall see, each of these broad groups of stimuli may be registered by receptors with different properites. There are, for example, several kinds of mechanoreceptors and receptors responding to chemical substances in the tissue fluid.

When a particular kind of receptor is stimulated with sufficient intensity to cause a consciously perceived sensation, we always get the same kind or *modality*[1] of sensory experience (for example, light, touch, pressure, warmth, pain, sound). This does not imply, however, that the receptor necessarily has been subjected to its adequate stimulus. Thus, most receptors can respond also to stimuli of other kinds (inadequate stimuli), although the threshold then is much higher for evoking a response. As an example, we can mention the perception of light upon a blow to the eye (mechanical stimulus of the receptors rather than the normal light stimulus), and perception of sound upon chemical, rather than the normal mechanical, irritation of the receptors for hearing. *The kind of perceived sensation—the quality or modality of sensation—is thus characteristic for each type of receptor* (the "law of specific nerve energies" of Müller). Irritation of the axon leading from the receptor will also evoke the same sensory modality as when the receptor is stimulated by its adequate stimulus.

Receptors differ not only with regard to their adequate stimulus or specificity. Many receptors send action potentials only when a stimulus starts (or stops). If the stimulus is continuous, this kind of receptor ceases to respond and thus provides information about changes in stimulation only. Such receptors are called *rapidly adapting*. When after a short time we cease noticing that something touches the skin, this is partly because so many of the receptors in the skin are of the rapidly adapting type. Other receptors, however, go on responding (and thus sending action potentials) as long as the stimulus continues. Such receptors are called *slowly adapting*. One example of slowly adapting receptors is those that are responsible for the sensation of pain. It would not be appropriate if the body were to adapt to painful stimuli since these usually signal danger and threat of tissue damage. Receptors signaling the position of the body in space and the position of our bodily parts in relation to each other must also be slowly adapting; if not, we would lose this kind of information after a few seconds if no movement took place. Adaptation is a property of the receptors themselves, and not (only) of processing within the central nervous system, as can be verified by recording the action potentials from sensory fibers supplying various kinds of receptors. For example, afferent fibers from receptors excited by warming of the skin stop sending impulses if the same stimulus is maintained for some time, whereas afferent nerve fibers from sense organs in a muscle continue to send impulses as long as the muscle is held in a stretched position.

Many receptors respond more vigorously to rapid changes in the stimulus than to slow ones. For example, rapid stretch of a muscle produces much higher firing frequency in the sensory nerve fibers leading from the muscle than when the same stretch is applied slowly (see Fig. 7.6). Such a receptor can therefore inform about the *velocity* of stretching—not only its magnitude. This property of a receptor is called *dynamic sensitivity*. A receptor that continues to produce action potentials with a constant frequency as long as the stimulus is constant (slowly adapting or non-adapting) is said to have *static sensitivity*. Often, one receptor has both kinds of sensitivity (Fig. 7.6). The majority of receptors, however, have dynamic sensitivity and are rapidly adapting. This helps to explain the everyday experience that we are much more aware of changing stimuli than those that are constant—such as an insect moving on the skin or a moving light as opposed to stationary ones.

Classification of Receptors on the Basis of Their Properties

Receptors can be characterized and classified in accordance with the nature of their *adequate stimulus*. A large group of receptors, the *mechanore-*

ceptors, responds primarily to distortion of the tissue in which they lie and thus informs the central nervous system about mechanical stimuli. Such receptors are numerous in the skin, deep tissues like muscles and joint capsules, and in internal organs. Many mechanoreceptors have a low threshold and send impulses even on the slightest touch of the skin or a just barely perceptible movement of a joint. Other mechanoreceptors require very strong stimulation to respond; such stimuli are usually perceived as painful. Depending on their location, mechanoreceptors may give information of very different events (even though all are mechanical): A low-threshold mechanoreceptor in the wall of the urinary bladder provides information about its degree of distension, and mechanoreceptors in the inner ear inform us about sound (movement of air molecules), whereas mechanoreceptors around the root of a hair respond to the slightest bending of the hair.

Another large group of receptors, *chemoreceptors*, responds primarily to certain chemical substances in the interstitial fluid surrounding the receptor. Many chemoreceptors respond to substances produced by or released from cells as a result of tissue damage and inflammation, regardless of the cause (mechanical trauma, burns, infection, and so forth). Other kinds of chemoreceptors are the receptors for taste and smell.

Receptors in the retina responding (with an extremely low threshold) to *visible light* are called *photoreceptors. Thermoreceptors* respond most easily to warming or cooling of the tissue in which they lie.

Receptors can also be classified on the basis of the *origin of their adequate stimulus.* This system for classification of receptors is convenient and functionally meaningful. We usually distinguish between *exteroceptors, proprioceptors*, and *enteroceptors. Exteroceptive impulses* reach the body from the outside, from our environment. Most exteroceptors are located in the skin, whereas the receptors in the eye and the internal ear represent important special kinds of exteroceptors responding to teleceptive impulses. *Proprioceptive impulses* originate in the body itself. The term is mostly restricted, however, to impulses arising in the musculoskeletal system, including the joints. *Enteroceptive impulses* arise from the internal (visceral) organs.

By the description above, we can classify receptors depending upon which characteristics we want to emphasize. We can also give a complete description of the receptor by mentioning all the characteristic properties, for example a proprioceptive, fast-adapting, low-threshold mechanoreceptor (informing about joint rotation), or an enteroceptive, slowly-adapting chemoreceptor (in the wall of an artery and informing about the oxygen tension of the blood).

Classification of Receptors on the Basis of Subjective Sensory Experience

Although more problematic than the above kinds of classification, receptors are also commonly classified by the conscious sensory experience they are believed to evoke. Thus, we use the term *pain receptor* to describe receptors that, when stimulated, produce pain. Stimulation of *cold receptors* causes a feeling of coldness, stimulation of *warm receptors* gives a feeling of warmth, and so on. Only exceptionally is it possible, however, to know whether a sensory experience is caused by one receptor type only, or by the simultaneous activation of several kinds. The connection between the conscious sensory experience and the responsible receptors is therefore often uncertain. Since only human beings can inform the observer directly of what they feel, animal experiments alone cannot resolve the question of the relation between receptors and conscious sensations. On the other hand, the very same receptors examined physiologically cannot be examined anatomically in human beings. Important insight has nevertheless emerged from correlation of observations obtained in animals with psychophysical observation in humans (see Chapter 7, *Microneurography*).

Not all impulses reaching the central nervous system from the receptors are consciously perceived. In particular, enteroceptive impulses are mostly processed only at a subconscious level. For impulses from all kinds of receptors, however, a considerable selection and suppression of signals take place at all levels of the sensory pathways in the spinal cord and the brain, to leave out "irrelevant" information. At the same time, "relevant" signals may be enhanced in the central nervous system—for example, to increase the contrasts in a visual scene (see Chapter 7, *Inhibitory Interneurons Improve Discriminative Sensation*).

We cannot explain how it happens that action potentials, which are of the same kind in all nerve fibers, evoke entirely different conscious sensations depending on where the stimulus arises. One prerequisite is that different kinds of sensory information are analyzed by different neurons (that is, neurons located in anatomically distinct parts of the central nervous system). A complete mixing of information from different receptor types would not be compatible with our discriminative abilities. It is equally, clear, however, that there must be ways in which the brain can bring the different kinds of information together and make a synthesis. Such a synthesis may not necessarlily be due to convergence of all relevant information onto a single cell group. Rather, we now believe the final processing to depend on extensive interconnections among cortical areas dealing with different aspects of sensory information.

NOTES

1. The words *modality* and *quality* are both used to describe aspects of sensation but unfortunately somewhat differently by various authors. Quality is used here to describe further the nature of a sensory modality—for example, pain is a sensory modality that may have a burning quality.

CHAPTER 7

THE SOMATOSENSORY SYSTEM

The term *somatosensory* includes, strictly speaking, all sensations pertaining to the body (soma). It is therefore more comprehensive than the significance commonly assigned to it—namely, *sensory information from skin, joints, and muscles only.*

EXTEROCEPTORS: CUTANEOUS SENSATION

The skin and the subcutaneous tissue contain receptors that respond to stimuli from our surroundings. Among the almost indefinitely varied sensory experiences that can be evoked from the skin, we usually distinguish only a few, regarded as the basic modalities: *touch, pressure, heat, cold,* and *pain.* There is indirect evidence that each of these sensations can be evoked by stimulation of one receptor type. Yet it is important to realize that terms such as pain, cold, and touch refer to the quality of our subjective sensory experience evoked by certain kinds of stimuli. Thus, a classification of sensations on this basis does not enable us to conclude that for each subjective quality of sensation there exists one particular kind of receptor.

Sensations such as itch, tickle, dampness, or dryness, the texture of surfaces, and the firmness or softness of objects are thought to arise from the simultaneous stimulation of several kinds of receptors in the skin and also in deeper tissues. As mentioned earlier, our conscious sensory experience is the result of a synthesis in the brain of information from a multitude of receptors.

Functionally, skin receptors—as receptors in other parts of the body—can be classified by their adequate stimulus as *mechanoreceptors*, *thermoreceptors*, and *chemoreceptors*.

The Structure of the Skin

The skin consists of two layers (Fig. 7.1). The upper layer, the *epidermis*, consists of stratified squamous epithelium. Like all epithelia, the epidermis lacks vessels and is nourished by capillaries in the underlying dermis. This is built of relatively dense connective tissue with numerous collagen fibers. The dermis sends small projections, *dermal papillae*, upward into the epidermis. In the dermis and partly in the loose connective tissue beneath it—the subcutaneous layer—there are sweat glands and sebaceous glands. The hairs, obliquely oriented to the surface of the skin, have their roots in the upper parts of the subcutaneous layer. A tiny smooth muscle runs obliquely from the root of the hair upward to the upper part of the dermis (the arrector pili muscle). Contraction of this muscle straightens the hair so that it stands more perpendicular to the surface of the skin.

Free and Encapsulated Receptors

Receptors in the skin (and also in deep tissues) are conveniently subdivided on a structural basis into *free* and *encapsulated*, although there are numerous transitional forms. In encapsulated receptors, the terminal ramifications of the sensory axon are surrounded by a specialized capsule-like structure of connective tissue cells, whereas such a structure is lacking around the free receptors or endings (Fig. 7.1). The encapsulation serves as a filter, so that only certain kinds of stimuli reach the axon terminal inside. The axonal ramifications of the free receptors are covered by Schwann cells, except at their tips, where their receptor properties presumably reside. Free receptors are the most numerous and widespread, being present in virtually all parts of the body. In the *skin*, free receptors are particularly numerous in the upper parts of the dermis, and they also extend for a short distance between the cells of the deeper layers of the epidermis.

Free receptors that are structurally indistinguishable can nevertheless have different adequate stimuli. The cornea of the eye, for example, contains only free nerve endings but functionally there are at least four different receptors. *Thus, anatomically identical receptors can differ functionally.* This can be explained by their expression of different repertoires of membrane channels and receptor molecules.

Nociceptors

Nociceptors in the skin and as far as we know, in all other tissues from which painful sensations can be evoked, are *free receptors*. It is characteristic that most stimuli we experience as painful are so intense that they *produce tissue damage or will do so if the stimulus is continued*. Functionally, skin nociceptors are of two main kinds: One responds to intense mechanical stimulation only (such as pinching, cutting, stretching) and is therefore termed *high-threshold mechanoreceptor*. The other kind is also activated by intense mechanical stimuli but, in addition, by intense warming of the skin (above 45°C) and by chemical substances that are liberated by tissue damage and inflammation. Because they can be activated

Meissner's corpuscle   Merkel cell   Fr.

EPIDERMIS

DERMIS

Ruffini's corpuscle

SUBCUTIS

Pacinian corpuscle

A

B

Myelin sheath

Schwann cell

C   D   E

Figure 7.1 *Cutaneous receptors.* Schematic drawing of receptors as they appear in sections through the skin. Sensory nerve fibers and receptors in (**A**) glabrous skin (palms of the hands and soles of the feet) and (**B**) hairy skin. Nerve endings in hairy skin wind around the hair follicles and are activated by the slightest bending of the hair. **C.** Meissner corpuscle (from glabrous skin). The axon (red) follows a tortuous course between flat, specialized connective tissue cells. The whole sense organ is anchored to the epidermis with thin collagen fibers. **D.** A disk of Merkel (present in both glabrous and hairy skin). The axonal terminal is closely apposed to a Merkel cell in the epidermal cell layer. **E.** Free nerve endings are covered by Schwann cells except at their tips, where, presumably, the receptor properties reside.

by different sensory modalities, such receptors are termed *polymodal nociceptors*. Recent studies indicate, however, that there are in addition *many nociceptors that are purely sensitive to chemical substances* (see below).

A characteristic feature of nociceptors is their tendency to be *sensitized* by prolonged stimulation. This partly explains why even normally nonnoxious stimuli (such as touching the skin) may be felt as painful when the skin is inflamed (inflammation acitvates a large number of nociceptors). This condition of lowered threshold for evoking pain is called *hyperalgesia*. As we shall return to below, hyperalgesia may also be caused by altered properties of neurons in the central nervous system, especially in the spinal dorsal horn.

Not All Nociceptors May Signal Tissue Damage

Recent studies show that there are many sensory units in the skin and in deep tissues (muscles, joints, internal organs) that respond only to chemical substances liberated by *inflammation*. They therefore presumably contribute to the pain evoked by tissue damage, although they respond neither to mechanical stimuli nor high temperatures (above 45° C, which is known to activate polymodal nociceptors). Consequently, such receptors are not activated under most conditions used to study nociceptors. This probably explains why such "silent nociceptors" were not discovered earlier. It is possible that they do not function primarily as a warning system for impending tissue damage but rather "play a more general long-term role in evaluating and signaling the status of the microenvironment in peripheral tissue," as suggested by the British neurophysiologist McMahon. Information from tissue chemoreceptors or silent nociceptors presumably plays an important role in the cooperation between the nervous system and the immune system. Thus, we know that the nervous system can influence the properties of the cells of the immune system, as we shall return to in Chapter 18. To do this, the nervous system needs information from the "battlefield" of the immune system.

Itch and Tickle

Itching is a peculiar, unpleasant sensation evoked by stimulation of free nerve endings in superficial parts of the skin and mucous membranes. The signals are conducted in unmyelinated sensory fibers to the spinal cord. From the cord to higher levels, the signals follow the pathways for pain, since cutting these also abolishes the sensation of itching. Furthermore, itching is usually evoked by liberation of *histamine* in the skin, for example from mast cells in allergic reactions. The leaves of stinging nettle (*Urtica dioica*) provoke intense itching because they contain histamine. Microneurographic studies in humans have identified a subgroup of peripheral sensory units (with unmyelinated fibers) that react vigorously to histamine but also to noxious stimuli. Even at the level of the cerebral cortex, units responding to histamine appear always to respond to noxious stimuli as well. Many other sensory units—in the cord and in the cortex—respond to noxious stimuli but not to histamine. If, however, all units responding to histamine (evoking itching) also are activated by noxious stimuli, how can we then explain that we experience itching and pain as two distinct sensations? In fact, we also know that weakly painful stimuli—such as scratching the skin—*suppress* the sensation of itching. It is of course possible that "itch specific" receptors exist but have not yet been found, because they probably are very few compared to nociceptors. Other explanations are now considered more likely, however. One theory attributes the specific sensation of itching to a particular *pattern of impulses* in the sensory units responding both to histamine and to noxious stimuli. Another theory assumes that there are neurons in the cord that respond only to histamine-activated sensory units. Although these neurons would be activated by noxious stimuli as well, this would always occur in conjunction with activation of other neurons responding only to noxious stimuli. If itching stimuli were applied alone, only the central "itch neurons" would be activated. In this way, signals from *both* "itch neurons" and "pain neurons" would be interpreted as pain, whereas signals from the "itch neurons" alone would evoke a sensation of itching. This theory at least fits with the observation that pain suppresses the itching.

Tickling is another peculiar sensory phenomenon. It is evoked upon stimulation of low-threshold mechanoreceptors although we do not know which subgroup is involved. The sensation of tickling is strongly influenced by emotions: The same stimulus may be experienced as tickling in one situation and merely as light tough in another. This example may serve to emphasize a point we will return to repeatedly, namely that the sensory messages sent from the receptors are subject to extensive processing before a conscious sensation is produced.

Thermoreceptors

It was previously believed that cold and warm stimuli were mediated by two kinds of encapsulated receptors (the Krause and Ruffini corpuscles, respectively). This cannot be the case, however, since sensations of both cold and heat can be perceived from regions of the skin containing only free receptors. Combined physiological and histological analysis has also strengthened the view that free endings are responsible for the perception of heat and cold. Nevertheless, there are two kinds of thermoreceptors, even though they look the same.

Cold receptors respond with an increase of firing frequency to cooling of the skin below the normal temperature (about 32° C). They stop responding, however, at very low skin temperatures. Surprisingly, cold receptors can also be excited by skin temperatures above 45° C. This explains why a hot shower may feel cold at the beginning (until we feel pain, as mentioned above, temperatures above 45° C excite polymodal nociceptors). This phenomenon is called *paradoxical cold (sensation)*.

Warm receptors respond to warming of the skin above the normal temperature up to about 45° C.

The *adequate stimulus* for thermoreceptors is the temperature of the tissue surrounding them or, rather, *changes* in the temperature. The receptors send action potentials with a relatively low frequency at a steady temperature, whereas a small change in the temperature elicits a marked change in the firing frequency. A heat receptor, for example, may at constant room temperature fire with a low frequency, but if the skin is warmed even slightly, there is a marked increase in the firing rate. The response is particularly brisk if the warming happens rapidly (thus, lukewarm water may be perceived as hot if the hand is cold when put into it). A change in skin temperature of 0.2° C is sufficient to cause a marked change in firing rate from a thermoreceptor. Thus, the *thermoreceptors do not give an objective measure of the actual skin temperature but rather signal changes that may be of significance for our adjustment to the environment (to keep the body temperature constant)*.

Mechanoreceptors of the Skin

The study of receptors for pain and temperature sensation is more difficult than the study of mechanoreceptors. These are therefore particularly well studied, and among them we know most about the *low-threshold mechanoreceptors*. The following account will mainly deal with low-threshold mechanoreceptors of the skin. *High-threshold mechanoreceptors* in the skin are nociceptors, and do not differ significantly from such receptors in muscles and around joints. As far as we know, they are always formed by free nerve endings (Fig. 7.1).

There are several kinds of low-threshold mechanoreceptors in the skin, ranging from free receptors to those with an elaborate capsule. Some adapt slowly or not at all; others adapt very rapidly. An example of rapidly adapting receptors is those found close to the roots of hairs (Fig. 7.1B). They are stimulated by even the slightest bending of a hair, as can be easily verified by touching the hairs on the back of one's own hand. If the hair is held in the new position, however, the sensation disappears immediately.

The thick, *glabrous skin* on the palm of the hand and on the sole of the foot lacks hair. Elaborate encapsulated receptors are, however, particularly abundant at these locations. They are obviously related to the superior sensory abilities of these parts, the fingers in particular. One such receptor is the *Meissner corpuscle*, mediating information about touch (Fig. 7.1C). These are small oval bodies located in the dermal papillae just beneath the epidermis (in fact, as close to the surface of the skin as possible without being directly exposed). Several axons approach the corpuscle and follow a tortuous course inside the capsule, between the lamellae formed by connective tissue cells. The Meissner corpuscles respond by sending action potentials even when the skin overlying the receptor is pressed down only a few micrometers. If the skin is kept in this position, however, the receptor stops sending action potentials, whereas a few action potentials are elicited on release of the pressure. The Meissner corpuscle is thus *rapidly adapting*, and it also obviously has a low threshold for its adequate stimulus. It is presumably well suited, among other things, to *signal direction and velocity of objects moving on the skin*.

The *Ruffini corpuscles* are also low-threshold mechanoreceptors and are most likely *slowly adapting*. They consist of a bundle of collagen fibrils with a sensory axon branching between the fibrils (Fig. 7.1A). The collagen fibrils are connected with those in the dermis, and stretching of the skin in the direction of the fibrils is the adequate stimulus for the receptor. This tightens the fibrils, which in turn leads to deformation and depolarization of the axonal ramifications, thus producing action potentials in the afferent fiber. It is therefore assumed that the Ruffini corpuscle functions as a low-threshold *stretch receptor of the skin*, informing us about the magnitude and direction of stretch.

Another kind of *slowly adapting*, low-threshold mechanoreceptor in the skin is the *Merkel's disk* (Fig. 7.1A and D), present particularly on the distal parts of the extremities, on the lips, and the external genitals. An axon ends in close contact with a large epithelial cell in the basal layer of the epidermis. Even after several minutes of constant pressure on the skin overlying the receptors, they continue to send action potentials at about the same rate.

Finally, a fourth type of low-threshold mechanoreceptor, the *Pacinian corpuscle* (Fig. 7.1A), is found at the junction between the dermis and the subcutaneous layer (it is also present at other locations, such as in the mesenteries, vessel walls, joint capsules, and in the periosteum). These are large (up to several millimeters long) ovoid bodies, which can be seen macroscopically at dissection. A thick, unbranched axon is surrounded by numerous lamellae formed by a special kind of connective tissue cell. Between the cellular lamellae there are fluid-filled spaces. The Pacininan corpuscle is *very rapidly adapting*, eliciting only one or two action potentials in the afferent fiber at the onset of indentation of the skin. The adequate stimulus is therefore extremely rapid indentation of the skin. In practice, this is achieved by *vibration* with a frequency of 100–400 Hz. If a vibrating probe is put in contact with the skin, the frequency of action potentials in the afferent fiber follows closely the frequency of vibration. Vibration with a frequency below 100 Hz appears to be signaled by the Meissner corpuscles.

What Information Is Signaled by Low-Threshold Cutaneous Mechanoreceptors?

Together, the four types of low-threshold mechanoreceptors described above are thought to mediate the different qualities of our sense of touch and pressure, which are so well developed in glabrous skin (fingers, toes, and lips). One important aspect is the ability to judge the speed and direction of a *moving object* in contact with the skin, as well as the *friction* between them. Thus, we may perceive quickly that an object is slipping from our grip and also judge from the friction the force needed to stop the movement. Two of the receptor types, the Merkel disks and the Ruffini corpuscles, are slowly adapting and, as long as the stimulus lasts, continue to provide information about slight pressure and stretching of the skin, respectively. The two others, the Meissner and the Pacinian corpuscles, are rapidly adapting and signal only the start and stop of stimuli. It seems likely that the Meissner corpuscles would be particularly well suited to signal the direction and speed of a moving stimulus (see *Microneurography*, below).

Free Receptors May Have Different Functional Properties

It was previously thought that each sensory modality has a corresponding morphologically distinct receptor. This simplistic view cannot be upheld, however. In particular, there are numerous examples of free receptors that are structurally indistinguishable but have quite different adequate stimuli, as mentioned above.

There is good evidence that all nociceptors are free endings of thin myelinated and unmyelinated axons, even though there are at least two subgroups of nociceptors (high-threshold and polymodal). Furthermore, low-threshold mechanoreceptors for touch are not always of the encapsulated type described above (Meissner, Ruffini, and others) but may also be of the free-ending type. Cold and heat receptors are also structurally free endings of axons, as mentioned above.

Punctate Localization of Cutaneous Sensation: Receptive Fields

It has been known for a long time that cutaneous sensation is punctate; that is, there are distinct tiny spots on the skin that are sensitive to different sensory modalities. We therefore use the terms cold, warm, touch, and pain spots. Cold spots are most easily demonstrated. Between the spots sensitive to cooling of the skin, there are others where contact with a cold object is felt only as pressure. This is so because each *sensory unit* distributes all its peripheral ramifications within a limited area of the skin. Thus, the sensory unit can be activated only from this part of the skin, called its *receptive field* (Fig. 7.2). Certain parts of the skin lack ramifications belonging to "cold" sensory units, and consequently sensations of cold cannot be evoked from such areas.

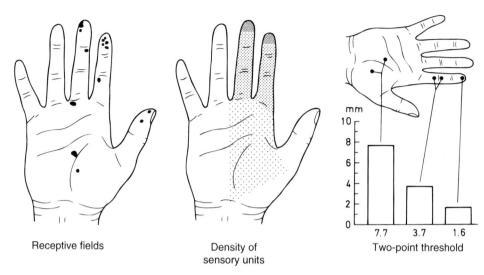

Receptive fields   Density of   Two-point threshold
                           sensory units

Figure 7.2 *Receptive fields*. **A**. Size and location of the receptive fields of 15 sensory units, determined by recording from the median nerve. All of these sensory units were rapidly adapting and were most likely conducting from Meissner corpuscles. Within each receptive field there are many Meissner corpuscles, all supplied by the same axon. **B**. Relative density of sensory units conducting from Meissner corpuscles (that is, number of sensory units supplying 1 cm²). Note that the density increases distally and is highest at the volar aspect of the fingertips. **C**. Two-point discrimination. The numbers give the shortest distance between two points touching the skin that can be identified by the experimental subject as two (reducing the distance further makes the person experience only one point touching the skin). Average of 10 subjects. Based on microneurographic studies by Vallbo and Johansson (1978).

Correspondingly, many small spots on proximal parts of the body, for example on the abdomen and the upper arm, lack nociceptors. Insertion of a sharp needle at such places is therefore only felt as touch. The receptive fields of nociceptive sensory units are so closely spaced, however, that one has to make a thorough search to find painless spots.

The size of the receptive field depends on the area of the skin receiving axonal branches from the sensory neuron. In general, the density of sensory units—that is, the number of units innervating, for example, 1 cm² of the skin—is highest in distal parts of the body (fingers, toes, and lips) (Fig. 7.2), and the receptive fields are smaller distally than proximally. This explains why the stimulus threshold is lower and the ability to localize a stimulus is more precise in the palm of the hand than at, for example, the upper arm.

Discriminative Sensation

The punctate arrangement of the cutaneous sensation is of importance for our *ability to localize stimuli*. Being able to determine that the skin is touched by two pointed objects (like the legs of a compass) rather than one must mean that the two spots are innervated by separate units. The distance between two points on the skin that, when touched, can be identified as two is not surprisingly shortest where the density of sensory units is highest, and the receptive fields are smallest—that is, on the fingertips (Fig. 7.2). Determining this distance gives a measure of what is called *two-point discrimination* and is often used clinically. The smallest distance at which two stimuli can be discriminated, is called the *two-point threshold* (Fig. 7.2). Another useful test for this kind of *discriminative sensation* is the writing of letters or figures on the skin (with the subject's eyes closed). The figures that can be interpreted are quite small on the fingertips, somewhat larger on the palms, much larger on the upper arm, and even larger on the trunk. The pathways conducting the sensory impulses from the spots on the skin are, as one might expect, arranged topographically so that impulses from different parts of the skin are kept separate at all levels up to the cerebral cortex.

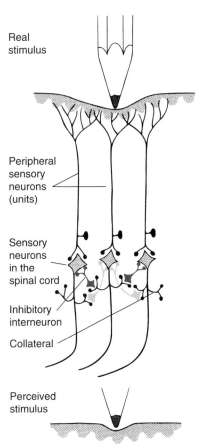

Real
stimulus

Peripheral
sensory
neurons
(units)

Sensory
neurons
in the
spinal cord

Inhibitory
interneuron

Collateral

Perceived
stimulus

Figure 7.3 *Lateral inhibition*. Simplified presentation of how inhibitory interneurons in the central nervous system can improve the precision of the sensory information reaching consciousness.

Lateral Inhibition: Inhibitory Interneurons Improve the Discriminative Sensation

The two-point threshold (Fig. 7.2) depends not only on the size and density of the cutaneous receptive fields. *Inhibitory interneurons* in the cord (and at higher levels) restrict the signal traffic from the periphery of a stimulated spot, thereby improving the discriminative ability compared with what might be expected from the anatomic arrangement of receptive fields (Fig. 7.3). This phenomenon is called *lateral inhibition*. The cutaneous sensory units (neurons) send off collaterals in the central nervous system that activate inhibitory interneurons that in turn inhibit sensory neurons in the vicinity. Figure 7.3 shows an example with a pencil pressed lightly onto the skin. The sensory units with receptive fields in the center of the stimulated spot receive the most intense stimulation. Therefore, they excite the inhibitory interneurons strongly, with consequent strong inhibition of sensory units leading from the periphery of the spot. Sensory units with receptive fields in the periphery are less strongly stimulated but receive strong inhibition. Thus, they cannot inhibit the transmission of signals from the center of the spot. Together, the impulse traffic from the periphery of the stimulated area is reduced, and we perceive the stimulated area as smaller and more sharply delimited than it really is. In this way, the central nervous system receives sensory information that is distorted.

Microneurography

Studies with techniques that enable recording from and stimulation of peripheral nerves in conscious human beings have provided important information with regard to the functional properties of receptors (Fig. 7.2). This technique was pioneered by the Swedish neurophysiologists Hagbarth, Vallbo, Johansson, and others. With the use of very thin needle electrodes, it has been possible to record the activity of single sensory axons within a nerve, such as the median nerve at the forearm. Thus, it is possible to determine the receptive field of this particular sensory unit, and also its adequate stimulus. In glabrous skin of the fingers and palms, *four types of low-threshold mechanoreceptors* have been so characterized. Most likely, they correspond to the four encapsulated types described above. Thus, there are two types of rapidly adapting sensory units, one with a small receptive field (most likely the Meissner corpuscle) and the other with a large and indistinct receptive field (Pacinian corpuscle). The two other types of sensory units are slowly adapting, and again one has a small receptive field (Merkel's disk) and the other a large but direction-specific receptive field (most likely the Ruffini corpuscle).

Stimulation of the axons of the sensory units that have just been recorded from enables correlations to be made between the conscious sensory experience evoked by stimulation of only one sensory unit. Stimulation of single sensory units most likely ending in Meissner corpuscles produces a feeling of light touch, like a tap on the skin with the point of a pencil. As a rule, the person localizes the feeling to exactly the point on the skin previously found to be the receptive field of the sensory unit. Activating a sensory unit that presumably leads off from Merkel's disks evokes a sensation of light, steady pressure (as long as the stimulus lasts). Stimulating axons that appear to end in Pacinian corpuscles gives a feeling of vibration. For unknown reasons, no conscious sensation has so far been evoked by stimulating slowly adapting, stretch-sensitive sensory units of the skin (presumably Ruffini corpuscles).

PROPRIOCEPTORS: DEEP SENSATION

As mentioned above, the term *proprioceptive* is used for sensations pertaining to the *musculoskeletal system*—that is, muscles, tendons, joint capsules, and ligaments. There are many similarities in structure and basic properties between proprioceptors and cutaneous receptors. There are, for example, numerous free receptors (belonging to thin myelinated and unmyelinated axons) in the muscles, the muscle fascia, and in the dense connective tissue of joint capsules and ligaments. Many of these are *nociceptors* as in the skin. Here, however, we are going to deal primarily with specialized, encapsulated sense organs in muscles and around joints. These are all *low-threshold mechanoreceptors*, and the signals from them are conducted centrally in thick, myelinated axons. The *adequate stimulus* of these receptors is *stretching of the tissue in which they lie*. Whether located in a muscle or in a joint capsule, joint movement is the natural stimulus that leads to activation of such receptors.

Nociceptors in Muscles

As mentioned, muscles are supplied with numerous free nerve endings of thin myelinated and unmyelinated axons (that is, the most slowly conducting fibers). Microscopic examination of muscle nerves in experimental animals shows that almost 40% of all the axons are either thin myelinated or unmyelinated sensory fibers, ending with free endings (Fig. 7.4). *Many—probably the majority—of the unmyelinated and thin myeli-*

nated axons lead from nociceptors in the muscle. This has been shown by recording the activity of single sensory units innervating a muscle while systematically exploring their adequate stimuli. Such units could be excited both by strong mechanical stimuli and substances liberated in inflamed tissue (such as bradykinin, known to provoke pain in humans). Inflammation also *sensitized* the nociceptive sensory units, making them respond to normal movements (this may partly explain the muscle soreness after heavy exercise). Like cutaneous nociceptors, those in muscle were sensitized also by prolonged stimulation. Some sensory units were activated by *ischemia*. It is well known that muscle ischemia, for example caused by a thrombotic artery, produces pain in humans.

Microneurography has shown the presence of sensory units with nociceptor-like properties also in human muscle nerves. Such units are slowly adapting, have high a threshold for mechanical stimuli, and can be activated by inflammatory substances (like those described above in experimental animals). Electrical stimulation of small nerve fascicles in human muscle nerves produces pain as the only sensory experience. The pain is felt to be deep (not in the skin) and has a *cramp-like quality*. The subject localizes the pain to the muscle supplied by the nerve, not to the site of nerve stimulation that is at a distance from the muscle. These findings have been confirmed by recording and stimulation of single sensory fibers. If the stimulation goes on, or is increased in intensity, the pain radiates to other regions than the muscle itself (this phenomenon is called *referred pain*; see below, *Spinothalamic Cells Receive Impulses from Both Somatic and Visceral Structures: Referred Pain*). Also, axons from nociceptors in a muscle *tendon* have been investigated with microneurography. Stimulation of such a sensory unit produced a sharp pain, different from the muscle pain described above. The pain was localized to the tendon by the subject.

Other Kinds of Free Receptors in Muscles

Not all the thin, slowly conducting sensory fibers in a muscle nerve are nociceptors. Thus, in experimental animals some of these fibers are activated by ordinary muscle contraction or gentle stretching of the muscle. Their maximal firing rate is reached by stimuli much weaker than those required to produce pain. Such receptors may be responsible for *circulatory and respiratory reflex effects* known to occur at the start of muscular activity. Thus, there is a slight increase of pulse and breathing rate that occurs too early to be caused by a rise in blood CO_2 or lowered pH. Although the receptors responsible for such reflex effects are not identified with certainty, they are called *ergoreceptors*.

Other non-nociceptor, slowly conducting sensory fibers in muscle nerves might mediate sensory signals responsible for the central effects of needle *acupuncture*, produced by rotating thin needles in a muscle. A further role suggested for such fibers is to mediate sensory signals that *inhibit the feeling of pain during physical exercise*. However, recent studies question whether there really is a direct link between physical exercise and inhibition of pain.

The Structure of the Muscle Spindle

The name muscle spindle is derived from the oblong shape of this sense organ. The muscle spindles are located within the muscle, among the striated muscle cells, and consist of a few (2–12) specialized muscle cells

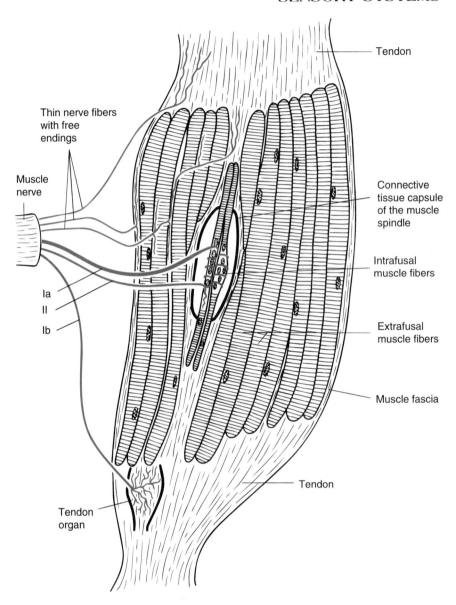

Figure 7.4 *Sensory innervation of skeletal muscles*. The size of the receptors relative to the muscle is exaggerated. Note that the muscle spindle is attached via connective tissue fibers to the tendons. Thus, the muscle spindle is stretched whenever the whole muscle is stretched. Many of the free nerve endings are nociceptors.

enclosed in a connective tissue capsule. The capsule is approximately 0.2 mm in diameter and 1–5 mm long. The muscle fibers (or muscle cells) of the spindle are called *intrafusal* and are much thinner than the ordinary, *extrafusal*, muscle fibers. In contrast to the extrafusal muscle fibers, the intrasfusal fibers show cross-striation only at their ends. This means that they are able to contract only these parts and not their middle portions. There are two main types of intrafusal fibers. One type is called the *nuclear bag fiber* because the nuclei are all collected in the middle part of the fiber (Fig. 7.5). In the other type, the *nuclear chain fiber*, the nuclei are evenly distributed along the fiber.

The number and density of muscle spindles vary from muscle to muscle, the *density being highest in muscles used for precision movements*, such as the extraocular muscles, the intrinsic muscles of the hand, and the small muscles around the joints of the neck. In large muscles like the latissimus dorsi, although the density is low, the total number of muscle spin-

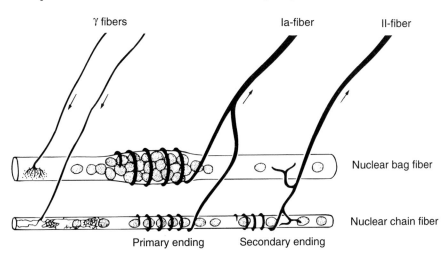

γ fibers   Ia-fiber   II-fiber

Nuclear bag fiber

Nuclear chain fiber

Primary ending   Secondary ending

Figure 7.5 *The muscle spindle.* Schematic representation of the two kinds of intrafusal muscle fibers and their innervation. Slightly changed from Matthews (1964).

dles is about 400, whereas the small abductor pollicis brevis with a much higher density contains about 80.

The *nerve supply* of the muscle spindles is highly complex, and only the main features will be treated here (Figs. 7.4 and 7.5). A thick afferent fiber ends with a spiraling course around the middle portion of the nuclear bag and nuclear chain fibers, forming the *primary sensory ending* of the muscle spindle. In addition, a thinner afferent fiber ends in relation to the nuclear chain fibers only, forming the *secondary sensory ending*. Afferent nerve fibers from muscles are classified with regard to thickness (and thus to conduction velocity) in groups I–IV, with group fibers comprising thick myelinated axons, and group IV unmyelinated ones. Group I is further divided into Ia and Ib, the former being the thickest. The primary sensory ending belongs to a *group Ia afferent fiber*, whereas the secondary sensory ending originates from a *group II afferent fiber*. Both types of sensory neuron have their perikarya in the spinal ganglia.

The *adequate stimulus* for the primary and secondary sensory endings is stretching of the intrafusal muscle fibers. This deforms the spiraling axonal branches and thus elicits depolarization and (if the depolarization is strong enough) action potentials in the group Ia and II sensory fibers.

The muscle spindle is also supplied with *motor axons*, called *fusimotor or γ fibers*, from γ motoneurons located in the ventral horn. The γ fibers end in the distal cross-striated parts of the intrafusal fibers and make them contract. This contraction leads to stretching of the noncontractile middle part of the intrafusal fibers, where the sensory endings are located. It should be emphasized that because the intrafusal fibers are so few and thin, their contraction does not contribute to the tension or shortening of the whole muscle.

The Properties of the Muscle Spindle

To understand how the muscle spindle functions, one must know that it is *arranged in parallel with the extrafusal muscle fibers*. Thus, both ends of the spindle are attached to the connective tissue within the muscle and are thereby indirectly anchored to the muscle tendons (Fig. 7.4). From

MUSCLE LENGTH

Dynamic phase (stretch)

Static phase

Static phase

Dynamic phase (shortening)

PRIMARY SENSORY ENDING
Ia

SECONDARY SENSORY ENDING
II

Action potentials

TIME ⟶

Figure 7.6 *The functional properties of the muscle spindle.* The diagram shows how both the primary and the secondary sensory endings signal the static length of the muscle (static sensitivity), whereas only the primary ending signals the length changes (movements) and their velocity (dynamic sensitivity). The diagram is based on recordings from single dorsal root fibers of anesthetized cats. The change of firing frequency of group Ia and group II fibers can then be related to static muscle length (static phase) and to stretch and shortening of the muscle (dynamic phases). The frequency of action potentials in the dorsal root fibers is indicated by the density of the vertical lines on the two lower rows. (The muscle spindle is not under the influence of γ motoneurons in this experiment.)

this structure one may deduce that *when the whole muscle shortens as a result of contraction of the extrafusal fibers, the intrafusal fibers will be shortened passively. Conversely, stretching of the whole muscle will stretch the intrafusal muscle fibers.* The rate of shortening or lengthening will be the same for the muscle spindle as for the whole muscle.

Action potentials can be recorded from single group Ia and II muscle afferent fibers in the dorsal roots of anesthetized animals (most often cats). It is then possible to study how the primary and secondary sensory endings behave in response to various stimuli. As expected from the anatomic facts described above, both types of afferent fibers increase their firing rate (that is, the frequency of action potentials) as the length of the muscle increases (Fig. 7.6). If the muscle shortens, the firing rate decreases (if the muscle is sufficently shortened, no action potentials can be recorded; see Fig. 7.7). When the length of the muscle is kept constant, the firing rate is also constant (static phase in Fig. 7.6)—the muscle spindle afferents are thus slowly adapting. This property of the muscle spindle is called *static sensitivity.* Since the firing rate of both the group Ia and the group II fiber depends on the length of the muscle, they both inform the central nervous system about the *length of the muscle at any time* (or the static length).

During the phase in which the *muscle length is changed,* however, the group Ia and group II afferent fibers behave differently (dynamic phase in Fig. 7.6). The firing rate of the group Ia fiber is much higher during the stretching than when the length is kept stationary in the stretched position, whereas the group II fiber does not show a similar change in firing rate. During the shortening phase, the Ia fiber becomes completely "silent." Although not shown in Figure 7.6, the firing rate of the group Ia fiber also depends on the velocity of the length change. Thus, the *Ia fiber signals that the length of the muscle is changing and the velocity with which it is occurring.* This property is called *dynamic sensitivity.*

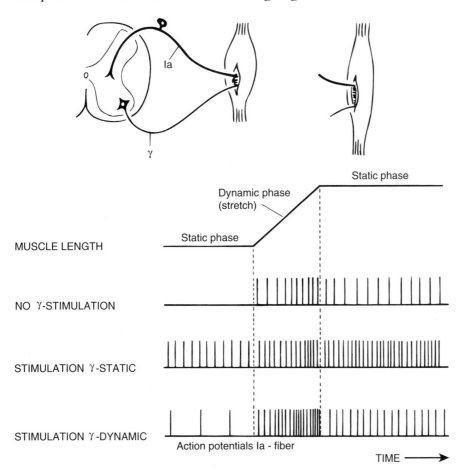

MUSCLE LENGTH

Static phase

Dynamic phase
(stretch)

Static phase

NO γ-STIMULATION

STIMULATION γ-STATIC

STIMULATION γ-DYNAMIC

Action potentials Ia - fiber

TIME ⟶

These facts indicate that the *primary sensory ending* of the muscle spindle has both static and dynamic sensitivity: It should be capable of informing about the actual length of the muscle (position of a joint), whether the length is constant or changing (joint movement), and the velocity of change (velocity of the movement). Since the *secondary sensory ending* almost totally lacks dynamic sensitivity, it should be able to inform primarily of the static length of the muscle.

That the primary and secondary sensory endings (and their afferent nerve fibers) have different properties is most likely due to differences in viscoelastic properties of the nuclear bag and nuclear chain intrafusal muscle fibers. There is much evidence to suggest that the *nuclear bag fibers are responsible for the dynamic sensitivity of the primary sensory ending, whereas the nuclear chain fibers are responsible for the static sensitivity of both the primary and secondary sensory endings.*[1]

Effects of Gamma Innervation on the Properties of the Muscle Spindle

What is described above of the properties of the muscle spindle derives from experiments in which there was no impulse traffic in the fusimotor γ axons (because the ventral roots were cut before recording from the dorsal roots). Impulses in γ fibers elicit contraction of the distal, cross-striated parts of the intrafusal muscle fibers, as mentioned above. This

Figure 7.7 *The action of γ motoneurons on the muscle spindle.* The experimental setup is as in Figure 7.6, except that in addition to recording the activity of group Ia fibers in the dorsal root, γ axons are isolated in the ventral roots so they can be electrically stimulated. In this example, there is no firing of the Ia fiber at the resting length of the muscle when the γ fibers are not stimulated. Stimulation of a static γ fiber (innervating the same spindle that the Ia fiber conducts from) makes the Ia fiber fire even at the static resting length, and stretching the muscle to a new static length increases the firing frequency to a new stable level. Stimulation of a dynamic γ fiber increases the firing frequency of the Ia fiber mainly during the stretching phase.

stretches the midportion of the intrafusal fibers with the sensory endings (Fig. 7.4). In addition, it also alters the stiffness of the intrafusal fibers so that their reaction to stretch is altered. In general, *the γ motoneurons and their γ fibers enable the brain to control the sensitivity of the muscle spindle to length and changes in length.*

In animal experiments (particularly in anesthetized cats), single γ fibers in the ventral roots have been stimulated while at the same time the activity of group Ia and group II afferent fibers in the dorsal roots were recorded. It has thus been shown that there are *two types of γ motoneurons* (Fig. 7.7). One type *increases the dynamic sensitivity of the muscle spindle* and is therefore called $γ_D$ (gamma dynamic). Upon a fairly rapid stretch of the muscle, the firing rate of a group Ia fiber increases more when the muscle spindle receives impulses from $γ_D$ motoneurons than without such influence. The firing rate during static length is, however, not significantly altered (Fig. 7.7). The muscle spindle's increased sensitivity to stretch enables the central nervous system to react more rapidly and forcefully to any unwanted change in muscle length (imposed, for example, by external forces upsetting body balance or ongoing movements).

Impulses from the other type of γ motoneurons *increase the static sensitivity of the muscle spindle*, and are therefore called $γ_S$ (gamma static). The activity of $γ_S$ motoneurons increases the firing rate of muscle spindle afferent fibers during constant length, as compared with a situation without γ activity. Although not shown in Figure 7.7, the firing rate of both group Ia and group II afferents increases. This influence of the γ system may be of importance to prevent the muscle spindles from becoming "silent"—that is, sending no action potentials—during the shortening of the muscle. In other words, the *length sensitivity* of the muscle spindle increases. Thus, the muscle spindle may signal the length of the muscle in its entire range of movements, which would seem important for precise movement control.[2]

Since the bag fibers appear to be solely responsible for the dynamic sensitivity of the muscle spindle, it has been assumed that dynamic γ fibers end on bag fibers and static γ fibers end on chain fibers. This is not fully clarified, however.

Even though the above description of the properties of muscle spindles is based on experiments in animals, there is evidence that it applies to the human muscle spindle. However, results from anesthetized animals, often with the spinal cord isolated from the rest of the brain, do not enable us to draw final conclusions as to the functions of the muscle spindle in intact organisms—for example, in human voluntary movements.

Muscle Spindles in Man and α–γ Coactivation

The activity of group Ia efferent fibers in the nerves of the arm and the leg has been recorded in conscious human subjects by *microneurographic* techniques. It appears (unexpectedly, on the basis of animal experiments) that in a resting muscle there is very little or no impulse traffic from the muscle spindle. Indirectly, this shows that there is no fusimotor (γ) activity either. If, however, the muscle contracts isometrically (that is, without change of length) there is a sharp increase of the firing frequency of Ia fibers. This must be caused by increased fusimotor activity, occurring simultaneously with the increase in α motoneuron activity (which evokes the contraction of the extrafusal fibers). This phenomenon of simultaneous activation of α and γ motoneurons is called α–γ *coactivation*. This ensures that the sensitivity of the muscle spindle is increased whenever the muscle is being used. In fact, the firing rate of the Ia fiber is upheld or increased even if the muscle is shortened during active contraction. This must mean that the fusimotor activity (firing rate of the γ motoneurons) *increases* during active shortening of the muscle.

The above example of α–γ coactivation does not mean that the γ motoneurons are activated only in conjunction with the γ motoneurons, even though direct proof of separate activation is lacking. There are situations in which it would be desirable to have increased sensitivity of the muscle spindle without simultaneous muscle contraction. One piece of indirect evidence comes from studies of stretch reflexes during mental imagery. In such a situation—when the subject imagines the performance of a movement—the stretch reflex response of the relevant muscles is increased without concomitant increase of α motoneuron excitablity. Thus, it appears that the sensitivity of the muscle spindle has been increased by selective acivation of γ motoneurons. It is also difficult to understand why the elaborate γ system has developed if its activity were always to reflect that of the α system. There are, in fact, some collaterals of α axons, socalled β (beta) axons, that innervate some intrafusal muscle fibers, and in submammalian species (for example, in the frog) there are only β fibers. During evolution, the β system appeared first in mammals.

Do Signals from Muscle Spindles Reach Consciousness?

As we will discuss below (*Changing Views of the Significance of Various Receptors for Kinesthesia*), there is convincing evidence that signals from muscle spindles can evoke a conscious, sensory experience. On the other hand, it appears that signals from a single receptor is not sufficient—in contrast to the situation with certain low-threshold mechanoreceptors in the skin and in the joint capsule. Microneurographic studies have been performed in humans with stimulation of single afferents from muscle spindles of the intrinsic hand muscles. Such stimulation did not evoke any sensation in the subjects. Perhaps several muscle spindles have to be activated at the same time to evoke a sensation. In a normal situation many—if not all—the muscle spindles are probably stimulated by stretching the muscle. Thus, it seems unnecessary and perhaps disturbing if every muscle spindle evokes a sensation alone (too much "noise").

The Tendon Organ

The other kind of proprioceptive receptor we will describe is the *tendon organ*, also called the *Golgi tendon organ*. It is built more simply than the muscle spindle and consists of a sensory nerve fiber that follows a convoluted course among collagen fibrils of the tendon, close to the musculotendinous junction (Fig. 7.4). The number of tendon organs in a muscle appears to be only slightly lower than the number of muscle spindles. The afferent fiber leading from the tendon organ belongs to group I and

Figure 7.8 *Functional properties of the tendon organ.* Action potentials are recorded from isolated Ib fibers in the dorsal roots. The firing frequency is indicated by vertical lines on the lower rows. Both passive stretching and active contraction of the muscle increases the firing frequency of the Ib fiber, but active contraction produces the greatest increase. The firing frequency of a Ia fiber during the same experiment is shown for comparison.

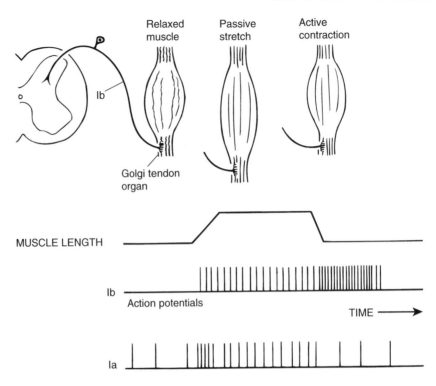

is called a *group Ib fiber* because it is somewhat thinner than the group Ia fiber forming the primary sensory ending of the muscle spindle. There is no efferent innervation of the tendon organ (in contrast to the muscle spindle)—its sensitivity cannot be controlled from the central nervous system.

The *adequate stimulus* of the tendon organ is stretching the part of the tendon in which it lies. Stretching tightens the collagen fibers, and thus the axonal branches between them are deformed (probably stretched, similar to the group Ia afferents). This depolarizes the receptor and, if the stimulus is of sufficient intensity, evokes action potentials in the afferent Ib fiber. Recording of the activity of Ib fibers shows that the receptor is *slowly adapting*. It is important to realize that the tendon organ, in contrast to the muscle spindle, is *coupled in series with the extrafusal muscle fibers*. Both passive stretch and active contraction of the muscle increase the tension of the tendon and thus activate the tendon organ receptor. The tendon organ, consequently, can inform the central nervous system about the *muscle tension*. In contrast, the activity of the muscle spindle depends on the muscle length and not on the tension.

Recording from single group Ib fibers in the dorsal root of anesthetized cats (Fig. 7.8) confirms what was expected on the basis of the structure of the tendon organ. In addition, however, such experiments have shown that the tendon organ is much *more sensitive to tension produced by active contraction than to that produced by passive stretch*. The tendon organ therefore appears to be primarily concerned with signaling how hard the muscle is contracting, rather than with how hard it is passively stretched.

Why Tendon Organs Are More Sensitive to Contraction Than to Passive Stretch

Structural details may explain why the tendon organ is more sensitive to active contraction than to passive stretch. Each tendon organ is directly attached to a small bundle of extrafusal muscle fibers. If one or a few of these contract, the tension set up in this particular small part of the tendon is very high compared with the tension measured for the whole muscle. To obtain the same tension in this particular tendon organ by passive stretch, much higher overall tension of the muscle would have to be produced. The muscle fibers attached to one tendon organ appear to belong to several motor units (see Chapter 11, *Motor Units*). Each tendon organ probably monitors the tension produced by only a few motor units. Thus the central nervous system is informed not only of the overall tension produced by the muscle but also of how the workload is distributed among the different motor units.

The Actions of Ib Afferents on Spinal Motoneurons

Activation of the group Ib afferents was shown a long time ago to inhibit (via interneurons) motoneurons of the muscle in which the tendon organs lie. Although these experiments were performed on anesthetized animals, and therefore should be interpreted with caution, the task of the tendon organ was said to be to prevent too strong contractions. More recent studies, however, have shown that the effects of the Ib afferents in the cord are not limited to inhibition. In awake animals, the effects on the motoneurons depend on the locomotor phase, and is reversed from inhibition to excitation when moving from the swing phase to the standing phase. Thus, tendon organs in hindlimb extensors excite extensor motoneurons when the leg is in the standing phase (via excitatory interneurons). In this case the signals from the tendon organ serve to amplify the contraction of the extensor muscles that keep the upright position. This is an example of how higher motor centers (in the brain stem and cerebral cortex) can switch the impulse traffic from one route to another in the cord, depending on the motor task. Further examples of this phenomenon are described in Chapter 11.

Low-Threshold Mechanoreceptors around the Joints

Not only muscle spindles and tendon organs provide information of importance for our awareness of movements and for motor control—receptors in the connective tissue around the joints also bring relevant information. The relative importance of information from joint and muscle receptors is not yet clear, however, and the view of the functional role of the joint receptors has changed considerably during the past 30 years.

Many sensory nerve fibers end in the joint capsules and in the ligaments around the joints (Fig. 7.9). Many are free-ending receptors; others are encapsulated endings corresponding anatomically and with regard to response properties to encapsulated receptors in glabrous skin. The encapsulated joint receptors are *low-threshold mechanoreceptors* and have been divided into four groups. The *type 1 joint receptor* resembles the *Ruffini corpuscle* in the dermis (Fig. 7.1). A myelinate axon ramifies among collagen fibrils, within a thin connective tissue capsule. They are found almost exclusively in the fibrous part of the joint capsules. The *ad-*

Figure 7.9 *Joint innervation.* **Right**, a knee joint, showing the distribution of the various kinds of joint receptors. To the **left**, the morphology of the four main receptor types is shown in more detail. From Brodal (1981).

equate stimulus of these Ruffini-like receptors is *increased tension* in the part of the capsule in which they lie. The higher the capsular tension, the higher the firing rate in the afferent sensory fiber from the receptor. Like the Ruffini corpuscle in the skin, this joint receptor is *slowly adapting*. Because the tension in various parts of the capsule depends on the joint position, type 1 receptors would appear suited to signal the position of the joint. For example, receptors in the posterior part of the elbow joint capsule would be highly active in a flexed position of the joint, which stretches the capsule, and less active in an extended position, which relaxes the capsule. The receptor also has dynamic sensitivity, giving a stronger response (higher firing rate) to a rapid movement than to a slow one. The *type 1 or Ruffini-like receptor thus seems capable of signaling static joint position, joint movements, and direction and speed of movements.* As will be discussed later, however, the ability of the type 1 receptor to signal static joint position appears to be limited.

The *type 2 joint* receptor resembles structurally and functionally the Pacinian corpuscle but is considerably smaller (it is also called *Paciniform receptor*). Type 2 receptors are present only in the fibrous part of the joint capsules. They are *rapidly adapting*, and their *adequate stimulus is stretching of the part of the capsule in which they lie.* Owing to their rapid adaptation, they can inform only of joint movements, not of static position. They appear particularly suited to signal movement velocity and have also been called "acceleration receptors."

A third kind of encapsulated receptor (type 3) resembles the tendon organ and is present in ligaments only. It is slowly adapting (like the tendon organ), but its functional role is unknown. A protective role in signaling overstretching of joints has been proposed but has not gained experimental support.

Microneurographic studies in humans with stimulation of single afferent fibers from finger joints, show that signals from low-threshold joint receptors can reach consciousness. Thus, when a fiber leading from a presumed type 1 receptor was stimulated, the subject reported the feeling of a movement of the relevant joint (the location and adequate stimulus of the receptor were determined before stimulation). In other instances of single unit stimulation, the subject reported only a non-painful, punctate feeling at the joint.

Joint Nociceptors

The fibrous part of the joint capsule and the ligaments are richly supplied with thin myelinated and unmyelinated axons ending in *free receptors*. These have been termed *type 4* joint receptors. Many of these, like free endings in other tissues, are *nociceptors*. The joint capsules and ligaments contain high-threshold mechanoreceptors, polymodal nociceptors, and "silent" nociceptors. Stimulation of the fibrous capsule and the ligaments during surgery of the knee joint confirms that pain can be evoked from both the capsule and ligaments. The sensation is punctate-like in the skin—so that certain spots when probed with a needle evoke pain while other spots evoke a feeling of pressure or no sensation at all.

Many of the thin fibers ending in the joint capsule contain neuropeptides, such as substance P (SP) and CGRP. Liberation of such peptides is believed to play a role in the development of inflammatory arthritis in humans (especially rheumatoid arthritis). Thus, the severity of induced inflammatory arthritis in experimental animals is reduced after depleting the joint sensory fibers of SP.

Other free joint receptors appear to play a role in *circulatory and respiratory reflexes* that are known to be elicited by passive joint movements (*ergoreceptors*).

The Innervation of the Synovial Membrane

Whether the *synovial membranes* of the joints receive sensory nerve fibers, has been a matter of dispute. Thus, such fibers were not convincingly shown by use of heavy metal impregnation, which reliably showed nerve fibers in the fibrous capsule. Recent immunocytochemical studies in humans show the presence of thin nerve fibers ending freely in the synovial membrane, which contain neuropeptides typical of primary sensory neurons. However, such fibers appear to be very sparse, leaving some doubt about their functional significance. Studies in humans with various ways of stimulating the synovial membrane (during surgery in local anesthesia) have given conflicting evidence—some reporting pain sensations to be evoked from the synovial membrane, others not. In probably the most careful study, however, pain (or any sensation at all) was only occasionally evoked from the synovial membrane of the knee joint with mechanical and chemical stimuli. This contrasted with the ease with which pain could be evoked from the fibrous capsule and ligaments, as described above.

In contrast to the sparse sensory innervation, there is a rich *efferent* (autonomic) innervation of the *synovial vessels*. These fibers contain norepinephrine and usually also neuropeptide Y (NPY). As mentioned above, SP may be involved in producing inflammation in arthritis, and release of norepinephrine can induce the release of SP from sensory nerve fibers in the vicinity. By removing the autonomic innervation of the joint, arthritic inflammation can be reduced in some animal models of arthritis. It should be emphasized, however, that norepinephrine and substance P are present also in the fibrous capsule.

Kinesthesia

The term *kinesthesia* (sometimes used synonymously with *joint sensation* and *proprioceptive sensation*) is commonly, and also here, used to refer to the perception of *joint position, joint movements, and the direction and velocity of joint movements.* Strictly speaking, however, the word kinesthesia (Greek: *kinesis* = movement) encompasses only the dynamic and not the static aspect of sensation. The term joint sensation is not a good alternative, however, since it may give the false impression that kinesthesia depends *only* on joint receptors. Some also include in the term kinesthesia the perception of force, effort, and heaviness in relation to muscle contractions.

Our ability to judge the position of a joint (without seeing it), even after a long period without movement, is usually fairly precise, as can be verified by trying to match the position of the joint to be tested with the joint of the other side (for example, finger or elbow joints). This is the static part of kinesthesia. Nevertheless, the precision of our judgment is increased considerably if movements are allowed, particularly active movements.

Changing Views of the Significance of Various Receptors for Kinesthesia

The views on which receptor types are responsible for kinesthesia have undergone considerable changes. At the beginning of this century, the newly discovered muscle spindle was held responsible for all aspects. Investigations during the 1950s and early 1960s, however, indicated that joint receptors had the necessary properties to signal all information needed for kinesthesia. It was also argued that the muscle spindle cannot give the necessary information, since the firing rate of its afferent nerve fibers depends not only on the actual position and movements of a joint but also on whether the γ motoneurons are active. It was also commonly held that impulses from the muscle spindles do not reach consciousness. Later, however, it was convincingly demonstrated that signals from the muscle spindles can reach consciousness, and that they contribute to our kinesthetic sense. A simple demonstration to this effect was performed by vibrating the muscle belly or the tendon of the biceps muscle in a normal subject. Vibration is known to be a powerful way to stimulate the primary sensory endings of muscle spindles (the stimulus consists of brief stretches of the muscle). The subject, who is blindfolded, feels that the forearm is moving downward even though no such movement is occurring—that is, there is an illusory extensory movement at the elbow joint. This corresponds to a *lengthening* of the biceps muscle, and under normal circumstances, of course, this would be the normal cause of an increased firing rate in muscle spindle afferents.

Reexamination of the *properties of joint receptors* showed a striking paucity of slowly adapting joint receptors (type 1) that are active in midrange positions of the joint—that is, the range in which the precision of kinesthesia is best. Most type 1 receptors appear to reach their maximal firing rate only toward extreme joint positions. Thus, it seems unlikely that joint receptors alone can give all the necessary information.

Furthermore, examination of *patients with artificial joints* who lack joint capsules (and thus presumably most of their joint receptors) show that their kinesthesia is only slightly reduced—at least with regard to the hip joint and the metacarpophalangeal joints. Presumably, muscle spindles (not tendon organs) are responsible for the remaining kinesthesia in such cases, even though skin receptors may contribute as well (particularly for the metacarpophalangeal joints). For the knee joint, however, elimination of presumably all afferent signals from the joint capsule and the overlying skin by local anesthesia did not impair kinesthesia appreciably. Local anesthesia of finger joint capsules and the skin of the fingers gives more marked reduction of kinesthesia, but not even in such cases is the loss of kinesthesia complete.

The *static aspect of kinesthesia* depends on slowly adapting receptors that change their firing rate with changing joint position. The *dynamic aspect of kinesthesia*—that is, the ability to perceive that a movement is taking place and to judge the direction and velocity of the movement—depends on receptors with dynamic sensitivity, many of them rapidly adapting. Receptors with such properties, which are influenced by joint movements, are found in the skin, muscles, and around the joints. The accumulated evidence today indicates that *muscle spindles, joint receptors, and skin receptors all contribute to kinesthesia.* Muscle spindles appear to provide their most important contribution to kinesthesia with regard to large joints, such as the hip and knee joints, whereas joint receptors and skin receptors may provide more significant contributions with regard to finger and toe joints.

Proprioceptors and Voluntary Movements

Patients with diseases causing loss of thick myelinated fibers in their peripheral nerves (neuropathies) have problems with voluntary movements, especially when they cannot see the moving parts. Their problems must be caused by the loss of information from *low-threshold mechanoreceptors*, presumably mainly *proprioceptors*. Most disturbed are movements requiring *coordination of several joints*, such as slicing bread, hitting a nail with a hammer, unlocking a door, and so forth. The regulation of muscular force is inaccurate, and they have particular problems with maintaining a constant force for some time. Presumably, information from proprioceptors is necessary for a continuous upgrading of the central motor program, so that the commands issued to the muscles are adapted to the actual position of the bodily parts. Thus, the influence of gravity changes continuously during a movement, and so do the mutual forces exerted by the parts (for example, between the arm and the forearm). The movements become inaccurate and insecure if the force of muscle contraction is not adapted to these changes—which may differ slightly every time we, for example, raise a glass of water. Such proprioceptive feedback is particularly important for small, precise movements, when unforeseen disturbances occur during the movement, and when we learn new movements. Vision may partially compensate for the loss of proprioceptive information.

Can such observations help to clarify the individual contribution of each kind of proprioceptor to movement control? As mentioned, kinesthesia depends not only on information from proprioceptors but also on information from cutaneous receptors. Also the latter kind is more or less affected in patients with peripheral neuropathies. Furthermore, when information of one kind is reduced, the patient will learn to rely more on information from other kinds of receptors. In addition, the analysis is complicated by the fact that the various proprioceptors differ regarding their contribution to kinesthesia in different joints, and this probably is so also for control of voluntary movements. *Thus, specifying the individual contribution of muscle spindles, tendon organs, joint receptors, and cutaneous receptors to the control of voluntary movements is very difficult.* The brain extracts what it needs for motor control from the *collective in-*

formation provided by all these receptors. If one source is reduced, we learn to rely more upon the remaining sources.

We will return to proprioceptors and their central actions later in this chapter, and their relation to motor control is further discussed in Chapter 11.

Clinical Examples of Loss of Somatosensory Information

The neurologist Oliver Sacks gives in his book *The Man who Mistook His Wife for a Hat* a vivid description of a young woman, Christina, who completely lost kinesthetic sensation. A sensory neuropathy of unknown origin deprived her suddenly of virtually all kinds of proprioceptive information. Her cutaneous sensation was only slightly reduced, and motor axons were essentially spared. Nevertheless, at first she could not stand without continuously watching her feet. She could not hold anything in her hands, and they wandered around without her awareness. When stretching out to grasp an object she usually missed—the movement stopping too soon or too late. "Something awful's happened, I can't feel my body. I feel weird—disembodied" she said, and ". . . I may 'lose' my arms. I think they're one place and I find they're another." After having proprioception explained, she said: "This 'proprioception' is like the eyes of the body, the way the body sees itself. And if it goes, as it's gone with me, *it's like the body is blind* . . . so I have to watch it—be its eyes. Right?"

Another example concerns a 36-year-old man who gradually lost both cutaneous and kinesthetic sensation of the extremities due to a sensory neuropathy (described by Rothwell and co-workers in 1982). His muscle power was hardly reduced, and he did surprisingly well on several routine tests of motor function. He did, for example, various finger movements that require cooperation between muscles in the forearm and the hand. He could move his thumb fairly precisely over three different distances and with three different velocities, and he could judge reasonably well the resistance to a movement. In spite of this, his hands were almost useless in daily life. He could not hold a cup with one hand, hold a pen and write, or button his shirt. Most likely, this can be explained by lack of automatic adjustment of ongoing movements, and by an inability to maintain constant muscle force for more than a few seconds (without seeing the part). The problems seemed to arise also because he was unable to do longer sequences of simple movements without constantly watching what he was doing.

THE SENSORY FIBERS AND THE DORSAL ROOTS

Afferent (sensory) fibers from the receptors follow the peripheral nerves toward the central nervous system. Close to the spinal cord, the sensory fibers are collected in the dorsal roots and enter the cord through these. The sensory fibers of the spinal nerves have their perikarya in the dorsal root ganglia (Figs. 3.3, 3.5 and 3.9). Likewise, the sensory fibers in the cranial nerves have their perikarya in ganglia close to the brain stem (Figs. 16.3 and 16.4).

As mentioned, the spinal ganglion cells are pseudounipolar and send one long process peripherally, ending freely or in encapsulated sense organs. Functionally and structurally, both the peripheral and the central processes are axons. The central process enters the cord and then divides into an ascending and a descending branch (Fig. 7.10). These branches give off several collaterals ventrally to the gray matter of the cord. *One sensory neuron, entering the cord through one dorsal root, can therefore influence spinal neurons at several segmental levels of the cord.*

Figure 7.10 *Terminal pattern of a dorsal root fiber.* A dorsal root fiber (in this case conducting from disks of Merkel) divides into an ascending and a descending branch after entering the cord. These branches give off several collaterals ending in the dorsal horn. The piece of the cord shown is about 1 cm long, but the axon continues beyond this in both directions. Corresponding reconstructions have been made for sensory units leading from several other kinds of receptors, and each sensory unit has a characteristic terminal pattern in the dorsal horn. Based on Brown (1981).

Are There Sensory Fibers in the Ventral Roots?

An old controversy concerns whether there are exceptions to the rule that sensory fibers enter the cord through the dorsal roots, and motor fibers through the ventral roots (the law of Magendie). Thus, the fact that cutting the dorsal roots (dorsal rhizotomy) does not always abolish pain, has been taken to indicate that some sensory fibers enter the cord through the ventral roots. Electron microscopic investigations have proved the presence of many unmyelinated fibers in the ventral roots of several species, including man. Many of these are efferent, preganglionic autonomic fibers, but physiological data show that many (30% in the rat) are sensory and react to stimulation of nociceptors. However, few, if any, of these have been proved actually to enter the cord through the ventral root. With retrograde transport methods their cell bodies have been shown to lie in the dorsal root ganglia. Some ventral root sensory fibers leave the ventral root to innervate the pia at the ventral aspect of the cord, others turn around before they enter the cord. Some of these then enter the cord through the dorsal root, whereas the further course of the others is unknown. Neither do we know whether these peculiar arrangements have some special biological meaning.

Classification of Dorsal Root Fibers in Accordance with Their Thickness

The dorsal root fibers vary in thickness, from the thickest myelinated ones, with a diameter of 20 μm and conduction velocity of 120 m/sec, to the thinnest unmyelinated fibers, with a diameter of less than 1 μm and conduction velocity of less than 1 m/sec. The thick fibers belong to the ganglion cells with large perikarya, and the thin fibers belong to those with small perikarya. We have previously mentioned classification of sensory axons from muscle mechanoreceptors by their thickness (conduction velocity) into groups I and II. Another classification of sensory neurons, on the basis of their conduction velocity, is also used (mainly for cutaneous afferents). *Myelinated fibers* fall within *group A*, and *group C* contains the *unmyelinated fibers*. In the A group, the fastest conducting (thickest) fibers are termed Aα, somewhat slower conducting fibers are Aβ, and the thinnest of the myelinated fibers are called Aδ.

Figure 7.11 *The terminal regions of the dorsal root fibers in the cord.* The thickest myelinated fibers (Aα, from muscle spindles and tendon organs) end in the deep parts of the dorsal horn and partly also in the ventral horn. Thick, myelinated fibers from cutaneous mechanoreceptors (Aβ) end in laminae III–VI. The thinnest myelinated and unmyelinated dorsal root fibers (Aδ and C)—many of them leading from nociceptors—end in laminae I, II, and parts of V. Based on experiments with axonal transport of tracer substances.

The different kinds of sensory receptors are supplied with axons of characteristic thickness. Impulses from *low-threshold mechanoreceptors* are, for example, conducted in thick myelinated fibers (Aα and Aβ). Impulses from *cold receptors* are conducted in thin myelinated fibers (Aδ), whereas unmyelinated (C) fibers conduct from *heat receptors*. Impulses from *nociceptors* are conducted in Aδ and C fibers. In the spinal cord, the terminations of the Aδ and C fibers are almost completely separated from those of the Aα and Aβ fibers (Fig. 7.11).

Fibers from Different Receptors End in Different Parts of the Dorsal Horn

Early physiological experiments showed that impulses from different receptor types activate neurons in somewhat different parts of the spinal gray matter. For example, neurons particularly in Rexed's *lamina VI* are activated by *joint movements*, whereas impulses from *cutaneous low-threshold mechanoreceptors* activate mostly neurons in *laminae III to V*. That afferent fibers from low-threshold mechanoreceptors—that is, Aα and Aβ fibers—end in deep layers of the dorsal horn has been verified with combined physiological and anatomic techniques (intra-axonal tracer injections after physiological characterization). Such experiments have also made it possible to study in detail the pattern of the spinal termination of individual sensory units. Figure 7.10 gives an example of this. Single axons in the dorsal root have been penetrated with thin glass microelectrodes (pipettes). After determination of the receptive field and adequate stimulus of the sensory unit, the same pipette is used to inject HRP intra-axonally. The axon and its ramifications can subsequently be followed in sections of the spinal cord. A remarkable degree of specificity has been shown in the pattern of termination of fibers belonging to functionally different receptors.

Thin *Aδ and C fibers* conducting impulses from nociceptors have been shown to end almost exclusively in the dorsalmost parts of the dorsal horn—that is, *laminae I and II* (substantia gelatinosa). The Aδ fibers, however, to some extent also terminate in *lamina V*. Whereas the thin afferent fibers (many coming from nociceptors) from the skin end in laminae I, II, and V, corresponding fibers from the *viscera* have been shown to end almost exclusively in laminae I and V, thus avoiding the substantia gelatinosa. Thin *muscle and joint afferents* appear to terminate in the same parts of the dorsal horn as the fibers from viscera (although there are some conflicting data). Another feature of afferents from muscles and joints is their extensive rostrocaudal distribution in the cord. For example, afferent fibers from a single facet joint of the back terminate in 7–8 segments of the cord (cat). It is a common experience that pain of visceral origin has different qualities than pain evoked from the skin—being much more diffuse and difficult to localize. Also pain arising in muscles and joints is less precisely localized than cutaneous pain, and radiates out from the site of the noxious stimulus. We also mentioned above that muscle pain has a cramp-like quality. Presumably, the anatomic arrangements in the dorsal horn may be partly responsible for such differences.

Fiber Categories and Conscious Sensations

Relations between impulses conducted in sensory fibers of various calibers and conscious sensations have been investigated primarily by graded electrical stimulation of peripheral nerves and selective block of axonal conduction. By *electrical stimulation* of peripheral nerves, the weakest stimulation evokes activity only in the thickest myelinated fibers, and with increasing intensity the thinner fibers are recruited progressively. Thus, the thickest fibers have the lowest electrical threshold for activation. In human subjects, pain is evoked by such stimulation only if the stimulus is strong enough to activate Aδ fibers. The person then typically reports that the pain is of a sharp, pricking quality. If the stimulus strength is increased to recruit C fibers as well, the person experiences an intense, often burning pain that continues after the stimulus stops. These experiments are in agreement with the common experience that one usually can distinguish two phases of pain after an acute injury: The first phase, or *fast pain*, is experienced immediately after the stimulus, is well localized, and not very intense; the second phase, or *slow pain*, occurs with a longer latency and is more unpleasant, is not well localized, and usually continues after the end of the stimulus. The slow pain is delayed because it is dependent on being conducted in C fibers with a conduction velocity of less than 1 m/sec.

Injection of *local anesthetics* around a peripheral nerve blocks the thinnest (C) fibers first and the thickest myelinated ones last. Accordingly, with local anesthetics the pain disappears first, whereas the tactile sensation is conserved considerably longer, and some may remain throughout the period of anesthesia. When peripheral nerves are subjected to *pressure*, conduction in thick fibers is blocked first, and, accordingly, there first occurs a reduction of the ability to perceive light touch and to judge the position of joints, whereas pain perception is still present.

The difference in conduction velocity between fibers giving rise to fast and slow pain is most easily observed when something hits the foot hard enough to cause pain (for example, when a toe is bumped against a hard object). The pathway from the toe to the cerebral cortex is longer than from any other part of the body, so the time lag between the impulses conducted in thick and thin fibers is greatest. The very first sensation is in fact only that something touched the foot, due to activation of low-threshold mechanoreceptors. Almost simultaneously, the sharp and well-localized fast pain is perceived, and we then know that the pain will soon be worse—the diffuse, burning, and intensely unpleasant slow pain continuing for some time.

Primary Sensory Fibers and Neurotransmitters

Probably all primary sensory neurons release a classical transmitter with fast synaptic actions in the spinal cord. Among other evidence, this is based on the observation that boutons originating from dorsal root afferents contain small, clear vesicles, which have been shown in other parts of the nervous system to contain this kind of neurotransmitter. The most likely candidate for dorsal root neurons is the excitatory amino acid *glutamate* with an excitatory action. There is also indirect evidence that some primary sensory fibers release the nucleotide *ATP*, shown in other parts of the nervous system to exert fast, excitatory synaptic actions.

Several *neuropeptides* have been demonstrated in the central and peripheral terminals and in the perikarya of spinal ganglion cells with immunocytochemical techniques. These include SP VIP, *cholecystokinin* (CCK), *somatostatin*, CGRP, *galanin*, and others. The functions of these peptides are largely unknown, but they presumably mediate slow, modulatory synaptic actions in the dorsal horn. The neuropeptides are probably always colocalized with a classical transmitter. Many ganglion cells contain more than one neuropeptide; for example, 80% of all SP-containing cells contain CGRP as well. Both of these neuropeptides—when applied locally in the dorsal horn—increase the release of glutamate. We do not know, however, whether this is due to direct action on glutamatergic boutons of dorsal root fibers, or on glutamatergic spinal interneurons. Furthermore, SP receptors (neurokinin receptors) and NMDA receptors (glutamate) interact, making the NMDA receptors more sensitive to glutamate. *Release of SP in the dorsal horn might therefore enhance and prolong the excitation produced by incoming signals from sensory receptors.* We return later in this chapter to how this phenomenon may relate to increased pain sensitivity (hyperalgesia).

Most of the neuropeptides are found only in *small ganglion cells*, which have thin axons. Substance P is present in most of the small ganglion cells (in about 20% of *all*, large and small together). With the demonstration that SP is released from dorsal root fibers in the dorsal horn on nociceptor activation, this has led to the assumption that SP is a neuro-transmitter for nociceptive sensory neurons. A clear correlation between the adequate stimulus for single ganglion cells and the kind of neuropeptide they contain, however, has not emerged from studies combining physiological and immunocytochemical characterization of single spinal ganglion cells. Thus, a SP containing ganglion cell is not necessarily nociceptive, and many nociceptive neurons do not contain SP. On the other hand, there may be a relationship between the kind of tissue a neuron innervates and its neuropeptide content. For example, many more of the ganglion cells innervating viscera contain SP and CGRP than of those innervating the skin. About two thirds of the ganglion cells supplying joints contain SP and CGRP. The evidence so far is too limited, however, to draw final conclusions regarding relations between neuropeptides, sensory modalities, and tissue or organ specificity.

Release of Neuropeptides from Peripheral Branches of Sensory Neurons

The function of neuropeptides present in the peripheral ramifications of primary sensory neurons is even less understood than their functions in the central terminals. It is not known, for example, whether these peptides are released under normal circumstances and take part in the normal homeostatic control. We know, however, that the peptides can be released in the peripheral tissue by noxious stimuli and by antidromic activation of the axon (see Chapter 17, *The Axonal Reflex.*). Several of these peptides, when liberated in the tissues, have profound effects on vessels, as shown in the skin and mucous membranes. SP and VIP both produce vasodilatation and thereby increased blood flow, and also increased extravasation of fluid from the capillaries and edema. SP can, furthermore, activate cells of the immune system, resulting in phagocytosis and release of mediators of inflammation. *Inhalation of irritating gases* may provoke release of SP from peripheral sensory fibers in the airways, and the same takes place in the skin upon strong mechanical stimulation, such as scratching. The liberation of SP in such cases is probably due to an axon reflex because afferent signals from the receptors are transmitted not only toward the spinal cord but also distally in branches of the sensory fibers (that is, distally in the branches that were not stimulated).

Injury to the nerve or the innervated tissue changes the neuropeptide content of the ganglion cells. For example, experimental arthritis leads to a marked increase of SP and CGRP in the cell bodies of the ganglion cells innervating the affected joint (the arthritis is produced in animals by injecting the joint with a local irritant). SP is apparently also released from the joint capsule into the synovial fluid. This leads to release of such substances as prostaglandins and collagenase from leukocytes, and their release may contribute to the damage of the joint cartilage in arthritis. Since blocking the SP receptors (neurokinin receptors), or depleting the nerves of SP reduce the inflammatory reaction, neuropeptides are now believed to play a role in several human diseases (rheumatoid arthritis, asthma, inflammatory bowel disease, and migraine).

The Segmental Innervation: The Dermatomes

The ventral branches (rami) of the spinal nerves form plexuses supplying the arms (Fig. 11.1) and the legs. Each of the nerves emerging from these plexuses contains sensory and motor fibers coming from several segments. In the peripheral distribution of the fibers, however, the segmental origin of the fibers is retained. Thus, sensory fibers of one spinal segment—that

Figure 7.12 *The dermatomes of the trunk and the upper extremity*. Dermatomes not supplied by neighboring spinal segments meet at the ventral axial line (C₅ and T₁). From Keegan and Garrett (1948).

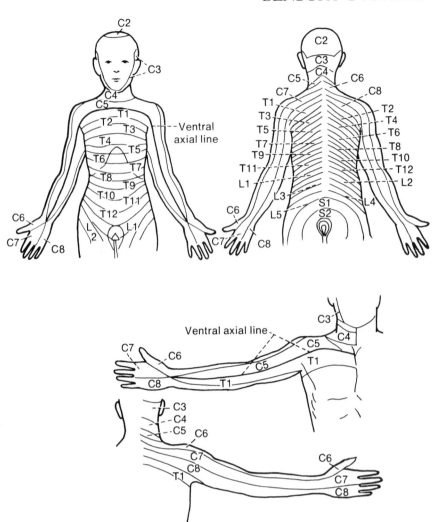

is, of one dorsal root—supply a distinct part of the skin. The area of the skin supplied with sensory fibers from one spinal segment is called a *dermatome*. In the thorax and abdomen, dermatomes are shaped like circular belts; in the extremities, however, conditions are more complicated (Figs. 7.12 and 7.13). Knowledge of the segmental innervation of the skin (and also of the segmental innervation of muscles and viscera, dealt with in Chapters 11 and 17) is of great practical value in clinical neurology. For example, if a dorsal root is interrupted, the skin sensation is reduced or abolished in the corresponding dermatome.

Because the dermatomes overlap, each spot on the skin is innervated by sensory fibers from at least two dorsal roots. Interruption of a single dorsal root therefore may not produce a clear-cut sensory deficit. Nevertheless, careful examination usually shows a narrow zone (centrally in the dermatome) where the cutaneous sensation to touch is slightly reduced and that for pain is abolished (analgesia). The usually more marked reduction in pain than in touch sensation is due to less extensive overlap of fibers coming from nociceptors than of fibers coming from low-threshold mechanoreceptors.

Figure 7.13 *The dermatomes of the lower extremity.* From Keegan and Garrett (1948).

When a dorsal root is subjected to irritation, as may happen by compression or stretching in connection with growth of an intraspinal tumor or protrusion of an intervertebral disk, this causes pain and other sensory phenomena (numbness, pricking, tingling, and so forth) in the territory of the dermatome. *Often the symptoms are felt only in smaller parts of the dermatome.* With a protruding (herniated) intervertebral disk in the lumbar spine, for example, most often the roots of the fifth lumbar or first sacral nerves are affected (Fig. 7.13), and the pain is felt in the leg (sciatica).

How the Dermatomes Have Been Determined

The oldest method for determining the dermatome is to follow the distribution of the nerves by dissection. To follow the course of fibers from a root through the plexuses is, of course, far from easy. Certain diseases may affect single dorsal roots and produce changes restricted to the dermatome. Shingles (herpes zoster), for example, is a viral infection of the spinal ganglion cells that produces skin eruptions in the dermatome of the affected dorsal roots. Examination of many patients with this disease served as a basis for maps showing the dermatome (Head). Electrical stimulation of dorsal roots during operations (Foerster) and comparison of observations during operations for herniated intervertebral disks with the information given previously by the patient of where the pain and sensory loss were localized also helped to determine the location of dermatomes. Local anesthesia of single or several dorsal roots in healthy volunteers has also been of value. The best method is to eliminate impulse conduction in several dorsal roots on each side of one that is left intact (method of remaining sensibility). This was done experimentally in monkeys by Sherrington but the results are not directly applicable to humans. The German neurosurgeon Foerster made more sporadic observations based on the method of remaining sensibility in patients in whom the dorsal roots were cut to relieve pain.

The dermatomal map presented here (Figs. 7.12 and 7.13, reproduced from Keegan and Garrett) is based on observations of a large number of patients with root compressions (usually due to a herniated intervertebral disk) and, in addition, on examination of the distribution of reduced sensation in volunteers subjected to local anesthesia of dorsal roots. The skin regions with reduced sensation (hypesthesia) were carefully mapped out before operation, and during operation it was determined which root was affected. Local anesthesia also produces a sensory loss much less extensive than the total distribution of sensory fibers of one dorsal root. Thus, the borders between dermatomes as presented in Figures 7.12 and 7.13 are imaginary. They ignore, for example, the great overlap between neighboring dermatomes, and on the other hand, that the dermatomes are much wider than the zones of hypesthesia occurring after damage to one dorsal root.

It should be kept in mind that all dermatomal maps are composites of many single observations—in no single person have more than one or a few dermatomes been determined. For this reason, *all maps showing dermatomes for the whole body can only be regarded as approximations*, not taking into account, for example, the considerable individual variations that exist. This, together with the fact that different methods have been used, probably explains why the dermatomal maps of different authors vary so much. For the student the main emphasis should therefore be on *learning certain main features of the dermatomal distribution rather than the artificial (and falsely accurate) borders indicated on the maps*.

Sensory Fibers Are Links in Reflex Arcs: Spinal Interneurons

Sensory information reaching the spinal cord through the dorsal roots is further conveyed to higher levels of the central nervous system, as will be described later. In addition, however, it should be observed that many of the spinal neurons that are contacted by dorsal root fibers are not links in ascending sensory pathways but have axons that ramify within the cord—that is, they are *spinal interneurons*. The axons of these interneurons establish synaptic contacts with other spinal neurons, among them motoneurons and neurons in the intermediolateral cell column, giving origin to efferent fibers to smooth muscles and glands (sympathetic preganglionic fibers). In this manner, *reflex arcs* for several important somatic (skeletal muscle) and autonomic (visceral) reflexes are established. Most, if not all, spinal interneurons also establish connections between neurons at different segmental levels (propriospinal fibers). Each spinal interneuron thus establishes synaptic contacts with a very large number of other neurons in the spinal cord. *Impulses entering the cord through one dorsal root may influence neurons at several segmental levels*, both via their own ascending and descending collaterals and via their influence on interneurons with propriospinal collaterals (Figs. 7.10 and 11.9). How far the impulses from one dorsal root fiber are propagated from interneuron to interneuron depends on what other synaptic influences these interneurons are subjected to. For example, higher levels of the central nervous system, such as the brain stem and the cerebral cortex, can selectively facilitate or inhibit spinal interneurons. This enables the impulse traffic from dorsal root fibers to be directed so that certain reflex arcs are used, whereas others are "turned off," in accordance with the need of the organism as a whole. *Presynaptic inhibition* is an important mechanism in this respect. For example, separate groups of interneurons mediate presynaptic inhibition of group I muscle afferents, group II muscle afferents, and group Ib tendon organ afferents. Spinal reflexes are treated in more detail in Chapter 11.

CENTRAL SOMATOSENSORY
PATHWAYS

So far in this chapter we have dealt with the peripheral parts of the somatosensory system—the receptors and the primary sensory neurons. We now turn to the tracts and nuclei conveying and processing somatosensory information within the central nervous system. The term somatosensory pathways is not entirely appropriate, however, because these pathways transmit signals not only from somatic structures, such as skin, muscles, and joints, but also from visceral organs. Most impulses from visceral organs are not consciously perceived, and visceral sensory processes have been less intensively investigated than somatosensory ones (see Chapter 17).

*Main Features of the Organization of
the Somatosensory Pathways*

There are several parallel somatosensory pathways, but most *consist of three neurons forming a chain from the receptors to the cerebral cortex.* The first, the primary sensory neuron, has its perikaryon in a spinal ganglion or a cranial nerve ganglion; the next, *the secondary sensory neuron*, has its perikaryon in the gray matter of the spinal cord or in the brain stem; and the third, *the tertiary sensory neuron*, has its perikaryon in the thalamus (Figs. 7.14 and 7.15). *All of the somatosensory pathways are crossed*, so that signals from one side of the body are brought to the cerebral hemisphere of the other side. The actual crossing over takes place at different levels for the various pathways, however. Another important point is that the pathways are *somatotopically organized*, which implies that neurons that conduct impulses from different parts of the body are kept separate. The pathways are also organized so that, to a large extent, neurons conveying signals related to different sensory modalities are kept separate.

Whereas axons of different thicknesses conducting from different kinds of receptors lie intermingled in the peripheral nerves and the dorsal roots, they are grouped in accordance with their thickness as soon as they enter the spinal cord. *The thick dorsal root fibers pass medially, whereas the thin ones follow a more lateral course into the dorsal horn* (Fig. 7.11). Their further course is also different: The medially located, thick dorsal root fibers continue without synaptic interruption rostrally in the dorsal funiculus, as part of the *dorsal column—medial lemniscus pathway* (Fig. 7.14). The perikarya of the secondary neurons in this pathway are located in the medulla oblongata, and the crossing of the pathway also takes place at the medullary level. Since the thickest dorsal root axons conduct impulses mainly from *low-threshold mechanoreceptors*, one might expect that the dorsal column—medial lemniscus pathway is of importance for perception of touch, pressure, vibration, and kinesthesia. As will be discussed below, this is largely correct. It should be emphasized, however, that the pathway is of primary importance for discriminatory aspects of sensation—that is, the ability to distinguish differently located

Figure 7.14 *The dorsal column–medial lemniscus pathway.* This is the main pathway for transmission of signals from low-threshold mechanoreceptors. Fibers leading impulses from mechanoreceptors in the face join the medial lemniscus in the brain stem.

and different kinds of stimuli. The pathway appears not to be necessary for the mere perception of, for example, light touch or movement of a joint.

The pathway followed by impulses conducted in the *thin dorsal root fibers* is different. The thin (Aδ and C) primary afferent fibers end in the gray matter of the dorsal horn, where most of the secondary sensory neurons of this pathway are located. The axons of the secondary neurons cross to the other side of the spinal cord and form the *spinothalamic tract* (Fig. 7.15). As the name implies, the fibers of this tract terminate in the thalamus. The spinothalamic tract is of primary importance for the perception of *pain and temperature*, which is consistent with the observation that it transmits information primarily from Aδ and C dorsal root afferents. (There are also some other, less important, pathways capable of transmitting somatosensory information.)

Leg

Arm

Face

Internal capsule

THALAMUS

Ventral posterior
lateral nucleus

Ventral posterior
medial nucleus

MESENCEPHALON

Trigeminal
ganglion

PONS

Spinal
trigeminal
nucleus

MEDULLA
OBLONGATA

Spinothalamic
tract

Spinal
ganglion

MEDULLA
SPINALIS

Figure 7.15 *The spinothalamic tract.* This is the main pathway for transmission of signals from nociceptors and thermoreceptors.

Before we describe the two major somatosensory pathways in more depth, a few basic features of the thalamus need to be emphasized.

The Thalamus—Relay Station for Sensory Pathways

Almost all pathways conducting sensory information from the receptors to the cerebral cortex—the somatosensory pathways among them—are synaptically interrupted in the thalamus. In addition, the thalamus has a decisive influence on the general level of neuronal activity of the cerebral cortex and thus on the level of consciousness. The macroscopic appearance of the thalamus is described and illustrated in Chapter 3 (Figs. 3.21, 3.26, and 7.20). Three major subdivisions, delimited by the Y-shaped *internal medullary lamina*, can be identified macroscopically (Figs. 3.23 and 3.26): the *anterior*, *medial*, and *lateral nuclear groups*. The lateral nucleus is usually divided into a dorsal and a ventral part (each consisting of several subnuclei; see also Figs. 7.20 and 20.7). Within and close to the internal medullary lamina are several less clearly defined groups of neurons, the *intralaminar thalamic nuclei*. These are of particular interest because of their relation to the thalamic influence on consciousness and sleep (this is further described in Chapter 15). The intralaminar nuclei are probably also of importance for the perception of pain.

Each of the three major thalamic subdivisions (the anterior, medial, and lateral nuclei) can be further subdivided into smaller parts on the basis of cytoarchitectonics. These are also called the *specific thalamic nuclei*, because most of them are relays in precisely organized, major pathways reaching certain parts of the cerebral cortex only.[3] The various specific nuclei have different functional tasks, and they receive fiber connections from the somatosensory nuclei, the retina, the nuclei of the auditory pathways, the cerebellum, the basal ganglia, and some other cell groups (see, for example, Fig. 14.14). Each nucleus as a rule receives afferents from only one of these sources.

The somatosensory pathways terminate in a subdivision of the lateral thalamic nucleus, as is dealt with in more detail later in this chapter.

The Dorsal Columns and the Medial Lemniscus

The thick, myelinated fibers in the medial portion of the dorsal roots curve rostrally within the dorsal columns just after entering the cord. Many of these fibers ascend to the dorsal column nuclei in the medulla, where they terminate and establish synaptic contacts (Fig. 7.14). As the fibers ascend in the dorsal columns, they send off collaterals ventrally to the spinal gray matter (Fig. 7.10). Most of these collaterals establish snyaptic contact with interneurons, but some reach as far as the ventral horn and contact α motoneurons.[4]

The fibers occupying the medial part of the dorsal columns, the *gracile fascicle* (fasciculus gracilis), conduct impulses from the lower part of the trunk and the legs (Figs. 7.14 and 7.16). These fibers end in the *gracile nucleus* (nucleus gracilis). Impulses from the upper part of the trunk and the arms are conducted in the lateral part of the dorsal columns, the *cuneate fascicle* (fasciculus cuneatus). The fibers of the cuneate fascicle terminate in the *cuneate nucleus* (nucleus cuneatus). Why the longest fibers of the dorsal columns are situated most medially is explained by the simple fact that they enter the cord at the lowermost level, where no other long ascending fibers are present. At higher levels, fibers entering from the dorsal root occupy positions lateral to those that have entered at more caudal levels. Initially the fibers of the dorsal columns are arranged *segmentally* (Fig. 7.16), but as they ascend, the fibers rearrange themselves so that they are organized *somatotopically* (Fig. 7.17)—that is, fibers conducting from the hand lie together, separated from those of the forearm, and so on (compare with the dermatomal map in Fig. 7.12). Thus, fibers from different dorsal roots are mixed at higher levels of the dorsal columns.

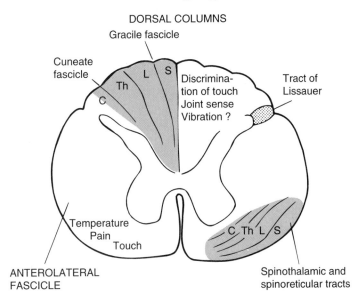

Figure 7.16 *Somatosensory pathways.*
Position and segmental arrangement in
the spinal cord white matter.

The primary afferent fibers ascending in the dorsal columns end in a
particular cytoarchitectonic subdivision of the dorsal column nuclei. The
morphology and arrangement of the neurons in these *cluster regions* ensure a particularly precise topographic arrangement of the afferent and efferent connections. The neurons of the cluster regions of the dorsal column nuclei send their axons rostrally to the thalamus, forming the *medial
lemniscus*. The fibers first course anteriorly and cross the midline to occupy a position just dorsal to the pyramid (Figs. 3.15 and 7.17). In the
pons and the mesencephalon, the medial lemniscus is placed more laterally (Figs. 3.17 and 7.17).

The medial lemniscus ends in the *ventral posterolateral nucleus* (nucleus ventralis posterior lateralis, VPL) (Figs. 7.14 and 7.20). The fibers
of the medial lemniscus are somatotopically organized,[5] and this pattern
is maintained as the fibers terminate in the VPL. Fibers from the gracile
nucleus (sensory impulses from the leg) terminate most laterally, with

Figure 7.17 *Somatosensory pathways.*
Position and somatotopic arrangement
in the medulla and the mesencephalon.

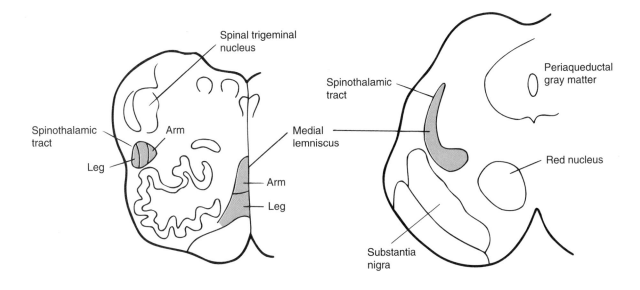

fibers from the cuneate nucleus (arm) terminating more medially. Most medially, in a separate nucleus, the *ventral posteromedial nucleus* (*VPM*), ends the fibers from the sensory trigeminal nucleus (relaying impulses from the face).

The neurons of the VPL and the VPM send their axons into the internal capsule (Figs. 3.26 and 7.14) and further through this to the *postcentral gyrus*. This part of the cortex, made up of cytoarchitectonic fields 3, 1, and 2 (after Brodmann; see Fig. 20.3), constitutes the *primary somatosensory area, SI* (Figs. 7.14, 7.20, and 7.21). In addition, some fibers from the VPL and the VPM end in the *secondary somatosensory area, SII*, situated in the upper wall of the lateral cerebral fissure (Fig. 7.21).

On electrical stimulation of SI or SII, human subjects (during operations with local anesthesia) report that they experience sensory phenomena (tingling, itching, numbness, and other). Just as the somatosensory pathways are somatotopically organized, this is also the case within SI and SII (Figs. 7.14 and 7.21). Fibers conducting impulses from the leg end most medially within the postcentral gyrus, then follow fibers conveying impulses from the trunk, arm, and face successively in the lateral direction. The parts of SI receiving sensory impulses from the feet, hands, and face are much larger than those receiving impulses from other parts of the body (see Fig. 7.22). Also, the region devoted to the thumb is larger than that devoted to the palm of the hand, which in turn is larger than that devoted to the forearm, and so on. This is mainly a reflection of the much higher density of sensory units that supply the skin at distal parts of the extremities (and parts of the face) than more proximal parts of the trunk. To utilize this very detailed information from the most densely innervated parts of the body, a large volume of cortical gray matter—that is, many neurons—has to be available for information processing.

Certain Kinds of Epilepsy Demonstrate the Cortical Somatotopic Pattern

On irritation of the cortex within the postcentral gyrus—for example, by a chip of bone from a skull fracture—the patient may experience fits of abnormal sensations. In the same person, the fits have the same characteristic pattern each time: The sensations are felt in one particular part of the body and then spread gradually to other parts. The spreading follows the known somatotopic pattern within SI (Fig. 7.22). For example, the patient may first experience a tingling sensation in the thumb, then it moves to the index finger and the other fingers, then to the forearm, upper arm, shoulder, and even further. Such epileptic seizures are called *Jacksonian fits* (after a famous British neurologist, Hughlings Jackson). They signify the presence of a local disease process of the brain, and the starting point of the abnormal sensations indicates the focus of the disease. Often the sensory phenomena are followed by muscle spasms (convulsions) due to spreading of the abnormal cortical electrical activity to the motor cortex of the precentral gyrus.

How Do We Study the Function of a Central Nervous Pathway?

Two types of investigations usually form the basis for our conclusions about the function of a particular tract or pathway in the central nervous system. One kind of data derives from the recording of the activity of the neurons of the pathway, to determine the factors that influence their activity. Most of our knowledge of the properties of single neurons in the somatosensory pathways thus derives from experiments in animals, even though recordings have sometimes been done in humans during brain surgery. The other type of investigation is to study the functional deficits that follow disruption of the tract of interest. In humans, diseases and injuries seldom affect one tract or pathway alone (for example only the dorsal columns), and furthermore, it is often not possible to determine the exact site of the damage.

With regard to the two major somatosensory pathways, there is agreement on most points that pertain to the adequate stimulus for single neurons at different levels of the central nervous system. When it comes to the deficits caused by their interruption, however, findings are partly conflicting. This is particularly true of the dorsal column–medial lemniscus system.

Why Similar Experiments May Produce Very Different Sensory Deficits

It may be difficult to understand why apparently identical experimental lesions of sensory tracts in the same species are in one laboratory reported to produce marked disturbances of movements and sensation, whereas in another laboratory hardly any deficits are observed. One explanation may be that, in spite of histological control of the lesions, they may have been of different magnitude and may have either included more than the tract under study or not interrupted all the fibers of the tract. Thus, experiments in cats have shown that sparing as little as 10% of the fibers of the dorsal columns may markedly reduce the sensory deficits with regard to, for example, the discrimination of surfaces with different roughness (as compared with a lesion comprising all fibers). Another reason for different results may be that sometimes the acute effects and the long-term effects of a lesion are not clearly distinguished. As a rule, the acute deficits—that is, those occurring immediately after a tract is cut—are much more severe than those present after some weeks or months. This is mainly due to the plasticity of the nervous system. One reason for functional recovery after brain damage is that other pathways take over. Thus, even if a functional capacity recovers, this does not mean that the destroyed pathway is unimportant for the function. On the other hand, functions that do *not* recover can more confidently be attributed to the destroyed pathway. A final reason for conflicting results may be that different tests are used for evaluating functional deficits. Some tests may be too crude to uncover such deficits, and although the experimental animal or the patient manages the test, the task is solved differently than before.

Single Unit Properties in the Dorsal Column–Medial Lemniscus System

As mentioned, *the dorsal columns contain primarily fibers coming from low-threshold mechanoreceptors in the skin, muscles, and joints.* Recording the activity of single units in the dorsal columns has confirmed this and has also shown that there is a predominance of rapidly adapting sensory units—relatively few are slowly adapting. Recordings from neurons in the *cluster regions of the dorsal column nuclei* show that many neurons are activated only by one kind of receptor and that they have small receptive fields, mostly at the distal parts of the extremities. Some are activated only by joint movement, others only by light touch of the skin, others only by vibration and so on. Such neurons are called *modality-*

specific (because they react only to one kind of stimulus) and *place-specific* (because they are activated only from one restricted part of the body).

Neurons in the *VPL* and *SI* also have the same characteristic response properties as those described for the neurons of the dorsal column nuclei, even though there is an increasing number of neurons that are activated by more than one kind of receptor. Also, the receptive field tends to be somewhat larger for neurons in SI than, for example, in the dorsal column nuclei.

Most of the axons at all levels of the dorsal column–medial lemniscus system are thick and rapidly conducting. This, together with the data from single-unit recordings briefly mentioned above, enable us to conclude that *the dorsal column–medial lemniscus system is particularly well suited to bring fast and precise information from the skin and musculoskeletal system about the type of stimulus, the exact site of the stimulus, and when it starts and stops.* Thus, it provides information about the sensory quality and the spatial and temporal characteristics of any stimulus of low intensity ("what," "where," and "when").

The Dorsal Columns Contain Postsynaptic Fibers Activated From Nociceptors

The fiber composition of the dorsal columns is more heterogeneous than was previously believed. Thus, some ascending axons that synapse in the dorsal column nuclei do not belong to spinal ganglion cells but to neurons with their perikarya in the dorsal horn (so-called postsynaptic dorsal column neurons). The functional properties of these are different from those of the primary sensory neurons with fibers in the dorsal columns. Thus, the postsynaptic units are often activated from several types of receptors. Some have a high stimulus threshold, suggesting that they are activated from nociceptors. It seems likely that they can influence the signals transmitted in the medial lemniscus to the VPL. Thus, in the monkey (in contrast to in the cat) many postsynaptic dorsal column fibers end in parts of the dorsal column nuclei sending fibers to the thalamus. Furthermore, neurons of the gracile nucleus cluster region have recently been shown to receive convergent inputs from low-threshold cutaneous receptors and high-threshold (nociceptive) pelvic visceral receptors, and similar convergence is described for many neurons in the VPL. Thus, although the dorsal column–medial lemniscus system is not primarily concerned with bringing painful stimuli to awareness, signals from nociceptors can nevertheless influence the signal transmission from low-threshold mechanoreceptors. The functional role, if any, of this kind of interaction is unknown. It seems, however, closely related to the well-known phenomenon that pain of visceral origin is usually projected to somatic structures (referred pain, see below).

The Tasks of the Dorsal Column– Medial Lemniscus System

As discussed, the properties of single sensory units of the dorsal column–medial lemniscus system enables it to provide fast and accurate information of sensory stimuli, especially about their temporal and spatial features. The next question is then *how* this information is used by the central nervous system. Unfortunately, on this point conclusions are largely based on the deficits observed when the system is *not* working. Furthermore, because of the adaptive changes taking place after an injury we have to distinguish between the acute and long-term functional deficits.

Most studies (with some exceptions) indicate that in monkeys, as in humans, *acute damage* to the dorsal columns produces severe *ataxia* (insecure and incoordinate movements), which recedes partly or completely within weeks to months after the damage. In some patients, the ataxia may be so severe that they cannot walk without support.

Observations some time after the damage indicate that the *dorsal column–medial lemniscus system is not necessary for all aspects of cutaneous sensation and kinesthesia*. First of all, temperature and pain perception appear to be unaltered by lesioning the dorsal columns. Secondly, light touch of the skin can easily be felt, as can passive joint movements. Two-point discrimination may not be appreciably reduced, and some reports even indicate that the ability to recognize objects by manipulation may be retained (clinical observations do not support the latter point, however). What appears to be *consistently impaired is the ability to solve tasks that require spatially and, in particular, temporally very accurate sensory information*. Thus, a coin pressed into the palm of the hand may perhaps be recognized, but the patient is unable to decide which is the larger of two coins. The patient may also correctly identify that something is moving on the skin, but not the direction of the movement. To ask the patient to identify figures written on the skin is, for example, one sensitive test of the function of the dorsal column–medial lemniscus system. Some careful clinical observations furthermore indicate that the perception of joint position and movement is abnormal after lesions of the dorsal columns.

The above-described sensory deficits occurring after lesions of the dorsal columns have in common that they concern spatial and temporal comparisons of stimuli, that is, what we call *discriminative sensation*. Such sensory information is of crucial importance for the performance of many voluntary movements and, indeed, disturbances of voluntary movements are characteristic of lesions affecting the dorsal column–medial lemniscus system.

After the acute phase, the *movement deficits* concern first and foremost movements that require fast and reliable feedback information from the moving parts. For example, the ability to adjust the grip when an object is slipping is clearly reduced. Delicate movements, such as writing and buttoning, are performed only with difficulty after lesions of the dorsal columns. It is not possible to throw an object accurately or to perform a precise jump, presumably because such activities require feedback information from skin receptors to judge the pressure exerted on the hand by the object or by the ground against the sole of the foot.

Many of the deficits that occur after damage to the dorsal column–medial lemniscus system may not be revealed by a routine neurological examination but may nevertheless render the patient severely handicapped in daily life. One example from a thorough clinical study by the British neurologist Nathan may serve to illustrate this point: A patient with damage to the dorsal columns was aware of a toe being passively moved by the examiner; nevertheless, his shoe would easily slip off his foot without his noticing, and he was unable to roll over in bed because he did not realize that one leg was hanging off the bed. We described earlier in this chapter similar symptoms occurring after loss of thick myelinated nerve fibers in the peripheral nerves. This is not surprising since many of these fibers continue into the dorsal columns (Fig. 7.14). The deficits may be more severe with peripheral loss, however, because also reflex effects from low-threshold mechanoreceptors (among other things) are lost.

In conclusion: *The dorsal column–medial lemniscus system is of primary importance for complex sensory tasks, such as determination (comparison) of direction and speed of moving stimuli. Furthermore, many precise voluntary movements—especially of the hand—depend on the fast sensory feedback provided only by this system. In fact, after damage to the system the motor deficits may be more disturbing than the purely sensory ones.*

The Dorsal Columns and Kinesthesia

Observations in humans have provided conflicting results as to whether lesions of the dorsal column–medial lemniscus system give impaired kinesthesia. A thorough clinical study by Nathan and co-workers, however, concludes that complete lesions of the dorsal columns *do* produce clearcut and enduring kinesthetic deficits. They emphasize, however, that "Routine examination of tactile sensibility does not show up these defects as well as everyday activities of living. The further one gets away from this testing situation, the easier it is to see the effects of these disturbances of sensibility." In monkeys, Vierck and co-workers describe deficient kinesthetic sensation of the hands after cutting the *cuneate fasciculus*, although the problems are only revealed by specific and detailed testing. Thus, the perception of passive finger movements was impaired only if the movements were small or slow. This is indeed what you would expect when eliminating a system devoted to very precise sensory information. It is worth noticing that the monkeys, in addition, had more obvious problems with accurate voluntary hand movements.

Fibers conveying impulses from slowly adapting low-threshold mechanoreceptors in muscles and joints are found only in the cuneate fasciculus and not in the gracile fasciculus, at least in the monkey. Primary afferent fibers with such impulses from the legs leave the gracile fasciculus at the low thoracic level and enter the dorsal horn, where they synapse on second-order sensory neurons. The axons of the latter continue in the dorsal part of the lateral funiculus. Since slowly adapting re-

Reliable Clinical Tests of Dorsal Column–Medial Lemniscus Function

Based on the above considerations, a routine examination of kinesthesia (asking the patient to indicate the direction of movement in a joint being passively moved) would not provide definite information. Thus such a test may be negative (that is, normal performance) in spite of damage to the dorsal columns or the medial lemniscus. Neither is testing the sense of vibration a reliable souce of information; several clinical studies show that it is not always reduced after damage to the dorsal columns. A routine testing of cutaneous sensation would not necessarily reveal the lesion. The most reliable information is presumably obtained by *testing the ability to judge the direction of a stimulus to the skin, and examine the patients ability to identify numbers written on the skin.*

ceptors are responsible for static aspects of kinesthesia, it makes sense that in monkeys no defect of static joint sense is observed in the legs after lesions of the dorsal columns at thoracic or cervical levels. However, the tests used after lesions of the gracile fasciculus did not address specifically small and slow movements, as described above. Whether the difference between the cuneate and the gracile fasciculi with regard to joint afferents pertains also to humans is not known, however.

Figure 7.18 *Signal transmission from nociceptors in the spinal cord.* The terminal region of thin dorsal root fibers leading from nociceptors, and the position of cells sending their axons to the opposite thalamus (spinothalamic neurons). Note that lamina II (the substantia gelatinosa) receives many C fibers, but the neurons of this lamina do not send their axons to the thalamus.

The Spinothalamic Tract

As mentioned, the fibers in the lateral portion of the dorsal roots are predominantly thin ($A\delta$ and C fibers). Immediately after entering the cord, such fibers divide into short ascending and descending branches—passing only for one or two segments in each direction. The collaterals and terminal branches of these fibers pass ventrally to end in the gray substance of the dorsal horn (Figs. 7.11 and 7.18), where they establish synaptic contacts with other neurons. The thinnest (largely C fibers) among the ascending and descending branches of the dorsal root fibers form a small bundle immediately dorsal to the dorsal horn, called the *tract of Lissauer* or the *dorsolateral fasciculus* (Figs. 3.10 and 7.16).[6]

Many neurons in the dorsal horn have long ascending axons. Most of these first course almost horizontally and somewhat ventrally across the midline through the gray substance. After having entered the lateral funiculus on the opposite side, the fibers curve sharply in the rostral direction (Figs. 7.15 and 7.18). As mentioned, some of these fibers ascend without interruption as far as the thalamus, thus forming the *spinothalamic tract.* The fibers of this tract are located anteriorly within the lateral funiculus (anterolateral fascicle) (Fig. 7.16). The spinothalamic fibers are intermingled in the anterolateral fascicle with other fibers that, for example, terminate in lower parts of the brain stem and numerous propriospinal fibers. In the brain stem, the spinothalamic tract is situated laterally and fairly superficially (Fig. 7.17).

The use of axonal transport methods in experimental animals has made it possible to determine the *location of the perikarya of the neurons that give rise to the spinothalamic tract* (Fig. 7.18). Such methods combined with physiological studies of the adequate stimuli and response characteristics of spinothalamic cells have provided new insight in recent years. Particularly, conditions in monkeys may be expected to correspond closely to those in humans (there are differences with regard to the organization of the spinothalamic tract among, for example, the rat, cat, and monkey). *Many spinothalamic cells are located in lamina I.* When we recall that many thin dorsal root afferents establish synapses in lamina I (Fig. 7.18), the relation between the spinothalamic tract and perception of pain becomes understandable. Another major group of spinothalamic cells is located in *lamina V* and particularly in those parts that receive Aδ fibers from the dorsal roots. In addition, scattered spinothalamic cells are found more ventrally in laminae VII and VIII (Fig. 7.18). It may appear surprising, however, that hardly any of the neurons in lamina II (substantia gelatinosa) send fibers into the spinothalamic tract, since most of the dorsal root C fibers terminate in this lamina.

The anatomic data indicate that *most thin dorsal root fibers do not synapse directly (monosynaptically) onto the spinothalamic cells but rather influence them indirectly via spinal interneurons.* The numerous small neurons in lamina II, which are contacted by dorsal root C fibers, send their axons in part dorsally into lamina I—where spinothalamic cells can be influenced—and in part ventrally in the dorsal horn to contact other interneurons, which in their turn form synapses on spinothalamic cells in laminae V, VII, and VIII. In addition, many of the neurons in lamina II send axon collaterals to spinal segments above and below their own (passing in the tract of Lissauer).

The synaptic arrangements underlying further transfer of signals transmitted in thin dorsal root afferents—many coming from nociceptors—must be very complicated. The large number of very small interneurons and the numerous neuroactive substances (for example, numerous neuropeptides) in the dorsal horn make it a difficult task to clarify how the impulses from nociceptors are processed in the spinal cord, and it is understandable that much remains in this respect. Generally, however, we can at least say that *the interneurons of the dorsal horn, especially those of the substantia gelatinosa, have a decisive influence on whether the signals from nociceptors will be transmitted to higher levels of the nervous system.* These interneurons can both inhibit and facilitate the impulse traffic that will ascend in the spinothalamic tract. Thus, they will determine to a large extent how intense the experience of pain will be on a certain stimulation of nociceptors. As we will discuss later in this chapter, the central nervous system can control impulse transmission from receptors in general to our consciousness by, among other things, descending fibers acting on the dorsal horn interneurons.

The *thalamic termination site* of the spinothalamic tract is more extensive than that of the medial lemniscus. Many of the fibers end in the *VPL* with a somatotopic pattern (Fig. 7.15), but not in exactly the same parts as the fibers of the medial lemniscus. The terminal ramifications are also different for the two pathways, reflecting their functional differences. In addition, fibers of the spinothalamic tract end in more posterior parts of the thalamus (in the so-called posterior complex, PO) and in some of the *intralaminar nuclei* (among them, the central lateral nucleus, CL, and the nucleus submedius). These three thalamic regions may possibly be related to somewhat different aspects of pain perception (see below).

The further transmission of impulses from the thalamus takes place—as for the dorsal column–medial lemniscus system—in thalamocortical fibers passing to the *primary and secondary somatosensory areas* (SI and SII). Recordings of single-unit activity in monkey SI indicate that neurons activated by high intensity—presumably noxious—cutaneous stimuli are concentrated in a narrow zone at the transition between Brodmann's areas 3 and 1. This may primarily concern impulses relayed through the VPL, whereas impulses from other parts of the thalamus receiving spinothalamic fibers may directly and indirectly influence other cortical areas as well, such as the *anterior cingulate gyrus* and the *insula*.

Single Unit Properties of Spinothalamic Neurons

As mentioned above, perception of pain and temperature are particularly dependent on the spinothalamic tract. A relatively crude sense of touch and pressure can also be mediated by this pathway, as witnessed by clinical observations. These conclusions fit well with physiological studies of single spinothalamic cells and of thalamic cells in the terminal regions of spinothalamic fibers. It also is in accord with the physiological observation that spinothalamic cells are preferentially activated from thin (Aδ and C) dorsal root fibers.

The *spinothalamic cells in the cord can be classified by their response properties*:

1. *low-threshold units*—cells that react only to light mechanical stimuli (for example, light touch of the skin);
2. *wide dynamic range units* (WDR)—cells that react to stimuli of high intensity (activating nociceptors) and to light stimuli. The impulse frequency of these cells increases with increasing stimulus intensity;
3. *high-threshold units* (HT)—cells that respond only to stimuli of an intensity sufficient to activate nociceptors; and
4. *thermosensitive units*—cells that respond only to either warming or cooling of the skin, indicating that they are activated by thermoreceptors.

The Function of the Spinothalamic Tract

The properties of spinothalamic cells, which have been determined in animal experiments, agree well with clinical observations in patients who have been subjected to therapeutic interruption of the anterolateral funiculus (containing the spinothalamic tract and other fibers). This operation, called *chordotomy*, is sometimes applied to alleviate intense pain that cannot be overcome in any other way (particularly pain caused by cancer of the lower abdominal and pelvic viscera). After such an operation, sensations of pain and temperature are almost totally abolished in the opposite side of the body in the parts supplied by sensory fibers from the spinal segments below the level of interruption.[7] Observations in patients with spinal injuries that leave only the anterolateral fascicle intact for the central transmission of sensory signals also indicate that some sensations of touch and kinesthesia remain.

Single-unit recordings in the *three main thalamic terminal regions* of the spinothalamic tract have suggested that there are certain functional differences among them. Schematically, the fibers ending most posteriorly (in PO) may be responsible for the immediate awareness of something painful ("ouch!"); those ending in the VPL signal where exactly the painful stimulus is ("my finger!"), whereas fibers ending in the intralaminar nuclei may be responsible for the intense discomfort and obligatory emotional aspects of pain sensation ("it hurts so—help me!"). Although this hypothesis probably captures some characteristic features, it is obviously an oversimplification. For example, recent evidence suggests that the emotional aspects of pain depend on all three terminal regions.

Spinothalamic Cells Receive Impulses from Both Somatic and Visceral Structures: Referred Pain

Recording from spinothalamic cells in the spinal cord has shown that many can be activated by nociceptive stimuli applied to visceral organs and to the skin. Impulses from the skin and viscera converge onto the same neuron, which then conveys the information to the thalamus. Nociceptive impulses from muscles and skin can also converge onto the same spinothalamic neuron. *Sensory convergence of this kind pertains to regions of the skin and deep tissues and to visceral organs that receive sensory innervation from the same segments of the cord.* The primary sensory fibers can activate the spinothalamic cells monosynaptically or via one or more interneurons (polysynaptically). In any case, presumably it will not be possible for higher levels of the central nervous system to decide whether the impulses arriving from a particular spinothalamic cell (receiving convergent inputs) originate in the skin or in a visceral organ. But because nociceptors in the skin are stimulated often during daily life, whereas those in the heart, for example, are activated only when the organ is diseased, we assume that the brain gets used to interpreting the signals as always coming from the skin. When signals arise for the first time in the heart, they are misinterpreted as coming from the skin. The pain is felt in the skin and perhaps deep structures, even though it arises elsewhere. This phenomenon, commonly experienced with diseases of visceral organs, is called *referred pain*. Infarction of the heart, for example, is usually accompanied by pain localized to the left arm, diseases of the gallbladder may manifest themselves with pain below the right shoulder blade, irritation of the diaphragm produces pain at the top of the shoulder, and so forth. Convergence on spinothalamic cells may also explain the phenomenon of *hyperesthesia*—that is, a region of skin becomes abnormally sensitive, such that even light touch may provoke pain. This is commonly observed with diseases of visceral organs, and careful examination to search for hyperesthetic skin regions may provide valuable diagnostic information. Thus, impulses from the visceral organ excite the spinothalamic cell so that less excitation from the skin is necessary to fire the cell (recall that many spinothalamic cells receive inputs from both low-threshold and high-threshold receptors—the wide dynamic range neurons).

Additional Pathways for Somatosensory Information

Many sensory spinal neurons send their axons to brain stem nuclei other than the dorsal column nuclei and the thalamus, and therefore do not belong to the two major somatosensory pathways described above. Yet they transmit somatosensory information. Some such brain stem nuclei supply the *cerebellum* and are not directly concerned with conscious sensation. Others are involved in reflex, *autonomic responses* (alterations of blood pressure and heart rate, sweating, breathing, muscle tension, control of the bladder and the bowel, and so forth). There remains, however, ascending fibers from the cord that end in cell groups projecting to the thalamus (among other targets). Most important are probably certain neuronal groups in the *reticular formation* in the pons and mesencephalon, such as the *parabrachial nucleus* (consisting of several subnuclei). Thus, a *spinoreticulothalamic pathway* may be capable of transmitting somatosensory signals to the cerebral cortex. The *spinoreticular fibers* are mixed with the spinothalamic fibers in the anterolateral fascicle (Fig. 15.8). Their cell bodies are located mainly in *lamina VII–VIII*, and some are activated by *noxius stimuli*. However, the parabrachial nucleus is special since it receives spinal afferents mainly from *lamina I*, which contains many neurons specifically activated from nociceptors.

Whereas the spinothalamic tract is mainly crossed, the spinoreticular pathways are bilateral. Thus, unilateral stimuli would reach the thalamus (and cerebral cortex) of both sides. Many reticulothalamic fibers end in the *intralaminar thalamic nuclei*, which has been taken to suggest that the spinoreticulothalamic pathway is of particular importance for the emotional (affective) component of pain perception (several studies indicate, however, that the affective aspect of pain is related to transmission through other parts of the thalamus as well). Detailed anatomic studies suggest that nociceptive spinoreticular neurons overlap only moderately with reticulothalamic neurons in the brain stem. This is not what one would expect if the spinoreticulothalamic pathway were important for transmission of nociceptive information. On the other hand, recordings during brain surgery in humans with chronic pain syndromes indicate abnormal activity of the spinoreticulothalamic pathway. Perhaps this pathway is involved in pain perception only under abnormal circumstances. In any case, the functional role of the spinoreticulothalamic pathway is difficult to ascertain. Thus, the spinoreticular axons are intermingled with the spinothalamic ones and cannot be lesioned alone. Chordotomy, for example, interrupts both spinothalamic and spinoreticular axons.

In animals such as cats and monkeys, another pathway for somatosensory signals has been discovered in addition to those described above. This is interrupted in a small cell group located in the lateral funiculus at cervical levels of the cord, the *lateral cervical nucleus*. The afferents to this nucleus come from neurons in the dorsal horn, located particularly in lamina IV. The neurons of the lateral cervical nucleus send their axons to end—after crossing the midline—in the VPL of the thalamus. This spinocervicothalamic pathway has been most intensively investigated in the cat, in which it conducts impulses both from nociceptors and from cutaneous low-threshold mechanoreceptors. The functional role of this pathway is not clear, however, and it is not established with certainty that it is present in man.

Some of the cell groups (included in the reticular formation) receiving somatosensory information from the cord, project to the *hypothalamus* and the *amygdala*. Such connections are probably involved in the varied affective, autonomic, endocrine, and behavioral responses to noxious stimuli, which will be discussed in Chapters 18 and 19. Suffice it here to emphasize that *signals from somatosensory receptors, and nociceptors in particular, reach many parts of the central nervous system and influence a number of processes in addition to evoking conscious sensations.*

Furthermore, it has been found that the peripheral nerve fiber of a few *spinal ganglion cells divides, with one branch going to the skin and another going to a visceral organ or a muscle.* This may also serve to explain the phenomenon of referred pain. Cutaneous hyperesthesia may in such instances be caused by a so-called axon reflex (see Chapter 17, *The Axonal Reflex*), since sensory impulses from the visceral organ are conducted not only into the cord but also peripherally in the branch to the skin. There neuropeptides, such as SP and VIP, may be liberated from the sensory fibers and cause changes of blood flow in the hyperesthetic area of the skin (see *Primary Sensory Fibers and Transmitter Substances*, above).

The data referred to above may not give a complete explanation of referred pain. Thus, recent studies show (contrary to earlier beliefs) also that *many neurons of the dorsal column–medial lemniscus pathway receive converging inputs from visceral organs and somatic structures* (especially the skin). This has been shown both in the dorsal column nuclei and in the thalamus, and usually concerns convergence of a low-threshold cutaneous input with a noxious visceral input (such as unphysiological distension of a hollow organ, or more moderate distension of an inflamed organ).

Alterations of *autonomically regulated processes of the skin*, such as blood flow and sweat secretion, may also be mediated by spinal reflexes. Thus, impulses from visceral nociceptors may activate sympathetic (preganglionic) neurons in the cord, which influence vessels and sweat glands. Again, the skin manifestations are localized to dermatomes that are supplied from the same spinal segments as the diseased visceral organ.

The Transmission of Sensory Impulses Can Be Controlled from the Brain

It has been known for a long time that there are descending fiber connections from the cerebral cortex and the brain stem ending in the various relay nuclei of the somatosensory pathways. One important group of such connections arises in the *SI and terminates in the thalamus (VPL and other nuclei), the dorsal column nuclei, the sensory trigeminal nucleus, and the dorsal horn of the cord.* These connections are somatotopically organized and enable selective control of sensory signal transmission from particular parts of the body and from particular receptor types (the fibers ending in the dorsal horn of the spinal cord constitute part of the pyramidal tract; see Chapter 12, *Termination of the Pyramidal Tract*). Physiological studies indicate that descending connections from the SI sometimes can facilitate impulse transmission through the sensory relay nuclei, but inhibitory effects appear to be most common. The latter effects are most likely mediated via inhibitory interneurons. Recordings from single units of the medial lemniscus in conscious monkeys have shown reduced impulse traffic from cutaneous receptors immediately before a voluntary movement. There is indirect evidence of the same phenomenon in man: The threshold for perceiving a vibratory stimulus is elevated immediately before a voluntary movement. Perhaps this happens because proprioceptive signals are of greater importance than cutaneous ones in this particular situation. We know from daily life that we have the ability to leave out sensory signals that are irrelevant at the moment. Without such filtering mechanisms, we would be flooded by sensory information. *The sensory information finally reaching the cerebral cortex is therefore "censored" and distorted compared with the stimuli received by the receptors.*

PAIN

Nociceptors and the Perception of Pain

It should be emphasized at this point that activation of nociceptors—provoked by noxious stimuli—and the conscious experience of pain may occur independently of each other. The usual definition of a *nociceptor* is purely physiological: *A receptor that is activated by stimuli that produce tissue damage, or would do so if the stimulus continued.* On the other hand, *pain* is a subjective experience with a psychological definition: *An unpleasant sensory and emotional experience, which occurs together with actual or threatening tissue damage, or is described as if it were caused by tissue damage.* Usually, of course, the pain we feel is caused by nociceptor activation by noxious stimuli, and when we feel pain we more or less automatically put it in conjunction with something that harms our body. Nevertheless, there are many examples of persons exposed to massive nociceptor stimulation who feel no pain, and, vice versa, a person may suffer the most intense pain, yet there may be no evidence of nociceptor stimulation. Examples of the first situation are seen in serious accidents in which the injured person may experience no pain immediately afterward, in spite of considerable tissue damage. This is most likely explained by mechanisms of the brain preventing signals from nociceptors from reaching consciousness (considered further below). The experience of pain without any signals from nociceptors is perhaps most dramatically exemplified in patients with injuries in which the dorsal roots are literally torn out of the cord. Even though no sensory signals at all can enter the cord, the patient often feels excruciating pain in the denervated parts of the body (called *deafferentation pain*). The so-called *phantom pain* that sometimes occurs after amputations is another example: In this case, the pain is felt in a part of the body that no longer exists. Thalamic lesions may sometimes be accompanied by the experience of severe pain, which is completely independent of what is going on in the painful part of the body (*thalamic pain*). There are also many examples from clinical practice of pain that continues or even gets more severe long after the injury that initially caused the pain is completely healed. In such cases there is evidence that alterations have occurred in the central nervous system itself—for example, in the dorsal horn or in the thalamus—that perpetuate without any external stimuli the neuronal activity in regions of the brain related to the experience of pain. Stimulation of intralaminar thalamic nuclei in some patients undergoing brain surgery for movement disorders (that is, without chronic pain) are reported not to produce pain (or any other sensation), whereas stimulation of corresponding sites in patients suffering from pain of the deafferentation type can provoke or intensify their usual type of pain.

Clinical experience and animal experiments indicate that many parts of the brain (among them, parts of the so-called limbic system) are of importance for our perception of pain and how we cope with it. After large lesions of the frontal lobes, for example, a peculiar indifference to pain may occur. The patient feels the pain, but the emotional coloring—which makes us describe pain more vividly than other sensations—is lacking. But in healthy persons, too, as most of us have experienced, the intensity of pain may vary considerably with our state of mind. For example, anxiety makes the pain much worse. If we do not know the cause and fear that it may be caused by a dangerous disease, the pain may be felt as intolerable. As soon as we are told that the cause is innocent and that the pain will soon pass, it feels less intense.

Chronic Pain and Plastic Changes in The Dorsal Horn

Many observations suggest that acute, "ordinary" pain differs from chronic pain regarding central mechanisms. The former is clearly related to nociceptor activation, and ends when (or shortly after) the stimulus ends. The threshold for eliciting acute pain is high (cf. the definition of a nociceptor above), and the pain serves a protective purpose. Chronic pain, on the other hand, is characterized by an abnormally lowered threshold, so that normal, innoxious stimuli (such as touching the skin) elicit pain (*allodynia*). Furthermore, the experience of pain upon nociceptor stimulation is more intense than normal (*hyperalgesia*). Thus, the somatosensory system is abnormally sensitive.

We all experience this altered state of the somatosensory system with, for example, a sprained ankle or a local infection—that is, in situations with *inflammation*. Even slight movement or touching of the injured part evokes intense pain, or it may be painful also at rest. Nevertheless, also in this situation the pain can be seen as biologically meaningful, since it ensures that the injured part gets the necessary rest. The lowered pain threshold, which may arise in minutes after an injury, is due to sensitization of both the receptors and of neurons in the dorsal horn. In addition, "silent" nociceptors become active when certain mediators of inflammation accumulate in the tissue. The increased sensitivity of the dorsal horn neurons is most likely caused by liberation of neuropeptides from the central terminals of dorsal root fibers. Neuropeptides, such as SP, increase the postsynaptic sensitivity to glutamate. For example, increased glutamate sensitivity of wide-dynamic range spinothalamic neurons would make them react more vigorously to inputs from low-threshold mechanoreceptors.

Normally, the pain subsides in parallel with the inflammation as the tissue heals. In some patients, however, *the pain continues in spite of complete healing*, as mentioned above. Such a condition can also be produced in experimental animals by provoking longstanding inflammatory reactions in the skin or a joint, or by damage to peripheral nerves. The continuation of the pain is related to persistence of the synaptic changes in the dorsal horn (and probably at other sites, such as the thalamus). Thus, a state persists in which there is an *abnormal reaction to stimulation of low-threshold mechanoreceptors* (with signals conducted centrally in thick $A\beta$ fibers). The traffic of such impulses apparently serves to perpetuate the pain. We do not know why such central changes persist in some patients and not in others. It typically occurs, however, when the healing process after a compound injury to an extremity is delayed and painful, for example due to inadequate initial treatment. For example, an apparently trivial fracture of the radius is sometimes followed by insufferable pain for years after the fracture has healed. The pain is usually characterized by a burning quality and is triggered by innoxious stimuli, such as light touch or a movement. The condition is called *causalgia* (other names are also used for this and related conditions of persistent posttraumatic pain). See also Chapter 17, *Pain Relief and Blockage of the Sympathetic System.*

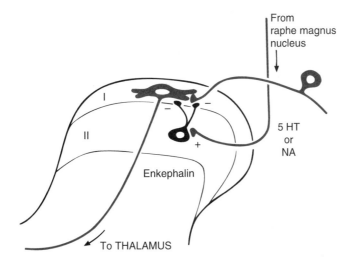

Central Control of Transmission from Nociceptors and Pain Sensation

Among the various aspects of central control of sensory impulse transmission, those related to pain in particular have received much attention in recent years. A dramatic observation by Reynolds in the late 1960s was the starting point for much later research. He showed that by electrical stimulation of a mesencephalic region, the *periaqueductal gray matter* (PAG) (substantia grisea centralis) (Figs. 3.19 and 7.17), conscious rats could be subjected to major surgery without apparently feeling any pain (as judged from their behavior and other observations). The stimulation produced *analgesia* (no experience of pain on noxious stimuli). In humans, too, electrical stimulation of regions close to the PAG has been tried, to treat patients with severe chronic pain, with some good results. Subsequent research with anatomic, physiological, and pharmacological methods indicates that the effect of PAG stimulation can be explained, at least in part, by activation of descending fiber connections to the dorsal horn. Although a sparse direct pathway from the PAG to the spinal cord exists, the main pathway appears to be synaptically interrupted in cell groups in the medulla, especially the *raphe magnus nucleus* (NRM) (Figs. 15.1 and 15.5) and other nearby cell groups in the medullary reticular formation (see Chapter 15). The descending fibers from these nuclei (raphespinal fibers) lie in the dorsal part of the lateral funiculus (dorsolateral fascicle) (Fig. 7.19), and cutting the latter abolishes the effects of PAG stimulation almost completely. Electrical stimulation of NRM inhibits spinothalamic cells so that they are less readily activated by impulses from nociceptors. We do not know in detail the neuronal interconnections in the spinal cord mediating these effects from the brain stem, but it is of interest that fibers from the NRM establish synapses in the dorsalmost part of the dorsal horn (laminae I and II), which receives most dorsal root fibers conveying impulses from nociceptors. Many of the NRM neurons contain *serotonin*, and this is apparently a transmitter at synapses established by the boutons of the raphespinal fibers in the cord.[8] The actions of serotonin are complex and not fully understood. Experiments with microinjections of serotonin indicate that it has an inhibitory effect on nociceptive spinothalamic cells. Probably, the inhibitory effects are mediated partly by direct synapses on spinothalamic cells of raphespinal fibers and partly by synapses on dorsal horn interneurons (Fig. 7.19).

Some of the dorsal horn interneurons contain *opioid peptides*. These neuropeptides, found in many parts of the brain, got their name because they have actions that resemble closely those of the opiate-type drugs (such as morphine). The naturally occurring (endogenous) peptides of this kind are also called *endorphins*—that is, endogenous morphine. Opioids, when injected locally in the dorsal horn, have inhibitory effects on spinothalamic cells, but it is not known whether the inhibition is caused by a direct action or is mediated by interneurons (or both). Three main groups of endorphins have so far been discovered, each with its characteristic distribution in the brain and spinal cord. Best characterized are *β endorphin*, two varieties of *enkephalin*, and *dynorphin*. Whereas *β* endorphin is restricted to one neuronal group in the hypothalamus (the arcuate nucleus), the enkephalins and dynorphin are present in interneurons in many parts of the central nervous system (among them, parts that are not concerned with aspects of pain sensation).

The effects of PAG stimulation on pain sensation are probably not only mediated by descending connections to the cord. There are also *ascending connections from the PAG*, which may influence impulse transmission at the thalamic level (intralaminar thalamic nuclei) or in other cell groups related to pain sensation.

We may conclude so far that the brain contains groups of neurons and fiber connections that, under appropriate circumstances, can effectively suppress the experience of pain (produce analgesia) or, in the case of animal experiments, suppress behavior that is normally linked with experience of pain. There is nevertheless much to be learned before we know the anatomic organization of the pain-suppressing systems and, in particular, the interactions between the numerous transmitters and neuropeptides involved.

The Functional Role of Pain-Suppressing Systems

We do not fully understand the functional role of the pain-suppressing systems and under which conditions they are normally activated. It is reasonable to assume, however, that they are active in situations with severe injuries and little or no experience of pain (as, for example, in war and major civil accidents). Suppression of pain may in such situations enable continuation of intense physical activity for a while, which may be of vital importance. Also, in more peaceful vigorous physical activities, such as sport competitions, it is obvious that pain sensitivity may be markedly reduced. Animal experiments further indicate that analgesia may be produced in certain stressful situations, characterized by the inability of the animal to escape a threatening or unpleasant situation ("stress-induced analgesia"). It has been suggested that *suppression of pain sensation is just one among several adjustments of the body, controlled by the nervous system, to certain kinds of extraordinary physical demands or stress.*

Analgesia Can Be Produced by Drugs, Nerve Stimulation, or Stress

That morphine and other opiates can alleviate severe pain has been known for hundreds of years. Today we know that there are *receptors in the brain to which opiates can bind* and exert their effects. These receptors are actually receptors for the endorphins, and at least five different receptors, each with affinity for a certain subgroup of endorphins, have so far been identified. Opiate receptors (binding morphine) are present in, among other places, the PAG, the NRM, and parts of the *spinal dorsal horn* (especially laminae I, II, and V; compare with Fig. 7.19). Microinjection of morphine in the PAG can produce analgesia in experimental animals that depend at least in part on connections from the NRM to the spinal cord. The actions of morphine appear thus to be exerted both in the spinal cord and in the PAG. In the cord, binding of morphine to opiate receptors on inhibitory interneurons in the substantia gelatinosa and, presumably, on primary afferent terminals, leads to inhibition of spinothalamic cells. The action in the PAG occurs most likely by activation of the descending pathway from NRM and probably also by activation of ascending connections from the PAG acting on higher levels of the central nervous system. Binding of morphine in other parts of the brain, such as nuclei of the limbic system, is probably also of importance to explain the actions of morphine.

Conditions are indeed complex, as witnessed by experiments indicating that stimulation of the *PAG may produce analgesia by two different mechanisms*. Stimulation of the ventral part of the PAG in rats produced analgesia that appeared to be mediated by opioids (endorphins) because the effect could be abolished by injections of *naloxone* (which prevents binding of some opioids to their receptors). Stimulation of dorsal parts of the PAG, on the other hand, produced an analgesia that could not be reversed by naloxone, suggesting that transmitters other than endorphins were responsible for the analgesia.

Analgesia may also be produced by *stimulation of peripheral nerves*. When done with surface electrodes, the procedure is called *transcutaneous nerve stimulation* (TNS). One kind of analgesia occurs immediately and is mediated by activity of thick myelinated fibers in the stimulated nerves (that is, fibers leading from low-threshold mechanoreceptors). Selective stimulation of such fibers is elicited by electrical stimulation with high frequency and low intensity or by natural stimuli such as vibration, light touch, or pressure. The analgesia is restricted to parts of the body innervated by the peripheral nerves, and it usually disappears when the stimulation stops. This kind of analgesia is thought to be mediated by activity in collaterals of the thick dorsal root fibers that can inhibit impulse transmission from the thin (Aδ and C) fibers in the dorsal horn (most likely via inhibitory interneurons). This mechanism is presumably the basis of the everyday observation that it helps to blow at a finger that hurts, that it may help to move the part that has received an acute injury, that the pains of labor may be alleviated by rubbing over the lower back, and so forth.

Another kind of stimulation-induced analgesia requires that thin sensory fibers be activated. This can be achieved by electrical stimulation of low frequency with relative high intensity. Classical *acupuncture* probably obtains the same effect by rotation of thin needles in the tissue. The analgesia produced by this kind of stimulation occurs with a latency after the stimulation has started, and it may last for hours after termination of the stimulation. If analgesia occurs (it does not always happen), it is not limited to the parts of the body that were stimulated. This kind of stimulation-induced analgesia is most likely due to, at least in part, activation of the descending connections from the brain stem described above. This may happen by way of collaterals from spinothalamic and spinoreticular cells to the PAG and adjacent parts of the reticular formation, assuming that activation of thin dorsal root afferents first activate spinothalamic cells in the cord. The analgesia has been reported to be reversed or prevented by intravenous injection of naloxone, and in animal experiments it has been blocked by sectioning the dorsolateral fascicle. The results of such control experiments are, however, in part contradictory and indicate that not all aspects of stimulation-induced analgesia can be explained by liberation of endorphins.

Various kinds of *stressful situations can also produce analgesia* in experimental animals (rats in particular have been used for this kind of research). Depending on the nature of the stress, the analgesia may be mediated by liberation of endorphins or by apparently endorphin-independent mechanisms. There is also evidence to suggest that the *emotional state* of the animal is of importance for whether analgesia is produced or not. Thus, if the animal is frightened instead of calm and relaxed at the start of the period of stress (which may constitute vibration, mild electrical shocks, and so forth), hyperalgesia (increased pain sensitivity) rather than analgesia may occur. Thus, the same stimulus may produce either hyperalgesia or analgesia depending on the state of the animal. It is perhaps of relevance to compare the well-known effects of anxiety on pain perception in humans.

Thus, the distribution in the brain of the opioid peptides shows that they are of importance for functions of the autonomic system, with, for example, marked effects on circulatory and respiratory control.

Detailed anatomic and physiological studies of the *PAG* suggest that this complex of smaller subdivisions plays a pivotal role in *coordinating bodily reactions to painful and potentially harmful somatosensory stimuli*. Interestingly, two main kinds of responses to painful and other

Placebo

The word *placebo* (literally: "I shall please") has been used for a long time about mock medicine; that is, drugs and procedures that the doctor knows have no effect. In clinical trials, for example, salt tablets are given as a placebo to decide whether a drug has a *specific* effect on a disease. Thus, it is well known that a treatment without any specific effect may influence the disease and the experience of pain. The *placebo effect* has attracted special interest in connection with the treatment of pain. We know that the effect is only present if the patient expects the treatment to work. Furthermore, surgery produces a larger placebo effect than drugs, and injection of a drug is more efficient than oral administration. An operation introduced in the 1950s to cure angina pectoris exemplifies the placebo effect of surgery. On a dubious theoretical basis the internal mammary arteries were ligated to improve the blood supply to the ailing heart. Many patients noted improvement in their condition after the surgery. Later pathological examinations showed, however, that no improvement of the blood supply had occurred. Therefore, a study was initiated to compare two groups of patients with angina pectoris: one group underwent ligation of the artery, the other group underwent the same procedure but without ligation (a sham operation). Most of the patients in both groups noted improvement, and the improvement lasted for the observation period of six months. Remarkably, the improvement did not only concern reduction of pain but also objectively measurable variables, such as walking distance, drug consumption, and (in some) even the electrocardiogram. Several later studies have shown similar results. For example, in one study the effect of ultrasound on pain after tooth extractions was compared with placebo. Not only did the patients receiving the probe without any ultrasound (the placebo group) feel less pain, they also got less local edema, and could open their mouths wider than patients receiving no treatment. Thus, *the placebo effect is not limited to subjective experiences related to disease but can also affect physiological processes*. It follows that the placebo effect is not merely a question of imagination, and its presence in a patient is not related to whether the disease is organic or imaginary.

The examples above illustrate that the *expectation* of a positive effect influences markedly how the brain treats signals from nociceptors, and also its control of bodily functions. Thus, the placebo effect depends on whether the patient believes that the doctor can help. In fact, the opposite effect, called *nocebo*, can occur if the patient expects no help, or believes that the treatment may be harmful. In such instances, a neutral substance may worsen the pain and produce unwanted biologic effects. These facts will inevitably influence every therapeutic situation. Besides the specific therapeutic effect of the treatment initiated by the doctor, the outcome for the patient depends on whether the (unspecific) placebo effect is achieved.

A common misconception is that the placebo effect works only with moderate pains, and only in comparison with "weak" drugs. However, if the patient believes that the drug he gets is morphine, the placebo effect is much greater than if he believes it to be aspirin.

What is the *neurobiological basis* of the placebo (and nocebo) effect? The "endorphin hypothesis" became popular when it was reported that the placebo effect could be prevented by an opiate antagonist (naloxone). These results have been criticized. Anyway, as emphasized by Wall, "...it is not clear what insight into the overall placebo phenomenon is provided by showing that some link in the machinery involves endorphins." The placebo and nocebo phenomena should be viewed in a broader context of how the brain handles challenges that threaten the organism or our emotional stability. As with other complex behavioral reactions, many parts (and systems) of the central nervous system are involved, and the total behavior cannot be explained by the actions of one system or one neurotransmitter alone.

stressful stimuli appear to be mediated by different parts of the PAG. One is an active, defensive behavior elicited by external (cutaneous) stimuli, the other is an immobility (freezing) reaction caused by pain arising in visceral organs and joints. This corresponds to typical human reactions to pain originating from skin and from the viscera, respectively. Pain of cutaneous origin typically produces movements and increased heart rate and respiration, whereas pain arising in deep structures is often accompanied by immobility, lowered heart rate, sweating, and nausea.

Modern Views on Pain and Pain Treatment

Recent years of intensive interdisciplinary research have led to important new insights in pain mechanisms, and improved pain therapy. Some aspects have been mentioned above. We now realize that many more parts of the brain are involved in pain processing than believed only 10 years ago. Although we are still far from a complete understanding, we know many of the pieces that form the basis of subjective pain experience and the physical and mental reactions to pain. We also have learned that the central pain system is plastic, so that its behavior can change quickly. This has led to a better understanding of the differences between acute and chronic pain. Some pain conditions, previously rejected as "imaginations" or ignored because they were incomprehensible, can now be at least partly explained in a neurobiological context. Such advances in basic pain research have influenced clinical practice; for example, new drugs are designed to attack the central synaptic changes in chronic pain directly. Furthermore, an important aim for modern pain therapy is to *prevent* the occurrence of the plastic changes in the dorsal horn and elsewhere. Thus, analgesic drugs are often administered *before* surgery, and afterwards the dosage is individualized according to the need of the patient rather than to a fixed scheme. In addition, the importance of quick and adequate pain relief in patients with injuries that are apt to produce persisting pain is being realized.

Better insight in the neurobiology of pain has also led us to abandon the traditional distinction between "organic" and "psychological" pain. Previously, pain states that could not be attributed to a known organic disease with nociceptor activation were often defined as psychological—sometimes with the tacit assumption that the pain was not real. The search was directed toward finding traits of personality that correlated with psychological pain, rather than towards understanding pain as a multifarious phenomenon. It seems more fruitful, however, to focus on what chronic pain—whatever its cause—produces of altered behavior and mood, and on the biological correlates in the central nervous system. It may, furthermore, often be impossible to decide what comes first—the altered psychology or the altered biology. Rather than explaining pain states by putting them into pigeonholes like "bodily" or "mental," we should realize that pain always includes both aspects.

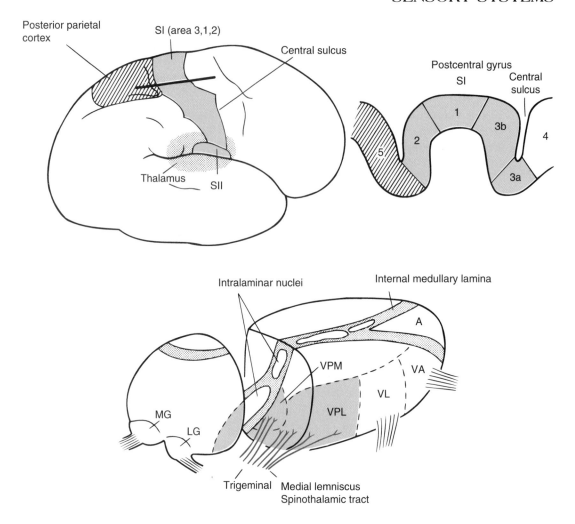

Figure 7.20 *The somatosensory cortex and its thalamic afferent nucleus.* **Upper left** drawing shows the location of the SI and SII and parts of the posterior parietal cortex in the human brain. The extension of the various cytoarchitectonic areas of the central region is shown in the **upper right** drawing.
Below, the VPL—supplying the SI and SII with somatosensory signals—is marked on a schematic drawing of the right thalamus. The main afferent pathways to the VPL are also indicated. A = anterior thalamic nucleus; LG = lateral geniculate body; MG = medical geniculate body; VA = ventral anterior nucleus; VL = ventral lateral nucleus.

THE SOMATOSENSORY CORTICAL REGIONS

As mentioned, the sensory impulses conducted in the medial lemniscus and the spinothalamic tract finally reach the two somatosensory areas, SI and SII. Both of these cortical regions receive somatotopically organized projections from the VPL and VPM (Figs. 7.20, 7.21, and 7.22). Somatosensory impulses also reach other cortical regions, however, such as the MI in the precentral gyrus. Not unexpectedly, primarily signals from proprioceptors are conveyed to the motor cortex.

The Primary Somatosensory Area

The primary somatosensory area (SI) in particular has been the subject of intense anatomic and physiological investigations. The subdivision of SI into different cytoarchitectonic areas—3, 1, and 2 of Brodmann (Figs. 12.3 and 20.2)—corresponds to functional differences. These areas extend as narrow strips from the midline laterally along the postcentral gyrus—that is, perpendicular to the somatotopic arrangement (Figs. 7.20 and 20.3). Animal experiments, particularly by the American neurophys-

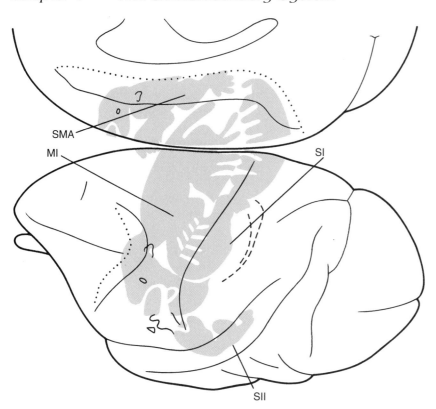

Figure 7.21 *The somatosensory regions SI and SII and their somatotopic organization* (monkey). Motor areas are also shown. Redrawn from Woolsey (1964).

iologist Mountcastle, show that the cytoarchitectonic subdivisions differ with regard to the kinds of receptor from which they receive information. *Area 3a*, on the transition to the MI[9] (Fig. 12.3), receives sensory signals from *muscle spindles* in particular. Neurons in *area 3b* are first and fore-

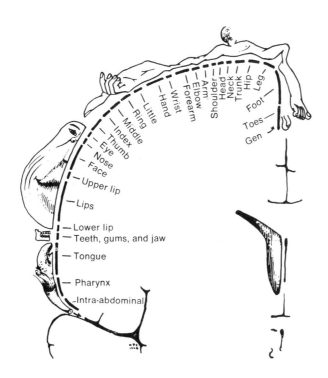

Figure 7.22 *Relative size of the cortical regions representing various body parts.* Schematic section through the postcentral gyrus (SI) of the human brain. Based on electrical stimulation during brain surgery under local anesthesia. From Penfield and Rasmussen (1950).

most activated by stimulation of *cutaneous receptors* (predominantly by low-threshold mechanoreceptors). Neurons receiving information from rapidly adapting receptors appear to be separated from those receiving from slowly adapting receptors. *Area 2* is influenced by proprioceptors to a larger extent than area 3b—for example, many neurons are most easily activated by bending of a joint. *Within each of the cytoarchitectonic subdivisions it appears that the whole body has its representation*; thus there are probably three body maps within SI. The map in Figure 7.21 therefore gives a somewhat misleadingly simplified presentation.

Even though many neurons in SI are activated only or most easily from one receptor type—that is, they are *modality-specific*—there are also neurons in SI with more complex properties. Many neurons have, for example, large receptive fields, indicating that they receive convergent inputs from many primary sensory neurons. Even though many neurons are activated by movement of just one joint in one direction, others are activated by several joints. Some neurons in SI require specific combinations of receptor inputs to be activated. Thus, *some processing of the "raw" sensory information also takes place in SI—it is not merely a simple receiver of sensory information.*

Efferent association connections from SI pass posteriorly to the posterior parital cortex, which further processes the sensory information, and anteriorly to the motor cortex (MI). The latter connections appear to be of particular importance while learning new movements, whereas they are not crucial for the performance of well-rehearsed movements (as judging from lesion experiments in monkeys). This may be explained by an extra need for fast and precise feedback from the moving parts during learning. The connections from SI to MI are, furthermore, necessary for motor recovery after cutting the connections from the cerebellum to MI. This may also be regarded as a learning situation.

Further Processing of Sensory Information Outside SI

Even though some processing takes place already in SI, clinical and experimental observations show that the cortex posterior to SI is necessary for comprehensive utilization of the sensory information reaching the cerebral cortex. The *posterior parietal cortex comprises areas 5 and 7* (Figs. 7.20 and 20.12) and belongs to the so-called association areas of the cerebral cortex, which will be treated in Chapter 20. Areas 5 and 7 do not receive direct sensory information from the large somatosensory pathways but via numerous association fibers from SI and SII. They also receive numerous connections from other parts of the cortex. Neurons in area 5, for example, often have large receptive fields and respond only to complex combinations of stimuli, as shown in monkeys. Their activity may depend not only on what is occurring in the periphery but also on whether the *attention* of the monkey is directed toward the actual stimulus. Some neurons are only active in conjunction with the monkey stretching its arm toward something it wants. Broadly speaking, *in areas 5 and 7 the bits of information reaching SI are put together and compared with other inputs* (such as visual information, and information about the mental state of the animal).

Which Cortical Regions Receive Information
from Nociceptors?

The number of neurons in SI activated from nociceptors has been found in animal experiments to be surprisingly low, considering that no other area appears to contain more of them than SI. Although pain sensations have been elicited by electrical stimulation of SI in humans, this is an infrequent effect of such stimulation. Ablations of SI do not necessarily reduce pain perception, and only occasionally has it been reported to relieve chronic pain. It is fair to say that the central processing of signals from nociceptors is far less understood than the processing of signals from other kinds of receptors. Some have even questioned the importance of the cerebral cortex for pain perception. However, recent studies in humans show that painful stimuli to the hand is accompanied by a clearcut increase of blood flow in the SI hand representation. Such studies have given partly conflicting results as to activation of other parts of the cortex. Several authors have, however, reported increased blood flow in the *anterior part of the cingulate gyrus*. This part of the cortex appears to be related to emotions, and surgical removal of the anterior cingulate gyrus has been used in the treatment of certain pain conditions. For the patients helped by the operation, especially if the affective aspect of pain perception is reduced—the pain is still there but less unpleasant and bothersome (this is similar to pain perception after large lesions of the frontal lobe). Activation of the *insula* has also been reported to be associated with painful stimuli in humans.

Lesions of the Somatosensory Areas

Lesions of SI in humans entail reduced sensation in the opposite half of the body. A localized destruction of the SI, or of the fibers reaching it from the thalamus, may produce loss of sensation in a restricted area (corresponding to the somatotopic localization within SI). Not all sensory qualities are affected equally, however. *Discriminative cutaneous sensation* and *kinesthesia* are particularly disturbed; much less reduced (if at all) is pain sensation. As is the case with lesions of the dorsal columns, the sensory deficits gradually diminish after the time of the lesion. The least improvement is seen, however, in the discriminative aspects of sensation, and is the most pronounced for pain. This can perhaps be explained by the fact that the pathways for signals from nociceptors are to a larger extent bilateral than the pathways from low-threshold mechanoreceptors. It might also be explained by signals from nociceptors being distributed to areas outside the SI.

Whereas lesions of the posterior parietal cortex produce difficulties with the *use of objects* (apraxia), lesions of SII and neighboring regions in the insula impair the ability to *recognize* objects by touch (tactile agnosia). Similar problems with the visual recognition of objects occur after lesions of dorsal and ventral divisions of the extrastriatal visual areas, respectively.

NOTES

1. In reality, the conditions are even more complex. There are, among other things, two types of nuclear bag fibers differing ultrastructurally and histochemically, and only one of them, called bag$_1$, appears to be responsible for the dynamic sensitivity of the primary sensory ending. The other type, called bag$_2$, behaves more like a nuclear chain fiber and contributes presumably only to the static sensitivity.

2. Figure 7.7 shows that stimulation of γ_s in fact reduces the dynamic sensitivity of the primary sensory ending, since there is no extra increase in firing rate of the Ia fiber during the stretch phase. Under the influence of γ_s, the primary sensory ending behaves more like a secondary one.

3. The intralaminar thalamic nuclei were formerly often called the unspecific thalamic nuclei, because their connections with the cerebral cortex were thought to be diffusely distributed, in contrast to the connections of the specific thalamic nuclei. More recent studies have, however, questioned the unspecific nature of the intralaminar nuclei.

4. Many of the primary afferent fibers in the dorsal columns do not reach the dorsal column nuclei, even though they may pass through many segments—for example, from the lumbar to the cervical levels. Furthermore, not all fibers of the dorsal columns are primary afferents. Thus, the dorsal columns contain a large number of *propriospinal axons*— that is, from neurons located in the spinal gray matter interconnecting spinal segments. Furthermore, some dorsal horn neurons (especialy in lamina 3 and 4) send their axons as far as to the dorsal column nuclei (postsynaptic dorsal column fibers).

Finally, at least in experimental animals, the dorsal columns also contain some *descending axons* coming from neurons in parts of the dorsal column nuclei and making synaptic contacts in the dorsal horn. Thus, the dorsal column nuclei may be able to influence the processing of sensory information at the spinal level.

5. That fibers carrying impulses from the leg are located more anteriorly within the medial lemniscus than those related to the arm (Fig. 7.14) is simply because the gracile nucleus is situated more caudally than the cuneate nucleus. When fibers from the cuneate nucleus join those from the gracile nucleus, the most anterior position is already occupied.

6. There has been a long-standing controversy with regard to the fiber composition of the tract of Lissauer, largely because of difficulties in tracing unmyelinated fibers. Recent investigations with improved methods indicate that about 80% of the fibers of the tract of Lissauer are primary afferent (dorsal root) fibers. The other fibers are propriospinal fibers ensuring cooperation between neighboring segments. This concerns in particular Rexed's laminae I and II, which also receive most of the synapses formed by the thin primary afferent fibers.

7. Usually, however, the pain returns during some months to a year after chordotomy. The reason for this is so far unknown, but possibly other pathways that under normal conditions are not of importance for transmission of painful stimuli take over.

8. Transmitters other than serotonin, such as norepinephrine, apparently also contribute to the effects on pain transmission obtained by stimulation of NRM and nearby structures. Conditions are complex, with several brain stem cell groups that can, in their own way, influence the transfer of nociceptive impulses to spinothalamic cells. Many of the NRM neurons contain one or more neuropeptides in addition to serotonin.

9. Some have argued that area 3a should be considered a part of the MI rather than of SI. In certain respects, anatomically and physiologically, it represents at least a transitional zone.

CHAPTER 8

THE VISUAL SYSTEM

Vision is the most important of the special senses of humans. There are approximately 1 million axons in the optic nerve, constituting almost 40% of the total number of axons in the cranial nerves. A correspondingly large part of the cerebral cortex is devoted to the analysis of visual information. The receptors for sight, *photoreceptors*, are the *rods* and *cones* of the *retina*. Their adequate stimulus is electromagnetic waves with a wavelength between 400 and 700 nm. The photoreceptors do not react to light with shorter (ultraviolet light) or longer (infrared light) wavelengths. The rods are responsible for vision in dim light, whereas the cones are responsible for vision in daylight and for color vision.

In this chapter we deal with the pathways for visual impulses from the eye to various parts of the central nervous system and also with how visual information is processed at various levels of the visual pathways. To understand the visual system, it is not sufficient to know the *conscious use of visual information*; the many *reflex effects* elicited by visual stimuli must also be taken into account. Among the reflex effects are those ensuring that our gaze is fixed on the object we want to examine and follows it if it moves, and those ensuring that the visual images formed at the retina are always in focus. Such visual reflexes, however, are only briefly mentioned in this chapter. They are discussed more thoroughly in Chapter 16 in relation to the innervation of the eye muscles and the vestibular apparatus.

THE EYEBALL AND THE REFRACTING MEDIA

The Eye and a Camera Have Certain Features in Common

The eyeball (bulbus oculi) (Figs. 8.1 and 8.2) has a firm outer wall of dense connective tissue covered on the inside by the light-sensitive retina. Between these two layers is a vascular layer, the choroid, which is highly

Figure 8.1 *The left eye.* The eye is divided in two along the visual axis.

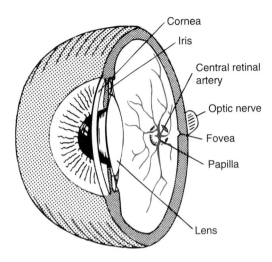

pigmented, thus ensuring that light enters the eye only through the pupil and also preventing reflection of light (compare with the dull black inside a camera). The diameter of the pupil (the shutter) controls the amount of light allowed into the eye. Refraction of the light takes place on its way through the cornea and the lens. The curvature of the lens can be varied by the use of the ciliary muscles, so that the retinal image is always sharply focused (in a camera, the focusing is brought about by varying the distance between the lens and the light-sensitive film). External eye muscles (extraocular muscles) are attached to the eyeballs and can move them to coordinate their positions, so that the visual images are formed at *corresponding points* of the two retinas (Fig. 8.3). This is a prerequisite for our perception of one image, and not two (two slightly different images are formed in the eyes).

Figure 8.2 *Transverse section through the right eye* (seen from above).

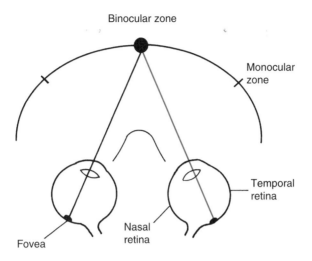

Figure 8.3 *The visual field*. The positions of the eyes ensure that the images fall on corresponding parts of the two retinae (**top**). The **lower** figure shows the visual fields of both eyes when the gaze is directed straight ahead.

Visual field

Binocular zone

Monocular zone

Temporal retina

Nasal retina

Fovea

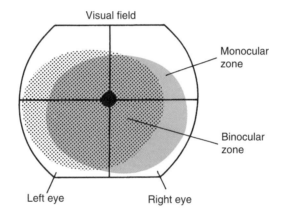

Visual field

Monocular zone

Binocular zone

Left eye

Right eye

Main Structural Features of the Eye

The wall of the eye consists of three layers. Outermost is the *sclera*; then follows the *choroid*, and the *retina* is the innermost layer. The eye keeps its spherical shape because the sclera has a certain stiffness, but mainly because the pressure inside the eye is higher than outside (15 cm H_2O).

Anteriorly, the sclera has a circular opening, in which the transparent *cornea* sits like a glass of a wristwatch. The cornea consists of a special kind of connective tissue with densely packed collagen fibrils arranged strictly geometrically. This arrangement is a prerequisite for the transparency of the cornea, as is also its lack of blood vessels. The cornea is nourished by the tear fluid and by the fluid inside the eye. The cornea contains numerous unmyelinated sensory nerve fibers, providing information about even the slightest touch to the cornea. The cornea is covered on the outside by stratified squamous epithelium that is only a few cells thick.

The *choroid* (the vascular coat) is rich in vessels that nourish the cells of the outer parts of the retina. In addition, the connective tissue of the choroid contains numerous highly pigmented cells. Anteriorly, close to the opening in the sclera, the choroid is thickened and forms a ring (Figs. 8.1 and 8.2) called the *ciliary body* (corpus ciliare). This contains smooth musculature, the *ciliary muscle*, which controls the curvature of the lens. From the anterior edge of the ciliary body, approximately at the junction between the sclera and the cornea, the choroid continues as the *iris*. This is a circular disk with a central opening, the *pupil*. The iris contains smooth musculature that serves to regulate the size of the pupil. Muscle fibers arranged circularly form the *pupillary sphincter muscle* (m. sphincter pupillae), which, when it contracts, makes the pupil smaller so that less light enters the interior of the eye. Muscle fibers that are arranged radially in the iris widen the pupil when they contract: the *pupillary dilatator muscle* (m. dilatator pupillae).

The space inside the eye in front of the lens and the iris is called the *anterior chamber* (camera anterior). It is filled with a clear watery fluid that is produced by small processes of the ciliary body. The space behind the lens, the *posterior chamber*, is filled with a clear jellylike substance called the *vitreous body* (corpus vitreum).

The eyeball is moved inside the orbit by six small striated muscles, the *extraocular muscles* (Figs. 16.23 and 16.24). The muscles originate in the wall of the orbit, and their tendons insert in the sclera. The muscles cooperate very precisely to produce the movements of the eyes that are necessary to ensure that the images of the objects we look at always fall on corresponding parts of the retina and to rapidly change our point of visual fixation. The extraocular muscles are discussed more comprehensively in Chapter 15 in connection with the cranial nerves innervating them (the third, fourth, and sixth cranial nerves).

The Visual Field

The visual field is the part of our surroundings from which the eyes can perceive light (without movement of the eyes or the head). Together the two eyes cover a large area (Fig. 8.3). Light from a particular point in the visual field falls on a particular point on the retina. Because of the refraction of the light when it passes the optic media of the eye, the image on the retina is upside down. The retina and the visual field can be conveniently divided vertically in two halves: the *temporal parts*—that is, lateral parts, toward the temple—and the *nasal parts*. The nasal halves of the retina receive light from the temporal halves of the visual field, and the temporal halves of the retina from the nasal visual field. The situation is the same for the upper and lower halves of the retina and the corresponding parts of the visual field. Thus, light from the lower half of the visual field reaches the upper half of the retina. The lateral 30° of the visual field is viewed by one eye only, and is therefore called the *monocular zone*. This is because the nose prevents light from reaching the most anterior part of the temporal retina (Fig. 8.3). The rest of the visual field, the *binocular zone*, is viewed by both eyes.

Damage to parts of the nasal retina in one eye produces a blind spot in the temporal visual field, with damage in the upper half of the retina in one eye the blind spot is in the lower visual field, and so forth. If however, the damage affects the binocular zone, it will usually not be noticed by the patient. Therefore, the visual field must be examined for each eye separately. This is done with the person fixating the gaze at a target straight ahead while one eye is covered. Often it suffices to test the outer borders of the visual field by moving an object (for example, the finger of the examiner) from well outside the visual field towards its center. An examination covering all parts of the visual field is done by so-called *perimetry*.

The Lens and the Far and Near Points of the Eye: Accommodation

The lens is transparent and built of a special kind of cell forming long fibers. It is elastic and, when loosened from the ciliary body to which it is attached with thin threads (see Fig. 8.2), it becomes rounder. Contraction of the ciliary muscle reduces the diameter of the ring formed by the ciliary body. This slackens the lens threads and enables the lens to become rounder; that is, its curvature (convexity) and thus also the refraction of the light increase. Contraction of the ciliary muscle is required to see sharply objects that are closer to the eye than approximately 6 m. This distance is called the *far point of the eye*. When viewing objects at distances greater than about 6 m, the lens maintains the same convexity, and yet the image is always focused on the retina. This is because the light rays entering the eye from points at such distances are all virtually parallel and are therefore collected in the plane of the retina (like a camera focused at infinite distance). The closer an object comes within the far point of the eye, the more the convexity of the lens must be increased by contraction of the ciliary muscle. Such adjustment of the lens for near sight is called accommodation. The closest distance from the eye at which we can see an object sharply is called the *near point of the eye*. One's own near point can be easily determined by fixing the eyes on an object (for example, a finger) that is gradually moved closer to the eye, until it no longer can be viewed sharply.

Whereas the far point of the eye depends on the curvature of the lens in its "relaxed" state—that is, with no contraction of the ciliary muscle— and remains stable throughout life, the near point depends on the ability of the lens to increase its curvature and moves gradually away from the eye from birth until about the age of 60. This happens because the lens becomes gradually stiffer and less elastic, so that the ability to increase its convexity is reduced. At about the age of 45 the accommodative ability is so much reduced—or, in other words, the near point is so far away— that it is difficult to read fine print. This condition, called *presbyopia*, can be corrected by the use of convex (+) glasses of appropriate strength.

THE RETINA

The retina forms the innermost layer of the eye (Fig. 8.2). The outer part of the retina, which adjoins the choroid, is called the *pigmented epithelium* and consists of one layer of cuboid cells with large amounts of pigmented granules in their cytoplasm. Internal to the pigmented eipthelium follows a layer with *photoreceptors*, and then two further layers with neurons (Fig. 8.4). The processes of the photoreceptors contact the *bipolar cells*, which in their turn transmit signals to the *retinal ganglion cells*. The axons of the ganglion cells leave the eye in the optic nerve to end in various nuclei in the diencephalon and the mesencephalon. The retinal layer with pigmented epithelium extends forward to the edge of the pupil (Fig. 8.2), whereas the photoreceptors, bipolars, and ganglion cells are present only in parts of the retina posterior to the ciliary body (pars nervosa retinae).

Unlike many other receptors, the photoreceptors are not of peripheral origin but belong to the central nervous system. The retina is formed in embryonic life as an evagination of the diencephalon (Figs. 4.3 and 4.5). Strictly speaking, the term retinal ganglion cell is not correct, but it is nevertheless maintained.

Figure 8.4 *The retina*. The main cell types and their interconnections (highly simplified).

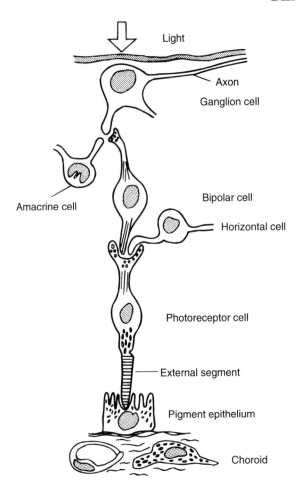

Since the photoreceptors are located external to the two other neuronal layers, the light has to pass through the latter to reach the photoreceptors. Because there are no myelinated axons in the retina, however, the layers internal to the photoreceptors are sufficiently translucent.

In addition to the neuronal types mentioned above, the retina also contains many *interneurons*, the *amacrine cells* and the *horizontal cells* (Fig. 8.4). The horizontal cells are, among other things, responsible for lateral inhibition. Altogether more processing of sensory information takes place in the retina than in any other sense organ. Thus, the visual information transmitted to higher centers of the brain from the retina is already "distorted" by enhancement of the contrast between light and darkness and by preference for signals caused by light from moving objects.

The Retina Has a Layered Structure

Under the microscope, several distinct layers of the retina can be identified in sections cut perpendicular to its surface (Figs. 8.5 and 8.11). Externally, toward the pigmented epithelium, lie the light-sensitive parts of the photoreceptors—their *external segments*. The two types of photoreceptors, the rods and the cones, can be distinguished because the exter-

— Axons

— Ganglion cell layer

— Inner plexiform layer

— Inner nuclear layer (bipolar cells)

— Outer plexiform layer

— Outer nuclear layer (photoreceptors)

— Outer segments of rods and cones

— Pigment epithelium

— Choroid

nal segments of the cones are thicker and usually somewhat shorter than those of the rods. Internal to the layer of the external segments, there are three distinct layers with cell nuclei. The *outer nuclear layer* consists of the nuclei of the photoreceptors. The *inner nuclear layer* is formed by the nuclei of the bipolar cells (and many of the interneurons). The innermost layer of nuclei belongs to the ganglion cells—the *ganglion cell layer*. Between the nuclear layers are found the processes of the neurons and their synapses, consequently termed the *outer and inner synaptic layers* (or plexiform layers). In the outer synaptic layer, the processes of the bipolar cells end in depressions in the processes of the photoreceptors (Fig. 8.4). The photoreceptor processes contain synaptic vesicles close to the presynaptic membrane.

A special kind of glial cell—the Müller cells—extends through the retina from the pigmented epithelium to the vitreous body. They are most likely a form of astrocyte.

Figure 8.5 *The retina.* Photomicrograph of a microscopic section showing the various layers (monkey). The section is from the peripheral part of the retina (this explains the low density of ganglion cells as compared with Fig. 8.11). The outer segment of a cone is marked with an asterisk. Magnification, ×175.

Figure 8.6 *The three different kinds of visual pigment.* The diagram shows the efficiency with which the three kinds of cones absorb light of different wavelengths. Note the marked overlapping of the absorbtion curves.

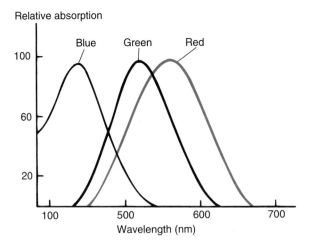

Photoreceptors and the Photopigment

Electron microscopically, the external segments of the rods and cones can be seen to be packed with folded membrane. Thereby a large surface containing the light-sensitive photopigment is formed. In the rods, the folds of membrane lie mostly intracellularly, whereas in the cones they are partly invaginations of the surface membrane. The folds of membrane are constantly removed and resynthesized.

The rods and the cones contain different kinds of photopigment. The *rods* contain *rhodopsin*, which has been the most studied. It consists of a protein part, *opsin*, and *retinal*, which is an aldehyde of the vitamin A molecule. Retinal is light-absorbing and is changed by light (absorption of photons). Simultaneously, the opsin part is changed and this leads to *alteration of the membrane potential of the photoreceptor* (hyperpolarization by closure of Na$^+$ channels). The transduction mechanism involves activation of G protein and intracellular signal molecules, and structurally the photopigments resemble closely other G-protein coupled receptors (for example, muscarinic receptors, and receptors for smell). The hyperpolarization of the photoreceptors by light stimuli affects the bipolar cells and retinal interneurons, which are synaptically connected with the photoreceptors. Eventually the frequency of action potentials conducted from the retinal ganglion cells in the optic nerve to the visual centers of the brain is altered.

The photopigment of the *cones* differs slightly from rhodopsin regarding the structure of the opsin molecules. Furthermore, there are three varieties of cone opsin molecules, which explains that we have three kinds of cones absorbing light of different wavelengths (Fig. 8.6). The opsin of the cones is also bound to retinal, but the wavelength sensitivity of retinal is determined by the opsin molecule.

Rods and Cones Have Different Properties

The rods are much more sensitive to light than the cones and react to extremely small amounts of light, whereas the cones need fairly strong light to react. This is partly because the outer (external) segment of the

Color Blindness

In most cases color blindness is an inheritable condition, due to lack of one kind of cones, or an error affecting one of the three cone photopigments. Green or red blindness (or weakness) are the most common forms, affecting about 3% of the male population, whereas blue blindness is very rare. The photopigments of the red and green sensitive cones are coded by genes at the X chromosome, whereas the genes for the blue-sensitive photopigment and for rhodopsin are at autosomal chromosomes. Since the condition is recessively heritable, it is understandable that almost only men are color blind.

Rarely two kinds of cones may be lacking, or even all three. Finally, deficient or absent color vision can sometimes be caused by disease of the retina or a lesion of the visual cortex.

rod is longer and contains more photopigment than that of the cone. The rods are thus responsible for vision when the light is dim—*scotopic vision*, whereas the cones are responsible in good light—*photopic vision.* (That vitamin A is necessary for the synthesis of rhodopsin explains why vitamin A deficiency causes night blindness.) The distribution of light sensitivity for different wavelengths of light is the same for all the rods (maximal sensitivity for wavelengths around 500 nm); hence they cannot help us discriminate between light of different wavelengths, a prerequisite for color vision. The cones, on the other hand, are as mentioned above of three kinds, each with a particular variety of photopigment with maximal light sensitivity to different wavelengths. One kind of cone responds best to light with wavelengths in the blue part of the spectrum, another in the red part, and the third kind in the green part (considerably fewer cones react to blue than to red and to green). One kind of cone cannot alone inform about color, however. Thus, each photopigment is not only bleached by light with wavelengths to which it is maximally sensitive but also stronger light with shorter and longer wavelengths (Fig. 8.6). Only by *comparing the degree of activation of the different kinds of cones*, the neurons receiving signals from them can extract information about the distribution of wavelengths in the light falling on the retina. The *cones are thus responsible for color vision.* As mentioned above, however, they are not very sensitive to light; from daily experience we know that we need fairly strong light to perceive the color of objects. In poor light, everything appears as a variation of gray.

Other important differences between rods and cones concern their connections with other neurons in the retina. For example, many rods are connected to one bipolar cell—that is, there is a high degree of *convergence.* For the cones, on the other hand, there is typically much less convergence, with a few cones connected to one bipolar cell. This means that the cones provide information with a higher *spatial resolution* than the rods—that is, two points must be farther apart to be perceived as two and not one when the rods are responsible for transmitting the information than when the cones are responsible (compare with our inability to perceive visual details, such as small letters, in dim light). *Thus, the cones are also responsible for our ability to perceive visual details.*

The different degrees of convergence also help us understand why less light is required to convey signals through the optic nerve from the rods than from the cones.

Signal Transduction in the Retina

The photoreceptors do not behave like other receptors when exposed to their adequate stimulus: They are *hyperpolarized* instead of depolarized. How hyperpolarization of the receptors can elicit action potentials in the neurons conducting the signals to the brain will be briefly discussed. One important point is that the photoreceptors are unusual also in another respect: They are in a depolarized state in the dark with a membrane potential around $-30mV$. This is probably caused by Na^+ channels that are open under such conditions. Like other receptors, the photoreceptors (and the bipolar cells) do not produce action potentials but only graded changes of the membrane potential. Because the distance is very short from the outer segment—where the membrane potential changes are produced—to the synapses between the photoreceptors and the bipolar cells, even small fluctuations of the membrane potential cause alterations of the transmitter release from the photoreceptors. (There is thus no need for the production of action potentials, which are important when signals are to be propagated over long distances.) Light falling on the retina most likely causes closure of the Na^+ channels of the photoreceptors via degradation of the photopigment and cyclic GMP. Closing of Na^+ channels hyperpolarizes the cell. Transmitter release from the photoreceptors (as from other neurons) is caused by membrane depolarization without any definite threshold that has to be exceeded. Thus, *in the dark the photoreceptors release transmitter continuously, whereas the release is reduced by light* (as if darkness were the adequate stimulus). Recording from *bipolar cells* has shown that they are of two kinds: *One is depolarized by light and the other is hyperpolarized.* Glutamate—which most likely is the transmitter released from the photoreceptors—has a depolarizing (and therefore excitatory) effect on neurons in other parts of the central nervous system. With regard to the bipolars, however, one kind appears to be hyperpolarized by glutamate, and another depolarized. This is presumably due to the existence of two different kinds of postsynaptic glutamate receptor.

We can *summarize* the events as follows: When light hyperpolarizes the photoreceptors, the release of glutamate is reduced, as mentioned above. This leads to less hyperpolarization—which is the same as depolarization—of one kind of bipolar. Thus, some of the bipolars are depolarized and therefore increase their own transmitter release. This is an example of disinhibition. The opposite happens with the other kind of bipolar cell, which is hyperpolarized (receives less depolarization) and therefore reduces its transmitter release. Thus, one kind of bipolar reacts with increased transmitter release when *light is turned on*, the other kind when the light is turned *off*. The bipolar cells have depolarizing (excitatory) effects on the retinal ganglion cells (and on amacrine cells), and we can then understand why there are also two kinds of ganglion cells: one that is excited, and one that is inhibited by light hitting the photoreceptors to

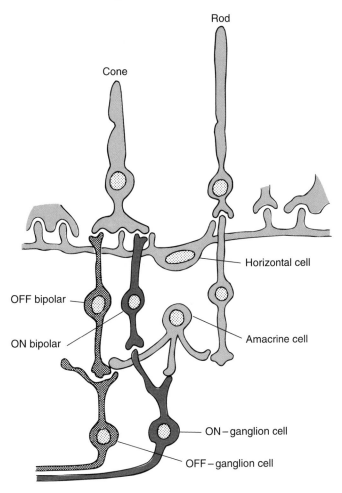

Rod

Cone

Horizontal cell

OFF bipolar

ON bipolar

Amacrine cell

ON – ganglion cell

OFF – ganglion cell

Figure 8.7 *ON and OFF bipolar and ganglion cells in the retina.* Simplified diagram showing the coupling of a cone to two different bipolar cells, and further coupling of the bopolars to ganglion cells that increase or decrease their activity, respecitvely, when light falls on their receptive fields. The diagram also shows that amacrine cells are intercalated in the coupling of rods to ganglion cells.

which they are coupled.We therefore use the terms *on* and *off bipolars* and *ganglion cells*.

In contrast to the photoreceptors and the bipolars, the ganglion cells produce action potentials (conducted in the optic nerve to the higher visual centers). Fig. 8.7 shows that there are two parallel signal pathways from the *cones*. The ON-ganglion cells increase their firing frequency with increasing intensity of light hitting the cones with which they are connected, whereas the OFF-ganglion cells increase their firing frequency with increasing darkness. These two channels enable the ganglion cells to inform of a much wider range of light intensities than if there were only one channel. However, the bipolars and the ganglion cells do not inform about the absolute light intensity but the intensity in a small spot on the retina in comparison to the surroundings. This is caused by lateral inhibition produced by horizontal cells (Fig. 8.7), which are electrically coupled.

The coupling from the rods to the ganglion cells is more complicated than from the cones. Thus, bipolars excited by rods do not influence ganglion cells directly but via a special kind of amacrine cells (Fig. 8.7). These amacrines excite ON bipolars and inhibit OFF bipolars. It should be noticed that the rods and cones are coupled to the same ganglion cells. Consequently, *a ganglion cell transmitting signals from cones in daylight, transmits from rods in the dusk.*

Dark Adaptation and Light Adaption

When looking into the eye (for example, through an ophthalmoscope), the color of the retina is a deep purple because of the content of rhodopsin. The reflection of light from the retina produces the red eyes of flash photography. The color bleaches quickly on illumination of the retina, but it returns slowly in the dark. The rhodopsin has been broken down by the light, and some time is needed to resynthesize it. The time taken for this process of dark adaptation can be experienced when entering a dark room from strong sunlight. In the beginning we can hardly see anything, but gradually the ability to see returns. This happens in two stages; first, there is a rapid stage of improvement of about 10 min and thereafter a slower stage of almost 1 h until full light sensitivity has been restored (if the initial illumination was very intense). Since the rods are responsible for vision in dim light (scotopic vision), the *dark adaptation depends on resynthesis of rhodopsin in the rods.*

The opposite phenomenon of dark adaptation, *light adaptation*, is experienced when going from darkness into strong light. Also then, after first seeing nothing, vision gradually returns. The strong light bleaches the photo pigment massively—that is, there is an intense, brief stimulation of many receptors producing the almost painful sensation of blinding light. The rhodopsin of the rods is kept bleached as long as they are exposed to strong light, and cannot contribute to vision under these conditions. The cones are first maximally hyperpolarized and are also unable to respond. This explains why we cannot discriminate forms and colors at first. However, *during a few seconds the outer segments of the cones depolarize to a level where they again can respond to changes of illumination.* Change of intracellular Ca^{2+} concentration is of crucial importance for this depolarization and thus for light adaptation (we will not go further into the mechanisms, however).

Also other adaptations occur when passing from darkness to light, such as *constriction of the pupils* to reduce light entering the eye (anyone having tried to enter a sunlit street after widening the pupils by atropine has experienced the importance of this adaptation).

Receptive Fields of Retinal Ganglion Cells

Most retinal ganglion cells have in common that they are excited most effectively by shining light on small circular spots on the retina. These are the *receptive fields* of the ganglion cells and can be defined as the *area of the retina from which a ganglion cell can be influenced.* The receptive field can of course be determined not only for ganglion cells but for neurons at all levels of the visual pathways. The ganglion cells are typically excited from a small central circle and inhibited from a peripheral circular zone, or vice versa (Fig. 8.8). This was first demonstrated by the American neurophysiologist Kuffler in the early 1950s. He introduced the terms *on-center* and *off-center* for ganglion cells that are activated and inhibited, respectively, by light hitting the central zone of the receptive field. These corresponds to *ON* and *OFF ganglion cells*, described above with reference to the center of their receptive fields (Fig. 8.7). Thus, as mentioned above, *illumination of a small spot on the retina can lead to increased activity in one chain of neurons—forming, as it were, a channel for signal transmission to the higher visual centers—and reduced activity in another.* (The arrangement of a central excitatory field and a peripheral inhibitory zone is not unique to neurons of the visual pathways but is found also in the somatosensory system.) For receptive fields of the retinal ganglion cells, the central excitatory or inhibitory part of the receptive field may be explained by direct coupling from photoreceptors to bipolars and further to ganglion cells, whereas the peripheral zone with

RETINAL GANGLION CELL   LATERAL GENICULATE BODY   STRIATE AREA

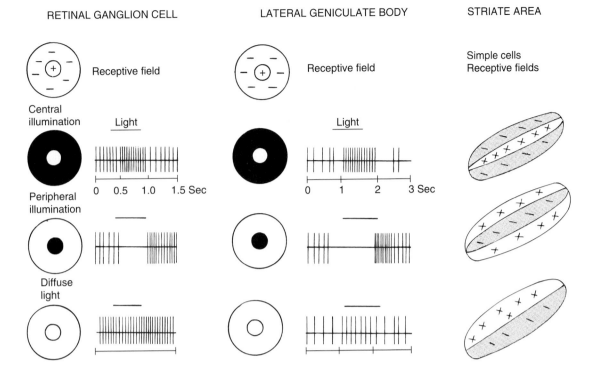

opposite effects must involve retinal interneurons (horizontal cells) producing *lateral inhibition*. As expected, illumination of the whole receptive field—the central and peripheral zones simultaneously—gives a much weaker response from the ganglion cells than illumination of only the central zone (Fig. 8.8).

In conclusion, *each ganglion cell brings information to higher visual centers about a particular small, round area in a definite position on the retina, and thus in the visual field. Together, the receptive fields of all ganglion cells cover the whole visual field with the same type of concentrically arranged receptive fields.* Ganglion cells that lie side by side in the retina have overlapping, but not identical, receptive fields.

As mentioned above, the retinal ganglion cells do not give information about *absolute light intensity*, as appears from recording of ganglion cell activity under different lighting conditions. Rather, their activity depends on the *contrast* of intensity between the light falling on the central and the peripheral parts of the receptive field. For example, for an on-center cell, maximal firing frequency would be achieved by a narrow beam of strong light hitting precisely the center of the receptive field while the peripheral zone is in darkness.

This preference of the visual system for contrast in light intensity can be demonstrated, for example, by looking at a gray circular spot surrounded by black (Fig. 8.9). Exchanging the black surrounding with a light gray makes the gray spot appear darker (even though the amount of light the eye receives from the central gray area is unchanged). This property of the visual system makes it particularly suited to detect *contours*—the latter being especially important for analysis of form. Our ability to judge contrasts of light intensities depends not only on retinal mechanisms, however. Thus, the brightness of an area compared with its neigh-

Figure 8.8 *Receptive fields of cells at various levels of the visual pathways.* Retinal ganglion cells and cells of the lateral geniculate body have similar receptive fields. The firing frequencies of the neurons when subjected to different kinds of light stimuli are also shown. Only cells that are excited by shining light on the central part of the receptive field are shown here (on-center field), but cells with the opposite properties—that is, inhibition from the central field and excitation from the periphery—also exist (off-center field). The receptive fields of simple cells of the area striata are typically oblong with an excitatory and an inhibitory zone. The cells are called orientation-specific because they respond preferentially to a stripe of light with a specific orientation. The figure shows only one orientation of the receptive fields, but all orientations are represented among cells of the striate area. Based on Kuffler et al. (1984).

Figure 8.9 Perceived light intensity depends on the contrast between lightness and darkness. The central circle reflects the same amount of light in both examples; yet we perceive the left one as darker than the right.

Interneurons in the Retina

As mentioned, the retina contains interneurons in addition to the photoreceptors, bipolars, and the ganglion cells (Figs. 8.4 and 8.7). The *horizontal cells* send their processes in the plane of the retina—that is, perpendicular to the orientation of the photoreceptors and the bipolars. The horizontal cell processes establish contact with the inner segments of the photoreceptors and with the dendrites of the bipolars. They therefore regulate the transmission from the photoreceptors to the bipolars. There is good evidence that the horizontal cells are responsible for the typical receptive fields of the bipolars and ganglion cells with central excitation and peripheral inhibition (or vice versa). This involves complex and unusual synaptic mechanisms that are not fully understood. The horizontal cells are interconnected with electric synapses, probably enabling transmission for several millimeters in the plane of the retina. They release GABA in their efferent synapses onto the inner segments of the photoreceptors. Each horizontal cell is depolarized by glutamate released from many photoreceptors. Thus, light hitting the photoreceptors leads to hyperpolarization of the horizontal cells, that is, they release less GABA so that the photoreceptors are disinhibited. Conversely, the horizontal cells hyperpolarize the photoreceptors in darkness.

The other kind of retinal interneuron, the *amacrine cell*, is located with its perikaryon in the inner nuclear layer and establishes contact both with the axons of the bipolar cells and with the dendrites of the ganglion cells (Fig. 8.7). They are thus intercalated between bipolar cells and the ganglion cells, and many bipolar cells exert their effect on ganglion cells only or mainly via amacrine cells. This is, as mentioned above, the rule for bipolar cells that are connected with rods (rod bipolars). Some of the processes of the amacrine cells also extend horizontally for considerable distances. The actions of the amacrine cells are varied and complex, and there are numerous morphological varieties. Some kinds establish both chemical and electric synapses. They are also heterogeneous with regard to their content of transmitter candidates. One subgroup of amacrines contains, for example, GABA; others contain acetylcholine or dopamine. At least seven different neuropeptides have been associated with amacrine cells. Twenty different kinds have so far been identified, considering differences both in synaptic connectivity and transmitter content. The amacrines play an important role in influencing the activity of many ganglion cells, the properties of which cannot be explained by transmission lines going directly from bipolars to ganglion cells. Thus, that certain ganglion cells are most sensitive to light stimuli (contrasts) with a specific orientation, may be partly due to the actions of amacrine cells.

Two kinds of photoreceptors with different sensitivities to light enable the visual system to give meaningful information even with being exposed to extreme variations of light intensities. Release of dopamine from one kind of amacrines seems actively to support the change from scotopic (rods) to photopic (cones) vision. Light induces release of dopamine that enhances the signal transmission from the cones compared with the rods. Furthermore, dopamine uncouples electric synapses so that signals are less widely distributed horizontally in the retina. This presumably contributes to the enhanced spatial resolution with photopic vision.

Nerve fiber layer
Ganglion cell layer
Bipolar cells
Photoreceptors
Pigment epithelium

Figure 8.10 *The fovea centralis.* Schematized drawing of microscopic section through the posterior pole of the eye. Note how the bipolar and the ganglion cells are "pushed" aside in the most central part of the fovea (the foveola), whereas the density of photoreceptors is at its highest.

bors depends on our (subconscious) judgmenet of how the light falls—that is, whether we assume that the area is in direct light or in shadow. This must be caused by processes at the cortical level, since it requires assumptions of the three dimensional form of the object and from where the light comes. If we misinterpret such conditions, we will make false judgements about relative light intensities.

The Size of Receptive Fields Is Different in Different Parts of the Retina: Visual Acuity

We know from everyday experience that, in order to perceive visual details, the eyes have to be directed toward the object we are looking at. The visual axes have to be oriented so that light from the object falls on a small region of the retina in the back of the eye, the *macula lutea*, corresponding to a small depression, the *fovea centralis* (Figs. 8.1–8.3, and 8.10). Here the *visual acuity* is maximal, and it decreases steeply when moving peripherally on the retina. The visual acuity can be expressed as the distance (in degrees)—two points in the visual field have to be apart to be perceived as two and not one. In clinical work, visual acuity is usually determined by viewing letters of different sizes at a fixed distance (at the far point of the eye). The macula is about 2 mm in diameter, and has a yellowish color when viewed through an ophthalmoscope, distinguishing it from the purple color of the surrounding retina. The central depression at the fovea exists because the bipolars and the ganglion cells are "pushed" aside, to enable maximal access for light to the photoreceptors. The small region is also devoid of capillaries. *In the central part of the macula, only cones are present*, and only in the macular part of the retina is the visual acuity sufficient to enable us to read ordinary print (for example, a newspaper). The farther we move peripherally from the macula, the lower the visual acuity. One can demonstrate this easily by trying to determine how far out in the visual field one can recognize a face. *Closely linked with these differences in visual acuity are differences in the size of the receptive fields of ganglion cells in the central and peripheral parts of the retina.*

What is the basis for such striking differences in the size of the receptive fields of ganglion cells? One important factor is that the *degree of convergence* varies dramatically. There are about 100 million photoreceptors in the human retina and only 1 million ganglion cells; on the average, 100 photoreceptors must be connected to 1 ganglion cell. In peripheral parts of the retina, however, the convergence is much greater than

Central retina   Peripheral retina

Ganglion cell layer

Inner plexiform layer

Inner nuclear layer

Outer plexiform layer

Outer nuclear layer

Outer segments of
rods and cones

Choroid

Figure 8.11 *Central and peripheral parts of the retina.* Photomicrographs illustrating how the various retinal layers differ in thickness when moving from central to peripheral parts of the retina. Note especially the difference in the density of ganglion cells.

100:1, whereas it is much smaller in central parts (Fig. 8.11). In the central parts of the macula (*foveola*, Fig. 8.10) there are even 1:1 connections—that is, one photoreceptor connects to one bipolar, which is connected to only one ganglion cell. As mentioned, the rods show a greater convergence than the cones, which is in accordance with the distribution of the rods and cones: In the macula it is almost cones only, whereas in the most peripheral parts it is almost rods only. The relative absence of cones in the peripheral parts of the retina (receiving light from peripheral parts of the visual field) can be demonstrated by how far out in the visual field the color of an object can be perceived. It then appears that the visual field for color is considerably smaller than that within which we can perceive a moving object.

Another factor that contributes to the higher visual acuity in the central parts of the retina—particularly in the region of the fovea—is that the *density of photoreceptors* is higher there than more peripherally. Figure 8.13 illustrates a third contributing factor: The *dendritic arborizations of the ganglion cells* are more restricted in central than in peripheral parts of the retina, which is also of importance for the degree of convergence on each ganglion cell. Finally, differences between the retinal interneurons in central and peripheral parts of the retina also play an important role.

Where the optic nerve leaves the eye, there is a circular area devoid of photoreceptors, appropriately called the *blind spot* (Figs. 8.1, 8.2, and 8.12). We do not notice these blind areas of the two retinae, however, because they are not located at corresponding points (Fig. 8.3).

There Are Two Main Types of Retinal Ganglion Cells

We described above two kinds of retinal ganglion cells differing as to whether they signal light or darkness (ON and OFF ganglion cells). There are, however, further specializations among ganglion cells that we should

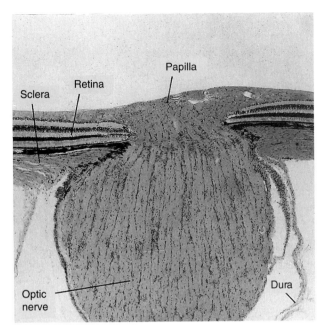

Figure 8.12 *The optic nerve and the optic papillae.* Photomicrograph of section through the posterior pole of the eye at the exit of the optic nerve (the blind spot). The optic nerve swells immediately outside the eye because the axons become myelinated (the ganglion cell axons are unmyelinated as long as they course through the innermost layer of the retina).

know to understand the information sent from the retina to higher visual centers.

Anatomic studies showed many years ago that the retinal ganglion cells differ greatly in size. One tendency, mentioned above, is that the dendrites of the ganglion cells are longer peripherally than centrally (Fig. 8.13). This is related to differences in the size of their receptive fields. But ganglion cells with the same placement with regard to eccentricity on the retina also vary in size. It is now customary to recognize two main kinds of retinal ganglion cells, together constituting about 90% of all—

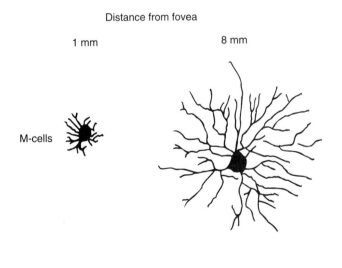

Figure 8.13 *Two main kinds of retinal ganglion cells* (monkey). Note how both types increase in size in the peripheral direction (distance from the fovea). The extension of the dendritic tree is related to the size of the receptive fields of the ganglion cells. The cells have been visualized by intracellular injection of HRP. Based on Shapley and Perry (1986).

the *M cells* and the *P cells*. As seen in Figure 8.13, the P cells are tiny compared with the M cells, but both types are much smaller centrally than peripherally. Physiological studies of their properties indicate that the *M cells primarily signal movement and contrasts of illumination, whereas the P cells are responsible for providing information about fine features (high visual acuity) and color.* Both kinds can have either ON or OFF properties, and can be activated both in scotopic and photopic light conditions. The latter is what one would expect, since signals from rods and cones converge on the same ganglion cells (Fig. 8.7). It is possible, however, that the M cells play a more important role than P cells in scotopic vision.

More About Retinal Ganglion Cells

The functional properties of the two main morphological types of ganglion cells have been clarified by intracellular staining of cells that first have been characterized by their response to various kinds of light stimuli. Particularly the cat's but also to some extent the monkey's retinal ganglion cells have been studied in depth. Even though cat and monkey (and presumably human) ganglion cells have several features in common—for example, with regard to the organization of their receptive fields—there are also important differences. This concerns both properties of the ganglion cells and the pathways conducting their signals to the visual cortex. One reason for such differences is that the cat has practically no ability to differentiate colors (that is, it is color-blind). Another difference concerns the visual acuity of the central parts of the retina, which is much higher in the monkey (and man) than in the cat (the cat has no macula). The subdivision of X, Y, and W retinal ganglion cells of the cat can therefore hardly be used without modifications for man. The monkey visual system is much more like the human in several respects, notably with regard to both color vision and visual acuity. Recent studies in the monkey indicate that the M cells described above correspond functionally to both the X and Y cells in the cat, whereas the P cells are not found in the cat (or in a very small number). What follows here is based on findings in the monkey.

The M cells (called A cells by some authors) have a large perikaryon and a fairly extensive dendritic tree (Fig. 8.13). The axon is relatively thick. The P cells (= B cells) have smaller perikarya, a less extensive dendritic tree, and a thinner axon than the M cells. The P cells are most numerous and probably constitute about 80% of all of the ganglion cells. A major difference is that many of the P cells respond preferentially to light with a particular wavelength—that is, they are color-specific—whereas M cells do not have such specificity. The M cells, however, are more sensitive than the P cells to contrasts in intensity of illumination. A third difference is that the M cells appear to respond better than the P cells to moving stimuli. Thus, in general the M cells tend to respond especially when a stimulus starts and stops, whereas the P cells tend to give a signal as long as the stimulus lasts. In spite of clear anatomic differences between M and P cells, however, each group contains a wide variety of properties. Thus, for most properties the two groups overlap so that some M cells are more like typical P cells with regard to certain functional properties, and vice versa.

A third kind of retinal ganglion cell does not fit into the two groups described so far. In the monkey, they constitute about 10% of all ganglion cells. Both anatomically and physiologically this group is heterogeneous, but the cells are predominantly smaller than the P cells and have thinner axons. The common feature of this group is that the cells send their axons to the *mesencephalon* rather than to the thalamus, like the M and P cells. A small fraction of the M cells sends an axon (most likely a collateral of the axon going to the thalamus) to the mesencephalon. It gives one some insight into the development of the visual system to compare the proportion of retinal ganglion cells that sends axons to the mesencephalon in various species. Thus, in the cat, about 50% of the axons in the optic nerve pass to the mesencephalon, and the proportion is most likely higher in lower mammals like the rat. In humans, there is reason to believe that even less than 10% pass to the mesencephalon. With increasing development of the cerebral cortex, more and more of the analysis of visual information takes place at the cortical level rather than in the brain stem visual centers.

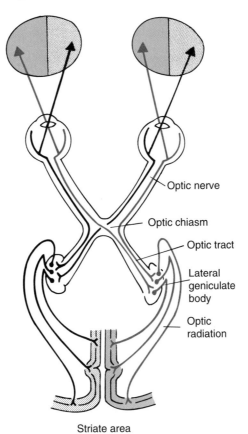

Figure 8.14 *The visual pathways.* For didactic reasons, the visual field of each eye is shown separately (cf. Fig. 8.3).

Optic nerve

Optic chiasm

Optic tract

Lateral geniculate body

Optic radiation

Striate area

In the following, we will discuss the organization of the pathways followed by the signals from the retina, and we will see that information from the two main types of ganglion cells is kept separate—at least to some extent—up to the cortical level.

ORGANIZATION OF THE VISUAL PATHWAYS

The axons of the retinal ganglion cells constitute the first link in the central visual pathways. All ganglion cell axons run toward the posterior pole of the eye, where they pass through the wall of the eyeball at the papilla (papilla nervi optici) (Fig. 8.12). They then form the *optic nerve*, which passes through the orbit and enters the cranial cavity. Here the two optic nerves unite to form the *optic chiasm* (Figs. 3.12 and 8.14). In the optic chiasm some of the axons cross, and crossed and uncrossed fibers continue in the *optic tract*, which curves around the crus cerebri to end in the *lateral geniculate body* (corpus geniculatum laterale) of the thalamus (Figs. 3.20, 3.21, 8.14, 8.16–8.17). Here the axon terminals of the retinal ganglion cells establish synaptic contact with neurons that send their axons posteriorly into the occipital lobe. These efferent fibers of the lateral geniculate body form the *optic radiation* (radiatio optica) (Fig. 8.15). The

Figure 8.15 *The optic radiation*. The course of the fibers from the lateral geniculate body to the striate area. Note how the fibers bend around the lateral ventricle and extend partly into the temporal lobe. Redrawn from Brodal (1981).

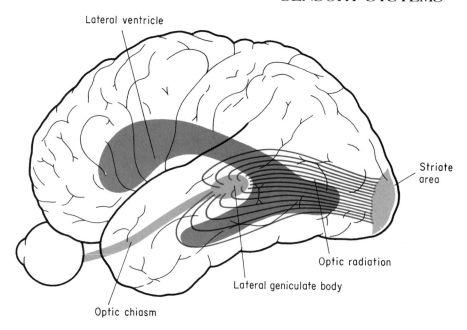

optic radiation curves anteriorly and laterally to the posterior horn of the lateral ventricle and ends in the *primary visual cortical area*, situated around the *calcarine sulcus* (Figs. 3.25 and 8.18–8.19). Some of the fibers of the optic radiation lie in the posterior part of the internal capsule, where they can be damaged together with the fibers of the pyramidal tract—for example, by bleeding or infarction—producing a combination of weakness (paresis) of the muscles of the opposite side of the body and blind areas in the opposite visual hemifield. The primary visual area is area 17 of Brodmann, which is also called the *striate area* (area striata). The latter name (which we will use here) refers to a white stripe in the cortex running parallel to the cortical surface. The stripe is made up of myelinated fibers and is therefore white in a freshly cut brain, whereas it appears dark in microscopic sections stained to show myelin (see Fig. 8.18).

Not all fibers of the optic nerve terminate in the lateral geniculate body. Some (about 10% in the monkey) terminate in certain *mesencephalic nuclei* (the superior colliculus and the pretectal nuclei). These fibers are of importance primarily for reflex adjustments of the position of the head and the eyes (this will be discussed in Chapter 16).

Axons from the M and P Cells Terminate in Different Layers of the Lateral Geniculate Body

The human lateral geniculate body (and that of other primates, like monkeys) consists of six cell layers (Figs. 8.16 and 8.17). The two ventralmost laminae (1 and 2) are composed of large cells and are therefore called the *magnocellular layers*, whereas the dorsal four are composed of small cells and are called the *parvocellular layers*. Anatomic and physiological studies have shown that the large retinal ganglion cells, *The M*

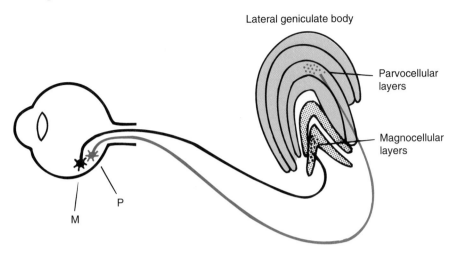

Figure 8.16 *The lateral geniculate body*. The two main kinds of retinal ganglion cells end in different layers of the lateral geniculate. Based on Shapley and Perry (1986).

cells, send their axons to the magnocellular layers of the lateral geniculate body, whereas the small ganglion cells, *the P cells*, send their axons (at least preferentially) to the parvocellular layers (Fig. 8.13). There is thus a division of the lateral geniculate body corresponding largely to the functional division among retinal ganglion cells. It is now usual to speak of the two parallel pathways—M and P—from the retina to the lateral geniculate and further to the visual cortex. The significance of this will be discussed in connection with the visual cortex.

Figure 8.17 *Fusion of the visual images*. The impulses from corresponding points on the two retinae end in different layers of the geniculate—that is, impulses from the two eyes are kept separate at this level. The convergence of impulses takes place in the striate area.

Figure 8.18 *The striate area.* Photograph of a section through the human occipital lobe showing the characteristic whitish stripe in layer 4 (the line of Gennari) of the striate area. The arrows mark the border between the striate area and neighboring extrastriate areas. (See also Fig. 20.4 for a thionine-stained section from the striate area.)

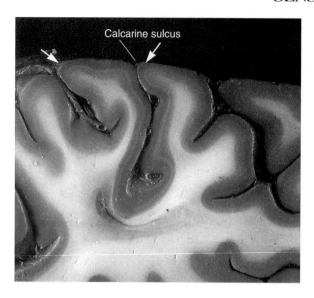

Visual Impulses from One Side of the Visual Field Reach the Hemisphere of the Other Side

Figure 8.14 shows how the fibers are arranged in the optic chiasm. The fibers coming from the nasal halves of the two retinae cross, whereas the fibers from the temporal halves pass through without crossing. In this way the left lateral geniculate body receives fibers from the temporal retina of the left eye and from the nasal retina of the right eye. *The lateral geniculate body thus receives light from the contralateral half of the visual field.* In functional terms, the crossing of signals corresponds to that taking place in the somatosensory system.

Optic nerve fibers from the two eyes are kept separate at the level of the lateral geniculate body, since three of the six layers receive fibers from the ipsilateral eye, and the three others from the contralateral eye (Fig. 8.17). After cutting one optic nerve, almost all cells in three of the layers degenerate (transneuronal degeneration), whereas the other three layers remain normal. Physiological experiments also show that neurons within each layer of the lateral geniculate body are influenced from one eye only—the cells are *monocular.* We first encounter cells that are influenced from both eyes—*binocular cells*—at the level of the striate area.

The Visual Pathways Are Retinotopically Organized

The arrangement of the visual pathways described above concerns merely retinal halves—that is, a crude retinotopic localization ensuring that signals from different parts of the visual field are kept separate (compare with somatotopic localization within the somatosensory pathways). The retinotopic localization is, however, much more fine-grained than what appears in Figure 8.19. Although many fiber systems of the brain are topographically organized, no one is as sharply localized as the visual pathways—they show a true point-to-point localization.

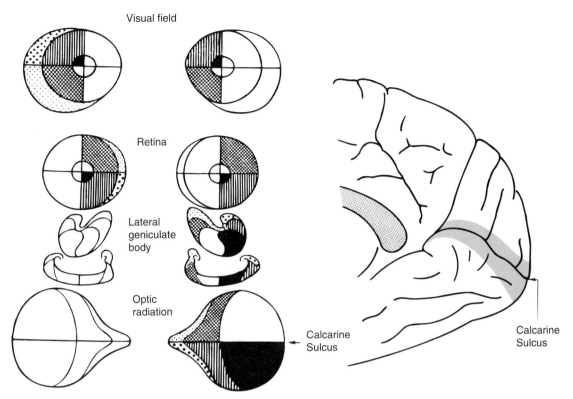

Visual field

Retina

Lateral
geniculate
body

Optic
radiation

Calcarine
Sulcus

Calcarine
Sulcus

In the *lateral geniculate body*, fibers from differently placed tiny parts of the retina end differently. Each small spot in the retina—and thus in the visual field—is "represented" in its own part of the lateral geniculate (Fig. 8.17). The retinotopic localization in the lateral geniculate is such that neurons influenced from the same part of the visual field—that is, from *corresponding points* on the retina—lie stacked in a column perpendicular to the layers. This has been demonstrated with various anatomic techniques, and physiologically by inserting microelectrodes perpendicular to the layers and determining the receptive fields of the cells that are encountered. The receptive fields of neurons in the lateral geniculate are quite similar to those of retinal ganglion cells (Fig. 8.8).

The connections from the lateral geniculate body to the striate area are also organized with a precise retinotopic arrangement. This has been demonstrated, for example, by injection of small amount of HRP in the striate area: Retrogradely labeled cells are then confined to a narrow column extending through all six layers of the lateral geniculate.

That all links of the visual pathways are retinotopically organized can be verified by shining light on a small spot on the retina. This evokes increased neuronal activity in a small region of the striate area, and when the light is shone on other parts of the retina, the evoked cortical activity changes position systematically. This kind of experiment has clarified how the visual field is represented in the cerebral cortex of animals. Careful examination of patients with circumscribed cortical lesions (often gunshot wounds) provides the basis for maps of the human visual cortex, as shown in Figure 8.19. Electrical stimulation of the human occipital lobe confirms the retinotopic arrangement within the striate area. Stimulation

Figure 8.19 *Retinotopic localization of the visual pathways*. The striate area has been unfolded. Note that information from the upper half of the visual field reaches the part of the striate area below the calcarine fissure, whereas the lower visual field projects above. Central parts of the visual field are represented most posteriorly and peripheral parts most anteriorly in the striate area. The **right** drawing illustrates the extension of the striate area on the surface of the occipital lobe; most of it is buried in the calcarine fissure. The striate area is similarly oriented in the **left** and the **right** figures.

with a needle electrode usually evokes the sensation of a flash of light in a certain part of the visual field. When the electrode is placed close to the occipital pole of the cerebral hemisphere, the person reports that the flash is located straight ahead, in agreement with the fact that fibers carrying signals from the macula end near the occipital pole. As the electrode is moved forward along the calcarine fissure, the light flash is perceived as occurring progressively more peripherally in the visual field (at the opposite side of the stimulated hemisphere). If the electrode is placed above (dorsal to) the calcarine fissure, the light occurs in the lower visual field, whereas stimulation below the calcarine fissure elicits a sensation of light in the upper visual field. Studies in healthy humans with PET have confirmed the main features of the retinotopic organization of the striate area.

Disease processes (for example, a tumor) involving the visual cortex may also at times elicit sensations of light because the neurons are abnormally irritated. Epileptic seizures originating in the visual cortex often start with a "visual aura"—that is, the muscular convulsions are preceded by bizarre patterns of light in the visual field opposite the diseased hemisphere.

Central Parts of the Visual Field Are Overrepresented in the Visual Pathways and in the Visual Cortex

In addition to the extremely precise retinotopic arrangement of the visual pathways, another important feature must be mentioned. We have described above that the density of retinal ganglion cells is considerably higher in central than in peripheral parts of the retina (particularly high in the macula). This corresponds to conditions in the somatosensory system, where the density of receptors is highest at the fingertips ("the somatosensory macula"). Figure 8.19 illustrates that axons from central parts

The Lateral Geniculate Body Is More Than a Simple Relay Station

Although the receptive fields of neurons in the lateral geniculate body are closely similar to those of retinal ganglion cells, the lateral geniculate is not merely a simple relay station. Anatomic and physiological studies indicate that signals from the retina are subject to modification before being forwarded to the striate area. There are, for example, a large number of *GABA-containing interneurons*. This presumably enables neurons with somewhat different receptive fields to influence each other. There are also complex synaptic arrangements and numerous dendrodendritic synapses, indicating that substantial interactions take place between neurons of the lateral geniculate.

In addition to its afferents from the retina, the lateral geniculate body also receives strong, retinotopically organized projections from the visual cortex itself. These connections most likely can control the impulse traffic through the lateral geniculate and have been shown physiologically to influence the properties of the neurons. Descending connections from the visual cortex may contribute to the suppression of vision of one eye in patients who are cross-eyed (strabismus). This has the obvious advantage of avoiding double vision. Finally, the lateral geniculate also receives fibers from other sources, notably from cholinergic cell groups of the pontine reticular formation. These connections probably regulate the signal transmission through the lateral geniculate to the striate area in accordance with the level of consciousness and attention.

of the retina end in a disproportionally large part of the lateral geniculate body and that this overrepresentation of the central parts of the retina becomes even more marked in the striate area. Again, conditions are similar to those in the somatosensory system (Fig. 7.22). Thus, *the parts of the body and the visual field in which we have the best somatosensory and visual abilities are provided with a higher density of receptors than other parts, and, furthermore, a much larger number of neurons at higher levels are devoted to the analysis of information from these parts.* A disproportionately large part of the striate area treats information from the small macular region. If information from all parts of the retina were to be treated with similar accuracy, the cerebral cortex would have to be several times larger. Precise control of eye movements, however, ensures that light from the most interesting part of the visual field always falls on the macula.

THE VISUAL CORTEX AND THE FINAL PROCESSING OF VISUAL INFORMATION

The retinotopic localization within the visual pathways may make it appear that a copy of the two retinal images is formed in the striate area. Indeed, the striate area was formerly sometimes called "the cortical retina." We now know, however, that such a view represents an undue oversimplification; considerable processing and integration of the visual information take place in the striate area. Thus, most neurons have properties that are different from those encountered at lower levels of the visual pathways. It should also be emphasized that, when using the term visual images, we do not mean images or pictures in the usual sense, either in the retina or in the visual cortex. Rather, there are temporally and spatially specific patterns of neuronal activity that represent the patterns of

Extrastriate Visual Areas

As mentioned, several areas around the striate area take part in visual processing. These are collectively called the extrastriate visual areas and consist mainly of *Brodmann's areas 18 and 19*, which in the monkey each consist of several subdivisions. Whereas V1 is often used for area 17 (the striate area), parts of the extrastriate areas are termed V2–V5. Other parts have specific names. In total, about 30 visual areas have been characterized so far in the monkey, each in some way involved in the processing of visual information. Many have a more or less complete representation of the visual field, and are retinotopically organized, although with different degrees of precision. Together, the visual areas occupy more than half of all cerebral cortex in the monkey. The interconnections between the striate area and the extrastriate areas, and among the extrastriate areas, are numerous and often reciprocal. The complete scheme of visual association connections is therefore extremely complex, and explains why it is hard to analyze the contribution of each individual area to the processing of visual information.

It is not immediately clear why the cerebral cortex is organized so that the visual field is represented repeatedly in different parts. It may perhaps be a result of the adoption of novel functions by the visual cortex during evolution; this probably occurs more easily by adding new areas (or duplicating an old one) than by already existing areas taking up new functions. It is presumably also a simpler solution to have several separate areas than one large area with regard to arrangement of the necessary fiber connections.

light falling on the retina. So far, however, we have only vague ideas about how the activityy of the neuronal populations engaged in visual processing at the cortical level is related to our subjective visual experiences.

We will now look at certain fundamental features of the functional organization of the striate area and also mention the regions surrounding the striate area, the so-called *extrastriate visual areas*. These take part in the further processing of visual information. Thus, the visual cortex consists of much more than just the *primary visual cortex* (V1), the striate area, even though most of the fibers from the lateral geniculate body terminate there. Schematically, the signals from the retina first reach the striate area and are then forwarded to other cortical areas. There is anatomic, physiological, and clinical evidence that different aspects of visual processing such as analysis of color, form, and movement take place in partly different subdivisions of the extrastriate areas. Thus, damage to the striate area produces complete blindness in a part of the visual field, whereas damage restricted to extrastriatal areas produce defects of restricted aspects of visual analysis. Many of the extrastriate areas receive only indirect projections from the striate area (Figs. 20.10 and 20.13).

Properties of Nerve Cells in the Striate Area

The retinal ganglion cells and cells of the lateral geniculate body have relatively simple, round receptive fields with a central zone that elicits excitation or inhibition when illuminated, and a peripheral zone with the opposite effect (Fig. 8.8). But round spots of light are not an effective stimulus for the neurons of the visual cortex. What constituted the adequate stimulus for the cortical cells remained a mystery for a long time. Diffuse light was not found to be effective, and neither was the kind of stimulus that so effectively affected the cells of the lateral geniculate. In 1962, however, the Nobel laureates (1981) Hubel and Wiesel from the United States were able to show that *many cells in the striate area respond briskly to elongated fields of light or elongated contrasts between light and darkness*. It was furthermore striking that many cells required that the light stimulus be oriented in a specific direction—turning a bar of light some degrees reduced the response markedly. This property was termed *orientation selectivity*. Some cells required a bar of light or a straight light/darkness transition of a specific orientation in a specific part of the visual field to respond, whereas other cells responded to a properly oriented stimulus within a larger area. Such cells thus appear to detect contours with a certain orientation regardless of their position within a larger part of the visual field. Hubel and Wiesel called the first type *simple cells* and the latter type *complex cells* (within each group there are several subtypes according to details of their properties). Why the properties of the complex cells are more complex than those of the simple ones may not be obvious, but presumably the terms were used because Hubel and Wiesel assumed that the properties of the complex cells could be explained by several simple cells acting on one complex cell. The properties of the simple cells, Hubel and Wiesel suggested, could be explained if several neurons in the lateral geniculate with round receptive fields in a row (together forming a stripe) converge on one cortical cell. It is, how-

Figure 8.20 *Ocular dominance columns.* Photomicrograph of a section cut tangentially to the cortical surface of the striate area and stained to reveal differences in cytochrome–oxidase activity. The section is from a monkey that was blind in one eye, causing reduced cytochrome–oxidase activity in the regions (light stripes) of the striate area connected mainly with the blind eye. The dark stripes receive their main input from the normal eye. Magnification, ×25. Courtesy of Dr. J. G. Bjaalie, Department of Anatomy, University of Oslo.

ever, not entirely clear which neuronal interconnections underlie the properties of cells in the striate cortex.

Hubel and Wiesel also discovered other fundamental properties of cells in the striate area. Among other things, *cells generally respond much better to a moving than to a stationary stimulus.* Many cells respond preferentially to a line or contour that is moving in a specific direction. Such *direction-selective cells* thus can detect not only the orientation of a contour but also in which direction it is moving. Other kinds of specificities have also been described for cells in the striate area.

In addition to single cells being specific or selective with regard to their adequate stimulus, there is also a *strong tendency for cells with similar properties in this respect to be located together*, more or less clearly separated from cells with other properties. This is called *modular organization* (Figs. 8.20 and 8.21) and concerns properties such as orientation selectivity, wavelength (color) selectivity, and ocular dominance (that is, which eye has the strongest influence). Such segregation of neurons in

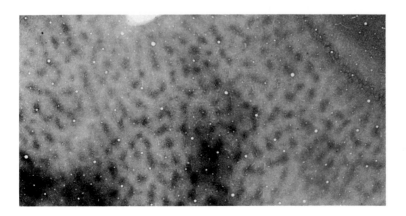

Figure 8.21 *Color-specific "blobs" in the striate area.* Photomicrograph of a section cut tangential to the surface of the striate area of a normal monkey stained to show differences in cytochrome–oxidase activity. The section passes through laminae 2–3 and shows numerous small, darkly stained patches or blobs, which correspond to regions with color-specific neurons. Magnification, ×25. Courtesy of Dr. J. G. Bjaalie.

the striate area requires that fibers carrying different aspects of visual information from the lateral geniculate end at least to some extent differentially in the cortex. In agreement with this, fibers from the parvocellular layers of the lateral geniculate (Fig. 8.16) terminate deeper in lamina 4 than fibers from the magnocellular layers.

Modular Organization of the Visual Cortex

The first example of modular organization discovered by Hubel and Wiesel was the tendency for cells with similar *orientation selectivity* to be grouped together in columns perpendicular to the cortical surface. If we imagine, however, that the striate area is unfolded and we are viewing it from above, the groups of cells with similar orientation selectivity are located in an irregular pattern of curving bands. This has been demonstrated with the deoxyglucose method (see Chapter 5, *Lesion and Stimulation Experiments are Used to Determine the Functions of Cell Groups*), which demonstrates the neurons that are most active at a certain time. When an experimental animal is exposed for some time to parallel stripes of light, increased glucose uptake takes place in cells distributed in bands in the striate area.

Another modular organization concerns *ocular dominance*. As mentioned, many cells in the striate area respond to light from corresponding points in the two retinas, but for most cells the influence is strongest from one of the eyes. The use of various tracer techniques and the deoxyglucose method has shown that neurons sharing ocular dominance are also distributed in bands within the striate area. Such *ocular dominance columns* can also be demonstrated in animals with monocular blindness (Fig. 8.20).

A final example of modular organization concerns cells that are *color-specific* (strictly speaking: wavelength specific). They are not aggregated in bands but rather in clumps or blobs in laminae 2–3 of the striate area of monkeys. For some unknown reason, these blobs have a higher cytochrome oxidase activity than the surrounding tissue and can thus be easily identified in sections with a simple histochemical procedure (Fig. 8.21).

See also Chapter 20 (*More About Intracortical Organization*) for a discussion of modular cortical organization in general.

Further Processing of Visual Information Outside the Striate Area

The properties of single neurons in the striate area suggest that these neurons together are the basis for the cortical analysis of form, depth, movement, and color. Their properties, for example, fit predictions made on the basis of psychophysical experiments in humans, such as the preference for contours and for moving stimuli. Nevertheless, what is taking place in the striate area appears to be mainly a first analysis and sorting of raw data, which must be further processed elsewhere to form the basis for our conscious visual experiences. For example, at some stage in the processing, different features of the visual image (such as form, color, movement, and location in the visual field) must be brought together and integrated. We will return to this below. It is, however, mainly the question of separate treatment of the various features of visual images that has been intensely investigated recently. We will mention here only a few examples.

It has been proposed that one stream of information concerning *object identification* ("what") passes downward from the occipital lobe to the temporal lobe, whereas another stream concerned with *spatial features and movement* ("where") passes upward to the parietal lobe (Fig.

20.10). This concept is partly based on results from experiments in monkeys with lesions restricted to "visual" parts of either the temporal lobe or the posterior parietal cortex. Monkeys with *bilateral lesions of temporal visual areas have reduced ability to identify objects*. They can, for example, no longer distinguish between a pyramid and a cube. On the other

Segregated Information Processing in the Extrastriatal Visual Areas

There is much evidence that different aspects of visual information are *segregated* in the striate area and in the further projections to the extrastriatal areas. Special attention has been paid to the possibility that informations originating from M and P cells are kept separate in the further processing outside the striate area. The degree of *convergence* of information in the extrastriate areas has been less studied. We will discuss a few salient points.

A striking feature of the projections from the striate area to other visual areas is that the fibers terminate in patches and bands. Closer examination of such patterns and correlation with the physiological properties of cells within the patches and bands indicate that *three functionally different pathways out of the striate area* may exist. One pathway comes from cells in the striate area that are predominantly influenced by the magnocellular layers of the lateral geniculate. The properties of these striate cells indicate that they signal movement and depth cues. Another pathway comes from cells that appear to be influenced by the parvocellular layers of the lateral geniculate. Accordingly, these striate cells have small receptive fields and are orientation-selective, and the pathway presumably signals forms and patterns and would seem particularly important for our ability to discern visual details. A third pathway originates in striate neurons also influenced by the parvocellular layers, but these neurons are, at least to a large extent, wavelength-specific.

These three pathways from the striate area appear to be kept separate, at least partly, also at the next station—that is, in area V2, which is adjacent to the striate area. From V2, information about *movement* appears to be channeled to *area V5* (also called MT, the middle temporal visual area), whereas information about *color* is channeled primarily to *area V4*. The major outflow from V5 has been traced to the posterior parietal cortex. How far the specialization goes within each of these areas is not clear, however. Single neurons in area V5, for example, are sensitive not only to movement but also to certain other visual features. Similarly, neurons in area V4 are not purely color-specific. Furthermore, the numerous interconnections among the extrastriate areas suggest that they cooperate extensively.

In spite of evidence showing that conditions cannot be that simple, it is often stated that the "temporal" and "parietal" streams out of the striate area segregate information from P and M cells, respectively. Textbook diagrams show two parallel pathways from the retina and far into the extrastriate areas (with further anatomic and functional segregation within each pathway). However, some convergence of information from M and P cells takes place already in the striate area (besides the more prominent segregation). Furthermore, although behavioral studies suggest that the "parietal" pathway be made nonfunctional by destruction of the magnocellular layers of the lateral geniculate nucleus, the "temporal" pathway is not correspondingly affected by destruction of the parvocellular layers (Fig. 8.16). Accordingly, the functional deficits differ after damage of the temporal pathway and the parvocellular layers, respectively. Thus, whereas destruction of the parvocellular layers affects color vision, acuity and contrast sensitivity, destruction of the temporal visual areas affects primarily form recognition and discrimination. In short, the *temporal extrastriate visual areas appear to receive information from both M and P cells, whereas the parietal areas receive only or mainly M cell information.* Selective lesions of the magnocellular layers produce reduced perception of contrasts with fast-moving stimuli. This defect does not occur after lesions of the parietal visual areas, however. Parietal lesions give reduced ability to judge movements in the visual field and disturbed eye movements. Finally, experiments with lesions of the magnocellular layers suggest that *depth perception* does not depend on information from M cells alone.

In summary, only poor correlations exist between the deficits following elimination of M or P cells, and elimination of the parietal or temporal visual areas, respectively. The reported deficits rather suggest, as emphasized by the US neurobiologists Maunsell and Merigan, that *the subcortical pathways from the retina to the striate area are specialized for signalling simple stimulus features, whereas the further pathways do more advanced analysis and processing using as, a rule, information from both M and P cells.*

hand, lesions of visual parts of the *posterior parietal cortex reduce the ability to localize an object in space and in relation to other objects.* It suffices with a unilateral lesion of the parietal lobe to produce deficits in the contralateral half of the visual field. This resembles the symptoms occurring in humans after damage to the posterior parietal cortex (See Chapter 20, *More About Symptoms after Lesions of the Posterior Parietal Cortex*). The pathways taken by the impulses from the striate area to the temporal and posterior parietal visual regions are not known in detail, but several visual areas are intercalated in the pathways.

Clinical observations indicate that separate processing of different aspects of visual information also occurs in humans. Thus, after restricted cortical lesions, several selective visual deficits have been described, for example, with regard to object identification. A patient may be unable to *recognize faces*, another may have no problem with faces but cannot recognize *fingers* (finger agnosia), and so on. Recordings with multiple surface electrodes in patients (to localize epileptic foci) show that several, separate small areas in the inferior temporal cortex are specialized for face recognition. These areas appear to be parts of a mosaic of areas with different specializations. This agrees with observations after lesions of extensive parts of the inferotemporal extrastriatal areas: Such patients are deficient concerning several speicific kinds of object recognition and not only faces. *Selective loss of color vision* (achromatopsia) after lesions restricted to a region below the calcarine fissure (in the lingual and fusiform gyri) has been convincingly documented. Patients with unilateral lesions in this region are reported to see everything in the opposite half of the visual field in black and white, whereas the other half has normal colors. Other aspects of vision (such as visual acuity and depth perception) appear to be completely normal.

Damage at the junction between the occipital and the parietal lobes can produce selective impairment of the *ability to recognize movements* (akinetopsia). A patient with a bilateral lesion of this region could not see moving objects. When the same objects were stationary, however, he could easily describe their form and color, and also judge depth in the visual scene.

Patients with *selective loss of depth perception* after cortical damage have been described. To such patients other people look completely flat, as made from cardboard, although they can recognize their color, contours, and shading. The exact site of the lesion in such patients has not been determined.

Color Vision

We have discussed parts of the elements responsible for color vision, namely the *three kinds of cones with sensitivities for light of different wavelengths* (Fig. 8.6). We have also emphasized that the brain must compare the degree of stimulation of three kinds of cone to "know" the wavelength composition of the light (and therefore the color of an object). Figure 8.6 shows the large overlap between the sensitivity curves of the three kinds of cone, especially between those with sensitivities in the red and green parts of the spectrum, respectively. How can we then perceive so many nuances of each color? Part of the explanation is found in how the cones are coupled to the next links in the pathway to the cortex. Thus, *retinal ganglion cells and neurons in the lateral geniculate have narrower sensitivity curves than the cones*, making them better at discriminating wavelengths. Many ganglion cells and lateral geniculate cells respond to light of different wavelengths but with opposite signs—one wavelength exciting the cell, the other inhibiting it. This phenomenon is called *color opponency* and must be due to convergence on one ganglion cell (or lateral geniculate cell) of signals from cones with different wavelength sensitivities. Some neurons are excited (ON response) by red light in the central zone of the receptive field (Fig. 8.8) and inhibited (OFF response) by green light in the peripheral zone, others are inhibited by red light centrally and excited by green peripherally, and so forth. Such combinations improve the ability to discriminate wavelengths in the red-green part of the spectrum. Some neurons exhibit color opponency to blue and yellow light (a combination of red and green), others to white light (stimulation of all three kinds of cones) and darkness.

Even more complex kinds of color opponency are found among neurons in the visual cortex. For example, a neuron may respond with an ON response to red light and an OFF response to green light in the center of its receptive field, whereas the reverse responses are evoked from the peripheral zone (double opponency). Such neurons are found in the cytochrome-rich patches in the lamina 2-3 of the striate area (Fig. 8.21). *Together, all the color opponency neurons provide accurate information of the wavelength composition of the light hitting any spot on the retina.*

We are used to, and take for granted, that an object has a certain color, regardless of whether we see it in direct sunlight , in the shadow, or in artificial light. For example, we consistently identify a banana as yellow, an apple as red, the grass as green, and so forth (although we perceive differences in nuances). This property of our visual system, called *color constancy*, is by no means self-evident. Thus, the wavelength composition of the light reflected from an object depends not only on the physical properies of the surface but also on the light shining on the object. Different light sources produce light with quite different wavelength composition. The light received by the eye from an object thus differs markedly under different lighting conditions. Color constancy is obviously of great biologic importance. The color of an object gives us essential information as to its nature, but only if the color is an invariant, typical property. For example, we know that a yellow banana is edible, whereas green or brown ones are not. Even under quite different illuminations, we easily make this kind of choice based on color.

We do not fully understand how the brain accomplishes this remarkable task, although it must depend on processing at the cortical level. Color constancy occurs only if the object we look at is part of a complex, multicolored scene. Experiments with patterned, multicolored surfaces show that the composition of the light reflected from one part of the visual scene may be changed considerably without changing the color perceived by an observer. If, however, the same square is seen against an evenly dark background, its perceived color changes according to the composition of the reflected light—for example from green to white. This must mean that *under natural conditions the brain determines the color of an object by comparing the wavelength composition of the light from its surface with the composition of light from all other surfaces in the visual field.*

If we look at a red surface for a few seconds and then move to a white, we see a green surface where we just saw the red. This is called an *after image.* The after image of yellow is blue, and for white it is black. This phenomenon can be partly explained by selective bleaching of a particular kind of cone. For example, a red light bleaches mainly the cones with wavelength sensitivity in the red part of the spectrum. When the eye then receives white light, the "red" cones are, for a short while, less sensitive than the others. This creates a relative dominance of signals from "green" cones, and the surface is perceived as green. What we have said so far might suggest that the color of the after image depends only on the light first hitting the retina. It is not that simple, however. The after image depends on the color *perceived* by the subject, not the absolute wavelength composition—that is, color constancy occurs also for after images.

Even this fragmentary discussion of color vision may give some thoughts as to the real meaning of the term color. *Color is, strictly speaking, not a property of an object but a subjective experience of a person seeing the object.* The experience is based on how the brain processes information about the wavelength composition of the light reflected from the object (and from all other objects in the same visual scene). That we also can *imagine* colors raises the question of where and how colors (as percepts) are represented in our memory. Now we can only give fragmentary answers to this and other questions about how the brain creates colors, or even visual images at all. Nevertheless, the above considerations might serve to emphasize that there is no absolute correlation between a visual stimulus and the perception it evokes. Of course, this is not specific to seeing, but pertains to the other senses as well. Fortunately, relationships between certain patterns of stimuli and external events are reasonably constant. Therefore, we usually take the right decisions by relying upon our brain's interpretation (our percept) of the stimuli (the color of a traffic light, the movements of a snake, the contours of a horse, and so forth).

How Are Data from Different Visual Areas Integrated?

The fact that there is much evidence of separate processing in the visual cortex of different aspects of visual information must not make us forget that at some level a synthesis has to occur. Information about form, position, movement, and color must in some way be linked together. After all, the color "belongs" to a certain object, with a certain form and position, and speed and direction of movement. Our percept is unitary, although the brain first has "dissected" out and analyzed the bits and pieces of information in the light falling on the retina. What does integration of information mean in the context of sensory processing? One might think that there must exist *one* final, site (area) in which all aspects of visual information are brought together. However, anatomic data do not favor the existence of such cortical areas. Thus, even in the prefrontal cortex visual information about "what" and "where" are treated separately (in conjunction with coupling of visual features of objects to voluntary movements). Also, there are theoretical problems with the notion of a final integrative area. Thus, although our conscious experience is unitary, it consists of components to which we have separate, conscious access. For example, a car may be characterized by its color, by its shape, or by its movements. The components are kept separate yet linked in such a way that we perceive them as belonging together. Another theoretical problem with a final integrative area is where to "place" awareness of the visual image. As expressed by the British neurobiologist Zeki: "If all the visual areas report to a single master cortical area, who or what does that single area report to? Put more visually, who is 'looking' at the visual image provided by that master area?" We have treated integration at early stages of the visual processing, such as cells in the striate area responding to contours with a certain orientation regardless where it occurs within a larger part of the visual field. Further integration produces more complex properties, so that cells respond only when several characteristics co-

Consciousness and Visual Experience

We will illustrate the problems with determining the structural basis of conscious visual experience with a few examples. The first example was published by Goodale and co-workers in 1991. A woman suffered damage to parts of her occipital lobes (with sparing of the striate cortex) because of carbon monoxide poisoning. Afterwards she was unable to recognize objects (visual agnosia). She could, for example, not decide whether an object was oriented vertically or horizontally, nor could she show the size of the object with her fingers. When asked to grasp it, however, this was done easily, and with normal preparatory adjustment of the fingers. Thus, she could adapt her grip to specific visual features, yet she had no awareness of these features. Obviously, the parts of the brain preparing voluntary, goal directed movements have access to information about shape, size, and orientation, no matter whether these features are consciously perceived or not.

Some patients with damage of the striate area have retained some ability to respond to moving stimuli in the blind visual field. They nevertheless have no conscious awareness of having seen anything. This phenomenon is called *blindsight*. In such cases, visual information must reach the extrastriate areas specialized for analysis of movements without going through the striate area (possible pathways are discussed below). We may then ask whether conscious visual experience requires that visual information first goes through striate area, or whether it requires synchronized activity in the striate area and certain extrastriate areas? Another approach to these questions is to study brain activity with the PET technique while subjects *imagine* visual scenes, such as a red Ford or their home street. In such situations the subject has retrieved the information from memory and "sees" the scene with closed eyes. Which parts of the brain are then specifically activated? It appears that largely the same extrastriate areas are activated during visual imagery as when seeing. The PET data are conflicting as to whether the striate area is activated with visual imagery. However, the fact that patients with cortical blindness (damage to the striate area) are able to imagine visual scenes, strongly suggests that the striate area is not necessary for visual imagery. Also other clinical observations suggest that visual imagery and seeing may not use identical cortical structures. Thus, a few patients have been reported who could recognize objects when seeing them, but could not imagine the same objects. Also, the reverse situation has been described.

In short, both clinical and PET studies clearly show that extensive parts of the cerebral cortex are involved in conscious visual experience. Furthermore, visual information that is not consciously perceived may nevertheless be used for preparation of voluntary (conscious) movements.

incide (such as a contour with a specific orientation moving in a certain direction). Such and more complex integration of data need not occur on single cells, however; It may also occur by coordinated activity in separate neurons that are synaptically linked. As mentioned, it is noteworthy that the many visual areas are so extensively interconnected. For example, the striate area receives connections from most of the areas to which it projects, and the same holds for many extrastriate areas and their relations to other cortical areas. *Presumably, our conscious visual image is a product of the total, synchronized pattern of impulses in many cortical areas at any moment.* Synchronized activity of neuronal groups receiving the same kind of information (for example, about movement direction) may play an important role, and has been shown to occur in cortical areas.

Visual Information Can Reach the Cortex via the Superior Colliculus and the Pulvinar

Not all fibers in the optic nerve end in the lateral geniculate body, as mentioned above. About 10% (in the monkey) leave the optic tract to terminate in the *pretectal nuclei* and in the *superior colliculus* (Figs. 3.18, 3.19, and 16.26). Some fibers end in the *pulvinar* (Figs. 3.20, 3.21, and 3.28), and this nucleus (and another thalamic nucleus, the lateral posterior nucleus, LP, Fig. 20.7) receives afferents from the superior colliculus. Like other thalamic nuclei, these send their efferents to the cortex, notably to the *extrastriate visual areas* (among other regions). Thus visual information may reach the cortex (through several links) even when the optic radiation or the striate area is damaged. Even though these visual pathways—circumventing the lateral geniculate body—are retinotopically organized, they are apparently capable of giving only very crude information about movement in the visual field. After bilateral damage of the striate area in monkeys, the animals react easily to moving stimuli, even though in other respects they behave as if they were blind. Studies of patients with damage at various levels of the visual pathways and of the visual cortex (localized with the use of MRI) indicate that, as long as parts of the extrastriate visual areas on the convexity are intact, the patients retain some capacity to recognize movements in the visual field. When sitting in front of a large screen with a random pattern of moving dots, patients with damage of the striate area (and surrounding areas on the medial aspect of the hemisphere) reacted with movements of the eyes, apparently following the moving objects. They reported that they felt something moving in front of them, and they had some ability to identify the movement direction. They had no feeling of seeing anything, however, and when tested with perimetry, they were completely blind.

The visual connections of the *superior colliculus* are primarily concerned with *reflex movements of the eyes and the head*, as already mentioned. Thus, most of the efferent connections from the superior colliculus pass to nuclei in the brain stem concerned with control of such movements. The pretectal nuclei constitute a link in the pathway for the light reflex (Fig. 16.26).

Fusion of Visual Images and Strabismus

Normally, we perceive one image of the objects we look at, even though two (slightly different) images are formed on the retina. The two images fuse into one, and the phenomenon is called *fusion*. Fusion requires that the optic axes of the two eyes be properly aligned, so that the images fall on *corresponding points* on the retina (Fig. 8.3). The two maculae are obviously corresponding points, and the images fall on them when we fix the gaze on a point to see it as sharply as possible. As mentioned, the signals from the two eyes are kept separate in the lateral geniculate body, but at the cortical level many cells are influenced from both eyes—that is, they are binocular (Fig. 8.17). Convergence in the cortex of signals from corresponding points in the two eyes is a prerequisite for fusion. Fusion is not present from birth but develops gradually from about the age of 3 to 7 months. During this period, the movements of the eyes become coordinated, so that all movements are conjugated and the images fall on corresponding points when the gaze is fixed.

Strabismus (cross-eyed) means that the optic axes of the eyes are not properly aligned, and, accordingly, the images do not fall on corresponding points. The lack of fusion in such cases leads to underdevelopment or suppression of vision for the eye not used for fixation. In this manner, bothersome double vision is avoided, but even a relatively brief period of strabismus in early childhood may lead to permanently reduced visual acuity (the underlying mechanisms are discussed in Chapter 4, *Critical Periods*). It has been shown in monkeys that strabismus (produced experimentally) leads to a reduced number of cells in the striate area that is influenced by both eyes. In one kind of squint, the two eyes are used alternatively for fixation, and in such patients the visual acuity is usually conserved for both eyes.

Development of Normal Vision Requires Proper Use

There may be causes for a lack of normal vision development other than a squint. If, for example, the eye does not receive proper stimulation because errors of refraction produce a retinal image that is out of focus or because light for some reason does not reach the retina, vision is not developed normally. In humans, the first 2–3 years (in particular the first year) are critical in this respect; lack of meaningful use of the eye even for a short period may then give permanently reduced visual acuity, as mentioned above. Animal experiments furthermore show that vision is better preserved if both eyes are covered for a period than if only one is covered. This is so because the two eyes "compete" during the early development of the visual system. If only one eye is used, it gets an advantage and takes over neurons in the visual cortex that normally would have been utilized by the other eye. For more data on the development of the visual system, see Chapter 4, (*Examples of Axonal Growth Guided by Chemotrophic Gradients and Local Cues*, and *The Role Played by the Environment in Development of the Nervous System*).

Interruption of the Visual Pathways

Partial damage to the visual pathways produces symptoms that confirm the arrangement of the cells and fibers at various levels of the optic system (Fig. 8.22).

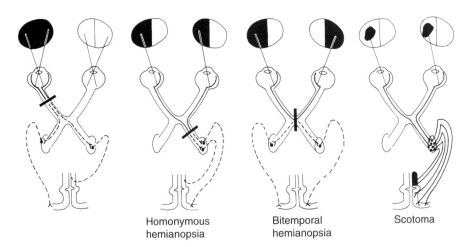

Homonymous
hemianopsia

Bitemporal
hemianopsia

Scotoma

Figure 8.22 *Visual field defects after lesions of the visual pathways.* The black areas indicate the blind parts of the visual field. The visual fields of the two eyes are shown separately for didactic reasons (cf. Figs. 8.14 and 8.19).

Interruption of the *optic nerve* prevents any visual signals from reaching the brain from that eye. On the other hand, if only the *crossing fibers* are damaged at the level of the *optic chiasm*, signals from the two nasal halves of the retinae are interrupted. The patient is blind in the temporal parts of the visual field on both sides (*bitemporal hemianopsia*). The patient may not notice this, however, because the blind part of the visual field is not experienced as darkness but rather as "nothing." The visual defect may be discovered incidentally by a tendency to bump into objects located a little to the side and perhaps by being hit by a car coming from the side when driving. This kind of visual defect may be caused by a tumor of the pituitary (located just below the optic chiasm). When the tumor grows, it has to expand upward since it is located in a bony excavation (the sella turcica) and thus first compresses the middle part of the chiasm. Damage to the optic tract produces a different clinical picture. If the damage is on the right side, visual signals from the temporal half of the right retina and the nasal half of the left retina are prevented from reaching the cortex—that is, the patient is blind in the left half of the visual field (*homonymous hemianopsia*). The same visual defect occurs when the *optic radiation*—or the striate area—is totally destroyed. More frequently, there are incomplete lesions of the optic radiation (note its position in the posterior part of the internal capsule) or of the striate area, producing blind spots or *scotoma* in the opposite visual field (at corresponding points). Because of the accurate retinotopic arrangement within the visual pathways (Fig. 8.19), mapping of such blind spots enables a precise determination of the site of the lesion.

CHAPTER 9

THE AUDITORY SYSTEM

The sense of hearing is of great importance in higher animals—not least in humans, for whom speech is the most important means of communication. The adequate stimulus for the auditory receptors is sound waves with frequencies between 20 and about 20,000 Hz. The sensitivity is greatest, however, between 1000 and 4000 Hz and declines steeply toward the highest and the lowest frequencies; that is, a tone of 15,000 Hz must be much stronger than a sound of 1000 Hz to be perceived. The range of frequencies to which the ear is most sensitive corresponds fairly well to the range of frequencies for human speech. The frequency of sound waves determines the pitch, whereas the amplitude of the waves determines the intensity. Many animals can perceive sound over a much wider range of frequencies than humans. For example, dogs can hear a whistle hardly noticed by humans, and bats use extremely high-pitched sounds for echolocation.

Sound waves pass through the air to the tympanic membrane, which transmits them via a chain of three tiny bones to the *cochlea*. The sensory cells of the cochlea are *low-threshold mechanoreceptors* sensitive to the bending of stereocilia on their surface. From the cochlea the signals are conducted to the brain stem through the eighth cranial nerve, the *vestibulocochlear nerve* (Figs. 3.14 and 3.18). This nerve also carries signals from the sense organ for equilibrium—the vestibular apparatus—which anatomically and evolutionarily is closely related to the cochlea. Functionally, however, these two parts have little in common, and we will describe the sense of equilibrium together with other aspects of vestibular function in Chapter 16.

THE COCHLEA

The Cochlea Is Part of the Labyrinth

The labyrinth consists of an outer bony part surrounding an irregular canal in the temporal bone, and an inner membranous part following and partly

Decibel

The most intense sound that the human ear can perceive is about 10^{12} times stronger than the weakest. A logarithmic scale is therefore used for sound intensity. One decibel (dB) represents the weakest perceptible sound and just below 130 dB represents the strongest (the pain threshold is at 130 dB). Ordinary speech produces about 65 dB. This scale gives relative measures of intensity, since the sensitivity of the ear differs for different frequencies.

filling the canal (Figs. 9.1, and 9.2). The membranous canal is filled with a fluid called the *endolymph* (Figs. 9.4 and 9.8). Between the membranous and the bony parts is a space filled with a fluid called the perilymph.

The labyrinth has two main parts. One is the *cochlea* and the other is the vestibular apparatus consisting of three semicircular ducts and two round dilatations (Fig. 9.2). Here we will consider only the organ of hearing, the cochlea.

The membranous part of the cochlea—the *cochlear duct*—forms a thin-walled tube with a triangular shape (in cross section), surrounded by the bony part of the cochlea. The duct forms a spiral with two and a half to three turns (Figs. 9.2–9.4). The lowermost wall of the cochlear duct is formed by the *basilar membrane* (membrana basilaris), which is suspended between the two facing sides of the bony canal (Figs. 9.5 and 9.7). At the inner side of the turns, the basilar membrane is attached to a bony prominence—the *bony spiral lamina* (lamina spiralis ossea), which follows the cochlea in its spiraling course (Figs. 9.3 and 9.7). The sensory epithelium, forming the *organ of Corti*, rests on the basilar membrane (Figs. 9.3, 9.5, and 9.7). The length of the cochlear duct—and thus of the basilar membrane—is about 3 cm (Fig. 9.8). The upper wall of the

Figure 9.1 *The ear*. Note the middle ear with the three ear ossicles and the inner ear with the membranous labyrinth (located in the temporal bone). The eustachian tube connects the middle ear with the pharynx.

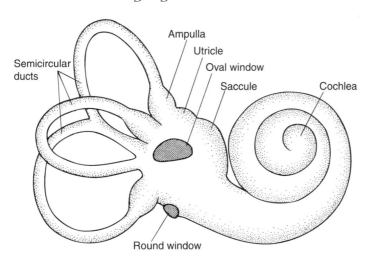

Figure 9.2 *The membranous labyrinth with its vestibular part* (the semicircular ducts, the saccule, and the utricle) and the auditory part (the cochlea). The stapes is attached in the oval window.

cochlear duct is formed by the thin *vestibular membrane* (Figs. 9.3 and 8.7). The third, lateral or outer wall of the cochlear duct lies on the bony wall of the canal and is formed by a specialized, stratified epithelium. The room outside the cochlear duct is thus divided into two parallel canals. The one situated below the basilar membrane is called the *scala tympani*; the one above the vestibular membrane is called the *scala vestibuli* (Figs. 9.3 and 9.8). Both have openings or windows in the bone facing the middle ear (Figs. 9.2 and 9.7). The *oval window* (fenestra vestibuli) sits at the end of the scala vestibuli, whereas the *round window* (fenestra cochleae) sits at the end of the scala tympani. The windows are closed by the stapes and a thin membrane of connective tissue, respectively (Fig. 9.8).

Figure 9.3 *Section through the cochlea.*

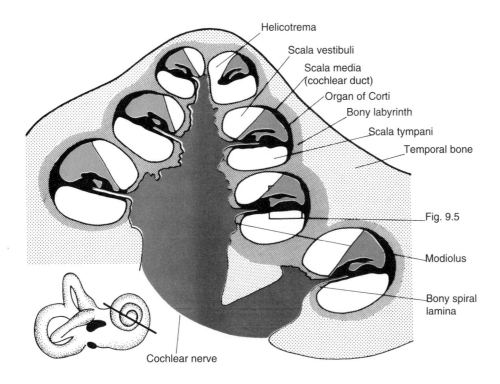

Figure 9.4 *The labyrinth*. Two closely spaced, frontal MRIs. The fluid-filled cochlea and semicircular canals are clearly seen just below the temporal lobe (the image is weighted so that water appears white).

Cochlea   Semicircular ducts

Figure 9.5 *The organ of Corti*. Compare with Figure 9.3.

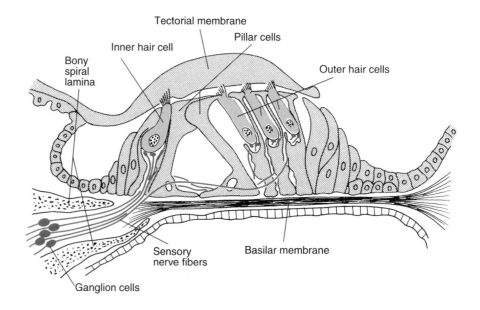

The Perilymph and the Endolymph

The composition of the endolymph and of the perilymph differs: The concentrations of sodium and potassium ions in the perilymph are similar to those in the cerebrospinal fluid (that is, similar to those in the extracellular fluid), whereas the concentrations of these ions in the endolymph are like those found intracellularly. Thus, the cilia of the sensory cells—surrounded by the endolymph (Fig. 9.7)—are embedded in an unusual extracellular fluid with K^+ as the dominating cation. The protein concentration, however, is much higher in the perilymph than in the endolymph and the cerebrospinal fluid.

How Sound Waves Are Transmitted to
the Sensory Cells in the Cochlea

Conduction of sound waves from the air to the receptor cells in the cochlea occurs through the *external ear* (the auricle and the external auditory meatus) and the *middle ear* or *tympanic cavity* (Fig. 9.1). Sound waves hitting the skull can also be transmitted through the bone directly to the receptors. This kind of transmission, however, is very inefficient with regard to airborne sound waves and therefore plays no role in normal hearing (such bone conduction of sound waves is used for testing the function of the cochlea and also for certain hearing aid devices).

Sound waves hit the *eardrum* or *tympanic membrane* located at the bottom of the external meatus (Fig. 9.1). The eardrum consists of a thin, tense connective tissue membrane covered by a thin layer of epithelium on both sides (it is richly supplied with nociceptors, like the tight skin of the inner part of the external meatus). The three ossicles form a chain through the middle ear and connect the eardrum with the oval window (Figs. 9.1, 9.2, and 9.8). The *malleus* (the hammer) has a shaft that is attached to the inner side of the eardrum. The head of the malleus is connected to the *incus* (the anvil) by a joint, and the incus is further connected to the *stapes* (the stirrup) by a joint. The basal plate of the stapes is inserted in the oval window, thus closing the scala vestibuli (Fig. 9.8). The sound waves make the eardrum and the ossicles vibrate with the frequency of the waves, and thus the movement is transmitted to the fluid in the cochlea. Because the area of the eardrum is so much larger than that of the basal plate of the stapes, the pressure per square unit is increased 20 times. This *amplification mechanism* of course increases the sensitivity for sound dramatically, compared to a situation without the ossicles. Normally, even the slightest movement of the eardrum is sufficient to cause stimulation of the receptors in the cochlea. If the sound waves were to be transmitted directly from the air to the fluid in the cochlea, a large proportion would be reflected without acting on the cochlea. The sound would have to be much stronger to be perceived in such a situation. This is the case when diseases of the middle ear destroy the ossicles or stiffen their joints and thus eliminate the amplification mechanism. The ensuing hearing loss is called *conduction deafness*. A prerequisite for the free movement of the eardrum is that the pressure be equal on the two sides. This is ensured by the *Eustachian tube* (tuba auditiva), which connects the middle ear cavity with the pharynx (Fig. 9.1).

When the stapes is pressed (slightly) into the oval window, the pressure of the sound waves is transmitted directly to the fluid (the perilymph) in the scala vestibuli. Since water is incompressible, the sound waves can cause movement of the fluid only because the room can expand at some other point. Such expansion is allowed by the thin, compliant membrane covering the round window, which is pressed outward (into the middle ear) each time the stapes is pressed into the oval window. Movement of the perilymph in the scala vestibuli is immediately transmitted to the endolymph in the cochlear duct through the thin vestibular membrane. The movement is thus propagated to the basilar membrane, which is pressed slightly downward, and transmits the movement to the perilymph in the

Figure 9.6 *Inner hair cell*. Compare
with Figure 9.5.

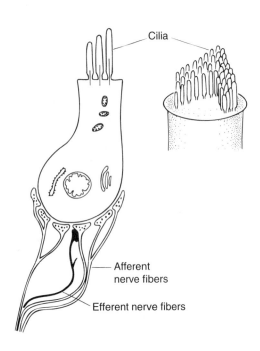

Cilia

Afferent
nerve fibers

Efferent nerve fibers

scala tympani. In short, *movements of the stapes in and out of the oval
window in pace with the sound waves produce corresponding movements
of the basilar membrane*. Movements of the basilar membrane stimulate
the receptor cells.

We will now describe how the receptor cells are arranged in the organ of Corti and the mechanism by which movements of the basilar membrane lead to excitation of the receptors.

The Organ of Corti

The receptor cells in the cochlea are called hair cells because they are
equipped with sensory hairs or stereocilia on their apical surface (Figs.
9.5 and 9.6). Along the basilar membrane there are two rows of receptor
cells—one row formed by the *outer hair cells*, the other row by the *inner hair cells* (Fig. 9.5). The hair cells are surrounded by supporting cells.
Two rows of especially large supporting cells, the pillar cells, separate
the inner and outer hair cells and form the *tunnel of Corti*. Above the hair
cells lies a thick plate, the tectorial membrane, which is indirectly attached
to the bony wall of the cochlea. *Sensory (afferent) nerve fibers* of the
eighth cranial nerve contact the basal parts of the hair cells (Fig. 9.5 and
9.6). The cell bodies of the sensory neurons are located in the *bony spiral lamina* (lamina spiralis ossea) close to the midportion of the cochlea
(the *modiolus*, Figs. 9.3, 9.5, and 9.7). The hair cells are also contacted
by efferent nerve fibers (Fig. 9.6), which enable the central nervous system to control the sensitivity of the auditory receptors.

The *mechanism by which the hair cells are stimulated* most likely
functions as follows: When the basilar membrane vibrates, the hair cells
are displaced relative to the tectorial membrane, which is relatively im-
mobile because it is anchored to the bony wall. The stereocilia, being

Scala vestibuli

Vestibular membrane

Cochlear duct

Tectorial membrane

Spiral ganglion

Organ of Corti

Basilar membrane

Scala tympani

embedded in the tectorial membrane, are thus moved back and forth in pace with the frequency of the sound waves. Bending of the cilia in one direction depolarizes the hair cell, whereas bending in the opposite direction hyperpolarizes it. Thus, the membrane potential of the hair cells oscillates in pace with the vibrations of the basilar membrane. Depolarization of the hair cells probably produces release of a neuroactive substance that transmits the signal to the sensory nerve endings. When sufficient amounts of the substance are released, action potentials are elicited in the sensory nerve fibers, and the signal is transmitted to the brain stem (Fig. 6.1).

Figure 9.7 *Section through the cochlea*. Photomicrograph. Compare with Figure 9.3.

Figure 9.8 *The cochlea*. The cochlear duct is pictured as if straightened. The oscillations of the stapes are transmitted to the fluid in the scala vestibuli and from there to the cochlear duct. Different tone frequencies set different parts of the basilar membrane in motion.

Scala vestibuli

Oval window

Endolymph

Cochlear duct (scala media)

Stapes

Helicotrema

Round window

Basilar membrane

Perilymph

Scala tympani

Inner and Outer Hair Cells Have Different Properties

As mentioned, there are two rows of hair cells (Fig. 9.5). The inner row—closest to the bony spiral lamina—consists of a single row of *inner hair cells*. The outer row consists of three parallel rows of *outer hair cells*. There are approximately 3500 inner and 15,000 outer hair cells in the human cochlea. The two kinds of cells differ with regard to both morphology and innervation. Many more sensory nerve fibers contact the inner than the outer hair cells, whereas the situation is reversed with efferent innervation. It is now believed that the *inner hair cells are responsible for signaling sound, whereas the outer hair cells regulate the sensitivity of the sense organ.*

The motion of the basilar membrane differs from that expected of a passive mechanical structure. There must be mechanisms intrinsic to the cochlea that can amplify the vibrations of the basilar membrane (almost 100 times). Much evidence points to the outer hair cells as the motors of the amplification—that is, they can rapidly transmit mechanical energy to a very narrow strip of the basilar membrane. The fast movements of the outer hair cells in turn move the basilar membrane, producing both an amplification of the vibrations and a narrowing of the vibrating part (sharper tuning of the frequency curve). Together, these changes ensure more precise signal transmission.

Different Frequencies Are Registered at Different Sites along the Basilar Membrane: Tonotopic Localization

The ordered arrangement of neurons and nerve fibers signaling different pitches of sound (frequencies) is called *tonotopic localization* (compare with somatotopic localization in the somatosensory system and retinotopic localization in the visual system). As we will discuss later, the auditory pathways are tonotopically organized all the way from the cochlea to the cerebral cortex. The tonotopic localization in the cochlea has been demonstrated in several ways. After lesions restricted to a small part of the organ of Corti (which extends along the full length of the basilar membrane), experimental animals no longer react to sound in a certain, narrow range of frequencies (pitches), whereas they react normally to sounds of other frequencies. In humans, similar selective deafness may occur after prolonged exposure to noise—for example, in factories. Anatomic examination of the cochlea after death in such pesons has shown that the hair cells have disappeared in a restricted region on the basilar membrane, the position of the region differing with the frequency to which the person was deaf. The tonotopic localization has been determined in great detail by recording the response of single hair cells to sounds of different frequencies. Each hair cell is best activated by tones within a very narrow range of frequencies. Together, the hair cells and the sensory fibers leading from them cover the total range of frequencies we can perceive.

The tonotopic localization is such that the *tones with the highest pitch (highest frequencies) are registered by the hair cells closest to the oval window—that is, on the basal part of the basilar membrane—whereas the lowest frequencies are registered at the top of the cochlea, that is, at the apical part of the basilar membrane.* This can be explained, at least partly, by the physical properties of the basilar membrane, as proposed by the German physicist Hermann Helmholtz in the nineteenth century. The basilar membrane is most narrow basally, and becomes progressively wider in the apical direction. The fibers of the basilar membrane are oriented transversely to the long axis of the basilar membrane (Fig. 9.5) and are therefore longer apically than basally. In analogy with the strings of an instrument (for example, a piano), basal parts would be expected to vibrate with a higher frequency than apical parts. This is the main basis of the resonance theory of Helmholtz, which postulates that each position along the basilar membrane corresponds to a certain frequency. Although later research has shown that even a pure tone makes large parts of the basilar membrane vibrate, the region in which the maximal amplitude occurs is very narrow. This appears to be caused by not fully understood *amplification mechanisms* in the cochlea (see above, *Inner and Outer Hair Cells Have Different Properties*). Thus, the hair cells differ in accordance with their position on the basilar membrane, so that their thresholds are lower for certain frequencies than for others.

Hearing Loss

The most common causes of hearing loss are diseases of the middle ear, either because they compromise the conduction of sounds to the cochlea, or because they destroy the neural elements of the cochlea. The first kind is called *conductive deafness*, the second *sensorineural (or nerve) deafness*. Transmission of sound to the cochlea can be reduced or abolished by middle ear infections damaging the eardrum or the ossicles. Less frequently hearing loss is caused by lesions of the central auditory pathways. This kind, called *central deafness*, is considered later in this chapter.

To distinguish between conductive and sensorineural deafness, one can compare the threshold for sounds conducted through the air with sound conducted through the bones of the skull. In the *Rinne test*, a vibrating tuning fork is first applied to the mastoid process and then a little away from the external ear. Normally, the sound is heard much better when conducted through the air than through the bone. However, in conductive deafness—caused by destruction of the eardrum or the ossicles—the bone conducted sound is heard best. In the *Weber test*, the vibrating tuning fork is applied to the forehead in the midline. Normally, the sound is heard equally in both ears. In conductive deafness, it is heard best in the deaf ear, whereas in sensorineural deafness it is heard best in the normal ear.

THE AUDITORY PATHWAYS

The anatomic organization of the central auditory pathways shows some unusual features, different from other sensory systems we have dealt with. More nuclei are intercalated in the auditory pathways and, furthermore, these nuclei have extensive and complicated interconnections. Finally, there are fibers crossing the midline at several levels of the auditory pathways. These features have made the auditory pathways more difficult to study than other sensory pathways. The crossing at several levels also renders hearing examinations of limited practical value for determining the site of lesions in the central nervous system.

The Cochlear Nerve and the Cochlear Nuclei

The part of the eighth cranial nerve conducting impulses from the cochlea is called the *cochlear nerve*. Most of the fibers are afferent and have their perikarya in the *spiral ganglion*, which is located in the bony spiral lamina (Figs. 9.3 and 9.7). From the spiral ganglion the fibers pass through

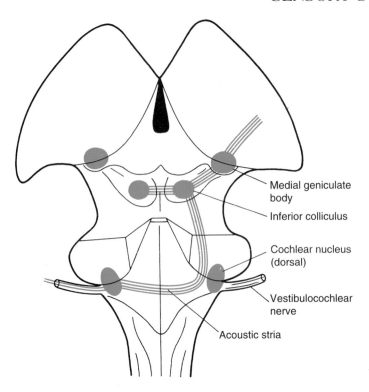

Medial geniculate body

Inferior colliculus

Cochlear nucleus (dorsal)

Vestibulocochlear nerve

Acoustic stria

the midportion of the cochlea (the modiolus, Fig. 9.3) and through the internal acoustic meatus (internal auditory canal) to the *cerebellopontine angle* (Fig. 9.9). There the nerve enters the *cochlear nuclei*, which are two large nuclei (the dorsal and the ventral cochlear nuclei) located laterally on the medulla (Figs. 9.9, 9.10, and 16.2), external to the inferior cerebellar peduncle (Fig. 14.1). After entering the nuclei, the cochlear nerve fibers divide and end in precise tonotopic order in several parts of the nuclei. The tonotopic localization has been demonstrated, for example, with microelectrode recordings that make it possible to determine the response of single fibers and neurons to tones of different frequencies.

The *efferent fibers* of the cochlear nerve arise in the *superior olivary complex*, located in the rostral part of the medulla (Fig. 9.10). The fibers end, as mentioned, predominantly around the outer hair cells and enable the central nervous system to control the sensitivity of the inner hair cells.

Ascending Pathways from the Cochlear Nuclei

From the cochlear nuclei the auditory impulses are transmitted to the *inferior colliculus* (mainly of the opposite side). The pathway formed by the ascending fibers from the cochlear nuclei is called the *lateral lemniscus* (Figs. 9.9 and 9.10). Many of the fibers end, however, in other nuclei—such as the superior olivary complex—that send fibers to the inferior colliculus. Neurons in the inferior colliculus send their axons to the *medial geniculate body* of the thalamus (Figs. 3.20, 3.21, 9.9, and 9.10). The fibers form an oblong elevation at the dorsal side of the mesencephalon, the *inferior collicular brachium* (brachium quadrigeminum inferius). The efferent fibers from the medial geniculate body end in the

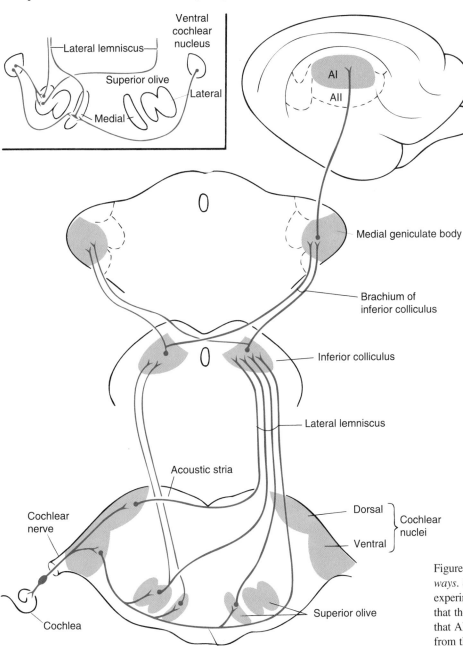

Figure 9.10 *Ascending auditory pathways.* Schematic presentation based on experimental studies of the cat. Note that the connections are bilateral, so that AI on one side receives impulses from the cochleae of both sides. **Inset:** *Connections of the superior olive.* Only some main connections are shown. Note that impulses from both ears reach the medial part of the superior olive. This arrangement is believed to be of importance for localization of sound.

auditory cortex located in the temporal lobe (in the superior temporal gyrus, Figs. 9.10 and 9.11). The ascending fibers from the medial geniculate body are located in the posterior part of the internal capsule. At all levels, the auditory pathway is precisely organized, with cells responding to sounds of different frequencies arranged in parallel lamellae.

Even though the central auditory pathways are predominantly crossed, there is a significant uncrossed component. Therefore, unilateral damage to the pathways does not produce a clear-cut hearing deficit. The ability to localize from where a sound comes may be reduced, however.

The Auditory Pathways Consist of Functionally Different Components

Efferent fibers from the two cochlear nuclei take different routes (Fig. 9.10). Fibers from the *dorsal cochlear nucleus* pass in the *stria acusticae* dorsal to the inferior cerebellar peduncle and then cross through the reticular formation and join the lateral lemniscus. Most fibers from the *ventral nucleus*, on the other hand, pass ventrally and cross to the other side in the *trapezoid body* in the lowermost part of the pons. Some of these fibers end in the superior olivary complex of both sides, whereas others continue rostrally in the lateral lemniscus to the inferior colliculus. The functional significance of these parallel paths out of the cochlear nuclei is not fully understood, but animal experiments (especially in the cat) show that single cells in the dorsal and ventral nuclei have different properties. Schematically, many cells in the ventral nucleus respond to sound stimuli much like the primary afferent fibers of the cochlear nerve, whereas cells in the dorsal nucleus have more complex response properties. Cells in the dorsal nucleus are, for example, often excited by sound with one particular frequency and inhibited by another frequency. It has been suggested that the dorsal nucleus forwards signals that are of importance for the direction of attention toward a sound, whereas information from the ventral nucleus is of importance for, among other things, localization of a sound.

Experimentally, two components of the ascending auditory pathways have been identified. One is called the *core projection* and is a pathway for auditory impulses only. It is precisely tonotopically localized at all levels and terminates in the primary auditory cortex, AI. The core projection is relayed through the central parts of the inferior colliculus and specific parts of the medial geniculate body. The other component is called the *belt projection*. It is relayed through peripheral parts of the inferior colliculus and terminates in the cortex surrounding the AI. The cells of this pathway are influenced by visual and somatosensory stimuli in addition to auditory ones. The belt projection is thought to be of importance for integration of auditory information with other kinds of sensory information.

Generalizations to conditions in humans on the basis of studies done in other species must, however, be made with particular caution for the auditory system. Species differences appear to be greater for the auditory system than for other sensory systems. This may be related presumably to the great differences that exist among species with how sound is used as a source of information. For example, certain nuclei that are large in the cat are very small in man, and vice versa.

Sound Localization

It is not enough that the central nervous system analyzes the sound frequencies, and on this basis interprets the meaning of the sound (for example, who or what produced the sound). Locating the source of a sound is another important but difficult task of the auditory system. To be able to judge the distance and direction to a sound source (potential prey or a danger) is obviously of vital importance to most animal species.

Unilateral damage to the auditory cortex reduces the ability of experimental animals to locate sounds coming from the opposite side. Thus, a cat with such a lesion does not move toward its prey sending out a brief sound (for example, a mouse). The head and eyes, however, move toward the prey—even after bilateral damage of the auditory cortex—showing that nuclei at lower levels of the auditory pathways can locate the sound and elicit appropriate reflex movements.

Concerning location of sounds in the *horizontal plane*, that is, to the right or left of the midsagittal plane, basic computations occur in the first synaptic relay after the cochlear nuclei, the *superior olive* (Fig. 9.10). We are less certain regarding mechanisms for location of sounds in the *vertical plane*, although the *dorsal cochlear nucleus* is probably involved. Neurons in the inferior colliculus respond specifically to sound from a certain direction, and the inferior colliculus probably contains a map of our auditory space.

Descending Control of the Auditory Pathways

There are descending fibers at all levels of the auditory pathways. There are numerous fibers passing from the auditory cortex to the medial geniculate body (like other thalamic nuclei) and to the inferior colliculus. There are also fibers descending from the inferior colliculus to nuclei at lower levels. As mentioned, there are also efferent fibers in the cochlear nerve ending in contact with the hair cells of the cochlea. Such fibers come from the superior olivary complex, and form the *olivocochlear bundle*. The descending connections are, at least in part, precisely organized and can therefore be expected to control selectively subgroups of neurons in the auditory pathways (for example, neurons transmitting information about a certain frequency).

There are many *inhibitory interneurons* in the nuclei of the auditory pathways, and both GABA and glycine appear to be used as transmitters for such interneurons. Physiological experiments show that the central transmission of auditory impulses can be inhibited, probably at all levels from the cochlea to the cerebral cortex. The censoring of the sensory information that is allowed to reach consciousness is perhaps even more pronounced in the auditory system than in other sensory systems. Selective suppression

The Superior Olive and Sound Localization

The superior olivary complex (superior olive) is located in the lower part of the pons, in the trapezoid body (Fig. 9.10). A striking feature is that most neurons are influenced from both ears, which led to the assumption that the superior olive is of particular importance for the ability to localize the origin of a sound. When a sound hits the head from the right side, it will reach the right ear slightly before it reaches the left, because the head is in the way. The sound will also be slightly weakened before reaching the left ear. Psychophysical experiments in humans indicate that side differences in both time and intensity are used by the auditory system to localize sounds. The time difference is most important for localizing sounds of low frequencies, whereas intensity differences are most important for sounds of higher frequencies (above 4000 Hz).

The superior olivary complex consists of several subdivisions. The *lateral part* receives afferents from the cochlear nuclei of both sides and projects bilaterally to the inferior colliculi. Most cells in the lateral part are excited by impulses from the ear of the same side and inhibited by impulses from the contralateral ear (via interneurons). The cells respond best when the sounds hitting the two ears are of different intensities. Consequently, the lateral part of the superior olive is assumed to use intensity differences for the analysis of sound localization.

The *medial part* of the superior olive appears to be of particular importance for localization of low-frequency sounds. It receives afferents from a particular subdivision of the ventral cochlear nucleus of both sides (Fig. 9.10A). Each cell has two long dendrites oriented transversely. One dendrite receives signals from the right ear, the other from the left. These cells are very sensitive to small time differences in synaptic inputs to the two dendrites and are most sensitive to sounds with low frequencies. The efferent fibers of the medial part pass to the central nucleus of the inferior colliculus on the same side.

of auditory information is a necessity if we are to select the relevant sounds among numerous irrelevant ones. Such mechanisms are most likely at work when, for example, at a cocktail party with numerous voices we nevertheless are able to select and pay attention to only one of them.

Auditory Reflexes

The ascending auditory pathways convey signals that enable the conscious perception of sounds. Auditory information is, however, also used at a subconscious level to elicit reflex responses. The reticular formation receives collaterals from the ascending auditory pathways, and such connections mediate the sudden muscle activity provoked by a strong, unexpected sound—that is, a *startle response*. Other auditory impulses are transmitted to the nuclei of the facial and trigeminal nerves, which innervate two small muscles in the middle ear, the *stapedius and tensor tympani muscles*. Contraction of these muscles dampens the movements of the middle ear ossicles and thereby protects the cochlea against sounds of high intensity. Paresis of the facial nerve often is accompanied by hypersensitivity to sounds (hyperacusis).

Other, more complex reflex arcs mediate *automatic movements of the head and eyes*, and even the body, in the direction of an unexpected sound.

Interruption of the Auditory Pathways

Restricted lesions of the auditory pathways or the auditory cortex—*central lesions*—usually produce no clear-cut symptoms. As mentioned, this is because the connections from the cochlear nuclei to the cerebral cortex are bilateral (although with a contralateral preponderance). After destruction of the auditory cortex on one side, a person can still hear with both ears.

Destruction of the cochlear nerve (or the cochlea)—*peripheral lesions*—produces deafness of the ear on the same side (the same happens, of course, with a lesion of the cochlear nuclei). Destruction of the cochlear nerve may be caused by a tumor, called *acoustic neuroma*, in the internal auditory meatus (arising from the Schwann cells of the eighth cranial nerve). As the tumor grows, it compresses the cochlear, the vestibular, and the facial nerves (all passing through the internal meatus). Symptoms may therefore be caused by irritation (in the early phase) or destruction of all of these nerves. Thus, the first symptoms are usually due to irritation of the cochlear nerve, causing ringing in the ear (tinnitus), but gradually deafness develops. The cochlear nerve may also be compressed or torn by skull fractures passing through the temporal bone. Peripheral lesions of the auditory system, in addition to unilateral deafness, also reduce or eliminate the ability to localize the source of a sound.

Figure 9.11 *The human auditory cortex.*

The reflex centers for such reflexes are probably located in the inferior and superior colliculi. The inferior colliculus sends fibers to the superior colliculus, which has connections with the relevant motor nuclei in the brain stem and spinal cord. Furthermore, in the superior colliculus integration of auditory, visual, and somatosensory information takes place, so that the final motor response is appropriate for the organism as a whole.

THE AUDITORY CORTEX

Each of the nuclei of the auditory pathways consists in reality of subdivisions that differ in morphology, connectivity, and functions. This concerns, as mentioned, the cochlear nuclei, the superior olive, the inferior colliculus, and the medial geniculate body. The highest level, the auditory cortex, also shows such parcellation. Fibers from the medial geniculate body end with precise tonotopic localization in the *primary auditory cortex, AI* (Figs. 9.10 and 9.11). This corresponds largely to the striate area of the visual system. Regions around the AI receive fibers from parts of the medial geniculate body other than from where AI receives fibers. The *second auditory area, AII,* appears to receive afferents that are not tonotopically organized, whereas other areas (in the cat at least four) receive connections with a less precise localization than AI. Thus, cells in AI respond to sounds within a narrower frequency range than cells in the other auditory areas. Many cells in AI, however, have complex properties. Some respond best to a sound when the frequency is increasing or decreasing. Many cells are influenced from both ears, but often such that they are excited by signals from one ear and inhibited from the other. The functions of the auditory areas surrounding AI are less well known than the functions of the corresponding areas in the visual cortex.

In humans, Brodmann's area 41 in the superior temporal gyrus (Fig. 9.11) is thought to correspond to area AI of monkeys and other animals. In humans (as in lower animals), the cortex around the primary auditory area most likely receives fibers from both the medial geniculate body and the AI. It is, furthermore, highly likely that these areas are of particular importance for the interpretation of auditory information. Patients with bilateral damage of the auditory cortex are reported to be able to perceive sounds and even discriminate tones with different pitches and intensities (even though not necessarily with normal speed and precision). This corresponds to findings made in monkeys. The ability to recognize and interpret tones in particular patterns, however, is reduced or abolished. Such patients are unable to recognize familiar sounds like laughter, a bell that tolls, sounds of various animals, and so forth. They are furthermore unable to understand the speech of other people, even though they can speak and read themselves. This is called *acoustic agnosia.*

CHAPTER 10

OLFACTION AND TASTE

The chemical senses of smell and taste enable us to recognize a vast number of different molecules in our surroundings. Obviously, this gives us information of great importance—from avoiding poisonous food to enjoying the fragrance of a rose. Both senses depend on binding of *molecules to specific chemoreceptors*. These receptors are very sensitive, thus permitting recognition and discrimination of molecules in extremely low concentrations (in air or in fluids). *Stereospecificity*— that is, the shape of the ligand determines which receptor it binds to—is another common property of the chemoreceptors for taste and smell. The *transduction mechanisms*—that is, how the stimuli translate to graded receptor potentials—are similar for receptors for taste and smell since they (with some exceptions) are coupled to G proteins (like photoreceptors, and many neurotransmitter receptors).

As to the *organization of the pathways* for signal transmission from olfactory and gustatory receptors, however, there are few similarities. The olfactory pathway differs in this respect from all other sensory systems.

THE OLFACTORY SYSTEM

The sense of smell does not play the same important role for adult humans as the senses of hearing and vision. This does not mean, however, that the sense of smell is insignificant in daily life. The perception of odors is special by its close association with memories, and with emotions and moods. An enormous industry devoted to producing perfumes and other fragrances, shows that for humans the sense of smell plays an important role in interpersonal communication.

Going back in the evolution of the species, we find that smell is the most primitive of the senses. It is also the most important one at the early stages of evolution.To understand the evolution of the brain, knowledge of the "olfactory brain" or *rhinencephalon* has been important because in the early, primitive vertebrates almost the whole cerebrum is devoted to the processing of olfactory impulses. In higher vertebrates, new parts of the cerebrum emerge that gradually overshadow completely the phylogenetically old parts. The organization of the central pathways and nuclei processing olfactory information reflects that this system developed earlier than the parts of the cortex (the neocortex) treating other sensory modalities. The terms olfactory brain or rhinencephalon for these old parts are unfortunate, however. In higher vertebrates, large parts of the regions corresponding to the rhinencephalon in lower animals have nothing to do with the sense of smell but have taken on other important functions, the hippocampus (Chapter 18) being the most striking example. This is a common occurrence during evolution; structures that are no longer used for one function may form the basis for the development of new capacities. Thus, the parts treating olfactory impulses have not developed in pace with the rest of the brain during the evolution, and are therefore relatively much smaller in humans than in, for example, cats and dogs. In absolute terms, however, the differences are not so marked.

How Can We Discriminate so Many Different Odors?

What is the basis of our ability to discriminate several thousand different odors? One theory postulates that there are only a few specific olfactory receptors, and that further specificity is caused by combined activations of these few receptors (analogous to color vision). Seven primary qualities of smell have been proposed—among the innumerable nuances we can perceive—from experiments with a large number of odorous substances. It seems more likely, however, that there are many—probably about 1000—specific receptors. This is based upon studies providing evidence of a large gene family coding for olfactory receptors. Only the immune system can recognize more different molecules.

We do not know, however, how specific each olfactory cell is; that is, whether it expresses one, a few or many types of olfactory receptors in the membrane of its cilia. Electrophysiological recordings show that the individual olfactory cell responds to more than one odorant, although the number of effective odorants decreases as the stimulus becomes weaker. Probably, each cell expresses only a few out of the total repertoire of receptors. A patchy distribution in the olfactory epithelium of genes coding for different receptors has been shown in rodents with the in-situ hybridization technique. There is also evidence of some localization in the olfactory bulb: One odorant activates only a restricted set of neurons.

Receptors for Smell

The special receptor cells for smell are located in the mucous membrane of the upper part of the nasal cavity, the *olfactory epithelium*, within an area of about 1 cm^2 (the total surface of the nasal cavity is about 60 cm^2 on each side). The total number of receptor cells has been estimated to about 10 million in humans, and the cells are constantly renewed. Since they are in fact primitive neurons, they are exceptions to the rule that neurons that die are not replaced. The olfactory epithelium is pseudostratified and consists of supporting cells and so-called basal cells besides the receptor cells. The *supporting cells* probably insulate the receptor cells electrically, so that impulses are not propagated from one cell to another. The *basal cells* divide mitotically and probably give rise to the receptor cells. The receptor cells are bipolar and send a dendritelike branch toward the epithelial surface, and an axon through the base of the skull to the olfactory bulb. The dendrite ends with an expansion densely covered with cilia. The cilia are embedded in the mucus covering the epithelium. Only substances dissolved in the mucus can therefore act on the receptor cells. Many odorous substances are, however, hydrophobic, that is, they do not dissolve easily in water. Therefore, we assume that there must exist mechanisms—such as transport proteins-bringing hydrophobic odorants through the mucus. Specialized glands produce the mucus, which consists of several layers.

Experiments with a large number of odorants suggest that the *shape of the molecule*, rather than its chemical composition, determines how it smells (stereospecificity). This *stereochemical theory* of smell proposes that the receptor sites on the receptor cells have different shapes, and only molecules with a complementary shape fit into the receptor site. Binding of the odorant to receptors in the membrane of the cilia evokes a receptor potential. This involves activation of G proteins and cyclic AMP. Increased intracellular cyclic AMP opens Na^+-selective cation channels and thus depolarizes the cell, corresponding to the situation in photoreceptors. In contrast to photoreceptors, however, the olfactory receptors produce action potentials. The action potential arises in the initial segment of the axon and is transmitted to the olfactory bulb.

Central Pathways for Olfactory Impulses

Like other sensory cells—for example, those in the inner ear and in the taste buds—the olfactory receptor cells are surrounded by supporting cells. In other respects, however, the olfactory receptor cells are different from

The Olfactory Bulb

The structure of the olfactory bulb is complex. It is not a simple relay station but rather a small "brain" in itself, carrying out substantial processing of the sensory information reaching it. In this sense there are similarities with the retina—and both are parts of the central nervous system that have been moved outside the brain. Different odors appear to be represented somewhat differently in the olfactory bulb—that is, there is an "odorotopical localization." There is some evidence that the olfactory bulb is of decisive importance for the *discriminative aspect of olfaction*—that is, the ability to distinguish different odors. Thus, lesions of nuclei in which the fibers from the olfactory bulb terminate have been reported not to impair seriously simple olfactory discrimination.

As mentioned above, the unmyelinated axons from the receptor cells synapse with the dendrites of the mitral cells. The sites of contact are called *glomeruli* (glomerulus; latin: small ball of thread), because they form complex arrangements involving several dendrites and processes of local neurons. The number of glomeruli in the olfactory bulb declines with age, and only few are said to be left in very old persons. Besides mitral cells, the olfactory bulb contains numerous small *granule cells*, forming a separate layer. They are local neurons interconnecting mitral cells by way of dendrodendritic synapses (the granule cells lack axons). The granule cells are believed to mediate *lateral inhibition* in the olfactory bulb, analogous to the horizontal cells of the retina. Like the horizontal cells, the granule cells are electrically coupled.

Many *neurotransmitters* are found in the olfactory bulb. The mitral cells use most likely glutamate, whereas the granule cells release GABA. Another group of interneurons are believed to be dopaminergic. In addition, norepinephrine and glycin are present in some neuronal processes.

There are also *efferent fibers* in the olfactory tract, as shown with anatomic methods. Accordingly, electrical stimulation of the olfactory cortex can influence (primarily inhibit) the signal transmission through the olfactory bulb. Some of the efferent fibers release norepinephrine and are involved in synaptic changes in the olfactory bulb related to a certain kind of learning (see below).

Figure 10.1 *The olfactory pathways.* Schematic illustration of some main connections. To the **upper left** are the olfactory receptors in the nasal mucosa, sending their central processes to the olfactory bulb. The neurons of the olfactory bulb send their axons to the cortex and various nuclei in the vicinity of the tip of the temporal lobe.

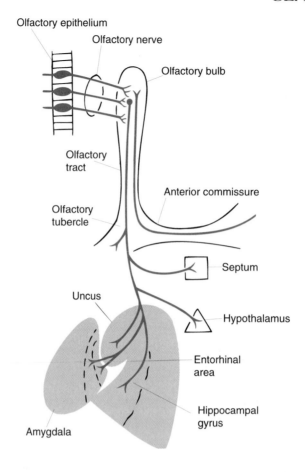

other sensory receptors, showing a more primitive arrangement. Thus, the olfactory cells themselves send a process (an axon) centrally, whereas in the inner ear, for example, a peripheral process of a ganglion cell contacts the receptor cell. The axons of the olfactory cells form many small bundles, together constituting the *olfactory nerve* (the first cranial nerve; Fig. 10.1). The bundles pass through the base of the skull close to the midline in the anterior cranial fossa (through the lamina cribrosa of the ethmoid bone). The olfactory nerve enters the *olfactory bulb* (Figs. 3.14 and 10.2), located just above the nasal cavity under the frontal lobe. In the olfactory bulb, the olfactory nerve fibers establish synaptic contacts with the *mitral cells*, which in their turn send axons to the brain through the *olfactory tract* (Figs. 3.14, 10.1, and 10.2). The fibers in the olfactory tract eventually take various directions, ending in different nuclei, most of which are located close to the tip of the temporal lobe.

The Terminal Areas of the Olfactory Tract

Most of the efferent fibers from the olfactory bulb end at the medial aspect of the temporal lobe, partly in the cortex and partly in the *amygdala* (Figs. 10.1 and 10.2). The latter is located just below the cortex in the tip of the temporal lobe (Figs. 10.1, 19.1, and 19.4). In the cortex, fibers terminate both in the so-called *piriform cortex* in the uncus and in the ad-

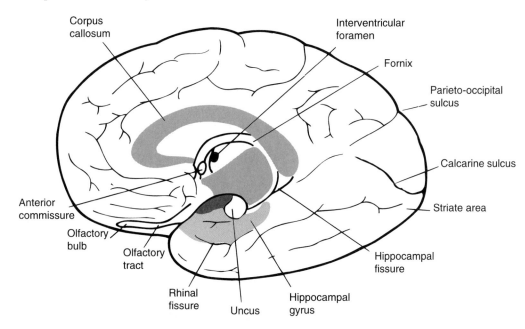

Figure 10.2 *The olfactory cortex.* The medial aspect of the cerebral hemisphere. The primary olfactory cortex is located in the uncus (dark red). The olfactory cortex in humans most likely also encompasses parts of the entorhinal area (light red).

joining parts of the *entorhinal cortex* (area 28). The fibers to the amygdala end only in the corticomedial nucleus, which sends efferent fibers to the hypothalamus (the amygdala will be discussed further in Chapter 19). The cortical regions in the temporal lobe that receive direct fibers from the olfactory bulb are called the *primary olfactory cortex*. It is believed that olfactory impulses come to consciousness in these and nearby cortical areas. Lesions affecting the uncus and the immediately surrounding cortex can be accompanied by subjective olfactory experiences (often unpleasant). Such sensations often occur as so-called *uncinate fits*, which frequently also include a peculiar feeling of experiencing the events in a dream (*dreamy state*). Often the patients feel that they have experienced the event before (*déjà vu*). Such uncinate fits may develop into an epileptic seizure, and the condition is regarded as a form of epilepsy.

The olfactory nuclei on the two sides are interconnected by fibers running through the anterior commissure.

Further Processing Outside the Primary Olfactory Cortex

The olfactory cortex and the amygdala forward olfactory impulses to other parts of the brain. Connections to other parts of the *cortex* serve the integration of olfactory with other kinds of sensory information, and the analysis of its meaning. From the primary olfactory cortex direct fibers reach nearby areas on the underside of the frontal lobe, the *orbitofrontal cortex*. (In addition, this part of the cortex might receive olfactory information indirectly by way of connections from the mediodorsal thalamic nucleus, which receives fibers from the amygdala.) The orbitofrontal cortex receives converging projections from many cortical areas, such as *visual and somatosensory* association areas, parts of the insula in receipt of *taste information*, and areas related to *emotions, motivation,* and *memory*.

Such connections are generally reciprocal; that is, the sending areas receive information from the orbitofrontal cortex, which presumably concerns the broader meaning of the olfactory information.

One important pathway for olfactory signals reaches parts of the *hypothalamus* (see Chapters 18 and 19). These hypothalamic parts are involved in control of appetite, digestion, and feeding behavior (among other functions). Since the orbitofrontal cortex sends efferents to the *hypothalamus* (among other areas), this part of the brain receives both relatively "pure" olfactory information from the amygdala, and highly processed information that has been analyzed regarding its meaning for the organism.

Olfactory Impulses and Behavior

Olfactory connections to the hypothalamus—both direct and indirect ones via the amygdala—are of importance for eating and for *behavior directed at acquiring food. Sexual reflexes* and *sexually related behavior* are also influenced by olfactory impulses, although more so in lower mammals than in man. The structural basis for such reflexes and behavior is very complex and not known in detail. Olfactory connections to the amygdala are most likely of importance, not only because the amygdala acts on the hypothalamus but also because it acts on other parts of the limbic structures. Among these, amygdala is closely related to emotions (see Chapter 19, *The Amygdala and Emotions*).

Olfaction and Learning

Olfactory sensations in certain sensitive phases of development can induce lasting changes of behavior; that is, learning. This phenomenon is called *olfactory imprinting*.

One example concerns *sheep that establish a strong bond to the lamb* shortly after the birth. This depends on odors of the lamb that are present in the amniotic fluid. The mother must be exposed to the odor(s) during the first 4 to 12 hours for the bond to develop. The *migration of salmons* for thousands of miles is an almost incredible example of how memory of odors can control behavior. At two years of age the salmon is imprinted by odors at its birth place, and these odors guide it when returning "home" several years later. Imprinting by smell or taste can occur also *before birth*. If pregnant rabbits are fed a diet with certain aromatic substances, their offspring prefer foods containing these substances. This happens even if they grow up with a substitute mother on a different diet.

Olfactory imprinting is related to *synaptic changes in the olfactory bulb* (and most likely other places as well). Simultaneous arrival of olfactory impulses and impulses in norepinephrine-containing afferents seems to be necessary for lasting synaptic changes to occur. In the example with sheep mentioned above, more mitral cells responded to odors from the lamb after imprinting.

THE SENSE OF TASTE

The sense of taste is not among the most important of the special senses in humans, and much of what we usually call taste experience is in reality brought about by stimulation of olfactory receptors (compare the reduced sense of taste during a common cold). In addition, signals from oral thermoreceptors and mechanoreceptors contribute.

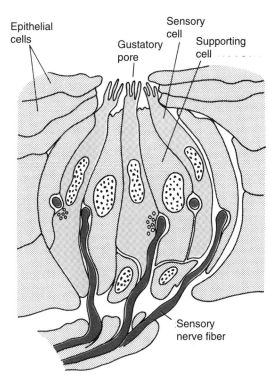

Epithelial
cells

Sensory
cell

Gustatory
pore

Supporting
cell

Sensory
nerve fiber

Figure 10.3 *Taste bud*. Semischematic drawing based on electron micrographs.

The Taste Receptors

The true taste impulses come from chemoreceptors in the *taste buds* located primarily in the epithelium of the tongue (Fig. 10.3). The taste buds are concentrated along the lateral margins of the tongue and the root of the tongue and are found in small elevations of the mucous membrane called *papillae*. The largest (vallate) papilla lies along a transverse line posteriorly on the tongue (Fig. 10.4).[1]

The taste buds are composed of approximately 100 elongated sensory cells and supporting cells (Fig. 10.3). The sensory cells of the taste buds are constantly renewed; each cell lives probably only about 10 days. They have long microvilli at their apical surface, protruding into a small opening in the epithelium, the *taste pore*. Here the membrane of the sensory cell comes in contact with substances that are dissolved in the saliva. Around the basal ends of the sensory cells are found terminal endings of sensory (afferent) axons. Binding of the tasty substances to receptors in the membrane of the sensory cells depolarizes the cell and thus produces a *receptor potential* (as in other sensory cells). An unknown transmitter, released from the basal aspect of the sensory cell, produces action potentials in the sensory nerve endings.

We usually distinguish only *four elementary taste qualities*: salt, sour, sweet, and bitter. Each of these are most easily perceived (have the lowest threshold for identification) in a particular region of the tongue (sweet at the tip of the tongue, then salty, sour, and bitter more posteriorly in that order). Such differences are only relative, however. Recordings of the activity of single afferent fibers from taste buds indicate that each sensory unit reacts to several of the four elementary qualities, but with the lowest threshold to only one.

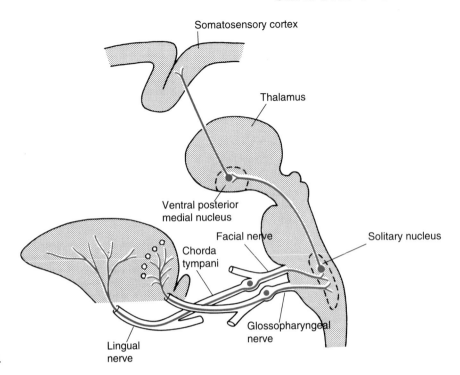

Figure 10.4 *Pathways for taste impulses.*

Flavors Act on Ion Channels and on G Protein–Coupled Receptors in the Apical Membrane

Studies of isolated sensory cells show that for some taste qualities there are no specific membrane receptors; the taste stimulus acts *directly on ordinary ion channels* in the apical membrane. This concerns salty and sour substances. The specificity of the sensory cell depends on the fact that the cell is exposed to the stimulus only at the apical membrane. The cells of the taste bud are interconnected with special cell contacts (zonula occludent) sealing the lateral membranes off from the taste pore. Thus, fluid in the mouth cannot penetrate between the cells.

Sour substances appear to act primarily by virtue of their concentration of hydrogen ions, which act by closing K^+ channels in the apical membrane. This depolarizes the cell. Hydrogen ions, however, act on various kinds of channels, such as channels for Na^+ and Ca^{2+}. One might think therefore that closure of such channels would counteract the effect on K^+ channels. Specificity is achieved because the concentration of K^+ channels is particularly high at the apical membrane, whereas the other kinds of channels are evenly distributed. Sour substances will therefore close many K^+ channels but only a few other channels.

Salty substances act primarily on passive Na^+ channels in the apical membrane. When the concentration of Na^+ increases in the fluid in contact with the apical membrane, Na^+ ions enter the cell and thereby depolarize it.

Sweet substances act probably both directly on membrane ion channels and on specific G protein-coupled receptors in the apical membrane. *Bitter substances* most likely act only via G proteins.

Some *amino acids* appear to have specific taste receptors (some directly acting, others indirectly). Arginine and alanine, for example, excite different sensory units leading from taste buds. *Glutamate* (the highly water soluble monosodium salt of glutamic acid) is used to add flavor to foods and has its distinct taste. It acts on an unspecific cationic channel.

The *sensitivity of the sensory cells* is influenced by various factors, such as hormones and neurotransmitters. The basal cells of the taste buds contain the neuropeptides serotonin and CCK. Serotonin increases the sensitivity of the sensory cells. The functional role of such control by the basal cells is unknown, however. Vasopressin (the antidiuretic hormone) and aldosterone—both protecting the blood volume by acting on ionic transport across the renal tubular epithelium—increase the response of the taste cells to sodium chloride (by acting on Na^+ channels).

There are probably more than only four specific receptors. Especially bitter tasting substances are detected by several specific receptors. This seems reasonable, since bitter taste often is associated with poisonous foods.

Pathways for Taste Impulses

The *intermediate nerve* (accompanying the facial nerve) contains the taste fibers from the anterior two-thirds of the tongue, whereas the fibers from the posterior third follow the *glossopharyngeal nerve* (Fig. 10.4). All taste fibers end in the rostral part of the solitary nucleus. The neurons in the solitary nucleus send their axons to several areas, thus mediating reflex effects, coordination of the activity of visceral organs, and perception of taste. Fibers pass to the *visceral efferent nuclei of the salivary glands* and to the *dorsal motor nucleus of the vagus*. Such connections mediate reflex secretion of saliva and gastric juice (and other digestive fluids). Some of the cells in the solitary nucleus send their axons to the *hypothalamus*. This enables taste impulses to influence the higher autonomic centers.

Fibers from the solitary nucleus also end in the *thalamus*, enabling taste impulses to reach the cerebral cortex. The synaptic interruption in the thalamus is in the *VPM nucleus* (Figs. 7.20 and 10.4), which serves as a relay for impulses from the face in general. Taste impulses are transmitted to the face region of the SI, close to the representation of the tongue (Fig. 7.21). Taste impulses reach, in addition, the anterior part of the *insula*, which also receives olfactory impulses.

Sensory units responding to the elementary taste qualities—at least to some degree—are anatomically segregated in the taste pathways. This is what one might expect since we can discriminate the elementary qualities. Each sensory unit is not specific for one quality, however, but rather responds more easily to one than to the others. Thus, the patterns of activity in many sensory units provide the information necessary for taste discrimination. This corresponds to conditions in other sensory systems (cf. color vision).

Cortical Processing of Taste

Our *conscious experience* of taste is due not only to stimulation of taste receptors, as mentioned above. Furthermore, many taste cells with different specificities are presumably always stimulated while eating or drinking. The synthesis in the cerebral cortex of all these varied impulses forms the basis of our subjective experience of taste. Convergence of olfactory and taste signals takes place in the anterior part of the insula. A higher level of integration occurs in the orbitofrontal cortex where taste, smell, and other sensory modalities meet. Thus, responses of neurons in the orbitofrontal cortex to flavors depend on whether the animal is hungry or not. This may be caused by connections from cortical areas related to motivation—that is, areas that may inform about the significance of a sensory stimulus. That our subjective sensory experience is determined not only by the stimulus holds for all sensory systems. Nevertheless, the emotional influence on the sensory experience is probably more marked for taste and smell than for other modalities. From everyday experience we know, for example, how the same smell or taste may be experienced as pleasant in one situation and nauseating in another.

NOTES

1. There are also some taste buds on the soft palate, which are innervated by the intermediate nerve. The few taste buds present on the most posterior part of the tongue and on the upper side of the epiglottis are innervated by the vagus nerve.

PART III

MOTOR SYSTEMS

The cell groups and tracts in the central nervous system that control the activity of the skeletal muscles compose the *motor systems*. We may also use the term *somatic motor systems* to distinguish them from systems controlling smooth muscles and glands.

The motor systems can be divided into several interconnected parts. First, the *peripheral motor neurons* (Chapter 11) and the *central motor pathways* (Chapter 12) are directly involved in mediating the commands from the motor centers to the muscles. These parts of the motor systems are necessary for the initiation of voluntary movements; paralysis ensues when they are damaged. Secondly, the *basal ganglia* (Chapter 13) and the *cerebellum* (Chapter 14) have their main connections with the central motor nuclei and are necessary for the proper execution of movements rather than for their initiation.

Motor and Sensory Systems Are Not Independent of Each Other

Although for didactic reasons we often treat the motor and sensory systems as independent entities, this is an oversimplification. For the motor systems to function, they must cooperate closely with the sensory systems. During most movements, the motor centers need constant information from receptors in muscles, around joints, and in the skin about whether the movement is progressing in accordance with the plan. Often visual information is also crucial for the proper execution of movements. Such *sensory feedback information* enables the central nervous system to adjust and correct the command signals issued to the muscles—either during the movement or the next time the movement is performed.

In addition, impulses from many other parts of the brain are necessary for movement—for example, those involved in the early stages of the movement planning and in the mediation of motivated behavior. Thus, large parts of the central nervous system may be considered motoric in the sense that they contribute to the activity of the more narrowly defined motor systems. On the other hand, such regions may also be considered sensory since they also take part in the processing of sensory information (cf. the posterior parietal assocation areas, discussed in Chapter 7, which process visual and somatosensory information and issue commands to motor areas). At the higher levels of the central nervous system it becomes meaningless to classify regions as sensory or motoric—these concepts are much too narrow "pigeon holes" to encompass the complex tasks undertaken by large parts of the cerebral cortex and many related subcortical nuclei.

Classification of Movements

Before we describe the motor systems, some comments on movements in general may be pertinent. First, muscle contraction may not necessarily elicit movement (that is, alter the position of one or more joints). Just as often, muscle activity is used to prevent movement: For example, muscles maintain our posture by counteracting the force of gravity. In the latter case, the muscles may be said to *stabilize* a joint (against external forces) and to have a *postural function.* Furthermore, movement in one part of the body—for example, in an arm—requires that muscles in other parts contract to prevent the body balance from being upset. A muscle in one situation may be used as a mover and in another situation as a stabilizer.

Whether or not a movement is to occur depends on the magnitude of the force produced by the muscle contraction and the external forces acting on the joint. When the external force is smaller than the muscle force, the muscle shortens and a movement occurs (isotonic contraction). When the external forces equal the force of the muscle contraction, no movement occurs (isometric contraction). When the external force is greater than the opposing force produced by the muscle contraction, the muscle lengthens. The latter is the case, for example, with the thigh muscles when we walk down a staircase. In the latter case the muscles *brake* a movement produced by the weight of the body.

Movements may be classified by the *speed* with which they are performed. *Ramp movements* are performed relatively slowly. The crucial point is that the movement is slow enough to enable sensory feedback information to influence the movement during its execution. *Ballistic movements* are very rapid, their characteristic feature being that they are too fast to enable feedback control (the name derives from analogy with a bullet shot out of a gun).

Movements may also be classified according to whether they are *voluntary* or *automatic*, the latter taking place without our conscious participation. This is in reality much too crude a distinction: There is a gradual transition from what Hughlings Jackson in the past century termed the *most automatic* to the *least automatic* movements. The most automatic movements are basic, simple reflexes like the retraction of the arm from a noxious stimulus. Locomotion is an example of a semiautomatic movement—that is, the basic pattern is automatic, whereas start and stop, and necessary adjustments, may require conscious (voluntary) control. The least automatic movements are precision grips with the fingers and delicate manipulatory or exploratory movements such as writing, drawing, playing a musical instrument, and so forth. Equally precise voluntary control exists for the muscles of the larynx, the tongue, and some of the facial muscles. We also know that the degree to which a movement is automatic changes with learning: In the beginning a new movement requires full voluntary control, whereas in the process of learning the movement becomes more automatic. When playing a well-rehearsed musical piece on the piano, for example, we do not need to pay attention to the fingers and their movements.

As a rule, the most automatic movements require only the use of relatively simple *reflex arcs at the spinal level*; participation of higher motor centers is not necessary. Somewhat less automatic and more complex movements such as ventilation, locomotion, and postural control depend in addition on the participation of *neuronal groups in the brain stem*. Such movements do not require our attention directed toward them but can also be subjected to voluntary control. The least automatic movements depend on the participation of the highest level—the *cerebral cortex*—to coordinate and control the activity of motor centers in the brain stem and spinal cord. The vast number of neurons and the plasticity of the human brain enable learning of an almost infinite repertoire of voluntary movements. Also, these features ensure great flexibility of how motor tasks are solved. The same task may be solved in different ways, and we can continuously adapt to novel challenges. The great adaptability and flexibility of movements distinguish humans from most animals. Most animals are highly specialized for a limited number of motor tasks, controlled by stereotyped motor programs that develope according to a fixed pattern.

THE PERIPHERAL MOTOR NEURONS

MOTONEURONS AND MUSCLES

The peripheral motor neurons are nerve cells that send their axons to skeletal muscles. Another term is *lower motor neurons*. These are the motoneurons in the ventral horn of the cord and in the somatic motor cranial nerve nuclei. As mentioned in Chapter 7, there are two kinds: The α *motoneurons* innervate the extrafusal muscle fibers, whereas the γ *motoneurons* innervate the intrafusal muscle fibers of the muscle spindle (Figs. 7.4 and 7.5).

The axons of the motoneurons leave the spinal cord through the ventral roots and continue into the ventral and dorsal branches (rami) of the spinal nerves (Figs. 3.5 and 3.7) to innervate skeletal muscles of the trunk and the extremities (Fig. 11.1). Correspondingly, the axons from the cranial nerve motor nuclei supply the muscles of the tongue, pharynx, palate, larynx, face, and the extraocular muscles. The axons of all the motoneurons located in one spinal segment leave the cord through one ventral root and continue into one spinal nerve. The ventral branches of the spinal nerves form plexuses so that the motor axons from one spinal segment are distributed to several peripheral nerves (Fig. 11.1).

Contraction of skeletal muscles can only be elicited by impulses conducted in the axons of motoneurons. If these axons are interrupted, the muscles become *paralyzed*. The peripheral motor neurons thus constitute the *final common path* for all signals from the central nervous system to skeletal muscles (the term final common path was introduced by the British neurophysiologist and Nobel laureate Sherrington). The motoneurons may be compared with the keys of a piano on which higher levels of the central nervous system can play. As we will describe later in this chapter, many parts of the central nervous system cooperate in determining the activity of the motoneurons and thus the contraction of our muscles.

Each motoneuron probably receives about 50,000 boutons—some forming excitatory synapses, others inhibitory; some with fast synaptic actions, others with slow modulatory ones. The sum of these influences determines whether and with what frequency the motoneurons will send action potentials to the muscles.

That we can perform such a wide variety of movements is due to the ability of the central nervous system to select precisely, by way of the motoneurons, the combinations of muscles to be used and to determine the speed and force with which they are to contract.

It is well established that the motoneurons use *acetylcholine* as transmitter substance, and the synthesizing enzyme choline acetyltransferase can be demonstrated with immunohistochemical techniques in the motoneurons and in their terminals. Motoneurons also contain the neuropeptide CGRP.[1]

The Motoneurons Are Somatotopically Organized

The motoneurons of the ventral horn and in the cranial nerve nuclei are easily recognized in microscopic sections because of their large size and the big clumps of rER (Nissl bodies) in the cytoplasm of their perikarya (Fig. 1.2). The rich content of rER indicates that the neurons have a high protein synthesis. These proteins are, for example, enzymes for transmitter synthesis and metabolism, and various kinds of membrane proteins (the vast surface of the motoneurons with their large dendritic tree and long axons presumably explains why motoneurons contain more rER than most other neuronal types).

The motoneurons are collected in groups, which form Rexed's lamina IX in the spinal cord (Fig. 11.2). *The dendrites of the motoneurons do not respect the boundaries of lamina IX*, however, and extend far in the transverse and in the rostrocaudal directions—for example, into lamina VII, where many interneurons are located (Fig. 3.11). The rostrocaudal (longitudinal) extension of the dendrites enables dorsal root fibers from several segments to act on each motoneuron. The dendritic tree increases the surface of the motoneurons enormously, and, not surprisingly, the vast majority of the boutons contacting motoneurons do so on the dendrites (forming axodendritic synapses).

When viewed three-dimensionally, the motoneurons are seen to be collected in *longitudinally oriented columns* (Fig. 11.2). Each column contains the α and γ motoneurons to one muscle (or a few functionally similar muscles). Within a column supplying more than one muscle, the motoneurons to each muscle are at least partly segregated. *Each column as a rule extends through more than one segment of the cord.* Consequently, each muscle receives motor fibers through more than one ventral root and spinal nerve. Destruction of one root or spinal nerve only—for example, by disk protrusion in sciatica or by a tumor growing in the spinal canal—will not produce paralysis of a muscle but only a more or less pronounced weakness (paresis).

The anatomic organization of motoneurons has been studied in part by transection of muscle nerves in experimental animals. A retrograde reaction, which is easily seen in the microscope, occurs in the perikarya of the motoneurons. Modern methods with retrograde transport of tracer substances such as HRP have detailed the picture considerably. Study of pa-

Figure 11.2 *Motoneurons.* **Left:** a photomicrograph and a drawing of a transverse section of the (lumbar) spinal cord. The motoneurons are collected in groups (columns) together forming the lamina IX of Rexed. **Right:** schematic drawing of the somatotopic localization of the motoneuronal groups innervating the arm, located in the spinal segments C_5–T_1. Motoneurons supplying the intrinsic muscles of the hand are located most caudally (C_8–T_1) and most dorsally in the ventral horn.

tients with poliomyelitis has provided information about conditions in the human cord (the poliovirus infects and kills motoneurons). Because the distribution of paralyzed muscles usually has been determined before death, it can be compared with the distribution of cell loss among the motoneuronal groups in the cord and brain stem.

Groups of motoneurons that supply axial muscles—that is, muscles of the back, neck, abdomen, and pelvis—are located most medially within the ventral horn, whereas motoneurons supplying muscles of the extremities are located more laterally. This explains why the ventral horn is broader (extends more laterally) in the segments of the cord that send fibers to the extremities (that is, C_5–T_1 and L_1–S_2; compare Figs. 3.8, 3.10, and 11.2). There is also a further somatotopic organization: Motoneurons supplying proximal muscles of the extremities (the shoulder and hip) are located more ventrally than those supplying the distal muscles (the hand and foot). This is shown in Figure 11.2, which also shows that the proximal muscles are supplied from motoneurons located more rostrally than those supplying the distal muscles. For example, the shoulder muscles are mainly innervated by the upper parts of the brachial plexus (C_5–C_6), whereas the intrinsic muscles of the hand are innervated by the lowermost segments (C_8–T_1).

Motoneurons Are of Functionally Different Kinds

As mentioned, the α and γ motoneurons supplying one muscle lie together within one column in the ventral horn. In a microscopic section of the cord it can be seen that the motoneuronal perikarya vary in size (Fig. 1.2). As in other parts of the nervous system, the neurons with the largest perikarya have the thickest (and thus fastest-conducting) axons. The smallest within a group are the γ motoneurons, whereas the size varies considerably among the α motoneurons. Such size differences among the α motoneurons are related to differences among the muscle cells supplied by the motoneurons. Briefly stated, the smallest α motoneurons control delicate movements with little force, whereas the largest motoneurons come into play only when a movement requires great force. The large α motoneurons also have a much higher maximal firing frequency than the small ones. On the other hand, the large ones tend to fire in brief bursts with a high frequency, whereas the small α motoneurons tend to go on firing for a long time with a low frequency. These differences in firing pattern reflect that the large motoneurons are used for forceful, rapid movements of short duration, whereas the small motoneurons can uphold a moderate muscular tension for a long time. For these reasons, we apply the term *phasic* α *motoneurons* to the large ones, and *tonic* α *motoneurons* to the small ones. The properties of the α motoneurons will be discussed further when dealing with the motor units.

The Motor End Plate

After entering the muscle, the axon of a motoneuron divides into many thin branches or collaterals. Each of these end or terminal branches con-

Figure 11.3 *Motor end plates*. Photomicrograph of skeletal muscle cells and a small bundle of nerve fibers innervating the cells. The tissue is stained with gold chloride to darken the nerve fibers and their terminal boutons. Each motor end plate consists of numerous small boutons. Four end plates are seen in the photomicrograph. Magnification, ×600.

tacts one muscle cell only. *Each muscle cell is thus contacted by only one branch from one* α *motoneuron.* Such a branch ends on the muscle cell approximately midway between its ends, forming the *motor end plate*, where the signal transfer from nerve to muscle takes place (Figs. 11.3 and 11.4). Within the end-plate region, the axonal branch divides further and forms up to about 50 boutons, each establishing synaptic contact with the muscle cell. The postsynaptic side at this *neuromuscular junction* is somewhat special compared with synapses in the central nervous system, since so-called junctional folds and a thin basal lamina are intercalated between the presynaptic and postsynaptic membranes (Fig. 11.4B). The boutons contain *acetylcholine*, and the postsynaptic membrane contains *acetylcholine receptors* of the nicotinic type. The density of acetylcholine receptors is much higher in the end-plate region than elsewhere on the muscle cell surface (this is appropriate since only at the end plate is the muscle cell normally exposed to acetylcholine).[2]

An action potential propagated along the axon of the motoneuron depolarizes all the boutons and elicits release of acetylcholine. The transmitter binds to the acetylcholine receptors, and—as at other excitatory synapses—this depolarizes the postsynaptic membrane. This change in

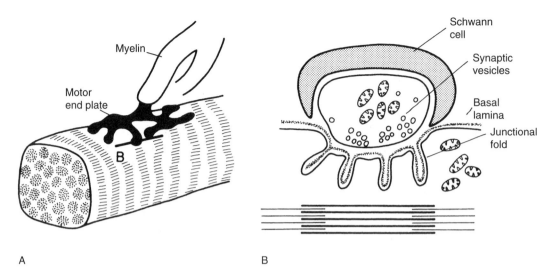

Figure 11.4 *The motor end plate.* **A.** Schematic drawing showing how the myelinated nerve fiber loses the myelin sheath before it ramifies in the end-plate area, each terminal branch ending in a bouton. Each muscle cell has only one end plate.

B. Drawing of a section through one of the boutons in **A**, based on electron microscopic observations. The synaptic cleft contains a thin basal lamina, and the postsynaptic membrane is thrown into deep folds (junctional folds).

the membrane potential is called the *end-plate potential*. Normally, enough transmitter is released by one action potential to depolarize the muscle cell membrane to the threshold for an action potential. The action potential is propagated over the whole surface of the muscle cell and elicits a brief contraction. The action of acetylcholine is rapidly terminated by the enzyme acetylcholine esterase present in the junctional folds.

Neuromuscular Transmission Can Be Disturbed by Poison and Disease

Various drugs and naturally occurring poisonous substances can influence the signal transmission at the neuromuscular junction and produce involuntary muscle contractions or muscle paralysis. The South American Indian poison *curare* and similar synthetic substances paralyze the muscle cells by blocking the Ach receptors. Such drugs are often used during abdominal surgery to obtain sufficient muscle relaxation. Several kinds of snake poisons act by blocking Ach receptors so that the victim is paralyzed. The *botulinum toxin* (produced by a microorganism growing in certain kinds of spoiled food) paralyzes the muscles by preventing the release of Ach from the boutons at the motor end plate. A similar mechanism sometimes produces muscle weakness in patients with *cancer*; apparently, substances preventing release of Ach are produced in the body.

The disease *myasthenia gravis* is characterized by excessive fatigability of the striated muscle cells, which is caused by autoantibodies binding to the Ach receptors. Thus, there are fewer than normal Ach receptors available at the neuromuscular junction, and fewer ion channels are opened by release of Ach, leading to less than normal depolarization. The probability of evoking an action potential in the muscle cell membrane is consequently reduced. The symptoms may be lessened by drugs that inhibit the acetylcholine esterase (neostigmine, physostigmine). Thus, the transmitter gets a longer time to act, and the probability of evoking an action potential is increased. Typically, the muscles of the head are most severely affected, producing symptoms such as double vision (due to paresis of extraocular muscles), and involuntary lowering of the upper eyelids (ptosis). The voice becomes weaker while speaking, and swallowing may become difficult. Also, the respiratory muscles are usually affected.

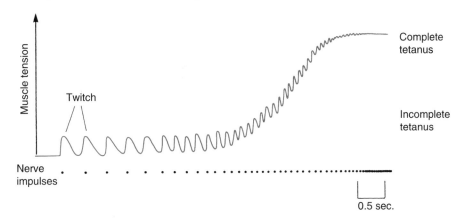

Figure 11.5 *Muscle contraction.* The muscle tension increases with increasing firing frequency of the motoneurons innervating the muscle cell. Redrawn from Kandel and Schwarz (1985).

The Force of Muscle Contraction Is Controlled by the Motoneurons

A single presynaptic action potential at the motor end plate elicits only a brief contraction, a *twitch*, of the muscle cell (Fig. 11.5). The twitch lasts only for about 1/10th of a second. If, however, another action potential follows shortly after the first one—that is, before the tension produced by the first twitch is over—the tension produced by the muscle may be sustained and, furthermore, increased considerably in magnitude. This is called *summation*. Up to a limit, the tension produced by the muscle cell increases with increasing frequency of action potentials; that is, the *force produced by the muscle cell is determined by the firing frequency of the motoneuron.* Whereas the twitch is the response of the muscle cell to a single nerve impulse, tetanic contraction is the term used of the muscle response to a train of impulses with the highest frequency to which the muscle cell can respond (Fig. 11.5). The tetanic tension is thus the maximal force the muscle cell can produce. (One may, as shown in Fig. 11.5, differentiate between unfused tetanus at submaximal firing frequencies and fused or full tetanus at the maximal firing frequency. The term tetanus, as used above, refers to the fused tetanus.)

There Are Functionally Different Kinds of Striated Muscle Fiber Types

In both animals and humans, the skeletal muscles are composed of different kinds of muscle cells or muscle fibers (these terms are used interchangeably). The most clear-cut evidence is provided by the fact that in some species certain muscles have a fairly dark color ("red" muscles), whereas other muscles are light ("white" muscles)—for example, the almost white breast muscles and the dark leg muscles of the chicken. Such muscles are composed of muscle fibers of only one (or predominantly one) kind—and the muscle cells are classified as either white or red. The color difference is due to differences in the content of myoglobin, which is red (closely related to hemoglobin) and is of importance for oxygen transport within the muscle cell. Further study showed that white and red muscle cells differ with regard to *endurance*—that is, how long they can

Figure 11.6 *Muscle fiber types*. Photomicrograph of cross sections of skeletal muscle (human). The sections are treated so that the color intensity of the muscle fibers depends on their myosin—ATPase activity. With this particular treatment the type 1 fibers are light, and the type 2 fibers are dark. The **lower** photomicrograph is from a "normal" person, whereas the **upper** is from a weight lifter. Note the difference in muscle fiber thickness. Magnification, ×200. Courtesy of Prof. H. A. Dahl, Norwegian University of Physical Education and Sport, Oslo.

maintain tension. This is mainly due to differences in the capacity to take up oxygen and to oxidative phosphorylation (aerobic ATP production). As one would expect, the red muscles have the highest endurance. In addition to containing more myoglobin than the white muscle fibers (cells), the red ones also contain more mitochondria (which are responsible for the aerobic ATP production). There are also other important differences: The white muscle fibers contract more rapidly and develop greater force than the red fibers. With physiological methods, muscle cells can be classified as *fast twitch* (FT), corresponding largely to white fibers, and *slow twitch* (ST), corresponding to the red fibers. The differences with regard to contraction velocity and maximal force development are related to differences in the amount and type of myosin ATPase (enzymes cleaving ATP, thus providing the energy for the muscle contraction). With histochemical staining methods, muscle fibers can be classified in accordance with their ATPase activity (Fig. 11.6). On the basis of ATPase staining, human muscle fibers are classified as *type 1*, corresponding largely to the red and the ST fibers mentioned above, and *type 2* fibers, corresponding largely to the white and FT fibers. The type 2 group is heterogeneous, however, and consists of *type 2A* fibers, which resemble the type 1 fibers in having a relatively high oxidative capacity, and the *type 2B* fibers, which are the most typical white fibers with low oxidative capacity. The central nervous system thus can select muscle fibers in accordance with the requirement of the task: One fiber type is best suited for contractions of moderate force that last for a long time, whereas the other type is used particularly for contractions with high force but short duration.

Human skeletal muscles are, with few exceptions, composed of a mixture of type 1 and type 2 muscle fibers. Histochemical examination of many different muscles in several individuals has indicated that the composition of fiber types is fairly constant when comparing muscles from one individual, whereas the interindividual differences are great. Thus, some persons have a high percentage of type 1 in most of their muscles, whereas others have a strong preponderance of type 2 fibers. Studies of fiber composition in successful athletes have shown that those engaged in endurance sports (such as marathons and cross-country skiing) usually have a high percentage of type 1 fibers, whereas a high percentage of type 2 fibers is found in those engaged in sports requiring explosive force (such as ice hockey and weight lifting).

Muscles Also Contain Connective Tissue

A muscle consists of a large number of muscle cells, stretching from tendon to tendon (usually at an angle to the longitudinal axis of the muscle). Bundles of muscle fibers are surrounded by connective tissue containing the vessels and nerves. The whole muscle is wrapped in a connective tissue sheath, the *muscle fascia*. In some muscles the fascia is thick and fairly tight; in others it is thin and loose. The connective tissue of the fascia and within the muscle is continuous with the tendons. Therefore, the *passive properties of a muscle*—that is, its consistency and resistance to being stretched—depend not only on the muscle cells but also on the amount and arrangement of the connective tissue.

Motor Units

As mentioned above, the axon of the motoneuron divides into numerous branches when entering the muscle, and each terminal branch makes synaptic contact with one muscle cell. Furthermore, each muscle cell is innervated by one motoneuron only. *When an α motoneuron sends action potentials to a muscle, all muscle cells innervated by that motoneuron contract simultaneously. An α motoneuron and all the muscle cells that it innervates* therefore in a sense constitute the smallest functional unit of the motor system and were called *a motor unit* by Sherrington (Fig. 11.7). (Compare with the term sensory unit, introduced in Chapter 6). The size of a motor unit—that is, the number of muscle cells supplied by one motoneuron—varies greatly. This has been studied by counting the axons in the muscle nerve (after destruction of the dorsal roots, to let the sensory axons degenerate) and counting the muscle cells. An average seems to be around 150 muscle cells per motoneuron, with a range of from less than 10 to more than 1000. As might be expected, the smallest motor units are found in muscles that are used for delicate movements,

Figure 11.7 *A motor unit.* Schematic drawing showing a motoneuron in the ventral horn and its axon, which branches to supply many muscle fibers. The muscle cells belonging to one unit (red) line intermingled with muscle cells belonging to other motor units.

which we must be able to control very precisely. Examples are the intrinsic muscles of the hand, the muscles of the larynx, the facial muscles, and, as mentioned earlier, the extraocular muscles. The largest motor units are found in large muscles used for movements of considerable force and with less precise control, such as the muscles of the back, the abdomen, and the thigh. Within one muscle, however, the motor units also vary in size.

The force of muscular contraction can, as we all know, be finely graded within very wide limits, from a barely perceptible contraction to a tension high enough to tear the muscle loose from its insertion. This depends on the ability of the central nervous system to control the activity (the level of excitation) of the motoneurons. *There are two means by which the force of muscle contraction can be increased in a graded manner.* One consists of making more and more α motoneurons send action potentials to the muscle. This is called *recruitment*, because more and more motor units—and thus muscle fibers—are called into action. The other means is by increasing the *firing frequency of the α motoneurons* already recruited and thereby increasing the force developed by each motor unit. Thus, the force exerted by each motor unit (as by each muscle cell) can be graded from the small and brief tension produced by a single twitch to full tetanic tension (Fig. 11.5).

Muscle cells belonging to the same motor unit are all of the same fiber type. Thus, they not only contract simultaneously but also share properties with regard to contraction velocity, maximal force, and endurance. Furthermore, there is a relationship between the size of the motor units and the fiber type of which they are composed. The smallest motor units consist of type 1 fibers, whereas the largest ones consist of type 2B fibers. This further increases the difference between large and small motor units with regard to their maximal force; not only are there more muscle cells in the large units, but each cell also develops more force. Recruitment of one extra motor unit with type 1 fibers adds just a little extra to the total tension of the muscle, which thus can be graded finely (like an electrical switch with many small steps to vary the heat of a stove). Such motor units are, not unexpectedly, used for precisely controlled movements of small force. Recruitment of a large motor unit consisting of type 2 fibers, on the other hand, gives a comparatively large increase in the total tension of the muscle (the switch has large steps). Such motor units are recruited only when large force production is needed. Often this concerns fast movements because high acceleration requires a large force.[3]

There is also a *relationship between the size of a motor unit (in terms of number of muscle fibers) and the size of its motoneuron*. Thus, the largest motor units have the motoneurons with the largest perikarya and the thickest axons. This fits with the use of large motor units for fast and forceful movements: The large motoneurons have the highest maximal firing frequencies, and their axons conduct the impulses to the muscles with a minimal delay.

When a muscle contraction is initiated, the small motoneurons are always recruited first, and with increasing force the larger ones are recruited successively. This is called the *size principle of recruitment* and was demonstrated by the American neurophysiologist Henneman in the 1960s. The excitability of the motoneurons is inversely related to their size; thus, the small motoneurons are more easily excited to the threshold for initiation of action potentials than the large ones. This is presumably related to differences both in membrane properties of the motoneurons and in the density of excitatory synapses. The size principle ensures selection of the motor units that are best suited for a particular kind of movement.[4]

Muscle cells belonging to different motor units lie intermingled in the muscle, as is obvious in sections stained to identify fiber types (Fig. 11.6). Correspondingly, muscle cells belonging to one motor unit are spread over a considerable part of the total cross-sectional area of the muscle (Fig. 11.7).

Recruitment Depends on the Required Force

The number of motor units that are recruited at the beginning of a voluntary contraction, depends on the force requirement. If maximal force is needed (as with a movement of maximal speed) most (all?) motor units are recruited almost simultaneously. Nevertheless, the small ones are activated slightly before the large ones because the small motoneurons reach the threshold for eliciting action potentials first. Thus, the order of recruitment is maintained (according to the size principle) when maximal force is required. To produce the maximal force, besides recruiting as many motor units as possible, the central motor centers must increase the firing frequencies of the motoneurons to the maximal: *A muscle develops maximal force when all motor units are recruited and contract tetanically (fused tetanus)*. Such a contraction, however, can only be maintained for a short period before the muscle fatigues.

The situation is different when the required force is low. Consider, for example, an isometric contraction of low force that should last as long as possible (that is, the force must be kept constant). Here, more than half the motor units are recruited at the beginning of the contraction (judging from animal experiments). Since a relatively large fraction of the motor units are recruited, the required force is achieved with a low firing frequency. Thus, the motor units can work for a long time without fatigue. However, if the contraction continues, some motor units fatigue and "fresh" ones are recruited to maintain constant force. Finally, however, so many small or medium large motor units are fatigued that the largest motor units must be recruited to prevent a drop of force. This recruitment pattern is only valid, however, when the contraction force is so low that the blood flow is not impeded (even at 25% of maximal voluntary contraction force the blood flow is significantly reduced).

Electromyography

As mentioned, muscle contraction is elicited by an action potential that is propagated along the muscle cell membrane. Like action potentials of nerve cells, the muscle cell action potential can be recorded with an electrode. This is called *electromyography* (EMG) and is performed either with an electrode placed on the skin overlying the muscle, or with a thin needle electrode inserted into the muscle. The first method gives an impression of the total electrical activity of the muscle, whereas needle electrodes sample the activity of a small part of the muscle. It should be understood, however, that the *EMG is a measure of the electrical activity and not of the mechanical activity of the muscle*. It is therefore not well suited to measure muscle force production. In some instances of prolonged activity, the muscle force may be declining in spite of constant or even increasing EMG activity—the declining force being caused by changed conditions in the muscle itself, whereas muscle action potentials are evoked normally by the nerve to the muscle. When recording from a normal muscle at the start of a very weak, voluntary contraction, the EMG shows regular, single potentials—presumably caused by the activity of one motor unit only. As the force increases, more potentials occur in the EMG, reflecting the recruitment of more motor units. At a certain level of force, the potentials are so frequent that the picture becomes unclear—that is, it is impossible to recognize a further increase of the EMG activity. This occurs not only because of recruitment but also because the frequency of action potentials for each motor unit increases.

EMG is a valuable tool for studying the participation of various muscles in *normal movements*: for example, to determine the timing of contraction in muscles of the leg during walking. EMG also aids in the *diagnosis of diseases* of the peripheral motor neurons and of the muscles themselves. For example, it can be determined whether a disease affects the motoneurons or the muscle. If the motoneurons are put out of action, the EMG activity will be reduced or absent, whereas in a disease affecting the contractile apparatus of the muscle, the EMG may be normal. Also, in cases of injury to peripheral nerves, it can be ascertained whether the lesion is complete (no EMG activity) or incomplete (even though there may be no visible movements).

REFLEXES

When a response to a stimulus is automatic (involuntary), and the response is mediated by the nervous system, we call it a reflex. There are numerous reflexes. Even though they differ in many respects, they nevertheless share some fundamental properties. Reflexes are stereotyped and constant because the same stimulus always gives the same kind of response. With increasing strength of the stimulus, however, the response usually increases in strength or magnitude. The reflexes are inborn—we do not need to learn them from experience (an example illustrating the need for inborn motor behavior is the sucking reflex in the newborn child). Many reflexes are found in large groups of animal species. All mammals, for example, have several reflexes in common. In general, the reflexes are appropriate and useful and ensure that the individual adapts to the environment. Reflexes are also fundamental for reproduction. Some reflexes are simple with regard to both the stimulus and the response, like the blink reflex (closing of the eye when something touches the cornea). Others are much more complex and require cooperation of many structures, like the swallowing reflex. Some reflexes involve lower parts of the central nervous system only (spinal cord, brain stem), whereas others involve the higher parts (even the cerebral cortex). Some reflexes are mediated by a chain of only two or three neurons, others by complicated and extensive neuronal networks. Many of the tasks of the nervous system are carried out reflexly—that is, independent of our consciousness. This, of course, frees the higher levels of the brain from handling numerous trivial everyday tasks.

Even though reflexes are independent of our will, some of them can be suppressed voluntarily (for example, the reflexes for emptying the bladder and the rectum). Other reflexes take place without our being aware of them, and with no possibility of influencing them voluntarily (like most of the reflexes related to the control of visceral functions). Reflexes involving skeletal muscles (those that participate in somatic motor control) have been most studied, and much of our knowledge of reflexes in general stems from such studies.

Conditioned Responses (Reflexes)

True reflexes should not be confused with another kind of automatic behavior, conditioned reflexes or, better, *conditioned responses*. In conditioned responses the stimulus evoking a true reflex response (the unconditioned stimulus) has been replaced—by *learning*—by another stimulus. This learning occurs when the unconditioned stimulus (for example, a puff of air on the cornea, eliciting a blink reflex) is regularly preceded by another kind of stimulus (for example, a tone; the conditioning stimulus). After some time, the conditioning stimulus will elicit the reflex response even when it is not followed by the unconditioned stimulus. The classical examples are the experiments of the Russian physiologist Pavlov, in which gastric secretion was produced by ringing a bell (conditioned stimulus). During the learning phase, the bell was always followed by food being presented (unconditioned stimulus). There are many examples from daily life of such conditioned behavioral responses, and conditioning is an important kind of learning.

The Reflex Arc and Basic Features of Reflexes

The structural basis of a reflex is a reflex arc, which consists of the following links:

1. A *receptor*, which records the stimulus and "translates" it to action potentials.
2. An *afferent link* (a primary sensory neuron), which conducts the action potentials to the central nervous system.
3. A *reflex center*, in which the signals from the receptor may be modified (increased or decreased) by signals from other receptors and other parts of the central nervous system, whereafter signals are issued to effectors.
4. An *efferent link* (neurons with axons passing out of the central nervous system), which conducts action potentials to the organ producing the response.
5. An *effector*, which may be skeletal (striated) muscle, cardiac muscle, smooth muscle (in the wall of vessels and visceral organs), or glands.

Figure 11.8 *A monosynaptic reflex.* The patellar reflex is used here as an example of a reflex with only one synapse intercalated between the afferent and the efferent link of the reflex arc. The stimulus is a tap on the patellar ligament below the patella, which stretches the muscle. The response is a brief muscle contraction. The **inset** shows that the Ia fiber from the muscle spindle contacts the motorneurons monosynaptically but also that it contacts many interneurons. Some of these are excitatory, mediating a polysynaptic activation of some motoneurons; other interneurons are inhibitory, mediating inhibition of other motoneurons.

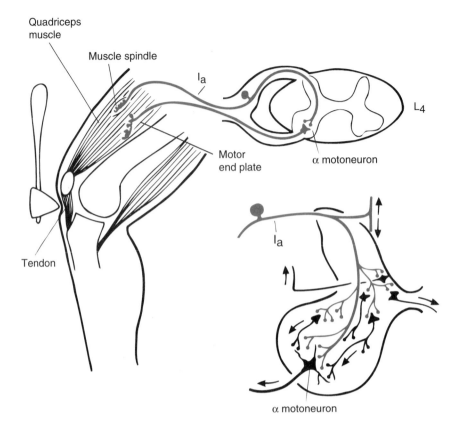

Some reflex *arcs* are simple; others are highly complex. Reflexes with their reflex center in the spinal cord are called *spinal reflexes*. *Brain stem* reflexes, as the name implies, have their center in the medulla, pons, or mesencephalon, whereas *cortical reflexes* have a reflex center that involves parts of the cerebral cortex.

We will now discuss two spinal reflexes as examples, both of them with skeletal muscles as effectors, although in other respects quite different. The first one has the simplest possible reflex arc, with only one synapse intercalated in the reflex center. Such a reflex is called *monosynaptic*. The other reflex to be discussed involves several synapses (coupled in series) in the reflex center and is therefore called a *polysynaptic reflex*. In the next chapter we will also discuss some reflexes in which cell groups in the brain stem coordinate the activity of spinal neurons (postural reflexes, neck and labyrinthine reflexes). Reflexes involving cranial nerve nuclei are discussed in Chapter 16, and examples of visceral reflexes in Chapter 17.

As an example of a monosynaptic reflex, we will use the *patellar reflex* (Fig. 11.8). The *stimulus* is a tap on the patellar ligament (the tendon of the quadriceps muscle). The *response* is a contraction of the quadriceps muscle, thus producing a brief extension movement at the knee joint. The reflex arc is shown schematically in Figure 11.8. The receptors are the muscle spindles in the muscle that is stretched; the afferent link is the Ia fiber, which ends in the spinal cord—notably with some collaterals ending directly (monosynaptically) on the α motoneurons supplying the quadriceps muscle. The axons of the α motoneurons constitute the efferent link, which at the motor end plate activates the extrafusal fibers of the quadriceps muscle (the effector).

Even a monosynaptic reflex is not quite as simple as Figure 11.8 indicates, however. Stretching of the muscle activates not one but presumably most of the muscle spindles of the muscle, and many motor units contribute to the response. The reflex center (the region with the coupling between the afferent and the efferent links) is not restricted to one spinal segment. Thus, α motoneurons supplying the quadriceps muscle are present in several lumbar segments (L₂–L₄). The motoneurons receive influences not only from the muscle spindle afferents but also from *other kinds of receptors* and *higher levels of the central nervous* system. Furthermore, the terminals of the Ia afferents are subject to *presynaptic inhibition*. This explains why the strength of the response—even when the stimulus is kept constant—may vary considerably from person to person and for one person depending on, for example, the level of anxiety. It also explains why—during learning of a motor task—the strength of the monosynaptic reflex response can be *modulated* up or down according to what is functionally appropriate. We will return to modulation of reflex responses below.

Most reflexes have a more complex reflex arc than the patellar reflex. As an example of a *polysynaptic* reflex, we will discuss the *flexion reflex* (withdrawal reflex). In this case one or more interneurons are intercalated between the terminals of the afferent sensory fiber and the motoneurons producing the response. When, for example, a foot hits a sharp object while walking, the whole leg is immediately withdrawn away from the object. That this is a reflex is clear from, among other things, the fact that it may be elicited even when the spinal cord is transected above the reflex center. The flexion reflex disappears in deep unconsciousness. For surgery, anesthesia has to be sufficiently deep to abolish flexion reflexes.

The *receptors for the flexion reflex* are nociceptors of the skin. The stimulus in this case hits a tiny spot on the skin, whereas the response involves a complex array of muscles (such as extensors of the ankle, flexors of the knee and the hip). Contraction of the muscles in the leg that is withdrawn, however, is not sufficient. Muscles of the other leg must also contract (primarily extensor muscles) to prevent loss of balance. Thus, the stimulus must be distributed to α motoneurons in many segments of the cord. This happens by way of ascending and descending collaterals of the primary sensory fibers, and spinal interneurons (Fig. 11.9). In response to a simple stimulus, a purposeful, harmonious movement occurs, requiring that all the muscles contract at the right time and with the right force. The synaptic couplings in the cord underlying this response must be both complex and precise.

The flexion reflex illustrates that *even an apparently simple reflex may depend on rather complex neural networks*. This means that the signal transmission through the reflex center is subject to modulation by impulses from other parts of the nervous system. As mentioned, this means that the strength of the response to a stimulus may vary. Because the excitability of the interneurons and motoneurons constituting the reflex center may vary, the extension of the reflex center may vary under different conditions. A reflex center should therefore not be imagined as a rigid set of interconnected neurons.

Figure 11.9 *A polysynaptic reflex*. The flexion reflex is used as an example. The diagram is highly simplified. In this case there is more than one synapse intercalated between the afferent and the efferent links of the reflex arc. In this example nociceptors in the sole of the foot are activated (walking on a sharp object). The impulses are conducted centrally in a sensory fiber (red), which branches and activates via interneurons α motoneurons at several segmental levels of the cord. This in turn makes many muscles contract to produce lifting of the foot off the ground (away from the painful stimulus). At the same time, extensor muscles are activated in the other leg to maintain balance.

Some reflexes are present only during certain *phases of development*, such as the *sucking reflex* and the *grasping reflex* in infants. When the reflexes disappear, they are no longer needed and would only disturb voluntary movements. The reflex arcs do not disappear, but the reflex response is suppressed by higher levels of the central nervous system. That the nervous apparatus persists is witnessed by the persistence or reappearance of primitive reflexes in brain-damaged children and adults.

Stretch Reflexes

We will now discuss in more detail reflexes of particular importance for motor control. The activity of motoneurons is partly determined by inputs from receptors in the skin, muscles, and around the joints. Also, when a movement is started and controlled from higher levels, spinal reflexes contribute more or less to the final result. *Stretch reflexes*—an example of which was described above—have been thoroughly investigated because of their importance for motor control. Receptors for all stretch reflexes are the muscle spindles. We speak of different stretch reflexes because *muscle contraction occurring as a result of muscle stretching* often consists of several distinct phases, each with a different latency as recorded by EMG. The *latency* of a reflex is *the time between the stimulus and the response* (between stretch and contraction). It results from the conduction time from the muscle spindles to the spinal cord, the delay at the synapse(s) intercalated between the Ia fibers and the α motoneurons, the conduction time from the motoneurons to the muscle, and, finally, the synaptic delay at the motor end plate. Measurement of the latency between the stimulus and the response makes it possible to decide whether a muscle contraction is the result of a monosynaptic stretch reflex, or whether other (polysynaptic) pathways are involved. Each intercalated synapse increases the latency. For each extra synapse intercalated in the reflex arc, the latency increases with a few milliseconds. Thus, *muscle contractions occurring with different latencies after stretching the muscle means that there are several pathways intercalated between the afferent link (the sensory fibers) and the motoneurons—not only the simple*

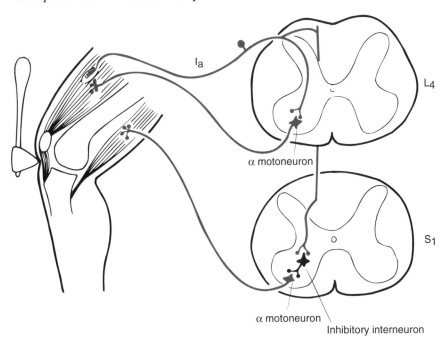

Ia

L4

α motoneuron

S₁

α motoneuron

Inhibitory interneuron

Figure 11.10 *Reciprocal inhibition.* Schematic illustration of how the stretching of one muscle—producing a reflex contraction—elicits inhibition of the antagonistic muscles via inhibitory interneurons.

monsynaptic one. We will discuss the monosynaptic and the polysynaptic stretch reflexes separately below. Much remains to be clarified, however, concerning the role of the stretch reflexes in movement control.

The effects of stretching a muscle are more complex than what appears from the above description. Thus, while the impulses from the muscle spindle excite the α motoneurons of the muscle that is being stretched, the motoneurons of the antagonists are inhibited. This phenomenon is called *reciprocal inhibition*, and is obviously functionally appropriate: It prevents a stretch reflex from being elicited in the antagonists when they are stretched by the reflex contraction of the agonists (this, in turn, would elicit a new stretch reflex of the agonists, and so on). In the case of the patellar reflex, the motoneurons of the knee flexors are inhibited (Fig. 11.10). The reciprocal inhibition reduces unwanted oscillatory movements. The inhibition of the α motoneurons of the antagonist is mediated by inhibitory interneurons (Ia-inhibitory interneurons), which are excited by Ia afferents from the agonist muscles.[5]

The Monosynaptic Stretch Reflex Is Phasic

The monosynaptic stretch reflex is described above (Fig. 11.8) To evoke a muscle contraction via this simple reflex arc, the muscle must be stretched rapidly—that is, by *phasic stretching.*The actual lengthening produced by the stimulus may be very little; the salient point is the *velocity* of stretching. As discussed in Chapter 7, the primary afferents of the muscle spindles are especially sensitive to the velocity of stretching, so that even such a brief stimulus, stretching the muscle only a fraction of a millimeter, produces a brisk repsonse. A tap on a tendon with a reflex hammer produces this kind of stimulus, although it is far from being a natural stimulus. Because both the stimulus and the response last only for a very short time, we also use the term *phasic stretch reflex*. This kind of stretch reflex can be elicited in most skeletal muscles but much more easily in some muscles than in others. There are also individual differences: In some healthy persons, phasic stretch reflexes cannot be elicited.

For the *patellar reflex*, the *latency* between the stimulus and the start of the contraction (as recorded with EMG) is about 30 msec, and a slightly shorter latency pertains to reflexes in the upper arm muscles because of a shorter peripheral pathway (for example, the biceps reflex has a latency of about 25 msec).

The Long Latency (Polysynaptic) Stretch Reflex

As mentioned above, stretching of a muscle may elicit reflex contraction via routes other than the monosynaptic reflex arc. The muscle spindle afferent fibers (Ia and II) contact not only α motoneurons but also many interneurons (Fig. 11.8; among them some that are inhibitory, as mentioned above). The British neurophysiologist Hammond showed already in 1956 that rapid stretching of the biceps muscle may elicit *two* reflex responses, as determined with EMG in human subjects. In addition to an early EMG activity with a latency of about 25 msec (the monosynaptic stretch reflex), another reflex contraction starts at about 50 msec—thus presumably mediated by a polysynaptic reflex pathway. It should be emphasized that this is not a voluntary response, since the earliest voluntary muscle contractions occur about 100 msec after the stretch (in the upper arm). This reflex response is called the *long-latency stretch reflex*, to distinguish it from the monosynaptic (short-latency) stretch reflex (other names are: the functional stretch reflex, the polysynaptic stretch reflex, and the long–loop stretch reflex).

A striking property of the long-latency stretch reflex is that the *strength of the response depends on whether the muscle is relaxed or active* at the time of stretching. If the muscle is relaxed or only slightly active when stretched, there is usually no long-latency reflex response at all. Furthermore, the strength of the response *depends on prior instruction to the subject* with regard to whether to resist the imposed stretch or to let go. When the person is asked to let go when an imposed movement (at an unpredictable time) stretches the muscle (for example, an imposed extension at the elbow that stretches the biceps muscle), the reflex response is much smaller than when the person is asked to resist the imposed movement. Thus, the magnitude of the reflex response can be adapted to what is functionally appropriate in a particular situation.

A further characteristic of the long-latency stretch reflex is that the *strength of the response may change during learning of a motor task*. Thus, by repeated trials, the reflex response becomes weaker in muscles in which a contraction in response to stretching is functionally inappropriate and stronger in muscles in which a contraction is appropriate. This learning effect or adaptation of the stretch reflex occurs only in connection with the particular learned movement; in connection with other movements, the reflex response of the muscle is unaltered. As mentioned, also the monosynaptic stretch reflex is subject to similar learned, task-related modulation, but the changes appear to be smaller than those obtained with the long latency reflex.

Such adaptation of the stretch reflex response is presumably mediated by descending connections from higher levels of the central nervous system (for example, from the motor cortex) that determine how readily the motoneurons react to a certain input. This appears to be exerted mostly by a precise control of the excitability of specific sets of spinal interneurons, which are intercalated in particular reflex arcs. Thus, reflex arcs may be "opened" or "closed" in accordance with the need of the organism.

It should be clear from the above that *stretching of a muscle does not necessarily elicit a reflex contraction.* Many factors influence whether there will be a response, such as the velocity of stretching, how long the stretch is, whether the muscle is active when being stretched, and whether a reflex contraction is functionally appropriate.

Examples of Stretch Reflex Modulation

Reflex modulation has been studied most during locomotion in humans, and is found in several muscle groups. Thus, the strength of reflex contractions in many leg muscles depends on whether the leg is in the swing or in the stance phase. In the ankle flexors (m. triceps surae), for example, stretch reflexes are weak or absent in the swing phase, whereas they are brisk in the stance phase. This seems appropriate, since in the stance phase the reflex contraction would strengthen the desired plantar flexion, whereas in the swing phase the appropriate movement is dorsal flexion of the foot to enable free swing of the leg.

Arm muscles also show marked reflex modulation in persons catching a ball. In a certain phase of the movement even the reciprocal inhibition is absent—that is, a stretch reflex can be elicited in a muscle without inhibition of its antagonists. This is functionally appropriate when agonists and antagonists are required to cocontract to stabilize the joint.

Is the Long-Latency Stretch Reflex Mediated via the Cerebral Cortex?

The exact central pathway followed by the impulses mediating the long-latency stretch reflex has been much debated. Indirect data indicate that the reflex pathway may involve the *motor cortex of the cerebral cortex* (therefore, the term long-loop stretch reflex is often used). In support of a transcortical route are the observations that the reflex is weakened or abolished by lesions of the descending motor pathways or by lesions of the dorsal columns (presumably carrying the signals from the muscle spindles to the cerebral cortex). Furthermore, the reflex is often weakened after lesions of the cerebellum. Such findings, however, may also be explained by a purely spinal reflex that is under strong supraspinal control.

More decisive evidence of a transcortical route for the long-latency stretch reflex —at least regarding certain muscle groups—comes from observations in a few patients with a peculiar inborn abnormality of the pyramidal tract. These persons always perform mirror movements of the hands; asked to flex the index finger of the left hand, they always flex the right index finger as well (more proximal movements, for example, of the shoulders, are performed normally). This behavior appears from electrophysiological studies to be caused by branching of individual pyramidal tract axons to supply motoneurons of both sides of the cord. Thus, stimulation of the hand region of the motor cortex of one hemisphere causes symmetrical movements of both hands (unlike the normal situation, in which such stimulation always cause movements of the opposite hand only). When eliciting stretch reflexes in such subjects, the monosynaptic reflex occurs only on the same side as the stretch is applied (as normal), whereas the long-latency stretch reflex occurs in both hands after a unilateral stimulus. The latter observation is hard to explain unless the reflex arc of the long-latency reflex involves the pyramidal tract.

It should be emphasized, however, that these findings may not pertain to long-latency stretch reflexes in *all* muscle groups. Thus, the long-latency stretch reflexes appear to differ in the forearm and calf muscles regarding its dependence on the pyramidal tract, and regarding whether group Ia or group II fibers are the main afferent link.

Many questions remain regarding the organization of the long-latency stretch reflex and its functional role—or rather *reflexes*—since there may exist several varieties.

Motoneurons Can Inhibit Their Own Activity: Renshaw Cells

The numerous different neural inputs to the motoneurons together determine their level of excitability—that is, these inputs also determine the activity of the skeletal muscles. Besides the inhibition of motoneurons by primary afferent fibers (via interneurons) described above, the motoneurons can also inhibit their own activity. Thus, the α motoneuron axons send off collaterals before they leave the ventral horn (Fig. 11.11). Because they turn back, they are called *recurrent collaterals*. The recurrent collaterals end primarily on a group of inhibitory interneurons, the *Renshaw cells*, located ventromedially in the ventral horn. The axons of the Renshaw cells ramify extensively and contact primarily the α motoneurons (but also certain kinds of inhibitory interneurons). In this manner, the activity of the α motoneurons excites the Renshaw cells, which in turn inhibit the same α motoneurons and other α motoneurons that supply muscles with the same action (agonists). Furthermore, the Renshaw cells inhibit the inhibitory interneurons mediating the reciprocal inhibition (Fig. 11.10)—that is, the inhibition of the α motoneurons supplying the antagonists is reduced (disinhibition). In case of a stretch reflex, the activity of the Renshaw cells shortens the reflex contraction of the agonists and at the same time shortens the reciprocal inhibition of the antagonists.

The Renshaw system seems important to prevent the α motoneurons from sending long trains of action potentials as a response to a brief stimulus. On the other hand, there are other situations, such as during voluntary movements, when prolonged motoneuronal activity is required. In such situations, descending connections from the brain stem and the cerebral cortex may inhibit the Renshaw cells supplying the working muscles. Thus, the activity of the Renshaw cells, as that of many other kinds of spinal interneurons, may be regulated in accordance with the overall plan for the movements being carried out.

The Function of Stretch Reflexes

One might think that the stretch reflexes, which after all are relatively simple, are well understood with regard to their functional roles. For example, the muscle spindles and the motoneurons are among the best characterized receptors and central neurons, respectively. Nevertheless, we still do not understand fully the role of the stretch reflexes in the control of voluntary movements and in the control of posture and muscle tone. We will discuss here only some possible functions.

One likely task of the stretch reflex is to *ensure that the length of a muscle is kept constant.* In many situations this is of obvious importance—for example, in the upright position when some external perturbation threatens the body balance. The sudden displacement of the center of gravity forward stretches the extensor muscles of the back and thus might elicit a stretch reflex tending to resume the former position. It is furthermore an obvious advantage that such a corrective contraction come as quickly as possible. Making such an adjustment dependent only on voluntary contraction would lengthen the latency fourfold, with the danger of the corrections coming too late. Also while walking, when external perturbations may disturb the programmed pattern of muscular activity, stretch reflexes may contribute to rapid adjustments. Nevertheless, it is not clear to what extent stretch reflexes really participate in such adjustments (see below).

Another situation in which stretch reflexes may be of importance is during *slow, precise voluntary movements when the external opposing forces change unpredictably.* Again, the advantage would be that the adjustment of muscle tension occurs much earlier than what can be achieved by voluntary action alone.

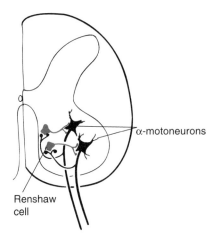

Figure 11.11 *Recurrent inhibition.* The α motoneurons inhibit their own activity by sending recurrent collaterals ending on the inhibitory Renshaw cells. The Renshaw cells are also influenced by other cell groups in the cord and at higher levels, which determine how strongly they will respond to a certain input from the α motoneurons.

Stretch Reflexes May Correct for Change in External Resistance during Precision Movements

Studies of slow movements of the thumb by the British neurologist Marsden have shed light on the contribution of stretch reflexes during precision movements. The subject is asked to flex the thumb with a constant speed against an external opposing force of constant magnitude. The EMG of the flexor pollicis longus muscle is recorded continuously. The external force is then changed suddenly at unpredictable times during the movement—either increased or reduced. When the external force is increased, the movement is immediately slowed down. Because of the α–γ coactivation (see p. 000), the frequency of impulses from the muscle spindle increases. The α–γ coactivation ensures that, as the muscle shortens owing to the activation of the α motoneurons, the spindle midportion is stretched. This upholds the firing of muscle spindle afferents in spite of the shortening, which otherwise would have led to reduced firing. To keep up with the steadily shortening muscle, the firing of the γ motoneurons must also increase steadily. When the movement is suddenly halted or slowed down, the firing frequency of the γ motoneurons continues increasing, in anticipation of further shortening of the muscle. Thus, for a moment, the firing of the muscle spindle afferents increases more than what is appropriate with regard to the actual length of the muscle. This increases the excitation of the motoneurons, and their firing increases, thus increasing the force of the muscle contraction. The result is that the increased external force is rapidly compensated for, and the original speed of the movement is resumed.

When the opposing external force is suddenly reduced, the opposite events take place. The speed of the flexion movement of the thumb increases, and the firing frequency of the spindle afferents decreases for a moment, thus reducing the firing of the α motoneurons and the force of contraction. The speed of movement is adjusted.

Probably, the stretch reflex functions in this manner especially during slow precision movements when we cannot predict accurately the external force at all times. The sensitivity of the muscle spindles is kept at a high level, so that they may record even the slightest perturbations and ensure that the activity of the α motoneurons is adjusted appropriately.

Automatic Adjustment of Muscle Contraction Is Not Only Due to Stretch Reflexes

Signals from receptors other than the muscle spindle can also influence the excitability of the motoneurons. When a reflex adjustment of muscle tension occurs (that is, the latency between the stimulus and the muscle contraction is too short for the contraction to be voluntary), we must therefore consider the possible contribution of signals from several kinds of receptors. Signals from the *tendon organ* (conducted in Ib afferent fibers) are known to influence the motoneurons via a spinal reflex arc. In anesthetized animals, it appears that signals from the tendon organs inhibit (via spinal interneurons) the motoneurons of the muscle in which the receptors lie (autogenic inhibition). We discussed in Chapter 7, however, that the effects on motoneurons of signals from tendon organs are modulated during natural movements. Thus, signals produced by increased muscle tension can have excitatory or inhibitory effects, depending on the situation. We still do not know the functional role of signals from tendon organs for reflex adjustments during natural movements in conscious human subjects.

We will now consider, as an example, a *situation in which we know reflex adjustment of muscle tension occurs with possible contributions from several receptors*. This situation occurs when the body balance in the upright position is disturbed. The contributions of various receptors have been studied in persons standing on a platform that can be tilted or moved forward or backward. When the platform is suddenly displaced backward (without tilting), the body first sways forward, with the movement primarily occurring at the ankle joints. The balance is regained mainly because the muscles at the back of the leg contract (the ankle flexors, primarily the triceps surae muscle; muscles of the hip, the back, and in the neck also contribute, however). The first part of the contraction of the leg muscles occurs so early after the perturbation that it must be mediated by a reflex. (Somewhat later there is also a voluntary contraction contributing to the final outcome of the postural adjustment.) But what causes the reflex contraction of the leg muscles? We have to consider at least the following possibilities:

1. that the stretching of the leg muscles elicits a *stretch reflex*;
2. that the muscle contraction is caused by signals from *receptors in the labyrinth* (vestibular apparatus) stimulated by the movement of the head;
3. that the muscle contraction is produced by signals from the *joint receptors* of the ankle joint;
4. that stimulation of *low-threshold mechanoreceptors in the skin* on the sole of the foot produces the reflex contraction of the leg muscles;
5. that *visual information* (presumably relayed via the vestibular nuclei and their connections to the spinal cord) elicits appropriate automatic adjustments.

All of these kinds of information most likely contribute, and the muscle spindles are certainly not responsible alone. There is even evidence that normal subjects differ with regard to which kind of information is used primarily for the reflex adjustment. For optimal postural stability, however, all kinds of sensory information mentioned above seems to be necessary. Nevertheless, elimination of either vestibular or somatosensory information in human subjects does not impair seriously their ability to automatically adjust body balance after moderate perturbations. However, the movement strategy—that is, the joints in which the major compensatory movements occur—is altered when one of the sensory inputs is removed.

In other situations, such as when the platform is suddenly tilted backward, the muscles at the back of the leg are stretched, as in the former example. The center of gravity is now displaced backward instead of forward, and consequently a contraction of the posterior leg muscles in this situation would not help to regain the balance but would rather worsen the situation. To regain balance, the muscles at the front of the leg (for example, the anterior tibial muscle) have to contract as rapidly as possible, and these are, of course, shortened by the tilting of the platform. The contraction of the anterior leg muscles, which in fact takes place, cannot be caused by a stretch reflex. In this situation one also gets an impression of the adaptability of the stretch reflexes—how inappropriate reflex responses to stretch may be suppressed. Thus, the reflex contraction occurring in the posterior leg muscles when the platform is tilted backward becomes weaker as the perturbation is repeated, so that the person knows that at some (unpredictable) moment the platform will be tilted.

In summary, it is clear that *the reflex adjustments that occur in numerous muscles of the body on perturbations of the balance are caused by signals from several kinds of receptors*. The information from the various receptors is integrated at the brain stem and spinal level, to ensure a coordinated and purposeful pattern of muscle activity. If necessary, voluntary activity follows and supplements the automatic, reflex adjustments. The more demanding the challenge to the balance becomes, the more important becomes the ability to use all kinds of receptors.

Cutaneous Receptors and the Precision Grip

There are also situations in which stimulation of low-threshold skin mechanoreceptors causes reflex muscular contraction. For example, when during a precision grip with the fingers the object slips, a reflex increase of the grip force occurs. The latency from the start of the slip to the muscular response is only 60–80 msec—that is, too short to be mediated by a voluntary command. Examination of patients with reduced skin sensation but normal motor apparatus suggests that loss of such rapid, reflex adjustment of the grip force is partly responsible for their difficulties with precision movements (see Chapter 6).

MUSCLE TONE

The term *muscle tone* usually refers to the slight tension that can be felt in a relaxed muscle (a more precise term is therefore *resting tone*). In pathological conditions, the resting tone may be changed—either increased or decreased. The term muscle tone is not unambiguous, however, as witnessed by its use by various authors. (Some authors have suggested that the term is too imprecise and should therefore be abandoned.)

Muscle tone is usually determined by *palpation* (judging the consistency and stiffness of the tissue by pressing the muscle belly between the fingers) and by *stretching* (judging the resistance offered to passive stretch). Some authors use the term only about the tone as judged by stretching. Palpation and stretching do not test identical properties of the muscle. For example, after a stroke giving central pareses (capsular hemiplegia), the muscle tone is commonly reduced when judged by palpation (the consistency is reduced), whereas the resistance offered to passive stretching is increased. Examination of muscle tone is of importance for the diagnosis of diseases affecting the motor system. It is therefore regrettable that we do not have a clear understanding of the basis of normal muscle tone and of the mechanisms behind changes of muscle tone in disease states.

Muscle Tone Is an Expression of the Stiffness of the Tissue

The confusion about the exact meaning of the term muscle tone stems partly from the fact that words like firmness, tension, stiffness, and elasticity are often used without definition. Different persons may therefore use them with different meanings. This is, unfortunately, often the case even when observations made by different examiners are compared. *Stiffness* and *tension* can, however, be defined in mathematical terms and can also be recorded and measured objectively. The definition of stiffness (K) is: $K = \Delta T/\Delta L$; that is, K expresses how much the muscles are stretched (ΔL) by a certain increase in tension (ΔT). The greater the stiffness, the higher the tension necessary to stretch the muscle. Note that this definition applies only to the component of muscle tension determined by passive stretching, and not to the consistency (firmness, elasticity) as judged by palpation. The latter can hardly be measured objectively and depends on the subjective assessment of the examiner.

Properties of the Muscle That May Contribute to Muscle Tone

From everyday experience we know that *contraction* of a muscle is the one factor that most markedly alters the muscle tone, as judged by both palpation and stretching. The purpose of the contraction, of course, is to increase the tension of the muscle. Under normal conditions, small contributions to the tension of the muscle stem from the *passive viscoelastic properties of the muscle cells and the connective tissue* of the muscle and its tendons. The elastic properties of the muscle explain why when the muscle is stretched passively beyond a certain length, the tension increases steeply (the slack is taken out of the elastic, as it were). This is experienced when a relaxed muscle becomes firmer on palpation and offers increasing resistance to stretching toward extreme joint positions (therefore, such positions should be avoided when examining muscle tone). Even in a relaxed muscle of medium length, however, properties of the muscle cells themselves can influence the muscle stiffness. Elastic *titin (connectin)* molecules of the cytoskeleton connect the Z discs with the myosin filaments. They extend from the Z disc to the middle of the A band of the sarcomere, and have been shown to contribute to the resistance to stretch offered by a relaxed muscle cell. The titins exist in several varieties (isoforms). For example, there are different isoforms in the soleus and the psoas muscles, and the resting tone differs greatly in these muscles (highest in the psoas). Furthermore, even in relaxed muscle a few crossbridges between actin and myosin filaments may exist. If the number of such cross bridges varies among muscles, it might contribute to differences in resting tone.

Which of the two factors—active contraction and passive viscoelastic properties—is responsible for the normal resting tone? It was formerly assumed that even relaxed muscle was in a state of slight contractile activity (caused by impulses from α motoneurons) and that this activity was maintained by a steady flow of impulses from the muscle spindles. This was based primarily on observations in animals with transection of the brain stem (decerebration), in which the activity of the γ motoneurons is enhanced. This increases the impulse traffic from the muscle spindles, and thereby the muscles are in a state of tonic contraction. In accordance with these observations, muscle tone in normal human subjects was assumed to be upheld by the long-latency stretch reflex ("tonic stretch reflex"). This view can hardly be upheld in the light of more recent data, however. In the first place, several EMG studies show that in persons who are able to relax properly, there is no electrical activity in their muscles (and, therefore, no contractile activity). Furthermore, microneurographical studies have not confirmed that there is impulse traffic in muscle spindle afferents conducting from relaxed muscles in human subjects. In relaxed subjects, the resistance against even rapid passive stretching of a muscle is very low (except when the monosynaptic stretch reflex is elicited by a tendon tap). There is thus no evidence of a "reflex tone" in relaxed muscles. The tone felt in a relaxed muscle, which shows no EMG activity, probably depends on the passive viscoelastic properties of the muscle. However, many healthy persons are unable to relax their muscles completely, at least during an examination. Thus, EMG would show a modest electric activity when the muscles are handled by the examiner. Even in such cases, however, the contraction is probably not of a reflex nature but produced by voluntary commands (that is, by signals issued from the cerebral cortex). Thus, in such persons there is usually muscle activity also in muscles that are shortened passively as the examiner produces a joint movement (the person "helps" the examiner).

The individual differences that can be observed with regard to resting muscle tone in healthy persons may presumably be explained to a large extent by differences in the degree of relaxation. In addition, there are probably also *individual differences with regard to the passive viscoelastic properties of the muscles.* Thus, there is evidence that even in persons who are able to relax their muscles completely (as judged by EMG), the muscle tone (as judged by palpation) may vary. Some possible factors contributing to such differences are discussed above.

INJURY OF PERIPHERAL MOTOR NEURONS

When all motoneurons (or their axons) supplying a muscle are destroyed, the muscle cannot be made to contract: It is *paralyzed*. Both voluntary and reflex movements are abolished. If not all of the motoneurons (or

Changes of Muscle Tone in Disease

Pathologically changed muscle tone is called *hypotonia* when it is lower than normal and *hypertonia* when higher than normal. To recognize abnormal muscle tone, one must by necessity first be able to decide what is normal. From the above discussion it should be clear, however, that "normal muscle tone" is not a precise, well-defined concept. The decision as to whether a muscle has a normal tone has to be based largely on the subjective judgment of the examiner. This judgment, of course, depends to a large extent on experience. Whereas hypertonus may be fairly easy to identify and even measure in semiquantitative terms by stretching the muscles, the decision as to whether a muscle has abnormally low tone (hypotonic) is more difficult. As mentioned, a normal, fully relaxed muscle will have a very low tension when tested by stretching. Some authors believe that when paretic or paralytic muscles feel softer and more flaccid than normal muscle, it is because of lack of voluntary contraction, which probably occurs to some extent during passive movements and palpation. Experiments measuring the resistance to passive stretching of normal and alleged hypotonic muscles did not show any consistent differences. The experiments were performed by measuring the falling time of the leg (passive flexion of the knee) in healthy persons with the ability to relax fully (EMG) and in patients with pareses of the quadriceps muscle (clinically judged as hypotonic). The individual differences in falling time—that is, muscle tone—among the normal subjects were fairly large, presumably because of differences in the passive viscoelastic properties.

It should be kept in mind, however, that with *peripheral pareses, rapid changes of the passive viscoelastic properties of the muscles may occur*, which may help explain why the paretic muscles feel softer on palpation. After damage to peripheral motoneurons, the muscles atrophy rapidly, reducing the muscle volume to sometimes only 20%–30% of normal in about 3 months. The metabolism of muscle cells is obviously dramatically altered by loss of contact between nerve and muscle.

Abnormally increased muscle tone, *hypertonus*, would imply that the muscles continuously have an increased tone, in spite of attempts to relax. As mentioned, many healthy persons are not able to relax completely, at least not in an examination situation, and the border between normal and pathologically increased muscle tone may not be easy to draw. In certain diseases of the central nervous system affecting the tracts and nuclei of the motor system, however, fairly characteristic disturbances of muscle tone occur. *Rigidity* is the term used to characterize the increased muscle tone occurring in Parkinson's disease (Chapter 13). Even with very slow, passive movements, an increased, "cogwheel"-like resistance is felt by the examiner. This may be caused by increased long-latency stretch reflexes that are elicited by abnormally slow movements.

The term *spasticity* is used in clinical neurology of a condition in which there is increased resistance only against *rapid stretching* of muscles. By palpation the muscles may feel normal or hypotonic, and there is not always increased resistance against slow, passive movements. Spasticity occurs after damage to the descending motor pathways from the cerebral cortex to the motoneurons and is probably caused primarily by changed excitability of spinal interneurons. The increased resistance to rapid stretch is most likely caused by *abnormally brisk monosynaptic stretch reflexes*, whereas the long-latency stretch reflexes are weaker than normal.

Also with rigidity and spasticity, there is evidence of *changed passive viscoelastic properties* (in addition to the changed stretch reflexes). Thus, in patients with moderately severe Parkinson's disease, increased resistance to slow elbow extension was found, even though there was no EMG activity of the biceps muscle (which was being stretched). In some spastic patients, increased resistance even to slow stretching of relaxed leg muscles was present, but only when the spasticity had lasted for more than a year. Thus, it seems as though an altered pattern of impulses from the motoneurons—like those occurring in diseases with rigidity or spasticity—may change the passive, viscoelastic properties of the muscles (rigidity and spasticity are discussed further in Chapters 12 and 13).

their axons) supplying a muscle are destroyed, the muscle can still contract, although with less speed and force than normal. This is called a *partial paralysis* or *paresis*. Typically, the paretic muscle feels soft and flaccid, and there is a marked reduction in the muscle mass. This is called *muscular atrophy* and is more marked the more complete the destruction of the motoneurons. The muscle cells that no longer receive impulses from the motoneurons become thinner and eventually disappear if no reinnervation takes place (see below).

This kind of muscle weakness, caused by the loss of the α motoneurons or their axons (lower motor neurons), is called a *peripheral paralysis* (paresis), to distinguish it from a *central paralysis* caused by interruption of the central motor pathways (the upper motor neurons; this is discussed further in Chapter 12). *Characteristic of peripheral pareses—apart from the weakened or abolished voluntary contractions—is that the muscles are flaccid, reflex movements are weakened or abolished, and muscular atrophy progresses rapidly and becomes marked.* In cases of peripheral pareses, the distribution of affected muscles may tell us where the disease process is located. For example, the distribution will differ depending on whether the lesion is located in the cord, in the plexuses formed by the spinal nerves, or in the peripheral nerves more peripherally (Fig. 11.1).

When a peripheral nerve is injured so that the axons are interrupted, the distal parts of the axons degenerate and are gradually removed (by macrophages). The perikarya (of the motoneurons and the spinal ganglion cells) show retrograde changes and, even though some of the cells die, many survive. The proximal parts of the axons of the surviving neurons start to grow. When possible, the growing axons follow the canals in the nerve left by the degenerated axons. The Schwann cells do not die and form a lining of the canals for the growing axons. The axons grow 1–2 mm per day, although the growth gets slower the farther peripherally the axon grows.

The final outcome of this *regeneration* of the axons depends on several factors, among them the conditions at the site of injury and the age of the person. If the continuity of the nerve is not lost—as when the nerve is crushed or damaged by compression—the growing axons have a fair chance of finding the right track and reaching the target they innervated formerly. If the nerve is completely severed (for example, by tearing or a cut), many axons will follow a wrong path even though the cut ends are meticulously stitched together. Thus, motor axons may innervate different muscles than previously, and, likewise, sensory axons may innervate different regions of the skin than before the injury. For example, motoneurons formerly supplying an extensor muscle may after the regeneration supply a flexor; sensory nerve fibers formerly supplying the thumb may innervate the index finger; and so forth. *The longer the distance an axon has to grow after the damage, the poorer the chances that it will reach its target.* Thus, one cannot expect full functional recovery after suture of a cut peripheral nerve. The results are better in children than in adults, however. This may be because children have a greater regenerative capacity, but presumably also because their brains adapt more easily to a novel pattern of innervation in the periphery.

In cases of incomplete severance of a nerve, the remaining motor axons usually send out new branches within the muscle. This is called *collateral sprouting* (See Chapter 4, *Collateral Sprouting Can Aid Recovery*). The sprouts grow into and make synaptic contacts at the "empty" motor end plates left by the degenerated axons. In this case, many of the muscle cells, which shortly after the injury were paralyzed, become reinnervated and some of the muscle power is regained. The remaining motor units of the muscle become larger, and therefore the control of the muscle may become less precise than before the injury. Animal experiments suggest that the remaining motor units may increase their size four to six times.

After suturing a cut muscle nerve, reflex contractions often show less recovery than voluntary contractions. This is probably because the sensory fibers (innervating muscle spindles and tendon organs) have greater difficulties in reaching their correct target than the motor axons. Thus, after crushing a nerve—when the regenerating axons more easily find the right path—the reflex contractions show better recovery.

NOTES

1. The level of CGRP in the motoneurons is under the influence of descending connections from higher levels of the central nervous system; when such connections are transected, the level of CGRP drops. In vitro studies indicate that CGRP influences the synthesis of acetylcholine receptors of the muscle cells. Since CGRP is present in the motoneuron terminals (in addition to in the perikarya), it seems possible that CGRP also has such an effect in vivo.

2. During development—before the muscle cells have received their innervation—the acetylcholine receptors are evenly distributed all over the muscle membrane. Only when properly functioning synaptic contacts have been established are the receptors redistributed to attain the mature pattern. The neuropeptide *galanin* is expressed transiently during development of spinal motoneurons and may possibly be related to interactions between the motoneurons and the muscle cells at the time of synapse formation.

3. The fiber type used for a particular kind of movement has been studied by the so-called *glycogen depletion technique*. By prolonged use, all of the muscle fibers of a motor unit deplete their stores of glycogen, and this may be shown histochemically in frozen sections of a small piece of muscle tissue obtained by biopsy. The type 1 muscle fibers are depleted first when the force exerted is low—that is, no type 2 fibers are recruited. When the force is very high, however, the type 2 fibers are depleted first. In the latter case, type 1 fibers are also recruited, but because of their high endurance they are not depleted during the short period in which a maximal force can be maintained.

4. In spite of the general validity of the size principle for recruitment of motoneurons, motoneurons with similar size may have quite different firing rates and innervate muscle cells with different contractile properties (the latter is presumably a reflection of the fact that the firing rate of motoneurons influences the contractile properties of the muscle cells). Furthermore, experiments with the use of biofeedback (EMG) during voluntary movements indicate that humans can to some degree select among the low-threshold motor units. This must depend on the ability of higher motor centers to focus excitation among motoneurons with presumably the same size.

5. Collaterals of the Ia afferents also contact other kinds of spinal interneurons. Thus, interneurons that inhibit the α motoneurons of the muscle being stretched are also contacted by Ia collaterals. This inhibitory effect is usually not evident when testing stretch reflexes—the excitatory, monosynaptic effect dominates. During natural movements, however, such autogenic inhibition may be of importance. Descending connections from higher levels of the central nervous system may direct transmission of the reflex arc, so that the excitatory or inhibitory effect dominates, depending on what is appropriate in the particular situation.

CENTRAL MOTOR PATHWAYS

Many parts of the brain are able to influence our movements because they send fibers that end in synaptic contact with the motoneurons (lower motor neurons) or with interneurons that in turn contact the motoneurons. These higher motor centers are neuronal groups (upper motor neurons) in the brain stem and in the cerebral cortex, which are highly interconnected. All of them participate (although to various extents) in most motor acts. The sharing of tasks among the higher motor centers is such that cell groups in the brain stem can by themselves control many automatic movements, whereas the participation of the cerebral cortex is necessary in less automatic movements. The importance of the cerebral cortex increases with the increasing degree of voluntary control of a movement.

Customarily, a division has been made between the pyramidal tract and all other nuclei and tracts more or less directly involved in motor control. The latter have often been collectively called the "extrapyramidal system." This term lacks a precise meaning, however, and can only be vaguely defined, a fact that has become more and more clear as our knowledge of the motor systems has improved. Thus, we will not use the term here. The pyramidal tract, however, is a well defined entity that can be described separately, even though it is just one of several motor pathways transmitting signals from higher levels to the motoneurons of the brain stem and the spinal cord. Figure 12.1 shows schematically the most important pathways descending from the cerebral cortex and the brain stem to the spinal cord. It should be noted, however, that such descending pathways not only serve motor tasks; some of them also participate in the control of signal transmission in the ascending sensory pathways (see Chapter 7).

Figure 12.1 *Descending motor pathways to the spinal cord*. In addition to the pyramidal tract, several tracts arise from brain stem nuclei.

THE PYRAMIDAL TRACT (THE CORTICOSPINAL TRACT)

The pyramidal tract is of crucial importance in our ability to perform precise, voluntary movements. The tract is formed by axons of neurons with their perikarya in the cerebral cortex, as indicated by its other name, the *corticospinal tract*. The axons descend through the internal capsule, the crus cerebri (cerebral peduncle), the pons, and the medulla (Figs. 12.2 and 12.5). Most of the fibers cross to the other side in the lowermost part of the medulla and continue downward in the lateral funiculus of the cord, to finally establish synaptic contacts in the spinal gray matter. *This is the only pathway that passes directly—that is, without synaptic interruption—from the cerebral cortex to the spinal cord.*

Fibers also leave the pyramidal tract on their way through the brain stem, to reach cranial nerve motor nuclei (Fig. 12.2). Such fibers form part of the *corticobulbar tract* (other corticobulbar fibers reach the red nucleus, the pontine nuclei, the recticular formation, the colliculi, the dorsal column nuclei, and other nuclei).

The pyramidal tract got its name from the pyramid of the medulla, which is formed by the fibers of the corticospinal tract (Figs. 3.14 and 3.15). Strictly speaking, therefore, the term *pyramidal tract* encompasses only the fibers destined for the spinal cord and not those destined for the cranial nerve motor nuclei. Nevertheless, for practical reasons both groups are usually included in the term.

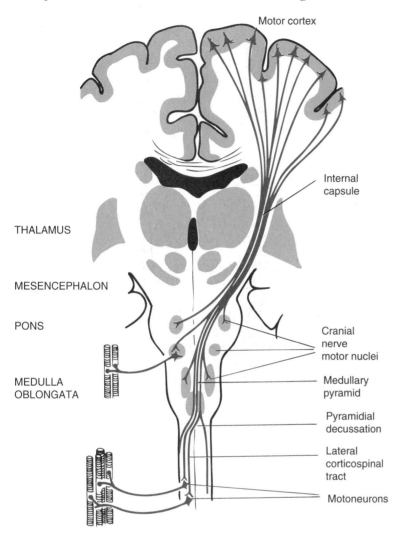

Motor cortex

Internal capsule

THALAMUS

MESENCEPHALON

PONS

Cranial nerve motor nuclei

MEDULLA OBLONGATA

Medullary pyramid

Pyramidial decussation

Lateral corticospinal tract

Motoneurons

Figure 12.2 *The course of the pyramidal tract.* Note that most of the fibers cross in the lower medulla.

Origin and Course of the Pyramidal Tract

A large proportion of the fibers of the pyramidal tract comes from neurons with their perikarya in the precentral gyrus—that is, area 4 of Brodmann (Figs. 12.3, 12.4, and 20.3). This region is called the *primary motor area (cortex) (MI).* In the last half of the nineteenth century, it was discovered in animal experiments that when the cerebral cortex was stimulated electrically, muscle contractions could most easily (with the weakest current) be elicted from area 4. Later, it was verified that this region in humans is located in the precentral gyrus. It was originally thought that *all* fibers of the pyramidal tract came from area 4, and, furthermore, only from the cells with the largest perikarya, the giant cells of Betz. The number of Betz cells is, however, much too low to account for the number of axons in the pyramidal tract (about 1 million in humans).

Recent studies with retrograde transport of tracer substances have largely clarified the origin of the pyramidal tract in various animals (Fig. 12.3). Findings in the monkey are presumably most relevant for humans.

Figure 12.3 *The central region with MI and SI.* Photomicrograph of a section perpendicular to the central sulcus (monkey). Note the difference in thickness between the MI and the SI. The dark dots in the deep parts of the cortex (in layer 5) are the perikarya of pyramidal tract cells that have been retrogradely labeled by an injection of HRP in the spinal cord. Note also that there are more labeled cells in the MI than in the SI.

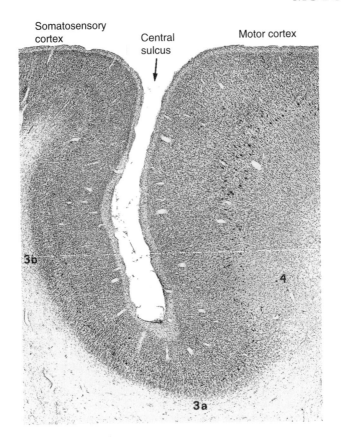

In the monkey, *numerous cells in area 4, in addition to the Betz cells, contribute to the pyramidal tract, as do also many cells in areas outside area 4.* With regard to the relative contribution from various areas, however, the results differ among authors: From less than half to three-fourths of the fibers of the pyramidal tract are reported to come from areas in front of the central sulcus—that is, MI (area 4) and area 6 (PMA and SMA in Fig. 12.7). The rest emanate from areas posterior to the central sulcus: SI (areas 3, 1, 2), SII, and parts of the posterior parietal cortex (area 5) (Figs. 7.20, 20.3, and 20.9). A fairly large proportion of the fibers from SI originate in area 3a (Fig. 12.3), which adjoins area 4 anteriorly (as mentioned in Chapter 7, area 3a is characterized by receiving sensory inputs from proprioceptors). The cell bodies of all neurons of the pyramidal tract lie in the *cortical fifth layer* (lamina 5; compare Figs. 12.3 and 20.2) and are called pyramidal cells. The name refers to the shape of the perikaryon (Figs. 1.1, 20.1, and 20.5). Muscle contractions can be elicited also from the areas outside MI, like SI, by electrical stimulation, but the stimulation has to be more intense than in area MI. This reflects that the pyramidal tract fibers from SI and the other regions outside area 4 have less direct access to the motoneurons than the neurons in area 4. The pyramidal tract fibers coming from SI and area 5 are probably more concerned with the control of sensory signal transmission than with the initiation of movements.

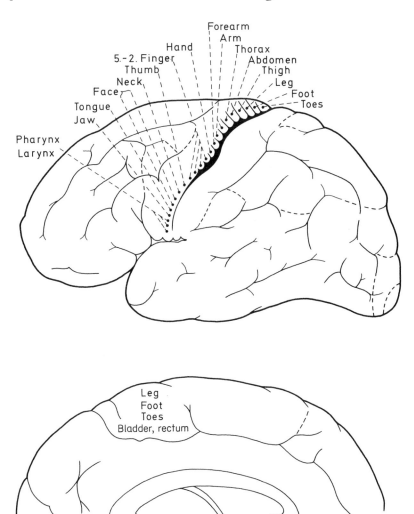

Forearm
Arm
Hand   Thorax
5.-2. Finger   Abdomen
Thumb   Thigh
Neck   Leg
Face   Foot
Tongue   Toes
Jaw
Pharynx
Larynx

Leg
Foot
Toes
Bladder, rectum

Figure 12.4 *The somatotopic organization of the motor cortex*. The points indicate the sites from which muscle contraction in a particular body part was produced by weak electrical stimulation. Based on Foerster (1936).

Electrical stimulation and localized lesions of the precentral gyrus (also in humans) have clarified the *somatotopic localization within MI* (Fig. 12.4). It corresponds closely to the localization in SI (Fig. 7.21).

As mentioned above, the pyramidal tract passes downward through the internal capsule, where it occupies a posterior position (Fig. 12.5). It was formerly assumed that the pyramidal tract fibers were spread over a large part of the "posterior leg" of the internal capsule (as seen in cross section in Figs. 3.30 and 12.5). Observations after small lesions (Fig. 12.9) and stimulation during brain surgery of the internal capsule in humans point to the more restricted region shown in Figure 12.5. Within this region, fibers governing the muscles of the face are believed to lie most anteriorly. Experimental studies in monkeys show that descending fibers from the PMA and supplementary motor area (SMA) are found in the "knee" region (genu) and the "anterior leg" of the internal capsule, respectively.

The internal capsule contains many other fibers than those of the pyramidal tract; the latter constitute only a minority. There are, for example,

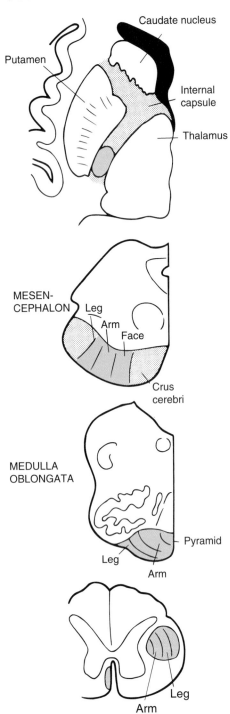

Figure 12.5 *The pyramidal tract*. Its position and somatotopic pattern are illustrated in sections from various levels of the brain stem and the cord. The **uppermost** drawing is of a horizontal section (cf. Fig. 3.28), whereas the other drawings are of transverse sections.

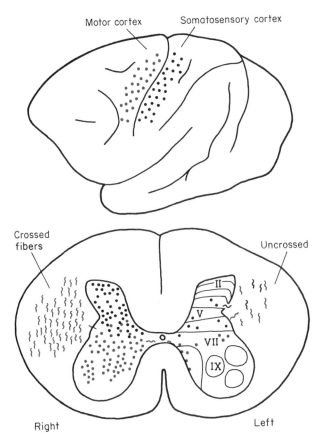

Figure 12.6 *The terminal region of the pyramidal tract*. Based on experiments in monkeys with anterograde transport of radioactively labeled amino acids after injections in various parts of the MI and the SI. Note that corticospinal fibers from the MI end more anteriorly in the gray matter of the cord than those from the SI. The uncrossed fibers end predominantly medially in the ventral horn—that is, in contact with motoneurons supplying axial and proximal muscles. Based on Ralston and Ralston (1985).

sensory fibers ascending from the thalamus to the cortex and descending fibers from the cortex to the reticular formation and other cell groups of the brain stem. In the anterior part of the internal capsule lie the pallidothalamic fibers (related to motor functions of the basal ganglia), and posteriorly (in the lower part) the optic radiation passes through on its way to the occipital lobe. Therefore, damage of the internal capsule—such as an infarction caused by occlusion of an artery—may produce various kinds of sensory deficits in addition to pareses of the muscles of the opposite body half (capsular hemiplegia).

In the *mesencephalon*, the pyramidal tract fibers appear to be spread out over the middle two-thirds of the crus and to be mixed with other fibers (Fig. 12.5). As mentioned, all of the corticospinal fibers are collected within the pyramid at the ventral side of the medulla (Figs. 3.14, 3.16, and 12.5). At the caudalmost level of the medulla, most of the corticospinal fibers cross the midline and continue in the lateral funiculus of the cord as the *lateral corticospinal tract* (Fig. 12.2). A small contingent continues, without crossing, downward in the ventral funiculus as the *ventral corticospinal tract*. Some uncrossed fibers may also pass in the lateral funiculus (Fig. 12.6). The pyramidal tract fibers that control the muscles of the head (the face, tongue, pharynx, and the larynx) leave the corticospinal fibers in the brain stem to end in or close to the motor and sensory cranial nerve nuclei (Fig. 12.2). *Apart from most of the facial muscles, other muscles of the head as a rule receive both crossed and uncrossed pyramidal tract fibers.* Thus, when the pyramidal tract fibers are interrupted in the internal capsule, there are seldom clear-cut pareses of the muscles of the tongue, the pharynx, and the larynx, whereas the corner of the mouth hangs down on the opposite side of the lesion.

Individual Variations of the Human Pyramidal Tract

There are considerable individual variations in both the *distribution* of the pyramidal tract fibers in the spinal white matter and the *percentage of uncrossed* fibers. These clinically important matters were recently reexamined by Nathan and co-workers. They found, for example, that the corticospinal fibers are more widely distributed in the lateral funiculus than usually depicted in textbooks. Thus, such fibers are usually found also ventral to the level of the central canal (Fig. 12.5 is fairly realistic in this respect). Equally important for the interpretation of symptoms in patients with spinal cord injuries is that the anteroposterior location of the whole lateral tract shows considerable individual variations. For example, in some subjects the whole lateral tract is confined to the dorsolateral fasciculus.

Although very rarely, the pyramidal tract can be *completely crossed* with *all* fibers found dorsally in the lateral funiculus, or *completely uncrossed* with all fibers in the ventral funiculus. In most individuals the majority of the corticospinal fibers cross, however, and it is customary to say that 15% of the fibers are uncrossed. The great individual variations emphasize that this is only an average number.

As a rule, most of the uncrossed fibers continue in the ventral funiculus as the ventral corticospinal tract (Fig. 12.5), whereas some join the crossed fibers from the other side in the lateral funiculus (Fig. 12.6). Some fibers cross twice, and many individuals have a small crossed, ventral component. The division of uncrossed fibers between the lateral and the ventral funiculi varies among individuals.

Finally, although usually not acknowledged, in about 75% of the population the *pyramidal tract is asymmetric*—the lateral and the ventral components both being larger on one side than on the other (most often on the right side). This asymmetry presumably arises because a larger proportion of the fibers from (usually) the left hemisphere cross than from the right hemisphere. Thus, the lateral (crossed) tract becomes larger on the right side than on the left, whereas the ventral (uncrossed) tract becomes smaller on the left side.

Such individual variations would influence the severity of motor symptoms after damage to the brain or spinal cord, and may help to explain why symptoms vary so much among patients with very similar lesions. Thus, occasionally an infarct of the internal capsule produces most severe pareses ipsilaterally (on the same side), and lesions of the cord may give motor symptoms that are unexpected from their location.

Termination of the Pyramidal Tract

The pyramidal tract fibers vary considerably in thickness, from the thickest myelinated kind to unmyelinated ones. Most are rather thin, with conduction velocities between 5 and 30 m/sec. In general, the thickest (and thus fastest conducting) fibers come from MI. In accordance with the somatotopic pattern within MI (Fig. 12.4), fibers from the medial parts of the precentral gyrus (leg representation) end in the lumbosacral part of the cord, whereas fibers from more lateral parts (arm representation) end in the cervical and upper thoracic cord.

Fibers from MI and SI also terminate differently in the cord (Fig. 12.6). Thus, fibers from SI end predominantly in the dorsal horn (laminae I–VI), whereas fibers from MI end more ventrally in laminae VII–IX. There are even differences with regard to the projections from individual cytoarchitectonic subdivisions within SI: area 3b—which receives primarily input from cutaneous low-threshold mechanoreceptors—sends fibers primarily to laminae III and IV, which receive the same kind of sensory input as area 3b. Fibers from area 3a end deeper in the dorsal horn, where primary afferents from proprioceptors end. Physiological experiments show that sensory cells in the dorsal horn are influenced from SI. Most often, neurons that are excited from low-threshold mechanoreceptors are inhibited from SI. It may be functionally important to be able to suppress selectively certain kinds of sensory information, for example, during movements.

Anatomic and physiological data show that *some of the pyramidal tract fibers coming from MI end monosynaptically on the motoneurons. This concerns primarily motoneuron groups that control the distal muscles of the extremities, in particular the intrinsic muscles of the hand.* During evolution the pyramidal tract has increased in size and also in the amount of monosynaptic connections with the motoneurons. This has taken place in parallel with increased versatility and precision of the movements of the hand, which are closely related to the increased size of the brain. In the rat and the rabbit, for example, the pyramidal tract is only slightly developed. It is more prominent in the cat, but there are no monosynaptic connections between pyramidal tract neurons in the motor cortex and motoneurons in the cord—all connections are with spinal interneurons. In monkeys, there is a modest proportion of monosynaptic connections, but the proportion is larger in the anthropoid apes (for example, the chimpanzee) and still larger in humans. The monosynaptic motoneuronal connections are of particular importance for the movements that require the highest degree of voluntary control (the least automatic movements) such as independent or fractionated finger movements. This relationship is witnessed by the fact that in certain lower mammals with an exceptional manual dexterity (and the ability to use the fingers individually), some monosynaptic motoneuronal connections are present.

The influence of the pyramidal tract on the muscles of the distal extremities is mediated almost exclusively by fibers that cross in the lower medulla. This is supported by studies in humans with magnetic stimulation of the motor cortex. The small contingent of uncrossed (and doubly crossed) fibers mentioned above can influence only proximal and axial muscles—in particular, muscles of the back, the thorax, and the abdomen. This is in accordance with their termination medially in the ventral horn (Figs. 11.2 and 12.6).

The Pyramidal Tract Fibers May Open and Close Spinal Reflex Arcs

Even in humans, a large proportion of the pyramidal tract fibers end in synaptic contact with interneurons in laminae VII and VIII (Figs. 3.12

and 12.6). Many—perhaps most—of these interneurons make synaptic contacts either on motoneurons or on other interneurons, in their turn contacting motoneurons. In this manner, the pyramidal tract may mediate varied effects on the motoneurons. This concerns not only the α motoneurons but also the γ motoneurons, so that the pyramidal tract can control the sensitivity of the muscle spindle. Because many of the interneurons contacted by pyramidal tract fibers are intercalated in reflex arcs, *the motor cortex can ensure that the various spinal reflexes are adapted to the overall aim of the movements*. For example (as described in Chapter 11), the strength of the long-latency stretch reflex can be increased or decreased depending on what is appropriate during motor learning. The interneurons mediating reciprocal inhibition during stretch reflexes (Fig. 11.10) can also be controlled by the pyramidal tract. Likewise, the Renshaw cells (Fig. 11.11) are subject to supraspinal control, so that the strength of the recurrent inhibition can be increased or decreased selectively in various motoneuronal groups. A final example are interneurons mediating inhibition of motoneurons evoked by stimulation of *tendon organs* (in the same muscle as supplied by the motoneurons). This reflex arc can also be "opened" or "closed" by the pyramidal tract. Thus, this *autogenic inhibition* elicited by stimulation of tendon organs can be reversed to excitation during voluntary contraction of the muscle, (whereas at the same time the inhibition of other muscles may be enhanced).

The Terminal Ramifications and Boutons of Corticospinal Fibers

The terminal ramifications in the cord of single pyramidal tract axons have been visualized by intra-axonal injection of HRP. The injection is done after the axon has been identified physiologically as belonging to a neuron with its perikaryon in the motor cortex. The ramifications of a single pyramidal tract axon can be very widespread, thus contacting many motoneurons in different segments of the cord, supplying several different muscles. This may appear surprising in light of the very discrete and precise movements the pyramidal tract is capable of producing. However, as a rule the various muscles have similar actions—that is, they are synergists. Furthermore, the *strength* of the influence of one pyramidal tract cell probably varies greatly among the motoneurons it contacts, depending on the number and location of synaptic contacts. Thus, pyramidal tract boutons are found both on the cell soma and on the dendrites (even the thin distal parts of the dendrites), and the former exert a stronger influence than the latter on the excitability of the motoneuron. So each pyramidal tract neuron in the motor cortex probably has a powerful influence on some motoneurons but only a weak one on many others.

The *transmitter* used by the pyramidal tract neurons is most likely *glutamate* (with a fast excitatory action). This is indicated by immunocytochemical studies and by physiological experiments. Under the electron microscope, most boutons of the pyramidal tract axons contain round, clear vesicles typical of excitatory synapses. Some boutons, however, contain so-called pleomorphic vesicles, which usually are associated with inhibitory synapses.

The Function of the Pyramidal Tract

As discussed in Chapters 5 and 7, to clarify the role played by a nucleus or a tract we study the synaptic connections and properties of single cells and the symptoms that ensue when the nucleus or tract is eliminated. In humans with lesions of the pyramidal tract, there is usually damage to other structures as well. As is well known, the fibers of the pyramidal tract are fairly isolated only in the pyramid (only very few patients have been described with infarcts limited to the medullary pyramid). In the internal capsule, the mesencephalon (crus), the pons, and in the cord, it is either mixed with or lies in close apposition to other tracts. In monkeys, however, it is possible to cut the pyramidal tract in the pyramid and to control the lesion microscopically later. Thus, the symptoms that occur when only the pyramidal tract is eliminated can be studied. It should be kept in mind, however, that the pyramidal tract is more developed in humans than in monkeys. Thus, the possibility cannot be excluded that symptoms would be somewhat more pronounced in humans after a corresponding lesion (as they are far more pronounced in a monkey than in a cat). Experiments in monkeys nevertheless provide good information about what the main tasks of the pyramidal tract are also in humans.

Shortly after unilateral transection of the pyramid, a monkey can move around apparently normally. Nevertheless, to use the hand to pick up a morsel of food, for example, is almost impossible for some time, even though the hand can be used effectively for climbing. Gradually, over some weeks, the ability to use the hand for grasping objects is regained, but the movements are clumsy and consist only of simultaneous flexion of all fingers (a sort of scraping movement). In the beginning, the fingers cannot be moved independently of the hand, but this improves over time. However, *the ability to move the fingers independently of each other— so-called fractionated movements—does not return* (even after 5 years). The precision grip, in which the thumb opposes the index finger, is permanently lost.

Monkeys in which the pyramid is cut shortly after birth never develop the precision grip. Thus, no other tracts can take over this task from the pyramidal tract. In humans with damage of the motor cortex or the pyramidal tract (often in the internal capsule), the most enduring symptom is difficulty with tasks requiring precise, fractionated finger movements, such as writing, tying shoelaces, buttoning a shirt, and picking up small objects (like a needle). Less precise movements involving larger muscle groups are usually less severely affected. In addition, lesions of the internal capsule in humans produce characteristic changes of muscle tone and reflexes (spasticity), which do not occur in monkeys with lesions restricted to the pyramidal tract. We will return to the symptoms produced by lesions of the descending motor pathways in humans at the end of this chapter.

OTHER DESCENDING PATHWAYS TO THE SPINAL CORD

There are several pathways in addition to the pyramidal tract that mediate impulses from higher levels of the central nervous system to the motoneurons in the cranial nerve nuclei and the spinal cord. The nuclei giving origin to these other tracts are located in the brain stem, but several of them receive afferents from the cerebral cortex—in particular from the motor cortex (Fig. 12.1). Thus, several pathways that are synaptically interrupted in the brain stem transmit impulses from the cortex to the motoneurons. Other cell groups with descending connections to motoneurons are not controlled from the motor cortex and are primarily involved in control of automatic muscle contractions, such as those aiming at maintaining body balance and the movements of locomotion and of respiration.

Broadly speaking, the pyramidal tract is of importance primarily for the least automatic movements—that is, those requiring a high degree of conscious, voluntary attention—whereas the other pathways are important mostly for more automatic movements. This agrees with the fact that the pyramidal tract is of prime importance for the movements of the distal parts of the extremities, whereas the other pathways are more concerned with movements of the proximal parts of the extremities and of the trunk. Such a task division does not imply, however, that these two "systems"—the direct and the indirect corticospinal pathways—operate independently. Most movements—even delicate finger movements—require that the hand is moved to the right position and kept in a specific posture. Furthermore, movements of the arm displace the center of gravity, requiring postural adjustments by many other muscles.

Corticoreticulospinal Tracts

The *reticular formation* is an important source of descending fibers that can influence the motoneurons. The reticular formation is discussed more completely in Chapter 15 (its functions are not restricted to motor control). *Reticulospinal fibers* arise primarily from the reticular formation of the pons and the medulla (Figs. 12.1, 15.1, and 15.7). These areas also receive fibers from the cerebral cortex—*corticoreticular fibers*—in particular from the motor areas (areas 4 and 6). Thus, there is a *corticoreticulospinal pathway* that can mediate signals from the cortical motor areas to the spinal motoneurons (Fig. 15.7).

It is impossible to transect the reticulospinal tracts in the white matter of the cord without at the same time involving other tracts. This has made it difficult to clarify the role of the reticulospinal tracts in control of movements. Nevertheless, experiments with relatively selective lesions of the reticular formation indicate that *the reticulospinal tracts are of importance for maintaining the upright position (posture), for movements that orient the body toward external events, and for fairly crude, stereotyped voluntary movements of the extremities* (such as extending the arm toward an object). The first two kinds are mostly automatic, reflex movements—called *postural reflexes*—that are relatively independent of descending connections to the reticular formation from the cerebral cortex. We will return to the postural reflexes below. Relatively crude, voluntary (less automatic) movements of the extremities, on the other hand, are most likely mediated by pathways from the motor cortex via the reticular formation and the reticulospinal tracts (Fig. 15.7). At least in monkeys, the pyramidal tract is not indispensable for such movements, as described above.

It should be noted that reticulospinal neurons receive inputs from sources besides the motor cortex, such as the vestibular nuclei, the colliculi, and the cerebellum. Thus, many cell groups cooperate to produce the final activity of reticulospinal neurons.

More About Reticulospinal Pathways

The actions in the cord of the reticulospinal fibers are multifarious. In Chapter 7, we described reticulospinal fibers coming from the raphe nuclei (Fig. 15.1) and adjoining parts of the reticular formation in the medulla. These fibers descend in the dorsal part of the lateral funiculus and end in the dorsalmost part of the spinal gray matter (Fig. 7.19), with powerful effects on the central transmission of signals from nociceptors. The reticulospinal fibers that are of interest in relation to motor control terminate more ventrally in the spinal gray matter, with effects on the motoneurons—monosynaptic and polysynaptic via interneurons. These fibers descend in the *ventral part of the lateral funiculus and in the ventral funiculus*. They belong to at least two tracts with different sites of origin in the reticular formation and somewhat different sites of termination in the cord.

Thus, fibers from the *pontine* and *medullary* parts of the reticular formation (Figs. 15.1 and 15.7) run in different parts of the white matter: The pontine fibers are located in the ventral funiculus, whereas the medullary fibers are in the ventral part of the lateral funiculus. The medullary fibers terminate somewhat more laterally in the ventral horn (particularly in lamina VII but to some extent also in lamina IX) than the pontine fibers. The latter terminate mostly more medially in laminae VII and VIII. The *medullary reticulospinal tract may thus be expected to have access to motoneurons innervating muscles of the extremities, whereas the pontine tract reaches mostly motoneurons of axial muscles* (neck, back, and abdomen). Together, reticulospinal fibers terminate in large parts of the ventral horn but primarily in medial parts, where motoneurons to axial muscles and proximal muscles of the extremities are located. Connections are particularly ample to motoneurons innervating neck muscles, which are of importance for movements of the head.

Many of the reticulospinal fibers send collaterals to both cervical and lumbar segments of the cord and often to the ventral horns of both sides. Thus, such neurons are capable of influencing numerous muscles at the same time. This may be functionally meaningful in relation to adjustment of posture and body balance. Nevertheless, there is also some degree of somatotopic organization among reticulospinal neurons, as demonstrated with retrograde axonal transport methods. Also, electrical stimulation of the reticular formation can elicit muscle contractions restricted to smaller parts of the body. Together, these data indicate that *the reticulospinal fibers can mediate both rather diffuse effects on large groups and muscles and more focused influences related to specific, goal-directed movements*.

Both *excitatory and inhibitory effects* on the motoneurons can be elicited by electrical stimulation of the reticular formation. Inhibition of reflex and voluntary movements can be produced by stimulation of a region in the lower part of the medulla (Fig. 12.10), whereas increased reflex movements and muscle tone can be elicited from a more rostral region. The reticulospinal fibers act on both the α *and* γ *motoneurons*. Thus, the reticular formation also controls the sensitivity of the muscle spindles, and in certain situations it is probable that it acts only on the γ motoneurons and not the α motoneurons. There is some evidence that the reticular formation may act selectively on either static or dynamic γ motoneurons.

The Rubrospinal Tract

The *red nucleus* (nucleus ruber) in the mesencephalon (Figs. 3.19 and 3.20) sends fibers to the spinal cord, forming the *rubrospinal tract*. The tract crosses the midline just below the red nucleus and descends in the lateral funiculus, mixed with the fibers of the pyramidal tract. The rubrospinal tract is somatotopically organized. In the cat and the monkey, the fibers terminate in largely the same parts of the spinal gray matter as the pyramidal tract.

The red nucleus receives fibers from the motor cortex of the same side. A pathway is thus established from the cerebral cortex to the spinal motoneurons, which is synaptically interrupted in the red nucleus. The rubrospinal tract has been most studied in the cat and monkey where it exerts its actions primarily on motoneurons supplying distal muscles, like the pyramidal tract. It thus supplements the pyramidal tract in the control of voluntary movements in these animals. Whether the corticorubrospinal tract plays such a role in humans, however, is not certain. Thus, most rubrospinal fibers in monkeys (and presumably also humans) come from the caudal, large-celled or *magnocellular part* of the nucleus, which is very small in humans (it is smaller in monkeys than in cats, and even smaller in humans than in monkeys). In monkeys, the ratio of corticospinal to rubrospinal fibers has been estimated to about 100:1, and this ratio is probably higher in humans. This is a major reason why the functional importance of the human rubrospinal tract is questionable.

When considering the functions of the red nucleus, it should be noted that in monkeys and humans most of the nucleus is made up of fairly small cells, forming the *parvocellular part*. This part receives its main afferents from the *cerebellum* (particularly the dentate nucleus). Many of the efferents from the parvocellular nucleus pass to the inferior olive, which is an important precerebellar nucleus—that is, it sends all its efferent axons to the contralateral cerebellum. Thus, it appears that the *major part of the red nucleus is related to motor functions indirectly via its influence on the cerebellum*. Efferents of the relevant parts of the cerebellum reach the thalamus and in particular the parts projecting to the motor cortical areas (Fig. 14.7). The red nucleus may therefore possibly influence motor control via the effects of the cerebellum on the motor cortex. The caudal, magnocellular part of the red nucleus receives many afferents from the anterior interpositus nucleus of the cerebellum and, as mentioned, projects to the spinal cord (Fig. 14.9). Thus, the information sent to the spinal cord from the motor cortex via the red nucleus is modified by the cerebellum.

The Tectospinal Tract

Several mesencephalic cell groups send axons to the spinal cord. A large number of fibers arise in the *superior colliculus* and form the *tectospinal tract*. The descending fibers cross the midline shortly below the superior colliculus, and most terminate at cervical levels of the cord. The superior colliculus receives numerous fibers from the retina, the visual cortex, and also from the so-called frontal eye field (area 8, Fig. 16.31), which are of particular importance for control of conjugate eye movements. Efferent fibers from the superior colliculus act not only on the cord; motoneurons in the brain stem innervating extraocular muscles are also influenced (although indirectly via the reticular formation). In agreement with these anatomic data, electrical stimulation of the superior colliculus in experimental animals produces coordinated movements of the eyes and the head. The tectospinal tract is of particular importance for *movements of the head and the eyes as parts of optic reflexes*—that is, the head and the eyes are directed toward something in the visual field. (Auditory impulses also reach the superior colliculus via the inferior colliculus and can thus elicit head movements.)

The superior colliculus receives afferents also from nonvisual parts of the cortex, like the SI and MI. Thus, a *corticotectospinal* pathway may also play a role in voluntary movements.

Vestibulospinal Tracts

Primary sensory fibers from the vestibular apparatus terminate in the *vestibular nuclei*, located in the pons and medulla (Fig. 16.16). Vestibular signals directly related to the position and movements of the head also indirectly provide information about the position of the body and about disturbances in balance. Two tracts, issued from the vestibular nuclei to the spinal cord, can contribute to the maintenance of body balance and posture. The largest is the *lateral vestibulospinal tract*, which comes from the lateral vestibular (Deiters) nucleus and reaches all levels of the cord. The tract lies in the ventral funiculus. The fibers exert an excitatory action on both α and γ motoneurons. Like the reticulospinal fibers, the vestibulospinal ones act primarily on motoneurons in the medial parts of the ventral horn—that is, axial muscles and proximal muscles of the extremities. Thus, the *lateral vestibulospinal tract can adjust the contraction of muscles that oppose the force of gravity* (antigravity muscles).

The other vestibulospinal tract is much smaller and reaches only the cervical and upper thoracic segments of the cord. This *medial vestibulospinal* tract is therefore primarily of importance for mediation of reflex head movements in response to vestibular stimuli. This conclusion is also supported by physiological experiments. Unlike the lateral vestibulospinal tract, many of the neurons of the medial tract are inhibitory (probably using glycine as a transmitter).

In contrast to the other cell groups in the brain stem sending fibers to the cord, the vestibular nuclei receive very few afferents from the cerebral cortex. The vestibulospinal neurons are therefore more independent of the cerebral cortex than, for example, the reticulospinal neurons. The vestibular nuclei mediate primarily automatic, reflex movements and adjustments of muscle tone. Nevertheless, the activity of the vestibular nuclei may be influenced indirectly from the cortex, since they receive afferents from the reticular formation. For example, the influence of vision on automatic adjustments of posture appears to be mediated via the vestibular nuclei.

Monoaminergic Pathways from the Brain Stem to the Spinal Cord

Although often included among the reticulospinal pathways, descending monoaminergic fibers to the cord from the raphe nuclei (Fig. 15.5), the nucleus locus coeruleus (Fig. 15.6), and scattered cell groups in their vicinity will be treated separately. Such monoaminergic fibers terminate in the ventral horn (in addition to in the dorsal horn, as described in Chapter 7). Many of the raphespinal fibers contain *serotonin*, whereas the coeruleospinal fibers contain *norepinephrine*. In addition, several peptides coexist with the monoamines. Both these tracts are diffusely distributed in the cord and can hardly mediate information related to specific movements. More likely, they exert general, *widespread facilitatory influences on the motoneurons*, as judged from the effects on spinal motoneurons of microinjections of serotonin and norepinephrine. Thus, the excitability of most motoneurons may be enhanced, so that they react more vigorously to an input from pathways mediating specific motor commands (such as the pyramidal tract). At the same time the descending monoaminergic connections to the dorsal horn may prevent "disturbing" signals from nociceptors from reaching consciousness.

Possibly, these monoaminergic pathways may contribute to the effects of *motivation* on the performance of voluntary movements—the muscle contractions may occur with increased speed and force. This may be related to the ability of the monoamines (serotonin in particular) to alter the excitability of the motoneurons by inducing a so-called *plateau potential*. Thus, serotonin can bring the motoneuron from a state of stable hyperpolarization with low excitability to stable depolarization (plateau potential) with tonic firing. In deep sleep (REM sleep; see Chapter 15), all movements are suppressed while the descending monoaminergic neurons show their lowest activity.

CONTROL OF AUTOMATIC MOVEMENTS

Postural Reflexes—An Overview

As mentioned above, the reticulospinal and vestibulospinal tracts mediate automatic, reflex muscle contractions that contribute to maintaining the upright position. We will now describe in more detail such reflexes, collectively called *postural reflexes*, and their overall control by higher levels of the central nervous system. (In Chapter 11 we made some comments on the role of stretch reflexes in postural tasks.)

The *tasks of these reflexes* are to maintain an appropriate posture of the body, to help regain equilibrium when it is disturbed, and to ensure optimal starting positions for the execution of specific movements. Postural reflexes produce the automatic movements that help us to regain equilibrium quickly, for example, when slipping on ice. It is a common experience that these compensatory movements happen so rapidly that only afterwards are we aware of which movements we performed.

The most important *receptors* for postural reflexes are the vestibular receptors in the inner ear, proprioceptors close to the upper cervical joints, and vision. Here, we will go more into the *overall control* of posture and balance.

The postural reflexes are difficult to study when the nervous system is functioning normally, and many parts from the cord to the cerebral cortex all cooperate in the production of movements. By transection of all descending tracts from higher levels (the cerebral cortex in particular) to the brain stem in animals, however, a condition with greatly exaggerated postural reflexes ensues. This is called *decerebrate rigidity* and is characterized by increased tone in the antigravity muscles—primarily extensors. In particular, two postural reflexes have been much studied, the *neck and labyrinthine reflexes*, which are elicited by stimulation of proprioceptors around the upper cervical joints and vestibular receptors, respectively.

Generally speaking, the *labyrinthine reflexes serve to keep the position of the head constant. The neck reflexes, on the other hand, serve to keep the position of the body constant in relation to the head.* The latter is a prerequisite for the labyrinthine reflexes to function properly; the vestibular apparatus can provide information only about the position of the head in space and not about its position relative to that of the body. Thus, *the labyrinthine reflexes work on the assumption that the head has a constant position relative to the body; this is ensured by the neck reflexes.*

As mentioned, in animals with an intact nervous system, many cell groups and tracts are of importance for the final muscle activity, and the postural reflexes are but one aspect of motor control. During voluntary movements, the postural reflexes—just like many other reflexes—can be suppressed or facilitated depending on what is appropriate for the task. After damage to higher levels of the central nervous system in humans,

Decerebrate Rigidity

In animals with transection of the brain stem just below the red nucleus (Figs. 3.19 and 12.1), the postural reflexes occur in an exaggerated and caricatured manner. As a result of loss of signals from higher levels, the animal persists in a state of increased extensor tone. Thus, such an animal—although deeply unconscious—can stand (with some support) with extended legs and the head and tail lifted. The animal is unable to walk, however, and, once fallen, it cannot get back on its feet. The animal does not die immediately from such *decerebration* because the control of respiration and circulation can be carried out by the lower brain stem independent of higher levels of the nervous system. The condition is called *decerebrate rigidity*. The name may seem misleading. There are no similarities to the condition called rigidity in clinical neurology, in which rigidity means the increased muscle tone in parkinsonism. There are, however, some similarities between decerebrate rigidity in animals and spasticity as occurring in humans after lesions of central motor pathways (see Chapter 11, *Changes of Muscle Tone in Disease*). In spasticity there may also be increased muscle tone in the extensor muscles of the legs (and in the flexor muscles of the arms, which in a sense may be regarded as postural muscles in humans).

The continuously increased muscle tension in decerebrate rigidity is caused by increased activity of motoneurons, but which nuclei and tracts are responsible? The *vestibular nuclei* and the *vestibulospinal tract* must contribute, since destruction of the lateral vestibular nucleus reduces the rigidity, whereas electrical stimulation of the nucleus increases it. In addition, the *reticular formation* and *reticulospinal tracts* play an important role. Since the corticobulbar and corticospinal neurons are excitatory, they must to a large extent influence neuronal groups in the brain stem that inhibit the vestibulospinal and reticulospinal neurons. The inhibitory region of the reticular formation in the lower medulla (Fig. 15.8) seems to be of particular importance in this connection. When this region loses its excitatory input from the cerebral cortex, the result is reduced inhibition of descending excitatory connections to the cord, producing increased α motoneuron firing. Since cutting the dorsal roots reduces or abolishes the decerebrate rigidity, the increased α motoneuron activity must also depend on increased muscle spindle afferent firing. This must be caused by increased firing of the γ motoneurons. Since increased activity of γ motoneurons plays a significant role, the decerebrate rigidity is also termed a γ rigidity (to distinguish it from α rigidity, in which there is no increased γ activity).

The *cerebellum* also influences the decerebrate rigidity in animals. Thus, electrical stimulation of the "spinal" parts of the cerebellum reduces the rigidity. This is because this part of the cerebellum sends inhibitory connections to the lateral vestibular nucleus.

however, the postural reflexes may be seen in exaggerated forms. In brain damaged infants, in particular, the postural reflexes may not be integrated in coordinated movement programs but are elicited in isolation, thereby disturbing normal movements.

Neck and Labyrinthine Reflexes

Studies of decerebrate animals have elucidated the postural reflexes, in particular the neck and labyrinthine reflexes. The latter reflexes, described below, may be either *tonic* or *phasic*. A phasic neck or labyrinthine reflex consists of a rapid, transient change of muscle tension in postural muscles as a response to a change of posture (usually a disturbance of the equilibrium). In a tonic reflex, the change of muscle tension lasts as long as the new position is maintained. Different receptors are responsible for evoking the neck and the labyrinthine reflexes.

In the *neck reflexes*, the response is a change of muscle tension—especially in the extremities—induced by a change in the position of the head relative to the body (such movements take place primarily in the upper cervical joints). To demonstrate clearly the neck reflexes in a decerebrate animal, the vestibular receptors must have been eliminated. When then the head is bent backward (extension of the neck), the muscle tension is increased in the extensor muscles of the forelimbs and decreased in the extensors of the hindlimbs. Forward bending of the head (flexion) induces the opposite pattern of changes (extension of the hindlimbs and flexion of the forelimbs). Tilting the head sideways increases the extensor tone on the same side and reduces it on the other side, as does turning the head sideways. These changes of the muscle tone aim at reestablishing the position of the body relative to the head. The receptors for these reflexes are located near the upper cervical joints, since they disappear after transection of the upper three cervical dorsal roots. Muscle spindles are the most likely candidates, but joint receptors may also contribute. The reflex center is located in the medulla, and the effects on the motoneurons are most likely mediated by both the reticulospinal and vestibulospinal tracts.

The functional role of the neck reflexes cannot be understood when observed in isolation; only in conjunction with the *labyrinthine reflexes* are their effects appropriate for the whole body. The labyrinthine reflexes are elicited by stimulation of the sensory receptors of the semicircular ducts and the utriculus of the labyrinth, which record the movements and the position of the head. To demonstrate clearly the labyrinthine reflexes, the neck reflexes must have been eliminated by cutting the upper dorsal roots (in a decerebrate animal). It then appears that the *effects produced by the labyrinthine reflexes are the opposite of those of the neck reflexes when the latter act alone*. Thus, bending the head backward elicits flexion of the forelimbs and extension of the hindlimbs, and vice versa when the head is bent forward. The purpose of these changes of muscle tone is to bring the head back to the position held before the movement—that is, to keep the position of the head in space constant. Provided the neck reflexes ensure that the body is kept in a constant position relative to the head, the labyrinthine reflexes will serve to maintain not only the position of the head in space but also the upright position of the whole body. The labyrinthine reflexes are shown clearly when the experimental animal stands on a platform that can be tilted in various directions. Tilting the platform forward increases the extensor tone in the forelimbs and decreases the tone in the hindlimbs. Tilting the platform sideways increases the muscle tone in the extensors on the side to which the tilt is directed. Both responses are obviously appropriate for the maintenance of body balance. When the platform is moved quickly in one direction and then back, the reflex response is transient (phasic reflex). When the platform is maintained in the new position, the altered muscle tone is upheld (tonic reflex). Vestibulospinal tracts are the most likely candidates for mediation of the labyrinthine reflexes (other reflexes are also elicited by stimulation of the labyrinth, as described in Chapter 16).

The neck reflexes are necessary because, as mentioned, the position of the head in space depends not only on the position of the body but also on the position of the head relative to the body. The vestibular receptors in the labyrinth can only inform about the position of the head in space, but since the neck receptors inform about the position of the head relative to the body, all necessary information is available to the central nervous system. When both reflexes work together in an intact organism, backward bending of the head, for example (with movement taking place only in the upper cervical joints and no change of body position), produces no change in muscle tension of the extremities. The tendency of the labyrinthine reflexes to produce forelimb flexion and hindlimb extension is canceled by the opposite tendency of the neck reflexes. On the other hand, when the same movement of the head is produced by a backward movement of the whole body (with no movement of the head relative to the body, like a horse that is rearing), the labyrinthine reflexes act alone to produce extension of the hindlimbs and flexion of the forelimbs. Another example is an animal standing on a platform tilting forward with no movement of the head taking place relative to the body. In that case the labyrinthine reflexes produce forelimb extension and hindlimb flexion. This is an appropriate response to maintain balance when standing on a downhill slope. If, on the other hand, the position of the head in space is kept constant and the body moved in relation to the head, the neck reflexes act alone. An example is a cat jumping down from a table: The neck is extended (keeping the head position fairly constant), producing extension of the forelimbs, which is appropriate for landing.

Other Postural Reflexes

We will now describe a few other reflexes that contribute to the maintenance of body equilibrium. An *unexpected fall* from some height elicits a contraction of the muscles of the leg as an appropriate preparation to the landing. The contraction begins about 75 msec after start of the fall and can therefore occur before landing (and thus before a stretch reflex can be elicited). The latency is also too short for the contraction to be voluntary. Animal experiments indicate that the receptors of this reflex are located in the labyrinth (probably in the macula sacculi, Figs. 16.10 and 16.11).

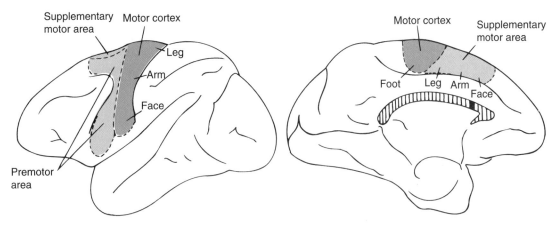

Figure 12.7 *The motor and the premotor areas.* The positions of MI, SMA, and PMA are shown in a drawing of the left hemisphere of a monkey.

Visual impulses also contribute to adjustment of muscle tone with the purpose of maintaining the equilibrium of the body. Experiments with humans standing on a platform that can be moved unexpectedly indicate that the muscle contractions in response to a movement of the platform depend on whether the subject can see that the body moves in relation to the surroundings. If the experimental setup is such that it appears as though the surroundings do not move (that is, they are made to move in the same direction as the head), the earliest reflex contractions of the legs are weaker than when the sense of vision also informs about the movement. With monkeys also the earliest muscle response is much weaker when visual information about the unexpected movement is excluded. We do not know which pathways are used by the visual impulses that influence the postural reflexes, but vestibulospinal pathways are probably of importance.

The *grasp reflex* is usually regarded as one of the postural reflexes. It is normally expressed only in infants during the first six months and has disappeared at twelve months. It consists of the fingers firmly grasping an object that touches the palm. The purpose of this reflex is to ensure that the baby can cling to the mother, but whereas this is of vital importance for monkeys, the reflex has lost much of its importance in humans. After damage of the frontal lobes (presumably in particular the so-called supplementary motor area, SMA; Fig. 12.7), the reflex may reappear in adults. The strength of the grasp reflex depends on the position of the body, reflecting that its purpose is to cling to the mother when she moves about (thus, the reflex is of less functional importance in humans than in monkeys).

Control of Locomotor Movements

The upright locomotion of man requires somewhat different movements than in animals walking on four legs. We should also keep in mind that the large size of the human brain has enabled many processes—which in lower animals are controlled from the spinal cord and the brain stem—to be controlled from the cerebral cortex. Nevertheless, with regard to basic mechanisms, the neural control of locomotion is probably very similar in humans and in other mammals. The following account is largely based on data obtained from animal experiments.

Fairly normal locomotion can be produced in animals (like cats) even when the spinal cord is isolated from the brain stem and the brain. This can be observed on a treadmill when the paws touch the moving ground (the animal has to be supported since there are no postural reflexes). Central rhythm generators must, therefore, exist in the cord, able to produce rhythmic, alternating leg movements in the absence of any command signals from higher levels. The rhythm generators consist of fairly complicated networks of interneurons with excitatory and inhibitory interconnections, eventually controlling the activity of the motoneurons. Some of the neurons within the network appear to have pacemaker properties; that is, they fire brief trains of action potentials with silent periods between, without receiving a rhythmically alternating input.

The rhythm generator is not dependent on sensory input from the moving parts to produce the motoneuron activity typical of locomotion. Thus, the rhythmic motoneuronal activity continues even after complete paralysis of the muscles (for example, after cutting of the ventral roots). This is called *fictive locomotion*, and the pattern of motoneuronal activity is strikingly similar to that observed during normal walking in intact animals.

This does not mean, however, that sensory inputs are without significance for locomotor control. The activity of the rhythm generators can indeed be modified by afferent signals from the peripheral receptors providing information about how the movements are proceeding. Inhibitory interneurons can contribute to the rhythmic pattern of activity by inhibiting the antagonists when the agonists have reached their maximal activity. *Renshaw cells* (Fig. 11.11) can probably also contribute by shortening impulse trains from the motoneurons and at the same time increasing the excitability of antagonist motoneurons.

There is probably one rhythm generator for each extremity. Long propriospinal fibers that interconnect the forelimb and hindlimb generators ensure that their activities are coordinated. The presence of *rhythm generators in the human* spinal cord is indicated by the occurrence of locomotionlike movements in anencephalic infants (born without most of the brain). In normal infants, walking movements of the legs can be elicited in the first few months (if the infant is held under the arms and the feet are made to touch the floor). This ability usually disappears, to reappear when the infant starts to crawl at about 8 months.

Several central cell groups contribute to the *control of the spinal rhythm generators*. Three regions have been identified physiologically in the brain stem: one in the so-called subthalamic region, one in the mesencephalic reticular formation, and one region in the pons. Continuous (nonrhythmic) stimulation of any of these regions can produce slow, walking movements in experimental animals. Most likely, the effects on spinal motoneurons from these regions are mediated by reticulospinal fibers, since they are abolished by cutting the ventral and ventrolateral funiculi. Furthermore, many reticulospinal neurons are rhythmically active in pace with walking movements. The connections of these locomotor regions, however, are not well known.

Connections from the cerebral cortex (especially the pyramidal tract) are of increasing importance for the control of locomotion as the ground becomes more uneven and unpredictable—that is, as each step has to be controlled individually. Thus, after destruction of the motor cortex, cats can still walk fairly normally on an even surface but are helpless when required to walk along a ladder or a narrow bar.

MOTOR CORTICAL AREAS AND THE CONTROL OF VOLUNTARY MOVEMENTS

Overview

As mentioned in the introduction to this chapter, there is no sharp division between the motor centers and other parts of the central nervous system. This is true also for the cerebral cortex. Improved methods have shown that large parts of the cortex are activated even in relation to a simple movement. When sensitive methods are used to record the electrical activity over the brain of a person asked to perform a simple flexion—extension movement of a finger, changes of activity over large parts of both hemispheres first occur. This is a slowly rising negative wave—a so-called *readiness potential*—starting about 850 msec before the movement. Approximately 60 msec before the movement, the activity is concentrated over the arm region of the motor cortex (on the side opposite the moving fingers). Studies of monkeys with implanted microelectrodes have shown that not only the cerebral cortex is activated before a voluntary movement; there is also increased neuronal activity in the cerebellum, the basal ganglia, the thalamus, and parts of the limbic structures. Thus, many parts of the brain cooperate in deciding and planning movements.

The decision as to whether a cytoarchitectonic cortical area (such as area 4) should be termed a "motor area," is to some extent arbitrary. New findings also neccessitate revision of former classifications. Thus, some of the motor areas—formerly thought to represent one functional unit—are now known to consist of several subunits. Since, in addition, the contribution of each area to overall control of movement is incompletely known, this is a difficult field to review.

The regions defined today as motor are largely confined to the cytoarchitectonic *areas 4 and 6* of the frontal lobe (Figs. 12.4 and 20.3). The *MI* (area 4) in the precentral gyrus has a special position, because it excerts the most direct and powerful effects on the motoneurons.[1] Thus, most or all corticospinal fibers ending monosynaptically on the motoneurons have their perikarya in area 4. Accordingly, the threshold for eliciting movements by electrical stimulation is lower here than in any other part of the cortex. (Near the end of the last century electrical stimulation of area 4 in dogs produced the first firm evidence of specializations within the cerebral cortex. Before that, the existence of functional localization in the cerebral cortex was hotly debated.) Furthermore, lesions of the MI produce clear-cut pareses, in contrast to lesions of other cortical regions.

Although several distinct motor areas are found within *area 6*, two main subdivsions are usually recognized: the medially situated *SMA*, and the lateral *PMA*.[2] Besides sending fibers to the spinal cord—thus contributing to the corticospinal tract—both the SMA and PMA send many fibers to the MI. They can therefore act on motoneurons in two fairly direct ways. Usually, however, the effect on MI has been considered most important, and consequently the SMA and PMA are often placed above the MI in a *hierarchy* of motor areas. Thus, SMA and PMA—sometimes termed *supramotor* areas—are believed to instruct the MI of what to do. Several observations support this assumption, for example that they usually become active in advance of MI during voluntary movements.

Clinical observations of patients with complete or partial lesions suggest that SMA and PMA are important for *precise movements of the hand, especially performance of rhythmic sequences* (there are no pareses). A pianist suffering from such a lesion could no longer play because he was unable to keep even intervals betwen the key strokes. The Russian neuroscientist Luria used the term *loss of movement melodies* to describe such symptoms. Among typical symptoms are, furthermore, difficulties with coordination of bilateral movements—such as swinging the arms in opposite directions.

Much is yet to be learned, however, before we have a full understanding of the roles of the PMA and SMA in motor control. Thus, recent studies show that both areas consist of subdivisions with different connections and single unit properties. For example, one part of SMA appears to be supramotor, whereas another probably operates in parallel with MI. We will discuss SMA and PMA in more depth below, after treating the organization and functions of MI.

The Primary Motor Area

The MI receives main afferents from SI (areas 3, 1, 2), SII, area 5, and area 6, in addition to afferents from "motor" parts of the thalamus (the ventrolateral nucleus, VL; Figs. 7.20 and 14.14). The cerebellum especially, sends important information about movement performance to MI via VL.

As mentioned above, many of the pyramidal tract fibers originate in the MI. It should be realized, however, that not all effects produced by stimulation of the MI are mediated by the pyramidal tract. Thus, *many efferent fibers from the MI reach other cortical areas and several subcortical nuclei involved in motor control*, such as the red nucleus, the reticular formation, the basal ganglia, and brain stem nuclei, which project to the cerebellum. Nevertheless, the movements evoked by very weak electrical stimulation of the motor cortex are mediated by the pyramidal tract. Such movements occur in the opposite body half and can be limited to a few muscles in distal parts of the extremities and the face. With increasing stimulus strength, more muscles are recruited, and also more proximal ones. As with SI, *a disproportionally large part of the MI is devoted to control of the hand* (especially the thumb and the index finger) and the lips and the tongue (Fig. 12.8). In comparison, very small parts of the MI contain neurons controlling muscles of the back and the abdomen. How many cortical neurons are related to the motor control of a

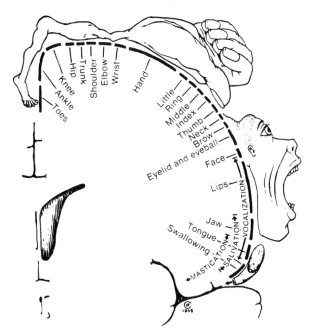

Figure 12.8 *The relative size of the regions of the MI representing various body parts.* Based on electrical stimulation of the exposed human MI. From Penfield and Rasmussen (1950).

particular body part depends on the variety and precision of the movements rather than on the size of the part.

The so-called Jackson epileptic fits (described in Chapter 7) illustrate the *somatotopic pattern within the MI.* The abnormal discharges of the neurons start at one site in the MI and spread out in a regular manner. Thus, the muscular cramps start in one part of the body—for example, the foot—and spread to the lower leg, then to the thigh, the abdomen, the shoulder, and so forth. Nearly always, the fits start around the mouth, in the tongue, the thumb, or the big toe. This is best explained by the fact that cortical neurons controlling these parts occupy the largest volume of the MI, and also have the largest proportion of monosynaptic corticomotoneuronal connections.

Muscles that are often used simultaneously on both sides of the body, like the muscles of the back and the abdomen, can be relatively easily activated on both sides (bilaterally) by stimulation of the MI of one side. Movements of the fingers, however, can only be evoked on the opposite (contralateral) side by stimulation of the MI, which reflects that the fingers are used independently and usually differently on the two sides. The anatomic basis of this is the complete crossing of the pyramidal tract fibers controlling distal muscles, mentioned earlier. Similar conditions are found for the commissural fibers interconnecting the MI of the two hemispheres: Only parts of the MI representing the trunk and the proximal parts of the extremities are interconnected. The large areas representing the distal muscles are devoid of commissural connections, presumably as an expression of the independent use of the two hands (Fig. 20.11).

Many cells in the MI become active (or increase their firing frequency) immediately before a voluntary movement starts, as shown with *microelectrode recordings.* In contrast, most cells in the SI become active after movement onset, indicating that they are activated by sensory signals from the moving parts but do not contribute to the initiation of the movement. Some pyramidal tract neurons (corticospinal neurons) increase their activity only in relation to the start of a movement, whereas others are active during the whole movement. The firing frequency of some neurons is related to the force of muscular contraction. In the MI of a relaxed monkey sitting quietly waiting for a signal to move, some corticospinal neurons fire continuously (that is, they are tonically active). This probably means that the motor cortex not only initiates and controls movements but also determines the "readiness" of selected motoneuronal groups by keeping them slightly depolarized (below the threshold for initiation of action potentials). This enables the motoneurons to respond more quickly to a "go" signal from the motor cortex, or from subcortical levels, such as the reticular formation, the vestibular nuclei, and sensory signals through the dorsal roots (for example, from muscle spindles).

At the same time as a corticospinal neuron has excitatory effects on motoneurons of synergistic muscles, *motoneurons of antagonistic muscles are inhibited* (via inhibitory interneurons).

Functional Organization of the Primary Motor Area

Focusing on the properties of single cells led to the view that pyramidal tract neurons were collected in groups controlling muscles around single joints (somewhat like the arrangement in the spinal cord where motoneurons are collected in groups related to single muscles; see Figure 11.2). However, further studies have not supported this interpretation. Thus, pyramidal tract neurons controlling motoneurons of one muscle are as a rule spread out over a relatively large cortical area (although respecting the rough somatotopic pattern shown in Figs. 12.4 and 12.8). Within, for example, the motor hand region, pyramidal tract neurons controlling different joints of the hand are intermingled. Thus, every small patch of the motor cortex would contain neurons controlling several different muscles. We also know that each pyramidal tract axon acts on more than one muscle (although with a stronger action on some than on others). Therefore, the explanation why we *can* do isolated movements of single joints cannot be that each pyramidal tract neuron is specified for one movement only. *A particular movement is specified by the collective activity of a large neuronal population*, rather than by a narrow tuning of a few neurons. Furthermore, such *populations appear to be related to initiation of purposeful movements involving several joints*, rather than to isolated, single-joint movements (consider how seldom our movements involve one joint only). In other words, the motor cortex is organized to optimize the performance of *tasks*, not to control individual muscles or joints. As an example, destruction of the cat's motor cortex does not affect single joint movements but complex, multi-joint movements, such as stretching the paw toward a goal.

We do not fully understand how the appropriate *corticospinal neurons are selected to produce a certain movement*. We do know, however, that the selection has to involve afferent connections to the MI from other cortical areas and from the thalamus. Cortical connections arise in parts of the *prefrontal cortex*, in the *SMA and PMA*, and in the *posterior parietal cortex* (see below). The decision to initiate a particular movement is certainly not made in the MI, neither is it likely to be related to activity in a particular cell group. In Chapter 8 we discussed that conscious, cognitive processes are expressions of activity in distributed networks of cortical neurons. The wide distribution of the readiness potential preceding movement initiation supports this view.

Several observations show that the selection of corticospinal neurons to be used can be extremely precise and varied. In the first place, one corticospinal neuron can be active when a certain hand muscle is used for a precision grip, whereas it is much less active or inactive when the muscle is used for a more crude grasping movement. Other corticospinal neurons must therefore be responsible for producing the required force from the muscle in the latter situation. Second, human subjects can quickly learn to recruit one specific motor unit among many others when allowed to see the EMG pattern of the muscle (biofeedback). This must be caused by an almost incredible ability to focus excitation from the motor cortex on certain spinal motoneurons. Considering the precision of movements required of a violinist, a watchmaker, or a neurosurgeon, the above observations become perhaps less surprising.

The Supplementary Motor Area

Located in front of the MI on the medial side of the hemisphere (Fig. 12.7), the SMA sends fibers to both the spinal cord and the reticular formation. Thus, the SMA contributes to both direct and indirect corticospinal pathways. The SMA also, however, sends many fibers to the MI, and this pathway is probably most important for its influence on motor control. This assumption is primarily based on results obtained by microelectrode recordings in monkeys showing the properties of single cells and on measurements of blood flow and metabolic activity in the human cerebral cortex. Afferents to the SMA come from—among other sources—the prefrontal association cortex (Fig. 20.13)

The neuronal activity in the SMA of humans appears to increase especially in relation to somewhat complex movements. When, for example, a person executes a series of simple flexion—extension movements of a finger, the activity is increased mainly in the MI hand area, not in the SMA. When the task is to perform a series of different movements in a specified sequence, however, there is also increased activity in the SMA. It appears that the activity increases first in the SMA and then in the MI. Increased activity in the SMA is not related to the movement itself, since it is sufficient that the person *imagines* the performance of a fairly complex movement. In such cases there is no increase of activity in the MI, which fits with the notion that the MI is instrumental in initiating the movement.

Damage of the SMA in monkeys produces striking difficulties with the simultaneous use of both hands to solve a task. When a piece of food is stuck in a hole in a Plexiglas plate, a normal monkey easily retrieves it by pushing with one finger from above and collecting the piece with the other hand from below. After damage to the SMA, both hands are used for pushing from above.

Recording of single-cell activity in the SMA has shown that many cells change their activity in relation to a sensory stimulus (light, passive movements, and so forth) that the animal knows is a signal to start a certain voluntary movement. SMA neurons respond to a visual stimulus, for example, only when the stimulus is connected with a movement response, and the SMA cells respond earlier than those in the MI.

Observations of the kinds discussed above have led to the suggestion that the *SMA is important for organizing and planning fairly complex movements and for mediating an appropriate motor response to sensory stimuli.* That the grasp reflex is disturbed (in adults it reappears) after damage to the SMA may possibly be explained by a disruption of normal integration of sensory stimuli and motor responses.

The Premotor Area

The PMA occupies the largest part of area 6 on the convexity of the hemisphere (Fig. 12.7). Like the SMA, the PMA receives its most important afferents from the prefrontal cortex, although not from identical parts. The PMA probably sends fewer fibers to the spinal cord than the SMA but has strong connections with the reticular formation, the red nucleus, the basal ganglia, and, indirectly, with the cerebellum. As with the SMA, however, the connections from the PMA to the MI are probably those most directly related to the motor functions of the PMA. Experiments in monkeys indicate that the *PMA is important for the control of visually guided movements*, such as the proper orientation of the hand and fingers when they approach an object to be grasped. Monkeys with lesions of the PMA also have difficulties with moving the hand around a transparent obstacle to reach an object: They persistently use the direct approach, bumping into the obstacle. After damage to the MI, the handling of an object is clumsy and insecure, but the ability to avoid an obstacle is not lost. Connections from the extrastriate areas in the occipital lobe to the PMA are necessary for the ability to perform such circumventive goal-directed movements.

In agreement with the above observations, *single-cell recordings* show that many cells in the PMA change their activity about 60 msec after a light signal that the monkey is trained to respond to with a certain movement. The activity of the PMA neurons continues until just before the movement starts, even when the monkey is trained to wait for many seconds after the signal before actually performing the movement.

Damage of the PMA often produces a peculiar tendency to continue a certain movement when first started, even though the movement is unsuccessful in achieving its goal. Thus, when the hand in one of the examples mentioned above bumps into an obstacle (in this case a transparent plate), the monkey nevertheless repeats the same movement over and over. This phenomenon is called *perseveration* and can occur also in humans after damage to the frontal lobes.

The Posterior Parietal Cortex and Voluntary Movements

Area 5 is of particular importance for processing somatosensory information (received from SI), whereas area 7 also receives information from visual cortical areas (Figs. 20.9 and 20.10). Many neurons in these areas are active in relation to movements, as shown by Mountcastle and others. One kind of neuron is active before *goal-directed, reaching movements*, such as when a monkey stretches its hand toward a banana. Such neurons do not become active, however, in relation to a movement in the same direction but without a specific aim, or in relation to a passive movement. Other kinds of neurons increase their activity in relation to *exploratory hand movements*, such as when a monkey studies a foreign object.

In area 7, some neurons increase their activity only when the monkey stretches the hand toward an object that it also looks at. Since there are ample connections from the posterior parietal cortex to the SMA and PMA (Fig. 20.12), it is likely that the behavior of cells in these motor areas is in part determined by the posterior parietal cortex.

Indeed, *damage to the posterior parietal cortex* also produces *motor disturbances*. There are no pareses, however, but rather difficulties with the execution of more complex movements. Thus, in humans, lesions of the posterior parietal cortex may, for example, make them unable to open a door or to handle previously familiar tools like a screwdriver or a can opener. Such persons also have difficulties with proper orientation of the hand in relation to an object, and they easily miss an object even though they see it clearly. This kind of symptom is called *apraxia* (see also Chapter 20). Interestingly, similar symptoms may occur after lesions of the frontal lobes in front of the MI in humans—presumably reflecting the intimate connections between the posterior parietal cortex and the frontal lobes.

SYMPTOMS CAUSED BY INTERRUPTION OF CENTRAL MOTOR PATHWAYS

The term *central pareses* is used for pareses that are caused by interruption of the central motor pathways conducting impulses from the cerebral

A

B

Figure 12.9 *Infarction in the internal capsule with degeneration of the pyramidal tract.* From a 19-year-old man who suddenly became hemiplegic, probably due to occlusion of a brain artery by an embolus from the heart. **A**. Drawing of a horizontal CT showing the localization of the infarction in the posterior limb of the internal capsule (cf. Fig. 12.5). Seven months after the stroke, the lesion measured 5 × 16 mm. **B**. Frontal MRI 4 months after the stroke, with the degenerated pyramidal tract (**arrowheads**) shown as whitish. It can be followed from the internal capsule through the pons and into the medulla. Immediately after the stroke the patient had pareses on the right side, most marked for finger movements. He recovered completely. PET studies in this patient after recovery showed that finger movements of the right hand were associated with increased activity in the left motor cortex and PMA, and bilaterally in the SMA, cingulate gyrus, and the insula (in normal controls only the motor cortex showed increased activity with isolated finger movements). The patient made involuntary mirror movements of the left fingers when using the right ones. From Danek et al. (1990). Reproduced with permission from Oxford University Press.

cortex (especially the MI) to the motoneurons. Only the pyramidal tract goes directly; the other pathways are indirect, with synaptic interruption in the brain stem. We have discussed above that the various pathways take care of somewhat different aspects of motor control. The term *upper motor syndrome* is often used for the clinical picture resulting from interruption of the central motor pathways, to differentiate it from the *lower motor syndrome* (peripheral pareses) resulting from destruction of the motoneurons (including their axons). Even though central pareses can be produced by lesions located anywhere between the motor cortex and the motoneurons, the commonest cause is interruption of the descending fibers by bleeding or a thrombosis in the internal capsule (Fig. 12.9). The pareses then affect the muscles of the opposite half of the body (hemipareses, hemiplegia). The term *capsular hemiplegia* is commonly used for this condition.

The pareses in capsular hemiplegia are clearly different from peripheral pareses. Thus, the motoneurons are not put out of action and can still be activated by impulses through the dorsal roots from various receptors.

Figure 12.10 *Hemiplegia of the left side*. Note the characterstic position of the arm with flexion in the elbow and wrist. The paretic leg is moved laterally in a semicircle during the swing phase to keep the foot off the ground (circumduction).

They can also be influenced by fibers descending from cell groups in the brain stem, such as the reticular formation and the vestibular nuclei. Stretch reflexes may be consequently elicited, and there is not a marked wasting of the muscles. Immediately after the stroke causing the capsular hemiplegia, the stretch reflexes are weak or absent, but within weeks or months they increase in strength and become stronger on the paretic than on the normal side (hyperreflexia). Typically, the increased reflex response is seen primarily when muscles are stretched rapidly; usually there is no increased muscle tone when judged by slow stretching. In certain muscles, however, even the resting tone may be increased, with a characteristic distribution (Fig. 12.10): In the arm the increased tone affects the flexors so that the arm is kept flexed at the elbow, whereas the extensors of the leg are affected (central pareses due to destruction in the spinal cord of motor pathways result in increased resting tone of flexors also in the leg). This condition with changed resting tone and increased phasic stretch reflexes is usually called *spasticity* (see also Chapter 11 for a discussion of altered muscle tone in disease). The most *constant and characteristic feature of spasticity is the velocity-dependent increased strength of stretch reflexes*, and some authors limit the definition of spasticity to this. Others use the term primarily for the characteristically increased resting tone in flexors of the arm and in extensors of the leg.

One important feature of central pareses, when compared with peripheral ones, is that the velocity with which voluntary movements can be performed is reduced more than the isometric force (that is, speed of movements is reduced more than strength). This phenomenon is called *retardation* of movements. It concerns particularly fine finger movements and movements of the lips and tongue, whereas larger movements are less severely affected. Writing, tying, buttoning, and similar movements may be impossible for a patient with capsular hemiplegia, or the movements are performed only very slowly and clumsily. The *fatigability* is also abnormally great—that is, the muscular force drops quickly when a voluntary movement is repeated several times. The patient also experiences a dramatic increase in the *mental effort* needed for voluntary movements: Movements that before the stroke required no mental effort can afterwards only be performed with the utmost concentration and strain.

Changes in the *contractile properties* of the paretic muscles have also been found in hemiplegic patients. Thus, in the intrinsic muscles of the hand the fatigability of type 1 muscle cells is increased, and the contraction velocity of the type 2 fibers is reduced. Such changes will presumably contribute to the retardation and increased fatigability in patients with central pareses.

Interruption of descending central motor pathways, as in capsular hemiplegia, also produces changes of reflexes other than the stretch reflexes. The so-called *plantar reflex*, elicited by stroking with a pointed object in a forward direction along the sole of the foot (especially the lateral margin), is inverted (Fig. 12.11). Instead of the normal response, which is a flexion movement of the great toe (and the other toes), the great toe extends (moves upward). This phenomenon, with extension instead of flexion of the great toe, is called the *sign of Babinski* and is a sensitive indicator of damage to the motor pathways leading from the cor-

Figure 12.11 *Inverted plantar reflex in central pareses (sign of Babinski).* **A.** The normal plantar reflex is plantar flexion of all the toes when a pointed instrument is moved along the sole of the foot (from the heel to the toes). **B.** In a patient with central pareses (damage of the pyramidal tract) the big toe moves upward (dorsilflexion).

Mechanisms Responsible for the Development of Spasticity

It is fair to say that the mechanisms underlying the development of spasticity are not fully understood. Conditions probably vary in different patients, even when the lesions appear to be similarly located. Studies of patients with central pareses (upper motor neuron syndromes) and spasticity indicate that the *monosynaptic reflex response to stretch* is enhanced, whereas the *long-latency (polysynaptic) stretch reflex* appears to be reduced in strength. This conclusion is based on EMG recordings in muscles subjected to accurately graded stretches and vibration.

It was formerly assumed that increased impulse traffic from the muscle spindles—as a result of increased γ motoneuron firing—explained the increased stretch reflex responses in spasticity. This has not been verified by microneurographic recordings, however, since the firing frequency of Ia afferent fibers was not increased. Only a few patients have been studied in this manner, however.

Several other factors may contribute to a decreased inhibition of α motoneurons, so that they react with abnormal firing frequency and duration to an excitatory stimulus. Probably most important are changes in the spinal cord itself. Thus, the loss of descending corticospinal fibers most likely results in *decreased activity of inhibitory interneurons*. There is some evidence, for example, of reduced activity in *inhibitory interneurons activated from tendon organs* (Ib afferents); thus, the normal inhibition of certain α motoneurons from tendon organs when the muscular tension increases may be missing in spastic patients. There is also evidence of reduced activity of GABAergic interneurons mediating *presynaptic inhibition of Ia afferent terminals*. This would lead to a stronger excitatory effect of muscle stretch than normal (particularly rapid stretch) on the α motoneurons (one study, however, found reduced presynaptic inhibition after spinal cord transections but not in hemiplegic patients). Another possible factor may be *reduced recurrent inhibition of α motoneurons* in spastic patients. The Renshaw cells, mediating the recurrent inhibition (Fig. 11.11), are known to be under supraspinal control. Thus, Renshaw cells acting on the motoneurons of the antagonists of a working muscle are excited by corticospinal fibers. When, for example, ankle extensors contract, the motoneurons to the ankle flexors are inhibited by Renshaw cells so there is less chance of eliciting an unwanted stretch reflex in the flexors. Some studies indicate that the recurrent inhibition in such instances is reduced in spastic patients. This may perhaps contribute to the occurrence of repeated reflex contractions as a response to a single stretch in spastic patients. This phenomenon is called *clonus*. The interneurons mediating *reciprocal inhibition* (Fig. 11.10) are also excited by descending supraspinal pathways, and there is some evidence that the activity of such interneurons is reduced. This would also help to explain the occurrence of hyperreflexia and of clonus. Thus, for example, when the Achilles reflex is tested with a tap on the tendon, a monosynaptic stretch reflex is elicited in the calf muscles (ankle flexors). Normally, the reciprocal inhibition prevents a stretch reflex from being elicited also in the antagonists—that is, the ankle extensors. If, however, the reciprocal inhibition is reduced, a reflex contraction of the ankle extensors may occur, and this may in turn produce a new reflex contraction in the flexors, and so forth.

As mentioned in Chapter 11, the passive viscoelastic properties change in spastic muscles. Thus, the resistance to stretching (the stiffness) can be increased even when no reflex contraction is elicited.

tex to the spinal cord. Thus, for example, increased intracranial pressure and unilateral herniation with compression of the descending motor fibers in the mesencephalon may invert the plantar reflex at a very early stage (this will occur with the foot contralateral to the herniation, owing to the crossing of the pyramidal tract in the lower medulla). An inverted plantar reflex may, however, also occur during general anesthesia and in other conditions with reduced cerebral activity.

See Chapter 4 for a discussion of mechanisms of recovery following a stroke.

The "Pyramidal Tract Syndrome"

Formerly, all of the motor symptoms occurring in capsular hemiplegia were thought to be caused by damage to the pyramidal tract, and the term "pyramidal tract syndrome" is still widely used. Closer study suggests, however, that only some symptoms can be explained by damage to the pyramidal tract. Both in monkeys and humans with lesions restricted to the medullary pyramid, difficulty with fractionate finger movements is the only constantly remaining symptom after some time. Otherwise, the recovery is almost complete—a patient with an infarction limited to the right medullar pyramid even learnt to play the cello afterwards (see caption to Figure 12.9). Hyperreflexia and spasticity have, however, been found in a few patients with (most likely) pure lesions of the pyramid. It is not clear, however, whether these symptoms were permanent or only transitory.

Other motor symptoms in capsular hemiplegia must be assumed to arise from destruction of other corticofugal pathways descending in the internal capsule. It seems likely that interruption of the *corticoreticulospinal pathways* is important for the more severe symptoms after a capsular lesion than after one limited to the medullary pyramid—including the development of spasticity. In monkeys, spasticity ensues after lesions of the motor and premotor cortex but not after complete lesions of the medullary pyramid.

We should also keep in mind that a lesion of the internal capsule may interrupt many tracts of importance for motor control other than the corticospinal and corticoreticular ones. Thus, many fibers acting (directly or indirectly) on the *cerebellum* and on the basal ganglia will usually be destroyed, and this probably contributes to the clumsiness of voluntary movements. Many patients with capsular hemiplegia have *sensory symptoms* in addition to the motor ones, because the thalamus itself may be partly affected, or the ascending fiber tracts conveying sensory signals from the thalamus to the cortex are interrupted (for example, visual field defects). Reduced or altered cutaneous sensation and kinesthesia may also contribute to the motor symptoms.

For patients without any sensory symptoms (pure motor hemiplegia), their difficulties with precise, voluntary movements—particularly of distal body parts—are most likely due largely, or solely, to destruction of the pyramidal tract. When, as is often the case, movements of more proximal body parts are also affected, this is most likely caused mainly by destruction of descending fibers to the reticular formation.

NOTES

1. It is not clear whether there is complete coincidence between the physiologically defined MI and the cytoarchitectonically defined area 4. Thus, some authors maintain that the MI extends anteriorly somewhat into area 6 with the representation of axial and proximal muscles. Such disagreement is probably caused by lack of clear-cut cytoarchitectonic changes when moving anteriorly from area 4 into area 6. Many cytoarchitectonic borders, as depicted so confidently in maps like that in Figure 20.3, are in reality seldom unequivocal. This is witnessed by the often great differences between maps published by different authors.

2. Assuming that area 6 of humans corresponds functionally to area 6 in monkeys, the supramotor areas have increased in size during evolution. Thus, areas 4 and 6 are of approximately the same size in monkeys (Fig. 12.7), whereas area 6 is much larger than area 4 in humans (Fig. 20.3).

3. The plantar reflex is normally extensor ("inverted") in infants and may be so for up to 2 years. This correlates well with the myelination period of the human pyramidal tract and the concomitant development of fractionated movements of the fingers.

CHAPTER 13

THE BASAL GANGLIA

In the previous chapter, we discussed descending pathways from the cerebral cortex, which (directly and indirectly) influence the motoneurons and thereby are crucial for the initiation and control of movements. It was formerly believed that the basal ganglia also have ample connections to the spinal cord, and such connections were regarded as an important part of the so-called *extrapyramidal system*. That the basal ganglia are related to the control of movement has been known for a long time; diseases affecting primarily the basal ganglia lead to characteristic *disturbances of movement* and of the *resting muscle tone*. Improved methods for tracing fiber connections have shown, however, that the *main efferent connections of the basal ganglia do not descend to motor nuclei in the brain stem and spinal cord but are rather directed "upstream" to the motor and other areas of the cerebral cortex.* The fact that diseases of the basal ganglia do not produce pareses is in keeping with the fact that they play a different role in motor control than the descending central motor pathways.

Broadly speaking, the *basal ganglia are intercalated in a loop of fiber connections from the cerebral cortex and back to the cerebral cortex via the thalamus.* In this respect, the basal ganglia resemble the cerebellum. Information from large parts of the cerebral cortex is processed in the basal ganglia (and in the cerebellum) before "answers" are sent back to, primarily, the motor areas of the cortex (Fig. 13.4). The nature of the processing that takes place in the basal ganglia is largely unknown, even though our knowledge about the internal "machinery" and the connections of the basal ganglia has increased enormously in the last few years.

The tasks of the basal ganglia are most likely not restricted to motor control, however. Even though the most obvious symptoms in diseases of the basal ganglia are related to the motor system, both clinical and experimental evidence indicates that the basal ganglia also play a role in higher mental functions. (This is another reminder that classification of parts of the brain into rigid functional categories such as "motor," "sensory," and "cognitive" must not be taken literally but rather as didactic oversimplifications.)

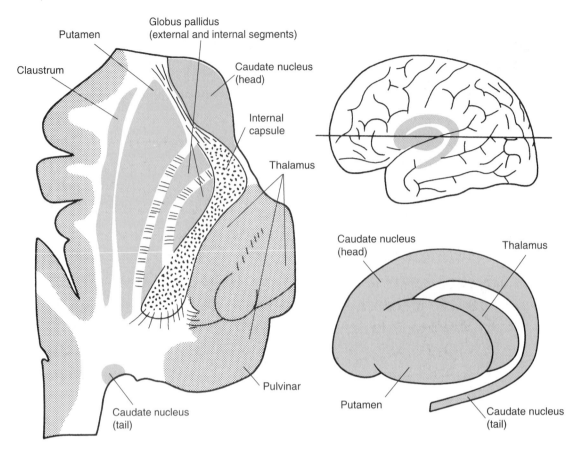

Figure 13.1 *The shape and position of the basal ganglia.*

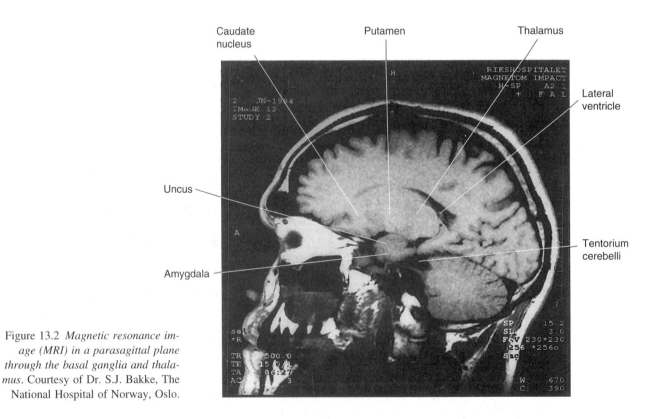

Figure 13.2 *Magnetic resonance image (MRI) in a parasagittal plane through the basal ganglia and thalamus.* Courtesy of Dr. S.J. Bakke, The National Hospital of Norway, Oslo.

372

Figure 13.3 *The basal ganglia in frontal sections.* The photomicrograph is of a myelin-stained section. The drawing to the **left** is from a slightly different anteroposterior level than the photomicrograph.

STRUCTURE AND CONNECTIONS OF THE BASAL GANGLIA

The term basal ganglia usually includes the *caudate nucleus, the putamen, and the globus pallidus* (Figs. 3.28, 3.30, and 13.1–13.4).[1] Because of their macroscopic shape, the putamen and globus pallidus together are called the *lentiform nucleus*. The caudate nucleus and the putamen are similarly built, with predominantly small perikarya. They are also functionally related and are collectively termed the *striatum* or *neostriatum*. The neostriatum con-

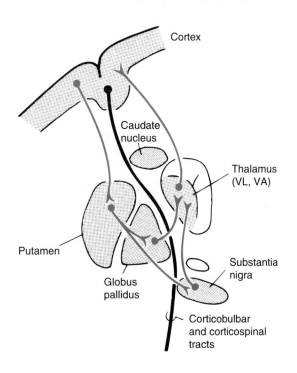

Figure 13.4 *Main connections of the basal ganglia.* Note the pathway from the cortex, through the basal ganglia, and back to the cortex via the thalamus.

tains several neuronal types that differ with regard both to where they send their axons and to which neurotransmitters they use (see below). Most of the neurons, however, send their axons out of the striatum (projection neurons), whereas a small group are interneurons with axons ramifying locally within the striatum (Fig. 13.8). The presence of such neurons, among other things, indicates that the striatum is not simply a relay station but also performs considerable processing of information.

The *globus pallidus* has a different internal structure than the striatum, with larger, more "motoneuron"-like cells, and is also called the *paleostriatum* or *pallidum*. The term *corpus striatum* includes both the pallidum and the neostriatum. Phylogenetically, the caudate nucleus and the putamen developed together and are younger than the pallidum (thus the names neostriatum and paleostriatum). As we will see, these two main divisions of the basal ganglia differ also with regard to connections.

When the term basal ganglia (as in the present account) is used of a set of *functionally related cell groups* rather than in a strictly topographic sense, we should also include the *substantia nigra* and the *subthalamic nucleus* because both are intimately connected with the corpus striatum. Cell groups that join the corpus striatum ventrally without sharp transitions—such as the *nucleus accumbens* and the olfactory tubercle—often are now also included among the basal ganglia. These cell groups are collectively termed the *ventral striatum*. They differ in some respects from the rest—that is, the *dorsal striatum*—and will be treated separately below (see Chapter 19).

Before going into detail about the connections of the basal ganglia, we may sum up the main features in the diagram below.

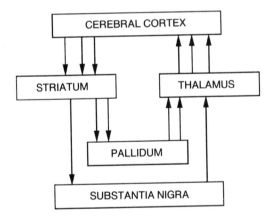

Afferent Connections of the Basal Ganglia

The *striatum*, which is largely the receiving part of the basal ganglia, is characterized by three sources of afferents: the *cerebral cortex*, the *intralaminar thalamic nuclei*, and *dopamine-containing cell groups in the mesencephalon* (Figs. 13.5 and 13.7). The largest contingent of afferents comes from the cerebral cortex. Almost all areas of the cortex send fibers to the striatum, but the caudate nucleus and the putamen receive from different parts of the cortex (Fig. 13.6). The *putamen* is dominated by somatotopically organized inputs from the SI and MI. The *caudate nucleus,*

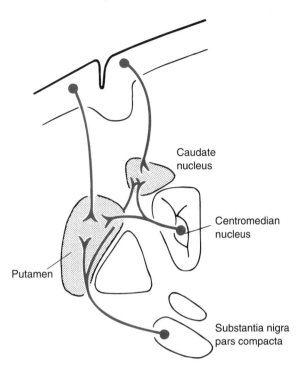

Figure 13.5 *The main afferent connections of the striatum.*

Caudate
nucleus

Centromedian
nucleus

Putamen

Substantia nigra
pars compacta

on the other hand, receives fibers predominantly from the association areas—that is, regions that perhaps are less directly concerned with motor control than with higher mental functions and emotions. Whereas the putamen receives relatively "raw," or unprocessed, information from sensory receptors via the SI and from motor cells in the MI, the caudate nucleus receives information that is a result of integration of signals from many

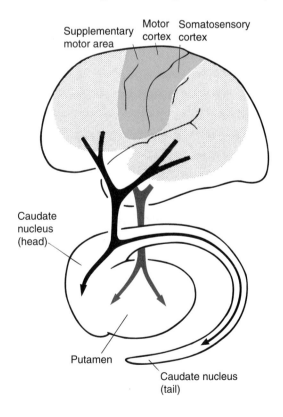

Figure 13.6 *The putamen and the caudate nucleus receive fibers from different parts of the cortex.*

Supplementary
motor area

Motor
cortex

Somatosensory
cortex

Caudate
nucleus
(head)

Putamen

Caudate nucleus
(tail)

Fig. 13.7 *Main connections of the substantia nigra* (see also Fig. 13.12).

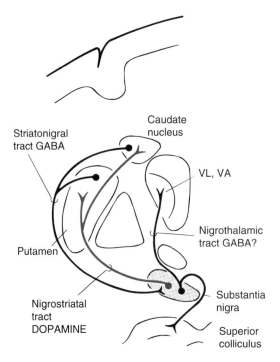

sources. Such information reaching the caudate nucleus may, for example, concern earlier stages in the chains of neural events eventually leading to voluntary movements.

In addition to cortical afferents, the striatum (including the ventral striatum) receives important connections from the *intralaminar thalamic nuclei* (Fig. 3.21), especially the *centromedian nucleus (CM)* (Fig. 13.5).

With regard to striatal afferents from *dopamine-containing cell groups in the mesencephalon*, the major contingent arises in the *substantia nigra*. More scattered dopaminergic cells outside the substantia nigra send their fibers primarily to the *ventral striatum*.

Additional afferents to the striatum come from the *raphe nuclei* in the brain stem (serotonin), among other cell groups.

Efferent Connections of the Basal Ganglia

The effects exerted by the basal ganglia on other parts of the nervous system are mediated primarily by efferent fibers from the pallidum and the substantia nigra. These nuclei receive their main efferents from the striatum, as shown in the diagram on p. 374 (and Figs. 13.4 and 13.7). In this manner, information from the striatum is processed in the pallidum and nigra before being forwarded to the thalamus. The connections are topographically organized, so that subdivisions of the striatum are connected with specific parts of the pallidum and the nigra.

The globus pallidus consists of two parts, an external (Gp$_e$) and an internal (Gp$_i$) segment (Figs. 13.1, 13.3, and 13.9). Both receive their main afferents from the striatum. The main part of the efferents from the internal segment goes to the thalamus (Fig. 13.4).[2] Many of the fibers pass through the internal capsule (Fig. 13.4) and can therefore be damaged by lesions in this region (this should be kept in mind when analyzing the symptoms occurring after the common infarctions in this region, as discussed in Chapter 12). In the thalamus the pallidal fibers end in the *ventral anterior nucleus (VA)* and in parts of the *VL* (Figs. 13.3, 13.4, 14.14, and 20.7). Some fibers also end in the *CM*. The VL and VA send their main efferents to the cerebral cortex (Fig. 13.14).[3] The CM, on the other hand, as part of the intralaminar thalamic nuclei, sends its main efferent projection back to the striatum. This is one of several examples of subcortical "side loops" used by the basal ganglia, which in some way influence the messages that are sent to the cerebral cortex.

The Striatum Has a Complex Intrinsic Organization: Projection Neurons, Interneurons, and Modules

Anatomically, at least six different cell types have been observed in the striatum. Some of these have been characterized with regard to connections and content of neurotransmitters. More than 90% of the neurons have relatively small perikarya and dendrites with numerous spines (Fig. 13.8). This cell type contains *GABA* and *sends its axon out of the striatum to the globus pallidus and the substantia nigra* (called medium-sized, densely spiny neuron, or medium spiny neuron for short). There appear to exist two main subtypes of this medium spiny neuron: One kind contains *SP* (and usually also dynorphin) in addition to GABA and projects primarily to the *internal segment of the pallidum* and/or to the *substantia nigra*; the other contains *enkephalin* in addition to GABA and projects mainly to the *external segment of the pallidum* (a third, less characterized kind of projection neuron contains neurokinin B in addition to substance P and enkephalin) . Although the relations between the peptides found in the projection neurons and where they send their axons are not absolute, those described here appear to be the most common.

The other cell types are most likely *interneurons*—that is, their axonal arborizations remain within the striatum. One conspicuous kind of interneuron has a large perikaryon and smooth dendrites and contains *acetylcholine*. The action of acetylcholine in the striatum seems to be predominantly excitatory (slow, modulatory action via muscarine receptors). Dopaminergic terminals of nigrostriatal neurons contact the cholinergic interneurons in addition to the projection neurons (Fig. 13.8). In agreement with this, both cell types express mRNA for dopamine receptors. The cholinergic interneurons contribute—in a yet uknown way—to the symptoms in Parkinson's diesease, since anticholinergic drugs can improve the condition.

The various cell types, and in particular the neurotransmitters, are not evenly distributed throughout the striatum. Rather, different smaller compartments can be defined with regard to connections and cytochemistry. In microscopic sections, a mosaic pattern appears after staining to demonstrate *acetylcholine esterase*. Poorly stained patches called *striosomes* are embedded in a heavily stained *matrix*. The matrix can be further subdivided by visualization of various transmitters and their receptors. GABAergic projection neurons are found within both the matrix and the striosomes, and the two main kinds do not appear to be clearly segregated either. Cholinergic interneurons also seem to be present in both compartments. Striatal afferent connections terminate in patches within the matrix. Each small part of the cortex, for example, projects divergently to many patches.

It is fair to say that, in spite of a wealth of interesting data, the functional significance of the division of the striatum into numerous minor compartments or *modules* is still a matter of speculation (and the interpretation of data is made more difficult by the existence of species differences). This should come as no surprise, considering the complexity of the striatum. To reveal for each neuronal type where it sends all its axonal branches and the cell types with which it establishes synaptic contacts, at the same time determine its content of transmitter candidates and other neuroactive substances, and furthermore correlate this with the distribution of receptors is a formidable task. It requires studies combining axonal tracing, Golgi impregnation of perikarya and dendrites, and immunocytochemistry (at the light and electron microscopic level). But this is not enough; we also need to know the physiological properties of the cell types, and this requires intracellular recording from single neurons, followed by intracellular staining. These kinds of data also have to be correlated in minute detail with the intricate patterns of afferent and efferent connections.

The substantia nigra also sends fibers to the thalamus, ending in slightly different parts than the pallidal fibers.

The parts of the VL that receive fibers from the pallidum and the nigra project primarily to the SMA, whereas the VA sends efferent fibers to the PMA and the *prefrontal cortex* (Fig. 13.14). *Thus, a large part of the impulse traffic from the basal ganglia is directed toward the motor cortical areas.* Physiological studies also indicate that the influence of the basal ganglia on motor control involves the corticospinal tract and indirect descending pathways from the cerebral cortex to the motoneurons (Fig. 13.4). It is worth noticing, however, that the caudate nucleus—which receives afferents mainly from association areas of the cortex—probably acts primarily on the prefrontal cortex, which is not directly involved in motor control but rather in *cognitive tasks*. Lesions of the caudate nucleus in monkeys produce symptoms similar to those seen after damage to the prefrontal cortex: among other things, reduced performance in tests requiring *spatial memory* (such as to recall where an object is located when it is out of sight; this is discussed further in Chapter 19).

In addition to the massive connections from the basal ganglia to the thalamus, there are also efferents reaching the *reticular formation* (especially in the mesencephalon) and the *superior colliculus*. Connections to a part of the mesencephalic reticular formation called the *pedunculopontine nucleus* (PPN) has attracted special interest because this region may be coexistent with the *mesencephalic locomotor region* (electrical stimulation of this region elicits walking movements in cats). One may therefore speculate whether these connections are of relevance for the characteristic disturbances of locomotion seen in Parkinson's disease (in which there is marked cell loss in the substantia nigra). Connections from the substantia nigra to the superior colliculus (Fig. 13.7) are probably of importance for the *control of coordinated head and eye movements*.

The main efferent connections of the basal ganglia may be summarized as follows: *The internal segment of the globus pallidus and the substantia nigra send the final product of basal ganglia processing toward premotor networks[4] in the mesencephalic tegmentum, superior colliculus, and thalamus* (Chevalier and Deniau).

Transmitters and Synaptic Actions of Neurons within the Cortex–Basal Ganglia–Cortex Loop: Disinhibition

To understand the processing going on within the basal ganglia and the effects of the ganglia on other parts of the brain, we need to know the transmitters and the synaptic actions of all the neurons involved. Hardly any other part of the brain has been as intensely investigated with regard to neurotransmitters and other neuroactive substances as the basal ganglia, and the conditions turn out to be extremely complex. More than 100 neuroactive substances have been found in the striatum so far, and more are undoubtedly still to be discovered. So far, however, only a few can be correlated with anatomic and physiological data (Figs. 13.7 and 13.8).

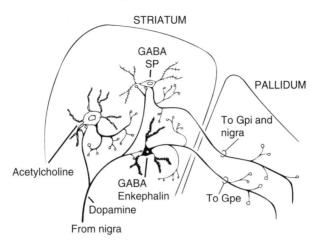

STRIATUM

GABA
SP

PALLIDUM

To Gpi and
nigra

Acetylcholine

GABA
Enkephalin

To Gpe

Dopamine

From nigra

Figure 13.8 *Three different cell types in the striatum.* Most or all striatal efferent neurons are GABAergic. Note the large, cholinergic interneurons. There are other cell types in the striatum than those shown here.

The *corticostriate connections* (Fig. 13.5) are excitatory, most likely due to release of glutamate (as is probably the case with all corticofugal fibers). The *striatopallidal* and *striatonigral fibers* (Figs. 13.3 and 13.6) contain GABA and have inhibitory effects. The *pallidothalamic* (and most likely also the *nigrothalamic*) fibers are also GABAergic and inhibitory. The *thalamocortical* fibers (from the VL and VA, as from other thalamic nuclei) are excitatory. Thus, the flow of information from the cerebral cortex through the basal ganglia and back is less straightforward than if all involved synapses were excitatory.

Theoretically, increased cortical input to the striatum would lead to decreased activity of the pallidal neurons (because excitation of striatal neurons produces increased inhibition in the pallidum). This in turn would increase the activity of thalamocortical neurons (because they would receive less inhibition from the pallidum). *Thus, excitatory impulses from the cortex would eventually produce disinhibition of the thalamocortical neurons* (and probably also of other "premotor" neurons in the reticular formation and the superior colliculus receiving fibers from the substantia nigra). Recordings of single-cell activity in the basal ganglia in awake monkeys are compatible with these considerations. At rest, most striatal neurons are "silent"—that is, they do not produce action potentials— whereas the pallidal neurons (and neurons in the pars reticulata of the substantia nigra) fire with a regular and high frequency. This would presumably *keep the premotor neurons in the thalamus in a state of inhibition when the animal is not moving.* Commands from the cortex to the basal ganglia in relation to the preparation or execution of movements would release the thalamocortical neurons from this inhibition. Indeed, electrophysiological experiments show that increased striatal activity reduces the activity of many pallidal and nigral neurons, followed by increased firing of thalamocortical neurons.

It has been proposed that the disinhibition of premotor neurons by the basal ganglia is a gating mechanism to control the access of other inputs (for example, sensory) to the motor cortex. Since the connections of the basal ganglia are topographically organized at all levels, this would be a specific and focused gating rather than a diffuse one, varying with the nature of the motor task.

The Subthalamic Nucleus Has Reciprocal Connections with the Pallidum and the Substantia Nigra

Whereas efferents of the internal pallidal segment primarily end in the thalamus, the GABAergic fibers from the external pallidal segment are directed toward the subthalamic nucleus (Fig. 13.9). Most of the *efferents from the subthalamic nucleus go back to both segments of the pallidum and to the pars reticulata of the substantia nigra*. Although the subthalamic nucleus also receives some afferents from the motor cortex, it is primarily a part of side loops of the pallidum and the nigra—perhaps assisting them in certain computations.

Recent studies show that the subthalamopallidal neurons are glutamatergic with excitatory actions (whereas they were formerly believed to use GABA). The efferents of the subthalamic nucleus are topographically organized in the monkey, as shown with axonal transport methods. Thus, different neuronal populations project to the substantia nigra and the pallidum, and there are also differences with the regard to projections to minor parts of the pallidum. Fibers from the subthalamic nucleus and the striatum converge on the same neurons in the internal pallidal segment (Gp$_i$). These data suggest that the activity of the GABAergic neurons in Gp$_i$ be determined largely by the sum of synaptic influences from the striatum ($-$) and the subthalamic nucleus ($+$). Since Gp$_i$ neurons inhibit thalamocortical neurons, increased subthalamic activity would be expected to produce reduced excitation of the motor cortex—that is, inhibition of voluntary movements. Thus, the subthalamic nucleus is believed to control or stop ongoing movements, rather than to select and initiate movements. Considering the somatotopical organization of its connections, the subthalamic nucleus presumably exerts rather specific actions, and not a diffuse inhibition of all motor activity.

Loss of influence from the subthalamic nucleus would produce disinhibition of thalamocortical neurons. Thus, the violent involuntary movements of the opposite body half after destruction of the subthalamic nucleus (*hemiballismus*) might be caused by hyperactivity among the thalamocortical neurons.

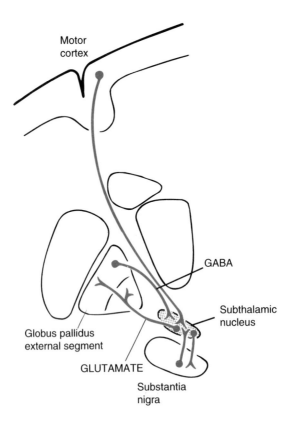

Figure 13.9 *Main connectious of the subthalamic nucleus.*

*The Basal Ganglia Are Probably Arranged in
Functionally Different, Parallel Circuits*

Anatomic studies with the use of axonal transport methods have shown
that the afferent and efferent connections of the basal ganglia have a high
degree of topographic order. Connections from functionally different parts
of the cortex end differently in the striatum, and this localization goes
much further than depicted in Figure 13.6. The next links from the striatum to the pallidum and the substantia nigra are also topographically
arranged. For example, by the use of two fluorescent tracers in the same
experiment, it has been shown in the monkey that the caudate nucleus
projects primarily to the nigra, whereas the putamen is more strongly connected with the pallidum. Accordingly, few cells in the striatum send axon
collaterals to both the nigra and the pallidum.

On the basis of such data, it has been suggested that there are four (or
more) lines or *circuits through the basal ganglia*, in which the flow of
information is kept segregated. Such circuits presumably handle different
kinds of information and participate in different tasks. Thus, recent studies indicate that the *basal ganglia process different kinds of information
in parallel, rather than being primarily concerned with integration of information from large parts of the cortex.* How far this segregation goes
is not clear, however. Thus, whereas some data indicate a high degree of
segregation, others are more compatible with considerable convergence
among the circuits.

Cortex–Basal Ganglia–Cortex Parallel Circuits

One circuit appears to arise in the *SMA, MI and SI*, passes through the putamen, and finally (via the pallidum and the
thalamus) ends in the SMA. This circuit is probably most directly involved in control of movements. Recordings of single-cell activity in the putamen support this assumption.

Another circuit arises in parts of the frontal and parietal lobes concerned with oculomotor control—that is, *area 8*
immediately in front of area 6, and *area 7* (Fig. 20.3). Via particular parts of the caudate nucleus, this circuit appears to
end in area 8. This area is also called the *frontal eye field* and is of particular importance for certain kinds of voluntary
eye movements.

Two circuits are postulated to arise in different parts of the *prefrontal cortex* and pass via the caudate nucleus, the
substantia nigra (to a lesser degree the pallidum), the VA, and the mediodorsal thalamic nucleus (MD in Figs. 13.3, 20.7,
and 20.8) and back to prefrontal cortical areas. This prefrontal circuit presumably enables the basal ganglia to influence
higher mental functions.

Finally, one postulated circuit arises in *"limbic" parts of the cortex* (the cingulate gyrus, orbitofrontal areas of the
frontal lobe, and parts of the temporal lobe cortex, which are parts of or closely connected with the limbic structures).
This "limbic" circuit passes through the ventral striatum, ventral pallidum, and the MD of the thalamus and back to the
cortical areas from which the circuit started. These connections are believed to be related to mood and emotions, and to
behavior directed to satisfy basal needs (such as eating and drinking), and to obtain rewards (See *The Ventral Striatum,
Psychosis, and Drug Addiction*, below).

The Substantia Nigra

The substantia nigra and some of its connections have been mentioned
several times, and we will also return to it when dealing with Parkinson's

Red nucleus

Pars compacta

Pars reticulata

Crus cerebri

Figure 13.10 *The substantia nigra.* Photomicrograph of transverse section through the mesencephalon (myelin stain). The cells of the pars compacta are clearly seen as dark dots. The dark color is due to their content of pigment. The photomicrograph is from the section shown in Figure 3.20.

disease, in which the nigra plays a crucial role. A collective treatment of the main features of the substantia nigra may therefore be pertinent at this stage.

The substantia nigra can be divided anatomically into two parts, the *pars compacta* and the *pars reticulata* (Figs. 13.10, 13.11, and 13.12). The compacta is richer in cells than the reticulata, whereas the latter (as the name implies) is dominated by dendritic arborizations. The reticulata also contains numerous neurons, however. The compacta neurons contain pigment (neuromelanin), which makes the nigra visible as a dark band in the freshly cut human mesencephalon. The pars reticulata, located ventral to the compacta, is lighter.

The *afferent* connections of the nigra (Fig. 13.4, 13.7, and 13.9) arise in numerous cell groups, but quantitatively the most important input comes from the *striatum*. Even though most striatonigral fibers terminate in the pars reticulata, cells in the compacta can also be influenced because their long dendrites extend into the reticulata (Fig. 13.10). GABA is the transmitter for the majority of the striatonigral fibers that exert an inhibitory effect on the cells in the nigra. Electrophysiological experiments show

Figure 13.11 *Dopaminergic cells in the substantia nigra.* Immunocytochemical demonstration of an enzyme used in the synthesis of dopamine (tyrosine hydroxylase). Magnification, ×180. Courtesy of Dr. J.-E. Aas, Department of Anatomy, University of Oslo.

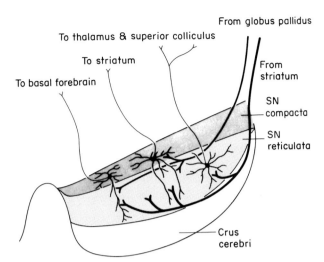

To basal forebrain

To striatum

To thalamus & superior colliculus

From globus pallidus

From striatum

SN compacta

SN reticulata

Crus cerebri

Figure 13.12 *The substantia nigra consists of two parts, which differ structurally and with regard to connections. Note that afferent fibers to the pars reticulata contact the dendrites of the dopaminergic neurons in the pars compacta.*

this inhibitory effect, but, in addition, many nigral cells are excited by electrical stimulation of the striatum. This double action is not fully understood.

Other afferents to the substantia nigra arise in the *pallidum* (probably GABA), in the *subthalamic nucleus* (probably glutamate), the *locus coeruleus* (norepinephrine), and the *raphe nuclei* (serotonin).

The *efferent* connections of the substantia nigra (Figs. 13.4, 13.5, 13.9, and 13.12) pass primarily to the striatum and the thalamus, with smaller contingents to cell groups in the reticular formation and the superior colliculus, as mentioned above. The dopaminergic nigrostriatal neurons are located in the pars compacta, whereas the GABAergic nigrothalamic neurons are located primarily in the pars reticulata (Fig. 13.12). The nigral neurons sending their axons to the superior colliculus are also found in largely separate parts of the nigra. Furthermore, the nigral afferents from different parts of the striatum (such as the putamen and caudate nucleus) end differently. Thus, the substantia nigra most likely consists of several functionally different parts, differing both with regard to afferents and the cell groups on which they exert their action.

The Actions of Dopamine in the Striatum

The most studied basal ganglia connection is the *dopaminergic nigrostriatal pathway*, which is the most massive dopaminergic pathway in the central nervous system. Striatal neurons contain, not unexpectedly, dopamine receptors. Dopamine has *modulatory* synaptic actions, altering the response of striatal neurons to specific inputs from the cerebral cortex and the thalamus. The latter are mediated by fast, directly acting transmitters like glutamate and GABA. In more detail, however, actions of dopamine on neuronal excitability in the striatum are multifarious and not fully understood. This is a question of great clinical interest because several diseases are related to disturbed dopamine-mediated synaptic transmission (Parkinson's disease, schizophrenia, Tourette's syndrome, and others).

Many studies find that dopamine has excitatory effects on certain striatal neuronal types but inhibitory effects on others. Thus, early electrophysiological studies suggested that dopamine has a weak excitatory effect on the GABAergic projection neurons of the striatum, whereas it has a strong inhibitory action on the cholinergic interneurons (Fig. 13.8). After the discovery of two main types of dopamine receptors, however, in-

The Ventral Striatum, Psychosis, and Drug Addiction

The term *ventral striatum* is used for rather diffusely distributed cell groups in the basal part of the hemispheres (the *basal forebrain*; see Chapter 19, for a discussion of its various constituting parts). The ventral striatum merges with the dorsal striatum without sharp boundaries. The *nucleus accumbens* represents a fairly distinct part of the ventral striatum, and connects the caudate nucleus and the putamen ventrally (Fig. 4.17). A similar diffuse cell group, the *ventral pallidum*, merges with the dorsal well-defined parts of the globus pallidus (Fig. 19.4). The *ventral striatopallidum* is used as a collective term.

Although the ventral striatopallidum has no sharp boundaries toward other cell groups in the basal forebrain, its relationship to the basal ganglia is witnessed by the similarities of their connections. We mentioned above one parallel circuit through the basal ganglia: from parts of the *prefrontal cortex and cingulate gyrus to the ventral striatum, from there to the ventral pallidum, then to the mediodorsal thalamic nucleus (MD), and finally back to the prefrontal cortex.* There is probably a further differentiation of connections through the ventral striatum (several circuits). Thus, it receives projections with some topographic localization from the *hippocampal formation*, the *amygdala*, the *orbitofrontal cortex*, and *parts of the temporal lobe* (all these sources are either parts of the limbic structures, or closely connected with them). Parts of the ventral striatum (nucleus accumbens) also send efferent fibers to the hypothalamus and the mesencephalic reticular formation (PPN).

Like the dorsal striatum, the ventral striatum receives many *dopaminergic* fibers. The dopaminergic cell bodies projecting to the ventral striatum are located mainly dorsomedial to the substantia nigra, in the so-called *ventral tegmental area* (VTA). Since the ventral striatum and other cell groups that are closely linked with limbic structures are the main targets of dopaminergic neurons in the ventral tegmental area, the term the *mesolimbic dopaminergic system* is now widely used. To use the word *system* about this is, however, hardly justified, since we do not know whether these rather widespread dopaminergic projections are functionally homogeneous.

The dopaminergic projection to the ventral striatum (especially to the nucleus accumbens) has attracted much interest, because *antipsychotic drugs*—which are dopamine receptor antagonists—appear to bind with particularly high density in the ventral striatum. Neurons in the nucleus accumbens of experimental animals change their pattern of activity during development of *drug addiction*—no matter whether the drug is amphetamine, cocaine, or morphine. The addictive behavior is reduced by lesions of the nucleus accumbens, or by removing its dopaminergic innervation. Thus, after giving a dopamine antagonist, the experimental animals stopped self administration of cocaine (they could easily obtain an intravenous dose by a movement). Furthermore, dopaminergic activity is increased in paranoid psychoses elicited by amphetamines or cocaine.

However interesting these observations are, we should realize that they provide only limited insight. By focusing on *one* transmitter and *one* part of the brain, one may even give the impression that there is a simple biologic explanation to complex mental phenomena. One theory suggests, for example, that the dopaminergic mesolimbic connections constitute a "reward pathway", and that the pleasurable feelings evoked by narcotic drugs are caused by release of dopamine in the nucleus accumbens. This is not generally accepted, however. The Canadian pharmacologist Edward Sellers expressed his scepticism like this: "It would be a great oversimplification and disservice to the elegance of the brain to postulate one system." Indeed, many parts of the brain other than the nucleus accumbens show altered activity in the conditions discussed here (see Chapter 20 for some comments on mental illness and the cerebral cortex). In drug addiction, for example, changes of neuronal activity occur in the locus coeruleus (norepinephrine) and in the intralaminar thalamic nuclei. It is not clear whether the nucleus accumbens or the ventral tegmental area is the primary target of narcotic drugs in the brain, neither is it known how such drugs alter the properties of dopaminergic neurotransmission.

tracellular recordings showed that they could mediate opposite effects on the same neuron. These and other data have been interpreted to show that most striatal projection neurons express both D_1 and D_2 receptors. This conclusion is controversial, however. The hypothesis with most current support states that *GABA and SP containing neurons* (projecting to the nigra and Gp_i) express D_1 receptors and are *excited* by dopamine, whereas the *GABA and enkephalin containing neurons* (projecting to Gp_e) express D_2 receptors and are *inhibited*.[7] The Gp_e sends (GABAergic, inhibitory) fibers to the subthalamic nucleus. Thus, by simultaneously acting on D_1 and D_2 receptors, dopamine in the striatum would inhibit Gp_i neurons via two routes: *Directly*, by D_1-mediated increased activity of SP-containing projection neurons, and *indirectly* by D_2-mediated reduced activity of enkephalin-containing neurons. Reduced activity of the latter neurons would give less inhibition of the subthalamic nucleus (disinhibition) and by that increased excitatory input to Gp_i. We return to the actions of dopamine below when discussing Parkinson's disease.

The complex organization of the striatum, the many transmitters acting on the same neurons, and the presence of several kinds of dopamine receptors, may explain why the actions of dopamine are hard to clarify. To complicate matters further, we know that the action of modulatory transmitters may depend on the state of the postsynaptic neuron. This concerns, for example, the effect of dopamine acting on D_1 receptors. Electrophysiological studies show that the *striatal projection neurons have two functional states*: In one state they are depolarized and fire bursts of action potentials, in the other state they are hyperpolarized and inactive. In the latter state, activation of D_1 receptors depolarizes the cell (by closure of K^+ channels) so that it reacts more easily with burst to an excitatory input from the cortex. If the neuron is in the active state, however, it appears that D_1 receptor activation closes a Na^+ channel that keeps the neuron depolarized by leakage of cations into the cell. Closing this channel would stabilize the membrane potential, perhaps to avoid excessive activation by glutamate from the cortex. In both cases, *dopamine probably serves to keep the membrane potential in the range where the cell is apt to fire in bursts—that is, in a state suited for efficient signal transmission.*

The two main kinds of dopamine receptors, D_1 and D_2, each comes in several varieties. Together, there are at least five different dopamine receptors. Although all dopamine receptors act via G proteins, D_1 receptors activate the enzyme adenylyl cyclase and thus give increased intracellular level of cyclic AMP, whereas D_2-receptor activation reduces the level of cyclic AMP.

FUNCTIONS OF THE BASAL GANGLIA

In spite of enormous research activity and rapid progress during recent years, the functions of the basal ganglia are still far from fully understood. Even the most voluminous textbooks often restrict themselves to vague statements, such as "movement control," "control of muscle tone," "assist in cognitive tasks," and "influence mood and motivation." We will here restrict ourselves to a discusssion of the role of the basal ganglia in movement control.

Taking the connections of the basal ganglia as a starting point, it is noteworthy that their major output goes to the SMA, PMA, and the prefrontal cortical areas. The properties of these areas suggest that the basal ganglia would be important in the *planning phase of a movement*, such as when several single-joint movements have to be put together to produce a complex movement, or when sensory stimuli or stored information has to be translated into an adequate motor response. It has been suggested, for example, that the basal ganglia participate when *movements are learned by pure repetition* and not by gaining insight into the nature of the task and, furthermore, that the basal ganglia enable automatic performance of well-rehearsed movements by the use of motor programs located elsewhere in the central nervous system. One model (Hallett) proposes that *". . . the purpose of the basal ganglia curcuits is to select and inhibit specific motor synergies to carry out a desired action."* Such statements are, however, too general to help sorting out the tasks specific to the basal ganglia, as distinct from other parts of the motor system.

It is also possible that the basal ganglia contribute to the *linking of motivation and emotions to the execution of movements*. Thus, recording the activity of single cells in the striatum indicates that many respond best when a stimulus is linked with memory of an event that has a particular significance for the animal. Certain cells in the substantia nigra are, for example, active just before a rapid eye movement, but only when the movement is directed toward a target the animal cannot see and therefore has to remember where the target is. It has also been suggested that the *nigrostriatal dopaminergic fibers* provide information about the *relevance* of a stimulus.

Judged from the symptoms occurring in humans with diseases of the basal ganglia, it seems likely that in some manner they contribute to the speed of movements, with regard to both their start and further execution. Observations of symptoms in monkeys with lesions of the globus pallidus indicate that *learned movements primarily are slower than normal, whereas the manner in which the task is performed is not significantly altered*. Therefore, neither the movement command nor the movement program appears to be located within the basal ganglia themselves.

Experiments with *stimulation* of parts of the basal ganglia have not helped much to clarify their functional role. A bewildering multitude of

Are the Basal Ganglia Concerned with Initiation of Movements?

In the example above, with an eye movement temporally linked with activity of neurons in the basal ganglia, a crucial question is whether the movement is triggered by the basal ganglia activity. In other words, is the disinhibition of premotor neurons brought about by basal ganglia outputs sufficient to elicit specific movements, or is the excitability of the premotor neurons merely increased so they can react with action potential to another input? The latter appears to be the case, as judged from experiments in behaving monkeys. Thus, microinjection of a GABA agonist (muscimol) in the substantia nigra did not evoke rapid eye movements but gave a strong tendency to direct the gaze toward a certain point in the environment. Thus, to elicit a specific movement, the disinhibition induced by the basal ganglia (in the thalamus or the superior colliculus) probably must coincide in time with a command signal from another source.

movements and other effects can be produced. So far, however, these cannot be put together in a coherent model. Regarding the complex connections and internal organization of the basal ganglia, this should not come as a surprise.

DISEASES OF THE BASAL GANGLIA

Since we do not understand the tasks of the basal ganglia and how they are carried out, it should come as no surprise that we are unable to explain fully the symptoms occurring in diseases of the basal ganglia. Nevertheless, considerable progress has been made recently with regard to the relationships between certain symptoms and the elements responsible within the basal ganglia.

As mentioned above, the most obvious symptoms in diseases of the basal ganglia are motor ones. As a rule, there is a mixture of symptoms due to *loss of neuronal activity* (compare with pareses after destruction of central motor pathways) and symptoms due to *abnormally increased neuronal activity* (compare with spasticity occurring after lesions of central motor pathways). The most frequent diseases of the basal ganglia impinge upon initiation of movement—*akinesia*—and when started, the movements are slower and smaller than normal—this is called *bradykinesia*. Since movements are difficult to initiate, there is also a conspicuous *paucity of movements*, usually implied in the term akinesia. In addition, there are more or less pronounced involuntary movements called *dyskinesia*.

The diseases of the basal ganglia fall into *two broad groups*: those characterized by *akinesia and rigidity* (Parkinson's disease is the most common example), and those dominated by *dyskinesia* (for example Huntington's disease).[8] The first group is, furthermore, characterized by loss of dopamine effects in the basal ganglia, whereas the second group shows signs of dopaminergic hyperactivity.

The most frequent disease affecting the basal ganglia is *Parkinson's disease* or *parkinsonism* (another name is paralysis agitans). Typically, voluntary movements are hard to initiate (akinesia) and they are slower and smaller than normal (bradykinesia). The akinesia also leads to a conspicuous lack of facial movements—the face becomes like a "mask." In addition, there is an increased muscular resting tone (rigidity) and involuntary, rhythmic, alternating movements at rest (resting tremor). Patients with Parkinson's disease have regularly been found to have a pronounced cell loss in the substantia nigra and a corresponding decrease of dopamine in the striatum.

In *Huntington's disease* (Huntington's chorea), in which there is a marked cell loss in the striatum, the most pronounced symptom is involuntary, jerky, often "dance-like" movements (chorea).

Violent, large involuntary movements of one side of the body, called *hemiballismus*, occur typically after damage to the subthalamic nucleus of the opposite side. Other diseases are also dominated by sudden, involuntary muscular contractions, occurring with uneven intervals (*tics*). One example is Tourette's syndrome, believed to be caused by dysfunction of the basal ganglia. The symptoms can be partially relieved by dopamine antagonists.

Parkinson's Disease

This disease of unknown etiology usually starts during the fifth or sixth decade of life. The syndrome includes, as mentioned, *akinesia, bradykinesia, tremor*, and *rigidity*. In addition, there are also disturbances of *postural reflexes*. Notably, the body balance during walking is disturbed, so that the patient appears to be "running after his center of gravity." The steps are typically very short, which is due to the bradykinesia (the movements are not only slower than normal but also reduced in amplitude). When being pushed from behind, the patient has difficulty stopping and continues to move forward. The normal pendulum movements of the arms during walking are absent. There is also a conspicuous loss of facial expression, as mentioned. There are disturbances of the autonomic nervous system, such as increased salivation and secretion from sebaceous glands of the skin. We do not know how the basal ganglia would influence the autonomic nervous system, and the autonomic symptoms perhaps may be caused by a more general disturbance of monoamine metabolism (not only dopaminergic cell groups are affected in Parkinson's disease).

The *tremor* is typical, with its frequency of 3–6 per second, and it is most pronounced at rest. When the patient uses the hand, the tremor disappears or is reduced in amplitude. The increased muscle tone, the rigidity, is different from the spasticity occurring after lesions of central motor pathways. The resistance to passive movements is equal in extensors and flexors and is independent of whether the muscle is stretched slowly or rapidly. There is no clear-cut increase in the strength of the monosynaptic stretch reflex (such as the patellar reflex), whereas the *long-latency stretch reflexes are increased*, and this may perhaps contribute to the difficulties with balance and locomotion. The rigidity is apparently not caused by overactivity of γ motoneurons but rather by descending influences increasing the excitability of the α motoneurons so that they fire continuously—perhaps like the situation in a nervous person who is unable to relax his muscles.

The plantar reflex is normal in patients with Parkinson's disease, indicating that there is no damage to the central motor pathways. It is an old clinical observation that the tremor and rigidity disappear if a patient with Parkinson's disease has a capsular hemiplegia, and corresponding observations are made in experimental animals. The last central link in the pathways mediating the tremor and rigidity must therefore be pathways from the cerebral cortex to the motoneurons.

Pathology and Medical Treatment

The most pronounced structural change in the brain of patients with Parkinson's disease is a profound loss of pigmented (melanin-containing) neurons in the pars compacta of the substantia nigra. These are the dopamine-containing neurons. As a consequence of the loss of dopaminergic nigrostriatal fibers, the dopamine content of the striatum is reduced (symptoms first appear when the dopamine content of the striatum is reduced by 80%–90%). This latter finding led to attempts to alleviate the symptoms by giving the patients dopamine, to substitute for the loss of dopaminergic neurons. For various reasons, a precursor of dopamine—*L-dopa*—has to be used. This is converted to dopamine in the brain. This treatment had a beneficial effect on the symptoms, particularly on the very troublesome bradykinesia. Even though L-dopa has proved to be a very helpful drug, the first hopes turned out be unrealistic. The course of the disease is not affected by the drug, and the therapeutic effect decreases as the disease progresses. There probably must be a certain number of remaining dopaminergic neurons in the nigra for L-dopa to be converted to dopamine in the striatal dopaminergic boutons. More profound changes of the striatal neurons and their ability to react to dopamine may also occur. One might perhaps think that when the brain is unable to produce enough dopamine itself, it would not be able to produce dopamine from a supplied precursor either. However, enzymes converting L-dopa to dopamine are present not only in dopaminergic neurons in the nigra but also in glial cells and in other types of neurons.

The L-dopa treatment has *side effects*, as one might expect when giving a drug that acts not only in the striatum but also in many cell groups in the brain. For example, dopamine is present in the hypothalamus, and side effects like nausea, loss of appetite, and reduced control of blood pressure may perhaps be caused by actions there. Other side effects are sleep disturbances and changes of mood. In some cases the treatment can precipitate a psychosis. Such side effects may perhaps be related to actions of dopamine on the prefrontal cortex and parts of the limbic structures. Long-term treatment may provoke motor symptoms that are different from those caused by the disease, such as chorealike and athetoid dyskinesias (*athetosis* is used of slow, "worm-like," involuntary movements of the fingers and toes).

Attempts at Explaining the Symptoms

Not all symptoms occurring in Parkinson's disease can be explained on the basis of our present knowledge. One diffi-culty is represented by the complex and not fully understood effects of dopamine in the striatum. Furthermore, patho-logical changes, although most marked in the pars compacta of the substantia nigra, also occur elsewhere, such as in the pars reticulata, in the nucleus locus coeruleus, and in some of the raphe nuclei. Dopaminergic projections from the mid-brain to the frontal lobe are also affected by the disease.

Accepting for the time being that the main actions of dopamine are as described above, *akinesia* and *bradykinesia* can be explained by lack of stimulation of striatal D_1 and D_2 receptors. This would lead to increased inhibition of thal-amocortical neurons in VL and VA. The premotor areas would receive less excitation, with resulting poverty of move-ments (bradykinesia) and increased threshold for movement initiation (akinesia). In support of this hypothesis, cerebral blood-flow measurements in Parkinsonian patients suggest that they have reduced activity in SMA compared with nor-mal controls during voluntary movements. We will describe in more detail the hypothetical chain of events caused by loss of dopamine. As mentioned, D_1 receptors—with excitatory actions—are predominantly found on neurons project-ing to the inner segment of the globus pallidus (Gp_i) and the nigra (*the direct pathway*). Reduced D_1 stimulation would produce less inhibition of Gp_i neurons projecting to the thalamus (VL and VA), and consequently the thalamocortical neurons would be more inhibited. The same effect would be produced via *the indirect pathway* through the subthalamic nucleus. Since D_2 receptor activation is assumed to inhibit striatal neurons projecting to the external segment of the globus pallidus (Gp_e), loss of dopamine would result in reduced inhibition of Gp_e neurons. The latter inhibit subthalamic neu-rons, which in their turn excite Gp_i neurons. Thus, the subthalamic nucleus receives less inhibition, and consequently the Gp_i receives more excitation, again leading to more inhibition of VL and VA. A monkey model of Parkinson's disease (with selective destruction of the pars compacta of the substantia nigra with the chemical methyl-phenyl-tetrahydropyri-dine, MPTP) supports that there *is* increased activity of the indirect pathway in Parkinson's disease. Thus, in such mon-keys increased neuronal activity occurs in the subthalamic nucleus and in the Gp_i.

The model described above does not readily explain the rigidity and tremor in Parkinson's disease, however. One hypothesis ascribes the rigidity to abnormal actions of the basal ganglia on the mesencephalic reticular formation (PPN), assuming that this region receives less inhibition from the substantia nigra (pars reticulata). However, other data suggest that the rigidity and the tremor depend on VL and VA. Thus, surgical interruption of the pallidothalamic fibers leads, as a rule, to substantial reduction of these symptoms, whereas akinesia and bradykinesia are much less improved. To com-plicate matters further, experimental data suggest that akinesia and rigidity depend on dopamine loss in the *ventral stria-tum* and the *putamen*, respectively.

Considering the complexity of the basal ganglia, the present models seeking to explain the symptoms of Parkinson's disease are obviously oversimplifications. They incorporate only the factors considered most important by our present knowledge, and not all symptoms are satisfactorily explained. For example, the effect of dopamine deficiency on the cholinergic interneurons is not taken into account (because it is still unknown), and mutual interactions between the stri-atal projection neurons are left out of the model. As mentioned above, transmitters other than dopamine are affected in Parkinson's disease, and the interactions between several transmitters and their receptors are probably disturbed. For ex-ample, dopamine loss leads to alterations of the peptide content of striatal projection neurons.

Treatment with Transplantation of Nervous Tissue

The possibility of replacing by transplantation the lost dopaminergic neurons in Parkinson's disease is now under intense investigation. Animal experiments—pioneered by, among others, the Swedish neurobiologist Björklund—show that trans-plantation can eliminate virtually all symptoms produced by lesions of the substantia nigra in adult rats. The transplanted cells must come from an embryo, and a sufficient number must be put into the striatum in the adult lesioned animal. The best results are obtained when embryonic cells in a suspension are injected rather than being implanted as a solid piece of tissue. Because the transplanted cells are embryonic, they are not rejected and start growing apparently normal processes in their new location. The cells synthesize and liberate dopamine. The method is now under trial for use in patients with Parkinson's disease, but it is not yet clear whether the method will work in humans. One major problem is presumably to obtain a sufficient number of transplanted embryonic cells for survival. Furthermore, the huge size of the human stria-tum poses problems that are not encountered in the small brain of the rat.

Huntington's Disease (Huntington's Chorea)

This disease is dominantly inherited and usually starts in the fourth decade of life. It has a steadily progressing course. The disease is characterized by rapid, jerky, involuntary movements of the face, arms, and legs. In advanced stages the patient is never at rest. The dancelike quality of the movements led to the terms chorea and choreatic movements (Greek: *chorea* = dance). The most prominent pathological change involves the striatum, with a marked reduction in the number of GABAergic projection neurons.

Observations suggest that in *early stages* of the disease, mostly neurons projecting to the Gp_e degenerate (the *indirect pathway*, see above under Parkinson's Disease). This would produce reduced inhibition of Gp_e neurons, and by that increased inhibition of the subthalamic nucleus. (Animal models support that reduced activity of the subthalamic nucleus may be crucial for development of choreatic movements.) This in turn leads to reduced excitation of Gp_i, and by that to reduced inhibition (disinhibition) of thalamocortical neurons in VL and VA. Thus, the choreatic movements may be causally related to increased excitatory input to motor cortical areas.

In *later stages* of the disease, also striatal neurons projecting to the Gp_i die (and many neurons in other parts of the brain). This leads to reduced inhibition of Gp_i with subsequent increased inhibition of thalamocortical neurons (as in Parkinson's disease). This is taken to explain why bradykinesia develops in later stages of Huntington's disease, while the choreatic movements continue. This is not obviously logical, however, if the effects of both the direct and indirect pathways are mediated via the Gp_i. Another explanatory model focuses on dopaminergic hyperactivity in the striatum, caused by loss of GABAergic inhibition in the substantia nigra (Fig. 13.7). Although there are also problems with this model, it fits with the observation that L-dopa worsens the choreatic movements of patients with Huntington's disease.

The disease also leads to mental deterioration with *dementia*, which probably may be explained by cell loss occurring also in the cerebral cortex (particularly the frontal lobes).

The etiology of the disease is unknown. One hypothesis is that the cell death is caused by a toxin produced in the brain, mimicking the action of glutamate on the striatal neurons, probably involving the NMDA receptor. It has recently been shown that the genetic defect is located on the short arm of chromosome 4, and this makes it possible to decide whether a person is a carrier of the disease long before the symptoms occur. This is of importance regarding the choice whether or not to have children. However, to provide individuals with such knowledge as long as there is no effective treatment poses obvious ethical questions.

Tourette's Syndrome

This is a peculiar and multifarious condition with *multiple tics* (quick involuntary movements that are repetitive at irregular intervals) associated with involuntary vocalization as central manifestations. The disease starts during childhood, usually between the ages of five and ten years, and affects boys more frequently than girls. Many patients have a repertoire of repetitive behavior, such as touching others, repeating their own words, or echoing the words or movements of others. Vocalizations (vocal tics) commonly include explosive cursing or compulsive utterance of obscenities, which interrupt normal speech. Many patients describe that an inner tension builds up, and this is temporarily relieved by the tic. Some people with Tourette's syndrome appear to have unusual energy and creativity. As children, they often show hyperactive behavior. This may lead to serious social problems, especially when—as often happens—the disease is misdiagnosed as a behavioral disorder of social origin.

Treatment with dopamine antagonists (especially haloperidol, a D_2-receptor antagonist) may reduce the involuntary movements and other troublesome symptoms. However, the patient's mental energy and self-perception may be severely affected by the treatment. As vividly described by Oliver Sacks in *The Man who Mistook his Wife for a Hat*, this may be experienced by some patients as worse than the symptoms.

NOTES

1. The claustrum and the amygdaloid nucleus were also included in the term basal ganglia by the early anatomists. The function of the claustrum is still largely unknown, even though it is known to receive its main afferents from the cerebral cortex and to send efferents directly back to the cortex. The amygdaloid nucleus differs with regard to both connections and function from the other parts of the basal ganglia and is now usually considered a part of the so-called limbic structures (Chapter 19).

2. The efferent fibers from the pallidum form two bundles, the *ansa lenticularis* and the *fasciculus lenticularis*. They arise from somewhat different parts of the internal pallidal segment and fuse to form the *fasciculus thalamicus* after having traversed the internal capsule.

3. The *thalamic nuclei VL and VA* are not just relay stations in which impulses from the pallidum and nigra directed to the cerebral cortex are synaptically interrupted. Considerable processing of information takes place in these nuclei; what goes out is not a mirror image of what goes in. Thus, like other thalamic nuclei, the VL and VA receive afferents from sources other than the basal ganglia. They both receive ample connections from the parts of the cortex to which they project. (The VL receives connections from the cerebellum, but such fibers appear in the monkey to end in other parts of the VL than the pallidal fibers, making the possibility of interactions small.) The VA receives fibers also from the reticular formation and the intralaminar thalamic nuclei (especially the large centromedian nucleus [CM]).

4. Here we use the terms *premotor* and *premotor networks* in a rather loose sense about neuronal groups acting either directly on motoneurons or on the motor cortex. Such premotor networks are found in the spinal cord, the reticular formation, and in the thalamus. Neurons of the thalamic VL nucleus are considered premotor due to their direct projection to the motor cortex. Premotor networks organize the activity of motoneurons to produce purposeful actions (not merely isolated movements).

5. The *cholinergic interneurons* constitute about 1% of all striatal neurons. Besides modulatory inputs from dopaminergic, nigrostriatal neurons, they receive excitation from the intralaminar nuclei and inhibition from GABAergic, striatal projection neurons (but perhaps only from those containing SP). They exert synaptic effects mainly on the striatal projection neurons by acting on a certain kind of K^+ channel. The membrane potential of the postsynaptic cell determines whether the channel is opened or closed by acetylcholine (as with the actions of dopamine). The overall effect of acetylcholine on the projection neurons is to ensure that they react with bursts of action potentials to excitatory inputs from the cerebral cortex—that is, the efficiency of signal transmission is enhanced.

6. Among other afferents to the striatum, most of the fibers from the raphe nuclei contain serotonin. Serotonin has most likely an inhibitory (modulatory) action in the striatum. The thalamostriatal neurons (in particular those from the CM) appear to be glutamatergic with an excitatory effect in the striatum.

7. More detailed studies indicate that D_1 and D_2 receptors are segregated (with regard to cell type) on distal dendrites but mixed on proximal dendrites and the cell soma. In quantitative terms, however, D_1 dominates on GABA + SP cells, whereas D_2 dominates on GABA + enkephalin cells.

8. Some authors use the terms *hyperkinetic* and *hypokinetic* disorders to distinguish the two main kinds of basal ganglia diseases. It should be noted, however, that the hypokinetic disorders are usually combined with rigidity and tremor (that is, signs of neuronal hyperactivity), whereas the hyperkinetic disorders are often combined with muscular hypotonia.

CHAPTER 14

THE CEREBELLUM

It has been known for a long time from clinical observations that the cerebellum is important for the execution of movements. Its fiber connections also suggest a motor function: It is mainly connected with parts of the central nervous system involved in motor control, such as the spinal cord and the motor cortex. There are certain similarities between the cerebellum and the basal ganglia; both are involved in motor control without being responsible for the initiation of movements, and both are built into "side loops" of the motor cortical areas and the central motor pathways.

Damage to the cerebellum produces characteristic symptoms primarily with respect to the execution of voluntary movements. Our normal movements are always *coordinated*—that is, the various muscles participating contract at the proper time and with the proper force. This is a prerequisite for our ability to hit a nail with a hammer, for writing even and rounded letters, for the words to follow each other with proper loudness and rhythm during speech, and so forth. After cerebellar damage such coordination is lacking, and the movements become uncertain and jerky.

The cerebellum *receives information* from many sources. Sensory impulses come from the skin, joints, muscles, the vestibular apparatus, and the eye. In most instances, this sensory information appears to be related to aspects of movements, such as signals from muscle and joint receptors about positions and ongoing movements. Information is also coming from other parts of the central nervous system, especially from the cerebral cortex—primarily from cortical areas treating information about movements or involved in planning or initiation of movements. The cerebellum *sends information* primarily to cell groups that give origin to the central motor pathways, like the motor cortical areas and the reticular formation of the brain stem. (Some cerebellar connections, however, suggest that it may also be involved in functions other than motor ones.)

It is a striking feature of cerebellar organization that the number of fibers leading to the cerebellum is much larger than the number of fibers leading out; the relationship is about 40:1 in humans. In Figure 14.1 the thickness of the arrows shows roughly the relative number of afferent and

Figure 14.1 *The cerebellar peduncles.* The brain stem seen from the left. The arrows indicate the peduncle used by the main afferent and efferent connections on entering or leaving the cerebellum. The thickness of the arrows indicates the magnitude of the various connections. Note the massive afferent pathway from the pontine nuclei entering through the middle cerebellar peduncle (the brachium pontis). The largest number of efferent fibers leave the cerebellum through the superior cerebellar peduncle (the brachium conjunctivum). From Brodal (1981).

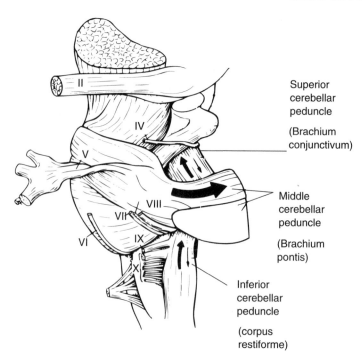

Superior cerebellar peduncle

(Brachium conjunctivum)

Middle cerebellar peduncle

(Brachium pontis)

Inferior cerebellar peduncle

(corpus restiforme)

efferent fibers in the three cerebellar peduncles. The major afferent contingent enters through the middle cerebellar peduncle (the brachium pontis), whereas most of the efferent fibers leave the cerebellum through the superior cerebellar peduncle (the brachium conjunctivum). The high degree of convergence shows that considerable integration and processing of information takes place in the cerebellum before an answer is issued. *How* the processing is done is still largely unknown, despite very detailed knowledge of the structure and properties of the neuronal elements of the cerebellum.

The afferent fibers end in segregated regions of the cerebellar cortex, and the efferents from these regions are also largely segregated. This suggests that the cerebellum consists of many functional units or *modules*, each carrying out a specific task. Due to the structural homogeneity of the cerebellar cortex, however, all modules have the same kind of machinery and, presumably, perform the same kind of information processing. Among several possibilities, the cerebellum may be specially designed for *accurate timing* of events—concerning not only movements but perhaps also certain cognitive tasks.

SUBDIVISIONS, STRUCTURE, AND CONNECTIONS OF THE CEREBELLUM

The macroscopic anatomy of the cerebellum was described in Chapter 3, but some points bear repetition here. The external part of the cerebellum is a thin, highly convoluted sheet of gray matter, the *cerebellar cortex*.

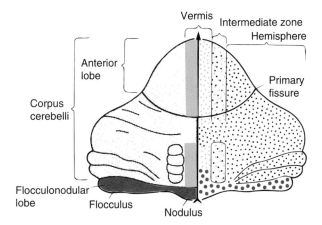

Figure 14.2 *Main cerebellar subdivisions*. **Above**, a schematic drawing of a partly unfolded cerebellum. The **lower** drawing shows how the unfolding was performed. The dots indicate roughly the cerebellar terminal regions of the main afferent contingents from the spinal cord, from the vestibular apparatus, and from the cerebral cortex via the pontine nuclei.

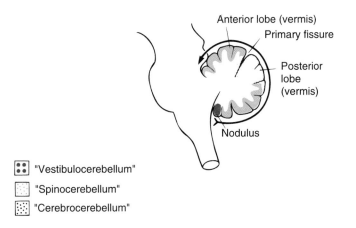

The folds are preponderantly arranged transversely and form *folia*. The underlying white matter contains the afferent and efferent fibers of the cerebellar cortex. In addition, masses of gray matter, the *intracerebellar nuclei*, are embedded in the white matter in the central parts of the cerebellum. These nuclei are relay stations in the efferent connections of the cerebellar cortex (Figs. 14.10 and 14.12).

The Cerebellum Consists of Three Functionally Different Parts

The structure of the cortex is the same all over the cerebellum. Various parts of the cerebellum differ in function because of differences in fiber connections: The various subdivisions of the cerebellum receive afferents from and act on different parts of the nervous system. A subdivision of the cerebellum on the basis of functional differences corresponds closely with a subdivision on the basis of differences in where the afferent fibers come from (Fig. 14.2). Furthermore, such a subdivision corresponds also with one based on the cerebellar phylogenetic development from lower to higher animals.

The most primitive part of the cerebellum—the part occurring first during phylogeny—is the small *flocculonodular lobe* (Fig. 14.2). With reference to its phylogenetic age, it is also called the *archicerebellum*. It consists of the nodulus in the midline (a part of the vermis) connected laterally with a thin stalk to the flocculus. The size of this part of the cerebellum varies little among mammals. The flocculonodular lobe receives afferents primarily from the vestibular apparatus and the vestibular nuclei and is therefore also called the *vestibulocerebellum*. The rest of the cerebellum is called the *corpus cerebelli*. This comprises all of the vermis (except the nodulus), which forms a narrow zone on both sides of the midline, and the large lateral parts called the *cerebellar hemispheres*. The medialmost part of the hemispheres, bordering the vermis medially, is called the *intermediate zone* (Fig. 14.2). This zone cannot be distinguished from the rest of the cerebellum on a macroscopic basis but only on the basis of fiber connections. The corpus cerebelli is divided by a deep, transversely oriented fissure, the *primary fissure*. The parts of the corpus cerebelli in front of and behind the primary fissure are called the *anterior lobe* and the *posterior lobe*, respectively. The anterior and posterior parts of the vermis constitute the phylogenetically oldest parts of the corpus cerebelli and are together called the *paleocerebellum*. The midportion of the vermis and the hemispheres are younger and are therefore called the *neocerebellum*. The anterior and posterior portions of the vermis and the adjoining parts of the intermediate zone of the corpus cerebelli receive afferents primarily from the spinal cord and are therefore also termed the *spinocerebellum*. The hemispheres receive their main input from the cerebral cortex, synaptically interrupted in the pontine nuclei, and are therefore termed the *cerebrocerebellum* or the *pontocerebellum*.

With regard to the *efferent connections* of the cerebellum, the three main subdivisions of the cerebellum *act on the parts of the central nervous system from which they receive their afferents*; that is, the vestibulocerebellum sends fibers mainly to the vestibular nuclei, the spinocerebellum influences the spinal cord, and the cerebrocerebellum acts on the cerebral cortex.

Afferent Connections from the Labyrinth and the Vestibular Nuclei

Primary vestibular afferents bring sensory impulses from the vestibular apparatus in the inner ear (the vestibular part of the labyrinth). They enter the cerebellum through the inferior cerebellar peduncle (Fig. 14.1) and end in the flocculonodular lobe and adjoining parts of the vermis (Fig. 14.3). Most of the primary vestibular afferents do not end in the cerebellum but in the vestibular nuclei. Many neurons in the latter send axons to the cerebellum. In this manner, the cerebellum receives vestibular information also via *secondary vestibular afferents*. The vestibular input provides the cerebellum with information about the *position and movements of the head*. Efferents from the flocculonodular lobe end in the vestibular nuclei and can thereby influence the body equilibrium (via the vestibulospinal tracts) and eye movements (Fig. 14.3). This is treated more fully in Chapter 16.

"VESTIBULOCEREBELLUM"

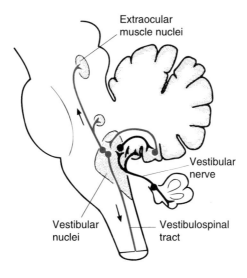

Extraocular
muscle nuclei

Vestibular
nerve

Vestibular
nuclei

Vestibulospinal
tract

Figure 14.3 *The main connections of the vestibulocerebellum.* Afferents are shown in black and efferents in red in a schematic drawing of a sagittal section through the brain stem. Note primary and secondary vestibulocerebellar fibers and the projection back to the vestibular nuclei. In addition to afferents from the vestibulocerebellum, the vestibular nuclei also receive cerebellar afferents from the anterior lobe vermis and from the fastigial nucleus.

Afferent Connections from the Spinal Cord

Several pathways bring impulses from the spinal cord to the cerebellum (Fig. 14.4). Some of these pathways go uninterrupted from the cord to the cerebellum and are called *direct spinocerebellar tracts*, whereas others are synaptically interrupted in brain stem nuclei and are therefore termed *indirect spinocerebellar tracts* (not shown in Fig. 14.4). The spinocerebellar tracts originate from neurons with their perikarya located in various lamina of the spinal cord (Fig. 14.6). They are therefore influenced by different kinds of receptors and spinal interneurons and bring different kinds of information to the cerebellum. *The spinocerebellar axons end mostly in the spinocerebellum of the same side* (as their perikarya). Some pass uncrossed; other fibers cross twice (first in the spinal cord and then back again in the brain stem). The fibers are located in the lateral

"SPINOCEREBELLUM"

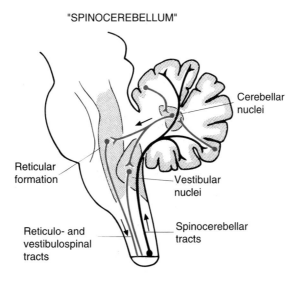

Cerebellar
nuclei

Reticular
formation

Vestibular
nuclei

Reticulo- and
vestibulospinal
tracts

Spinocerebellar
tracts

Figure 14.4 *The main connections of the spinocerebellum.* Note that the spinocerebellum can influence spinal motoneurons via reticulospinal and vestibulospinal pathways.

Figure 14.5 *Somatotopic localization of the cerebellar cortex*. Based on experiments with electrical stimulation of peripheral nerves and of various subdivisions of the SI and the MI.

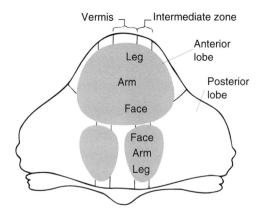

funiculus as they ascend. The tracts are *somatotopically organized*, so that signals from different body parts are kept segregated. The somatotopic pattern is maintained within the cerebellum (Fig. 14.5) so that the leg is represented anteriorly within the anterior lobe, with the arm and the face represented successively more posteriorly. In the posterior lobe the arrangement is the reverse, with the face represented anteriorly.

Functionally, the direct spinocerebellar tracts consist of two main groups. One group of tracts conveys information from *muscle spindles, tendon organs, and cutaneous low-threshold mechanoreceptors*. Physiological studies show that many of the neurons of the direct spinocerebellar tracts are activated monosynaptically by primary afferent (sensory) fibers. The tracts conduct very rapidly and appear to give precisely timed information about movements and skin stimuli (which also often are related to movements).

Another group of direct spinocerebellar tracts does not convey signals from receptors but provides information about the *level of activity among specific groups of spinal interneurons*. Such interneurons are as a rule intercalated in spinal reflex arcs and between descending motor pathways and motoneurons (that is, forming so-called premotor networks). Information about their activity is therefore presumably highly relevant for cerebellar operations.

Together, the spinocerebellar tracts provide the cerebellum with information about the activity both *before* and *after* the motoneurons—that is, about the *commands issued to the motoneurons and the movements produced by the motoneuronal activity*. The cerebellum can probably judge whether the command led to the desired result. When, for exam-

Figure 14.6 *The dorsal and ventral spinocerebellar tracts*. Schematic drawing of a transverse section through the thoracic cord, showing the position of the perikarya in the gray spinal matter and the tracts in the white matter. Most of the fibers of the ventral spinocerebellar tract cross twice (once in the cord and once in the brain stem), so that most spinocerebellar impulses reach the cerebellar half on the same side as the perikarya are located.

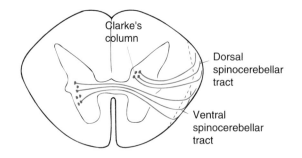

ple, an unexpected increase of external resistance to a movement reduces the velocity compared with what was intended, the cerebellum will be informed immediately. Via its connections to the spinal cord, the cerebellum can then help to adjust the firing of the motoneurons to the new situation, so that the correct velocity is regained.

The Dorsal, Ventral, and Some Other Spinocerebellar Tracts

Originally, two direct spinocerebellar tracts were described, differing with regard to the position of their fibers in the lateral funiculus of the cord. The fibers of one of the tracts are located dorsally and the tract was called the *dorsal spinocerebellar tract*; the fibers of the *ventral spinocerebellar tract* are located more ventrally (Fig. 14.6).

The *dorsal spinocerebellar tract* comes from a distinct cell group with fairly large cells at the base of the dorsal horn, forming the *column of Clarke* located in the spinal segments from T_1 to L_2 only. The axons of the cells in the column of Clarke ascend on the same side and enter the cerebellum through the inferior cerebellar peduncle. Primary afferent fibers entering the cord through spinal nerves below the L_2 ascend in the dorsal columns before entering the lowermost part of the column of Clarke. The dorsal spinocerebellar tract conveys information only from the trunk and the lower extremities and ends in the corresponding parts of the spinocerebellum. The same kind of information from the upper extremities is mediated by another cell group, the *external cuneate nucleus*, located laterally in the medulla oblongata. Functionally, this nucleus corresponds to the column of Clarke, and primary afferents from the arms ascend in the dorsal columns to end in the nucleus. The cells of the external cuneate nucleus send their axons to the arm regions of the spinocerebellum of the same side (forming the cuneocerebellar tract).

Since many primary afferent fibers from *muscle spindles and tendon organs end monosynaptically on the neurons of the column of Clarke* (and the external cuneate nucleus), it was assumed that the dorsal spinocerebellar tract mediates mainly receptor-specific information to the cerebellum. It was known, however, that the column of Clarke also receives *polysynaptic* information from the same kind of receptors, and from joint and cutaneous receptors. Recent physiological studies show that most of the column of Clarke neurons integrate information from various receptor types activated by a specific movement. Thus, the *dorsal spinocerebellar tract appears to inform primarily for more complex joint movements, for example such that involve the whole extremity.* This is another example that sensory relay nuclei do not merely transmit signals unchanged from receptors; they always process information in some way.

The *ventral spinocerebellar tract* originates from cells located mainly laterally in lamina VII (Figs. 7.11 and 14.6)—that is, in the lamina containing the largest number of interneurons. Most of the axons cross at the segmental level in the cord to the lateral funiculus of the opposite side. However, after having reached the cerebellum through the superior cerebellar peduncle (Fig. 14.1), many of the fibers cross once more. The perikarya of the neurons giving origin to the ventral spinocerebellar neurons are found only below the midthoracic level of the cord and have a rostral counterpart conveying information from higher levels of the cord (the rostral spinocerebellar tract). These tracts convey *information about the activity of the spinal interneurons*, as mentioned above. Physiological experiments indicate that they inform primarily about the activity of inhibitory interneurons.

In addition to the spinocerebellar tracts mentioned so far, other cell groups in the spinal cord also send fibers to the cerebellum. Among such cell groups is the *central cervical nucleus*, located in the upper cervical segments. The fibers end in the anteriormost folia of the anterior lobe and transmit signals primarily from *receptors around the cervical joints*.

An additional indirect spinocerebellar pathway is relayed in the *lateral reticular nucleus*, located in the medulla just lateral to the inferior olive. This spinoreticulocerebellar pathway, too, is mainly uncrossed and appears to convey information about the activity of certain *groups of spinal interneurons*. Since most of the spinal interneurons are strongly influenced by descending motor pathways, the ascending tract to the lateral reticular nucleus probably informs about their activity as well. The lateral reticular nucleus also receives afferents from sources other than the spinal cord, notably the red nucleus, the vestibular nuclei, and the motor cortex. Many cells, for example, are strongly influenced by tilting of the head (stimulating vestibular receptors).

Information from sensory receptors can reach the cerebellum not only through some of the spinocerebellar tracts but also through fibers sent to the spinocerebellum from the *dorsal column nuclei* and the *trigeminal nuclei*.

Figure 14.7 *The main connections of the cerebrocerebellum.* Note that the ascending connections to the cerebral cortex are synaptically interrupted in the dentate nucleus and in the thalamus. The projection to the cerebellar nuclei is GABAergic and inhibitory, whereas the thalamocortical fibers exert excitatory actions in the cortex.

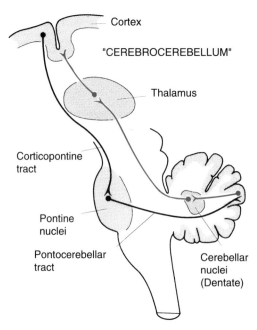

There are several *indirect spinocerebellar tracts*, but here we will only mention the one synaptically interrupted in the inferior olive in the medulla (Fig. 3.16). Neurons at all levels of the cord send fibers to the *inferior olive* of the opposite side. The spino-olivary fibers end in parts of the inferior olive that project to the spinocerebellum of the opposite side; thus, like the direct spinocerebellar tracts, the spino-olivocerebellar tract conveys information mainly from one side of the cord to the cerebellar half of the same side. This pathway, too, is precisely somatotopically organized. The kind of information conveyed by the spino-olivocerebellar tract appears to be different from that conveyed by the other spinocerebellar tracts. We will return to the inferior olive below, because this nucleus plays a unique role among cell groups sending fibers to the cerebellum.

Afferent Connections from the Cerebral Cortex

In humans, by far the largest number of cerebellar afferent fibers arises in the pontine nuclei (Figs. 3.17 and 14.7). The *pontocerebellar tract* ends primarily in the cerebellar hemispheres, which constitute the major part of the cerebellum in humans. The vast majority of afferents to the pontine nuclei arise in the cerebral cortex and form the corticopontine tract (Fig. 14.8).[1] The main task of the pontine nuclei therefore is to process information from the cerebral cortex and forward it to the cerebellar cortex. The corticopontine tract is uncrossed, whereas most of the pontocerebellar fibers cross; thus *the cerebral cortex of one side acts mainly on the cerebellar hemisphere of the opposite side.*

The corticopontine tract runs in the *internal capsule* and then in the *crus cerebri* (Fig. 3.20), where it occupies a large part; of the approximately 19 million fibers in the crus of the human brain, the corticopon-

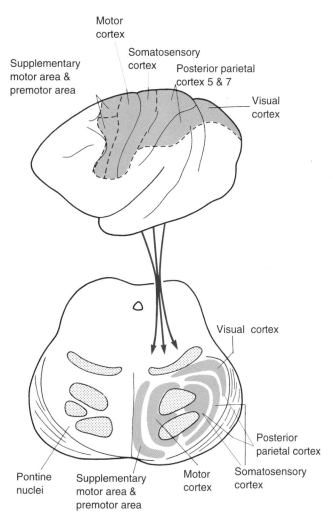

Motor cortex

Supplementary motor area & premotor area

Somatosensory cortex

Posterior parietal cortex 5 & 7

Visual cortex

Visual cortex

Posterior parietal cortex

Pontine nuclei

Supplementary motor area & premotor area

Motor cortex

Somatosensory cortex

Figure 14.8 *The corticopontine pathway*. Areas of the cerebral cortex that are strongly connected with the cerebellar hemispheres via the pontine nuclei are shown in red. Note the topographic arrangement of the corticopontine pathway in the pontine nuclei—each cortical region has its own territory.

tine fibers constitute the majority (the pyramidal tract, in comparison, contains only about 1 million fibers).

A large fraction of *the corticopontine fibers arise in the MI and SI*. There are, however, substantial contributions also from the *SMA and PMA* and from *areas 5 and 7* of the posterior parietal cortex (Fig. 14.8). All of these areas are, in various ways, active during or before movements (see Chapter 12). Presumably, the cerebellum thus receives information about movements that are being planned and about the commands that are sent out from the motor cortex; in response it can modulate the activity of the motor cortex so that the movements are performed smoothly and accurately. The pontine nuclei also receive afferents from the *visual cortex*, and physiological experiments indicate that these fibers inform primarily about moving objects in the visual field. Such connections may be of importance to the execution of visually guided movements.[2]

The pontine nuclei also receive connections from parts of the hypothalamus and limbic structures, particularly the *cingulate gyrus* and the *mammillary bodies*. The information conveyed from these regions is probably not directly related to movement, but may perhaps contribute to the well-known influence of motivation and emotions on movements. Both the corticopontine and the pontocerebellar projections are *topographically*

Figure 14.9 *The main connections of the intermediate zone.* Both the spinal cord (via the red nucleus) and the cerebral cortex (via the thalamus) can be influenced by the intermediate zone.

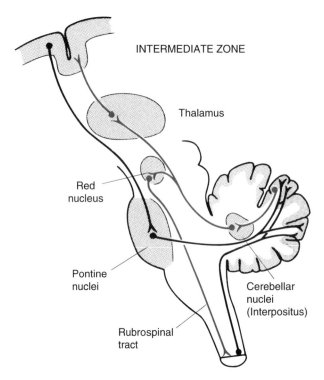

organized. This and other data indicate that there is a functional localization within the cerebellar hemispheres, so that smaller parts take care of specific tasks. In contrast to the cerebral cortex, the cerebellar cortex has no association and commissural connections—different parts of the cerebellum do not "talk" to each other. Thus, each subdivision of the cerebellar hemispheres that differs from its neighbors with regard to its afferent connections from the cerebral cortex may probably be considered a separate functional unit. In this respect, the *cerebellum resembles the basal ganglia, which appear to be organized in several parallel circuits starting and ending in the cerebral cortex.*

The Intermediate Zone Is a Meeting Place for Impulses from the Cord and the Cerebral Cortex

The intermediate zone of the cerebellum is mainly defined on the basis of its efferent connections. It also has special features with regard to afferents, however (Fig. 14.9). Whereas the lateral parts of the hemispheres are strongly dominated by inputs from the cerebral cortex, and the vermis is dominated by spinal inputs, the intermediate zone receives connections from both the cerebral cortex and the spinal cord (Fig. 14.2). Experiments in the cat indicate that the cortical input to the intermediate zone comes primarily from the MI and SI. Single neurons in the intermediate zone can be activated from both the cerebral cortex and the spinal cord. For example, in the "arm region" (Fig. 14.5) of the anterior lobe, intermediate-zone single neurons receive converging input from the arm region of the MI and SI and from sensory receptors in the arm. Perhaps the cerebellum in this case *compares copies of the motor commands sent from the cerebral cortex with the signals from the periphery providing information about the actual movement that was produced by the command.*

The Inferior Olive Also Conveys Information from the Spinal Cord, the Cerebral Cortex, and the Mesencephalon

The inferior olive consists of subdivisions that receive afferents primarily from the *spinal cord* via several precisely organized tracts and of other, larger parts (in humans) that receive fibers mainly from various mesencephalic nuclei, such as the *superior colliculus, the pretectal nuclei, the red nucleus, and several smaller nuclei.* These parts of the olive send most of their fibers to the cerebellar hemispheres. There is also a modest direct projection from the cerebral cortex (especially the MI) to the inferior olive. In addition, the red nucleus and several other mesencephalic nuclei receive cortical afferents from the MI, SMA, and PMA and may therefore mediate cortical influences on the inferior olive.

The *pretectal nuclei*, which receive visual signals from the retina, project to a small distinct part of the inferior olive, which in its turn projects to the flocculonodular lobe (Fig. 16.28). These connections are of importance for adaptations of the vestibulo-ocular reflex (See below, *The Cerebellum and Motor Learning*). The superior colliculus, also in receipt of visual signals from the retina and the cerebral cortex, influences other parts of the cerebellum via the inferior olive and contributes to control of eye movements. The kind of information sent from the red nucleus to the cerebellum via the inferior olive is largely unknown.

As we will return to later, the kind of information conveyed to the cerebellum from the inferior olive is most likely fundamentally different from that sent from the pontine nuclei.

Structure of the Cerebellar Cortex

Before discussing the efferent connections of the cerebellum, we need to know something about the cerebellar cortex (Figs. 14.10 and 14.11). Here, the vast amount of information provided by all of the afferents is processed. To some extent, different kinds of information are integrated, and then "answers" are issued to various motor centers of the brain and spinal cord.

As mentioned above, the cerebellar cortex has the same structure all over the cerebellum (it cannot be subdivided into cytoarchitectonic areas, differing also in this respect from the cerebral cortex). The structural arrangement of the neuronal elements is strictly geometric, so the individual elements can be distinguished fairly easily. This helps to explain why the structure and internal connections of the cerebellar cortex are much better known than that of the cerebral cortex.

The cerebellar cortex consists of *three layers*. The superficial, outermost layer is the *molecular layer.* It contains mainly dendrites and axons from cells in the deeper layers but only a few perikarya. The middle layer is dominated by the large, *Purkinje cells*, arranged in a monolayer (Fig.

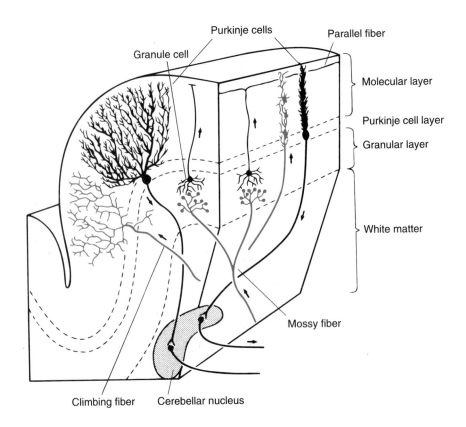

Figure 14.10 *The structure of the cerebellar cortex.* The three layers and the main cell types are shown schematically in a piece of cerebellar folium. Note the arrangement of the Purkinje cell dendrites perpendicular to the long axis of the folium and the parallel fibers. The two main kinds of afferent fibers (mossy and climbing fibers) are also shown. The mossy fibers end on the granule cells, whereas the climbing fibers enter the molecular layer to end on the Purkinje cell dendrites.

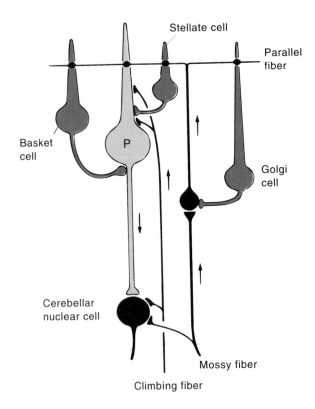

Figure 14.11 *The cerebellar cortex.* Schematic presentation of the main cell types and their synaptic arrangements. Red signifies inhibitory action; black, excitatory. Note the three kinds of inhibitory interneurons. Redrawn from Eccles, Ito, and Szentágothai (1967).

14.10), and is called the *Purkinje cell layer*. The deepest, lowermost layer is called the *granular layer* because it is packed with tiny *granule cells*. *The Purkinje cells are the only ones that send their axons out of the cerebellar cortex* and thus constitute the efferent channel. The axons of the granule cells ascend through the Purkinje cell layer into the molecular layer, in which they divide at a right angle into two branches running parallel with the surface of the cortex (Figs. 14.10 and 14.11). These branches are called *parallel fibers* and run in the direction of the long axis of the folia. The parallel fibers form numerous synapses with the Purkinje cell dendrites. The Purkinje cell dendritic tree is unusual: In the first place, it has an enormously rich branching pattern, and second, the whole dendritic tree is compressed into one plane, forming an espalier oriented perpendicular to the long axis of the folia and the parallel fibers. This arrangement ensures that each parallel fiber forms synapses with many Purkinje cells (the parallel fibers can be several millimeters long). At the same time, each Purkinje cell is contacted by an enormous number of parallel fibers. Thus, a Purkinje cell integrates the activity of a large number of granule cells. The *Purkinje cells contain GABA*, and they inhibit their target cells, as shown physiologically. The *granule cells* have an excitatory action on the Purkinje cells, releasing *glutamate*.

Afferents to the Cerebellar Cortex Are of Two Main Kinds: Mossy and Climbing Fibers

The numerous afferent fibers to the cerebellar cortex fall into two categories, which differ in how the fibers end in the cerebellar cortex. Both kinds have an excitatory synaptic action, mediated by an amino acid transmitter (most likely glutamate). The *climbing fibers* all come from the *inferior olive*, whereas afferents from nearly all other nuclei end as mossy fibers (such as the vestibulocerebellar, the spinocerebellar, and the pontocerebellar fibers).[3]

The *mossy fibers* conduct signals relatively rapidly and end in the granular layer, establishing synapses with the granule cell dendrites (Figs. 14.10 and 14.11). One mossy fiber branches extensively and contacts a large number of granule cells, each of which in its turn contacts many Purkinje cells. Thus, each mossy fiber influences many Purkinje cells, but the excitatory effect on each is weak, so that *many mossy fibers must be active together to provide sufficient excitation (via the parallel fibers) to fire a Purkinje cell* (as mentioned, the parallel fibers excite the Purkinje cells). A typical feature of the mossy fibers is that they transmit action potentials with a high frequency and produce Purkinje cell firing with a frequency of 50–100/sec.

The *climbing fibers* end very differently from the mossy fibers: The fibers ascend directly to the molecular layer and divide into several branches, each "climbing" along a Purkinje cell dendrite (Figs. 1.6B, 14.10, and 14.11). As they climb, they form numerous synapses with the dendrites. Each Purkinje cell receives branches from only one climbing fiber (that is, from only one cell in the inferior olive). Each olivary cell, however, innervates more than one Purkinje cell, since the number of Purkinje cells is higher than the number of olivary cells. Because each climbing fiber forms so many synapses with a Purkinje cell, the total excitatory action is strong. Thus, *even a single action potential in a climbing fiber elicits a burst of action potentials in the Purkinje cells it contacts* (Note the difference from the mossy fibers: Many of these have to be active simultaneously, and with a high frequency, to fire the Purkinje cells.). The firing frequency of the climbing fibers is very low under natural conditions (often less than one impulse per second). Even maximal stimulation does not bring the firing frequency above 10 sec.

In conclusion, the Purkinje cells receive excitation from both mossy and climbing fiber afferent inputs, but with very different spatial and temporal characteristics of their actions.

In addition, the signal traffic within the cerebellar cortex is influenced by several kinds of *inhibitory interneurons* (Fig. 14.11). These interneurons are also excited by afferent impulses to the cortex and serve in general to increase the precision of signal traffic through the cerebellar cortex (like inhibitory interneurons in the nuclei of the sensory pathways).

Mossy and Climbing Fibers Are Functionally Different

The great differences between the mossy and climbing fibers with regard to both structural and physiological properties strongly suggest that they convey different kinds of information and thus play different roles in cerebellar functions. Because of their ability to vary their impulse frequency over a wide range, the *mossy fibers* are presumably well suited for providing precisely graded information about movements (the muscles involved, and the direction, speed, and force of movements), localization and characteristics of skin stimuli, details concerning motor commands issued from the cerebral cortex, and so forth. Such assumptions also fit with the physiological properties of spinocerebellar fibers, known to end as mossy fibers (less is known about the corticopontocerebellar pathway in this respect).

The *climbing fibers*, because of their low range of firing frequency, are less likely to provide precisely graded information. Recording of the climbing fiber activity and the firing of the Purkinje cells in response to climbing fiber activation also suggests that the climbing fibers have a unique functional role. Thus, a single action potential in a climbing fiber is sufficient to trigger a burst of Purkinje cell action potentials (complex spikes). This would suggest an all-or-none action rather than a graded one. Several theories of cerebellar functions postulate that the *climbing fibers inform about errors in the execution of a movement* (giving an "error signal") when the movement does not correspond to what was intended). There is some experimental support for this hypothesis. Thus, some studies show that the firing frequency of climbing fibers increases in relation to a perturbation of an ongoing movement, whereas the firing frequency is unrelated to, for example, the direction and velocity of the movement. In experiments with walking cats, the firing frequency of climbing fibers leading from the forelimb increases when the foot meets an obstacle, so that the walking pattern has to be changed. In monkeys learning a new movement, there is increased climbing-fiber activity from the relevant body parts. When the movement is well rehearsed—that is, the learning phase is over—the climbing fiber firing frequency does not increase during execution of the movement (no more error signals?). A specific role of the climbing fibers during *motor learning* has been postulated on the basis of this and other kinds of experiments. The climbing fiber input is thought to alter for a long time (days, perhaps years) the responsiveness of the Purkinje cells to mossy fiber inputs. This appears to happen only when specific sets of climbing and mossy fibers simultaneously activate a Purkinje cell, leading to a change of Purkinje cell excitability, so that the following mossy fiber impulses have less effect than previously. This phenomenon, LTD, is discussed in Chapter 1. LTD depends on a rise in Ca^{2+} concentration in the Purkinje cell dendrites, which is produced by the binding of glutamate to AMPA and metabotropic glutamate receptors. Furthermore, the kind of result referred to above can be interpreted in various ways, and, consequently, the special role of the climbing fibers in motor learning is not generally accepted.

The Cerebellar Cortex Contains Three Kinds of Inhibitory Interneurons

All cerebellar interneurons contain GABA (some may also contain glycine, another inhibitory neurotransmitter). One main type of interneuron is the *stellate cell*, located in the molecular layer (Fig. 14.11). It receives afferent excitatory input from the granule cells (parallel fibers), and its axons form synapses with the Purkinje cell dendrites.

Another kind of interneuron, the *basket cell*, is located close to the Purkinje cell layer. Basket cells are also contacted by parallel fibers, whereas their axons end with synapses around the initial segment of the Purkinje cell axons— a location that enables the basket cells to inhibit the Purkinje cells very efficiently. The axonal branches of the basket cells are arranged perpendicular to the long axis of the folia, so that they inhibit Purkinje cells lateral to those that are being activated by parallel fiber excitation. Activation of a group of granule cells would lead to a narrow band of excitation of the Purkinje cells along the folium, flanked by a zone of inhibition on each side. Thus it appears to be a kind of lateral inhibition, which is common in sensory systems to increase the spatial precision of sensory transmission. Correspondingly, the cerebellar cortical region activated by each mossy fiber is reduced in extension.

The third kind of inhibitory interneuron, the *Golgi cell*, is located in the granular layer. The dendrites of the Golgi cells extend upward into the molecular layer and are therefore contacted by parallel fibers (like the stellate cells and the basket cells). The axonal branches form synapses with the dendrites of the granule cells and thus reduce the excitation received by the Purkinje cells after a mossy fiber input.

Efferent Connections of the Cerebellum: The Cerebellar Nuclei

As already mentioned, the three main subdivisions of the cerebellum act largely on the parts of the nervous system from which they receive afferent inputs (Figs. 14.2, 14.4, 14.7, and 14.9). *The axons of the Purkinje cells as a rule end in the cerebellar nuclei* (corticonuclear fibers). The neurons of these nuclei forward the information to the various targets of the cerebellum. The *cerebellar nuclei* (Figs. 14.12 and 14.13) are located in the deep white matter of the cerebellum, just above the roof of the fourth ventricle. In humans, there are four nuclei on each side. Close to the midline, under the vermis, lies the *fastigial nucleus* (medial cerebel-

Figure 14.12 *The cerebellar nuclei.* The photomicrograph (**right**) shows a myelin-stained section placed slightly more dorsally than the drawing at **left**. Therefore, only the dentate and the interposed nuclei are seen in the photomicrograph.

lar nucleus), then follow two small nuclei, and most laterally lies the large, folded *dentate nucleus* (lateral cerebellar nucleus). The two small nuclei have specific names in humans (the globose and the emboliform nuclei) and correspond to the *anterior and posterior interposed nuclei* in animals.

The *corticonuclear connections* are precisely organized with a *topographic pattern*, so that, for example, fibers from the anterior and posterior parts of the cerebellum end in anterior and posterior parts of the nuclei, respectively. There is a somatotopic pattern of the corticonuclear projections from parts of the cerebellum that receive somatotopically organized afferent input. Particularly marked is the *longitudinal localization*, with the *vermis sending fibers to the fastigial nucleus, the intermediate zone to the interposed nuclei, and the hemispheres to the dentate*

Figure 14.13 *Ascending connections from the cerebellum.* The Purkinje cells of the hemispheres send their axons to the dentate nucleus, which in turn projects to the thalamus (the VL nucleus) of the opposite side. The last link from the VL reaches primarily the MI. The connections are somatotopically organized. The figure also shows that the Purkinje cells of the intermediate zone and the vermis project to the interposed and the fastigial nuclei, respectively.

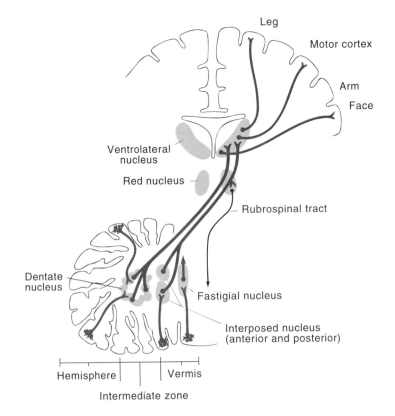

nucleus (Figs. 14.13 and 14.15). Each of the nuclei sends fibers to a separate target region, as shown in a very simplified manner in Figures 14.3, 14.4, 14.7, and 14.9. On the whole, impulses from different parts of the cerebellum are kept segregated through the nuclei and further on to other parts of the brain. However, there is a marked convergence of the corticonuclear connections, since the number of Purkinje cells is much higher than the number of nuclear cells.

Direct Projections from the Cerebellum to the Vestibular Nuclei

The Purkinje cells of the vestibulocerebellum send their axons directly to the vestibular nuclei as corticovestibular fibers (Fig. 14.3). The fibers from the vestibulocerebellum end primarily in parts of the vestibular nuclei that send ascending connections to the *external ocular muscles* (the medial longitudinal fasciculus, Fig. 16.17) and, to a lesser extent, in parts of the nuclei sending fibers to the spinal cord. The vestibulocerebellum thus contributes primarily to the *control of eye movements.*

The vestibular nuclei also receive direct projections from Purkinje cells of the vermis of the anterior and the posterior lobes; that is, outside the vestibulocerebellum as defined here. These fibers end primarily in the *lateral vestibular nucleus* (nucleus of Deiters; Figs. 16.16 and 16.17), which projects to the spinal cord. Thus, the cerebellar vermis can influence *postural mechanisms* via the lateral vestibulospinal tract (besides its effects mediated via the fastigial nucleus and its projections to the reticular formation).

The vestibular nuclei (mainly the nucleus of Deiters) also receive *indirect* cerebellar influences from the anterior and posterior lobe vermis. These are relayed in the the fastigial nucleus.

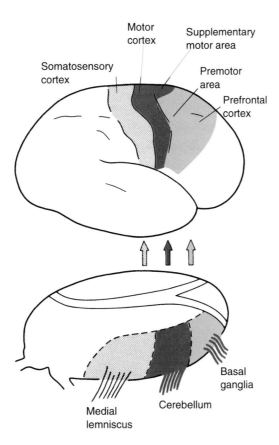

Figure 14.14 *Thalamocortical connections.* Schematic presentation of the arrangement within the ventral thalamic nucleus of afferents from the somatosensory pathways, the cerebellum, and the basal ganglia and their further projections to the SI, MI, and the premotor cortex.

Figure 14.15 *Zonal organization of the cerebellar cortex.* Very simplified illustration of the precise topographic pattern of cerebellar efferent and afferent connections. The cortex can be divided into longitudinal zones projecting to different parts of the cerebellar nuclei and receiving afferents from different parts of the inferior olive (**right** drawing). Note that each of the zones shown to the **left** can be further subdivided.

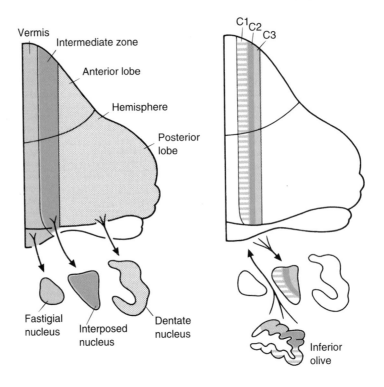

Neuronal Behavior in the Cerebellar Nuclei

The nuclear cells fire with a high frequency even in an animal sitting quietly. When neurons fire without any obvious excitatory input, they are said to be *spontaneously active*. Because all Purkinje cells are inhibitory (GABA), a continuous firing of the nuclear cells is a prerequisite for the information from the cerebellar cortex to be passed on (increased Purkinje cell activity leads to reduced nuclear cell firing). In vitro studies of cerebellar slices indicate that the nuclear neurons have intrinsic properties that depolarize the membrane even in the absence of an excitatory input (pacemaker properties). In addition, the nuclear cells receive other afferents than those coming from the Purkinje cells. Thus, some of the pathways ending in the cerebellar cortex, such as the spinocerebellar and olivocerebellar projections, give off collaterals to the cerebellar nuclei. As mentioned, these pathways are excitatory.

Increase or decrease in the firing frequency of the Purkinje cells immediately causes change in the activity of the nuclear cells. Even minute changes of Purkinje cell activity change the signals issued from the cerebellum to its target nuclei. Thus, the *outputs of the cerebellar nuclei reflect with a high temporal precision even very weak inputs to the cerebellar cortex.* This is presumably important for the cerebellar role in control of rhythm, as we will discuss later in this chapter.

Organization of Efferent Connections from the Cerebellar Nuclei

The fibers from the *dentate nucleus* leave the cerebellum through the *superior cerebellar peduncle* (Figs. 14.1 and 14.13). They cross the midline in the mesencephalon, and some fibers end in the red nucleus of the opposite side. Most fibers continue rostrally, however, to end in the *thalamus*. Here, the dentate fibers end primarily in the *VL* (some also reach the VA) (Figs. 14.13 and 14.14). These nuclei also receive fibers from the basal ganglia, but they end in different parts than the cerebellar fibers (as shown schematically in Fig. 14.14), which implies that the basal ganglia and the cerebellum also influence somewhat different parts of the cortex. Impulses from the *cerebellar hemispheres pass primarily to the MI, whereas the basal ganglia via the thalamus act mainly on premotor*

Sagittal Zones and Somatotopic Organization of the Cerebellum

We have so far described that the main subdivisions of the cerebellum—such as the flocculonodular lobe, the vermis, and the hemispheres—differ with regard to connectivity. Furthermore, we have seen that the lateral parts of the hemispheres, the intermediate zone, and the vermis differ with regard to their efferent connections (Fig. 14.15). This *organization of the cerebellum into three longitudinal zones*, each projecting to separate parts of the cerebellar nuclei, was first described by the Norwegian neuroanatomists Jansen and Brodal in the 1940s. But the localization within the cerebellum is far more sophisticated than what could be revealed by the fairly primitive methods 50 years ago. Each of the three longitudinal zones of Jansen and Brodal can thus be further subdivided, as shown by the Dutch neuroanatomist Voogd. Figure 14.15 shows the zones of the intermediate zone as an example.

The zonal pattern is especially sharp within the *olivocerebellar* and *corticonuclear* projections. The neurons located within a particular small part of the olive send their fibers to a narrow longitudinal zone, whereas the neighboring zones receive climbing fibers from other parts of the olive (Fig. 14.15). The Purkinje cells of the zones also send their axons to different parts of the cerebellar nuclei. The parcellation of the cortex into sagittal zones in fact goes further than shown in Figure 14.15. Physiological studies show that within the anterior lobe each zone consists of several *microzones* differing with regard to the information they receive. Apart from the parallel fibers, extending for a few millimeters perpendicular to the longitudinal zones, there are no association fibers interconnecting different parts of the cerebellar cortex. Thus, the cerebellar cortex and the cerebellar nuclei consist of numerous *compartments* or *modules* that function (at least largely) independently of each other. Some data suggest that each module takes care of a specific motor task. In this respect the cerebellar cortex differs from the cerebral cortex, which is characterized by extensive association connections and cooperation between different regions.

Another aspect of cerebellar localization is that cortical cell groups representing different body parts are spatially segregated—that is, there is a *somatotopic organization*, as already mentioned (Fig. 14.5). The mossy fiber projections to the cerebellum, carrying impulses from the spinal cord and the cerebral cortex, are somatotopically organized, as are the climbing fiber projections from the inferior olive. The somatotopic localization within the cerebellar cortex was first described by the British neurophysiologist Adrian and the Americans Snider and Stowell, using electrophysiological methods. Later investigations, also with anatomic methods, have verified their findings and provided further details. Lesions restricted to, for example, the forelimb region of the anterior lobe in experimental animals produce characteristic changes of muscle that are restricted to the forelimb of the same side as the lesion.

A novel aspect of the somatotopic localization within the cerebellum was described by the American neurophysiologist Welker and collaborators, using very precise micromapping methods. Thus, the mossy fibers, formerly thought to end with a fairly diffuse somatotopic pattern, were shown to end in numerous, discrete patches in the cortex, each patch being defined by its sensory input from a specific minor part of the body. Each patch is usually less than 1 mm in diameter (in the rat and cat). Thus, the leg region within the posterior lobe consists in reality of a mosaic of patches. A salient feature is that adjacent patches can receive inputs from body parts that are widely separated. Furthermore, the same body part is usually represented in several widely separated patches. This arrangement of the mossy fibers was termed *fractured somatotopy* by Welker. How this pattern of mossy fiber inputs is coordinated with the climbing fiber inputs is not clear. As mentioned, the climbing fibers terminate in narrow sagittal strips or zones, and one such strip is often related to one body part only.

areas and the prefrontal cortex. In addition, the cerbellum influences parts of the SMA and PMA that apparently differ from the parts influenced from the basal ganglia.

Because both the ascending fibers from the cerebellum to the motor cortex and the descending fibers from the cerebral cortex to the spinal cord are crossed, *the cerebellar hemisphere exerts its influence on the body half of the same side.* Consequently, with diseases of the cerebellum, the *symptoms occur on the same side as the lesion.*

As mentioned above, the efferents from the *intermediate zone* reach the *interposed nucleus.* This sends its efferents both to the contralateral *thalamus* (to the VL mainly, like the dentate) and the *red nucleus* (Figs. 14.9, 14.13, and 14.15). This enables the interposed nucleus to influence motorneurons via both the rubrospinal tract and the pyramidal tract. Since the rubrospinal tract is crossed, the interposed nucleus (and the intermediate zone) acts on the body half of the same side.

The *fastigial nucleus* (receiving Purkinje cell axons from the vermis) sends its efferents to both the *vestibular nuclei* and the *reticular formation.* Thus, motoneurons can be influenced via the vestibulospinal and the reticulospinal tracts. On the basis of what we discussed in Chapter 12, it seems likely that the cerebellum *via the fastigial nucleus can influence posture and relatively automatic movements like locomotion.* This is supported by the results of animal experiments and by clinical observations.

CEREBELLAR FUNCTIONS AND SYMPTOMS IN DISEASE

We will finally discuss the function of the cerebellum, with special reference to the motor disturbances occurring in humans after damage to the cerebellum. To some extent, the function of an organ is easier to discover when it does *not* work properly. Although not the ideal way of studying normal function, this approach is necessary since we do not understand the basic operations of the cerebellum.

Even though a multitude of symptoms have been produced in experimental animals after lesions of the cerebellum (among them, disturbances of autonomic functions) clinically, only certain motor symptoms can with certainty be referred to cerebellar lesions. This is probably explained by the fact that in humans the lesions that give clear-cut symptoms most often are large and not confined to particular functional or anatomic cerebellar subdivisions. Furthermore, they are usually combined with lesions in other parts of the central nervous system (for example, in parts of the brain stem). It is therefore often difficult to decide whether a particular symptom is caused by the cerebellar lesion. Modern imaging techniques (CT, MRI, PET; see Chapter 5), however, provide the opportunity to localize accurately even fairly small lesions in living subjects and, furthermore, to study cerebellar neuronal activity (indirectly) in healthy and diseased subjects performing specific tasks. As mentioned, derangement of motor functions dominates the clinical picture caused by cerebellar disorders. To judge from the cerebellar connections as we have discussed them above, it is clear that the cerebellum influences movements by acting on the neuronal groups that give origin to the central motor pathways (the pyramidal tract, the reticulospinal tracts, the rubrospinal tract, and the vestibulospinal tracts). These pathways, of course, control the activity of spinal and cranial nerve motoneurons. The three main subdivisions of the cerebellum (Fig. 14.2) act on different neuronal groups, and lesions restricted to each of the subdivisions give different symptoms. On this basis one usually distinguishes three cerebellar syndromes (a syndrome is a constellation of several symptoms that occur together): the *flocculonodular syndrome*, the *anterior lobe syndrome*, and the *neocerebellar syndrome*. The existence of three distinct syndromes is most clear-cut in experimental animals. In humans, the neocerebellar syndrome is most often seen, which is not surprising since the hemispheres (the neocerebellum) make up the major part of the human cerebellum.

*The Flocculonodular and
Anterior Lobe Syndromes*

Isolated damage to the flocculonodular lobe in animals produces *disturbances of the equilibrium*—that is, unsteadiness in standing and walking. When the body is supported, movements of the extremities can be performed normally, however. Sometimes, similar symptoms occur in humans with a special kind of tumor in the posterior cranial fossa, most often arising from the nodulus (*medulloblastoma*).

Eye movements may also be disturbed in patients with cerebellar lesions (particularly with affection of the vestibulocerebellum). This manifests itself as *spontaneous nystagmus*.[4] It is not quite clear, however, whether such symptoms are caused by the cerebellar damage itself or by concomitant damage to the vestibular nuclei or their connections.

Damage to the *anterior lobe in experimental animals* produces primarily *a change of the muscle tone*. In decerebrate animals, the decerebrate rigidity increases (See Chapter 12), as do the postural reflexes. This fits with the observation that electrical stimulation of the anterior lobe reduces the decerebrate rigidity (as mentioned, the Purkinje cells inhibit the cells of the cerebellar nuclei, whereas the nuclear cells have excitatory actions on reticulospinal and vestibulospinal neurons).[5] In addition, some Purkinje cells in the anterior lobe vermis send axons directly to the vestibular nuclei, and removal of this inhibitory action would also tend to increase the activity of the vestibulospinal neurons and thus the decerebrate rigidity.

In humans it is doubtful, however, whether increased muscle tone is produced by lesions including the anterior lobe. More marked is the *unsteadiness of walking* (gait ataxia) in patients with damage mainly affecting the anterior lobe vermis and intermediate zone (this occurs in cerebellar degeneration caused by alcohol abuse). Similarly, selective lesions of the fastigial nucleus in monkeys cause difficulties with walking, sitting, and maintaining the upright position. The anterior lobe vermis, via its efferent connections to the fastigial nucleus and from there to the reticular formation, must therefore be assumed to play a role in *coordination of the half-automatic movements of walking and postural adjustments*.

The Neocerebellar Syndrome

The neocerebellum plays a different functional role than the phylogenetically older parts of the cerebellum: It is primarily concerned with the *coordination of the (least automatic) voluntary movements*. This stands to reason, since the cerebellar hemispheres send their main output to the MI (via the dentate nucleus and the thalamus) and thus influence the neurons of the pyramidal tract. After removal of one cerebellar hemisphere in a monkey, the voluntary movements become uncertain on the same side of the body; they become *incoordinated* or *ataxic*. The same effect can be produced by cooling the dentate nucleus (by the use of a cooling electrode) in a monkey performing a well-rehearsed movement (as soon as the cooling is reversed, the movements again become normal). Movements that were performed quickly and smoothly become unsteady and jerky by the cooling. The monkey misses repeatedly when trying to grasp an object, even though it knows perfectly well where it is and what is demanded. Sometimes the hand is moved too far in relation to the object, sometimes too short. The movements tend to be *decomposed*; that is, instead of occurring simultaneously in several joints, they take place in one joint at a time, and the velocity is uneven—sometimes too high and sometimes too low. Selective damage or transient "uncoupling" of the dentate nucleus in monkeys indicates that the cerebellar hemispheres are particularly important when movements must take place in several joints at the same time. Picking up a raisin, for example, became impossible because the monkey could no longer coordinate the movements of the joints of the wrist, thumb, and index finger. Precise movements of one finger at the time could be done normally, however. Difficulties with hitting an object when trying to grasp it with the hand can probably be attributed to the same basic defect; that is, difficulties with coordinating the movements of the wrist, shoulder, and elbow joints.

Ataxia of this kind is also the most prominent symptom in humans with damage to the cerebellar hemispheres. For example, difficulty with the precision grip similar to that described above in monkeys has recently been observed in patients with unilateral infarcts of the cerebellar hemispheres. The increase of force when grasping an object is slower than normal, and the adjustment of the grip force when both grasping and lifting is deficient. In clinical neurology, the various elements of ataxia have particular names, such as *dysmetria* (movement is not stopped in time), *asynergia* (decomposition of complex movements), *dysdiadochokinesia* (reduced ability to perform rapidly alternating movements of, for example, the hand), and *intentional tremor* (tremor arising when trying to perform a movement, such as grasping an object). Speech is also often disturbed in cerebellar diseases. It has been called *speech ataxia*, to emphasize that it also appears to be caused by incoordination (in the respiratory muscles, the muscles of the larynx, and others), making the strength and velocity of the speech uneven.

All the elements of ataxia have been attributed to a *fundamental defect in control of the force and of the exact timing of the starting and stopping of movements*. It is not certain, however, that this suffices to explain why the symptoms are most marked when movements in two or more joints must be coordinated (such as moving the index finger quickly to the tip of the nose from a position with the arm stretched out).

As mentioned above, the *temporal aspect* appears to be central to the cerebellar contribution to motor control. This is evidenced by patients with cerebellar damage who are unable to perform sequences of finger movements in a particular rhythm. The movements are done by each finger without a fixed temporal relation to movements of the other fingers.

In *acute* damage to the cerebellar hemispheres in humans, the muscle tone often appears to be reduced when tested by passive stretch (the symptom is transient). This is called *cerebellar hypotonia*. The underlying mechanism is not clear although experiments in anesthetized animals suggested that it is caused by reduced γ motoneuron activity. Recent experiments in awake animals, however, show that the muscle-spindle sensitivity to stretch is not significantly altered by lesions of the dentate and interposed nuclei.

Does the Cerebellum Perform a Basic Operation Used in All Its Functions?

Even though the study of cerebellar symptoms provides reasonable insight into the functions of the cerebellum, we are far from understanding how the cerebellum performs its tasks. The striking uniformity and strictly geometric structure of the cerebellar cortex has led to comparison with a computer, which can perform the same kinds of computations on various kinds of information. The subdivision of the cerebellum into numerous, apparently independent units may fit such a concept. Several rather different theories have been put forward to explain how the cerebellum operates. None of them has so far been universally accepted, however, and there is disagreement with regard to interpretation of some experiments said to support one theory or the other.

The German neuroscientist Braitenberg proposed more than 30 years ago that the cerebellum functions as a kind of clock, measuring temporal intervals with great accuracy. The theory is based on, among other things, the regular arrangement of the parallel fibers. Action potentials conducted along the parallel fibers will excite the Purkinje cells in a fixed temporal sequence. We discussed above that a timing function may be crucial in the cerebellar contribution to motor control. Recent data furthermore suggest that the cerebellar timing function may be used also in non-motor tasks. Thus, patients with cerebellar damage were impaired not only in their ability to reproduce a certain rhythm by tapping their fingers but also in discriminating different sound rhythms. They had no problems with discriminating sounds of different intensities, however, which suggests that the defect be specific to discrimination of *temporal* intervals. Reduced ability to judge the velocity of visual stimuli has also been reported in patients with cerebellar lesions.

The inferior olive and the climbing fibers may play a crucial role in the timing function of the cerebellum. Thus, the olivary neurons fire rhythmically, and neurons that activate Purkinje cells within a narrow sagittal zone fire synchronously. One study, furthermore, found a correlation between the firing rhythm of olivary neurons and the rhythm of certain movements.

The Cerebellum and Motor Learning

Recent animal experiments suggest that long-lasting changes in synaptic efficacy may take place in the cerebellar cortex during motor learning. Thus, the cerebellum may not only be a machine used every time a movement is performed but may also be capable of remembering what was done and thereby adapting its influence on motoneurons in accordance with the outcome of a movement. In particular, the altered synaptic effects of the parallel fibers on the Purkinje cell dendrites have been thoroughly investigated. There is evidence that changed synaptic efficacy is produced by the simultaneous firing of mosssy and climbing fibers acting on the same Purkinje cell. The climbing fiber influence—although in itself excitatory—probably renders the Purkinje cells less excitable for a long time (LTD). Thus, the next time a certain mossy fiber input arrives, the Purkinje cell response is reduced (that is, it fires fewer action potentials). It has not been directly shown, however, that LTD *is* induced in the cerebellum during motor learning.

One example of synaptic changes in the cerebellum is the adaptability of the vestibulo-ocular reflex, as shown by the Japanese neurophysiologist Ito. The VOR ensures that when the head moves in one direction, the eyes move in the opposite direction with exactly the same speed. This makes it possible to keep the gaze fixed on a stationary object even though the head moves. The strength of the reflex response to a certain head movement (that is, the sensitivity of the reflex) needs to be adjusted when, for example, the head grows and alters its proportions. Via relay stations (Fig. 16.28), signals from the retina provide information about retinal slip (the image is not kept stationary on the retina but moves). Most likely, climbing fibers ending in the flocculus provide such signals and thus tell the cerebellum that the velocity of the eye movement is incorrect. Information about head movements from the vestibular apparatus is provided by mossy fibers, also ending in the flocculus. The sensitivity of the vestibulo-ocular reflex can be altered experimentally in a short time, as shown by making experimental animals wear prismatic glasses that displace the image on the retina. The most drastic experiment is when the movement of the surroundings appears to be the opposite of the real movement, leading to a complete reversal of the reflex response. Destruction of the cerebellar flocculus prevents adaptation of the reflex. It is disputed, however, whether the change in synaptic efficacy—that is, the learning—underlying the adaptability of the vestibulo-ocular reflex is caused by changes in the cerebellum or elsewhere.

Certain *conditioned responses* are examples of possible cerebellar participation during motor learning. Especially the so-called nictitating membrane reflex (a part of the blink reflex) in rabbits has been investigated. When a jet of air hits the eye, the nictitating membrane moves together with the eyelid. This is an unconditioned reflex, in which the trigeminal nerve is the afferent link, the reflex center is in the brain stem involving the sensory trigeminal nucleus, the reticular formation, and the facial nucleus, and the efferent link is the facial nerve to the muscles around the eye. If the jet of air is regularly preceded by a tone (conditioning stimulus), the rabbit will eventually react with a nictitating membrane movement even when the tone is presented alone. The impulse pathway for the conditioned response is much more complicated than that for the unconditioned reflex (for example, the auditory pathways and parts of the cerebral cortex are involved). What is interesting in this connection, however, is that after destruction of certain parts of the cerebellum, the reflex can no longer be conditioned (that is, only the unconditioned response occurs, and the animal can no longer be trained to react to the tone only). Damage to the cerebellum after having made the response conditioned abolishes the conditioned (but not the unconditioned) response. It is sufficient to remove a small part of the cerebellar "face area" of the intermediate zone to get these effects (this is a further example of the cerebellar functional localization). Other conditioned responses appear to be dependent on the integrity of the cerebellum, but they have been less rigorously studied than the nictitating reflex. As with the vestibulo-ocular reflex, however, it is not quite settled whether the learning of the conditioned response—that is, the memory traces coupling the conditioning stimulus to the response—is located in the cerebellum or elsewhere. If learning takes place in the cerebellum in such rather primitive motor responses, it is tempting to assume that corresponding changes occur in the cerebellar hemispheres when humans learn complex voluntary movements (such as learning to play a musical instrument). It should be emphasized, however, that the cerebellum is most certainly not the only place of plastic changes related to motor learning.

The Cerebellum and Cognitive Functions

Many isolated observations suggest that the cerebellar functions are not restricted to motor ones. This topic has attracted much interest recently. It is too early, however, to draw conclusions as to the importance of the cerebellum for mental tasks that are usually considered the domain of the cerebral cortex.

We mentioned above that the cerebellum might be important for the *perception* of rhythm—not only the proper execution of rhythmic movements. Furthermore, reduced ability to *shift the attention* from one kind of stimulus to another was found in six patients with lesions of the cerebellar hemispheres. The patients were only impaired, however, in *quick* shifts of attention. The patients' ability to maintain focused attention was not reduced, neither was their perception of the stimuli.

Although also other clinical studies report impairments in cognitive functions in patients with cerebellar lesions, establishing a causal relationship on this basis is difficult. Important supplementary information, however, comes from studies of cerebral blood flow in normals. Several studies report that blood flow increases in parts of the cerebellum during the performance of various cognitive tasks. For example, persons trying to solve a pegboard puzzle showed increased blood flow in the dentate nucleus. In such studies one tries to eliminate the possibility that the increase is caused by the movements alone (for example, moving the pegs). Another study reported increased blood flow in the cerebellar hemispheres in persons trying to *find verbs going with nouns*. Furthermore, increased blood flow in the hemispheres was observed in persons playing imaginary tennis, and in persons counting silently. Finally, the cerebellum may participate also in other kinds of learning than learning of movements. Thus, measurements of regional cerebral oxidative metabolism with PET in humans show that the posterior parts of the cerebellar hemispheres increase their neuronal activity when *learning a tactile recognition task* (more than during just tactile recognition of an object).

NOTES

1. Other precerebellar nuclei—that is, brain stem nuclei that send their efferents to the cerebellum—also receive afferents from the cerebral cortex. This concerns the reticular tegmental nucleus, located just dorsal to the pontine nuclei, and the lateral reticular nucleus. In quantitative terms, however, these pathways play minor roles compared with the corticopontocerebellar one.

2. There are modest connections to the pontine nuclei from the frontal eye field, area 8, and from parts of the auditory cortex. There are, however, few if any pontine fibers from prefrontal areas and major parts of the temporal lobe.

3. In addition to the climbing fibers and mossy fibers—demonstrated with the Golgi method a long time ago—a third kind of cerebellar afferent has been demonstrated with the histofluorescence method (that is, fibers containing catecholamines). Such fibers come from the raphe nuclei and from the nucleus locus coeruleus and contain serotonin and norepinephrine, respectively. They appear to end rather diffusely in both the granular and molecular layers. Fibers coming from the hypothalamus also end in this manner.

4. Nystagmus is movements in which the eyes move slowly in one direction (as when following a moving object with the gaze), and rapidly back. When nystagmus occurs in a person at rest with no kind of stimulation, it is called spontaneous. Nystagmus is discussed further in Chapter 16.

5. Electrical stimulation with electrodes surgically implanted at the cerebellar surface has been used in patients with neurological disorders such as epilepsy and cerebral palsy. The theoretical basis is the inhibitory action of the Purkinje cells with subsequent reduction of abnormally increased neuronal excitability and muscle tone. Even though some report favorable results with such stimulation, there is no agreement as to whether the effect is due to the cerebellar stimulation or some other factor.

PART IV

THE BRAIN STEM AND THE CRANIAL NERVES

The definition of the term *brain stem* varies. We use it here to refer to the *medulla oblongata, the pons, and the mesencephalon,* which together form a macroscopically distinct part of the brain. Often, however, also the diencephalon is included in the brain stem. Which definition is used is of no great importance, since the brain stem is a topographically and embryologically defined unit; it does not represent a functional "system." Neuronal groups within the brain stem take part in virtually all the tasks of the central nervous system.

Functionally, the brain stem may be said to have two levels of organization. On the one hand, most of the cranial nerves and their nuclei represent "the spinal cord of the head." On the other hand, many cell groups in the brain stem represent a superior level of control over the spinal cord and the cranial nerve nuclei. This section deals with both aspects. Chapter 15 deals with the reticular formation, which represents the superior level of control. Chapter 16 describes most of the cranial nerves and their nuclei.

CHAPTER 15

RETICULAR FORMATION

The reticular formation attends primarily to tasks involving the nervous system and the organism as a whole. Subdivisions of the reticular formation form premotor networks that organize several complex behaviors. This concerns, for example, control of body posture, orientation of the head and body toward external stimuli, control of eye movements, and coordination of the activity of the visceral organs. These tasks fit with the reticular formation being phylogenetically old and present even in lower vertebrates. Furthermore, to solve its tasks the reticular formation must have close relations with many other parts of the central nervous system. In this chapter we cannot avoid some reference to matters that are systematically treated in later chapters (particularly in Chapter 16 on the cranial nerves, and in Chapters 17 and 18 on the autonomic nervous system).

The reticular formation extends from the lower end of the medulla to the upper end of the mesencephalon, where it gradually fuses with certain thalamic cell groups.[1] At all levels it occupies the central parts (Figs. 3.17, 3.21, 15.1, 15.4, 15.7, and 15.10) and fills the territories not used by cranial nerve nuclei and other distinct nuclei (such as the dorsal column nuclei, the pontine nuclei, and the colliculi) and by the large fiber tracts (such as the medial lemniscus and the pyramidal tract).

Two cell groups that have close topographic and other relations with the reticular formation (and which are often considered a part of the reticular formation) have attracted much interest recently. These are the *raphe nuclei* (Figs. 15.1 and 15.5) and a small cell group called the *locus coeruleus* (Fig. 15.6). A characteristic feature of these nuclei is that their axons have extremely widespread ramifications, reaching many parts of

Figure 15.1 *The reticular formation.* Transverse sections through various levels of the brain stem (cat) showing the position of the reticular formation. The size of the black dots indicates the size of the neurons, which varies considerably among subdivisions of the reticular formation. Based on Brodal (1957).

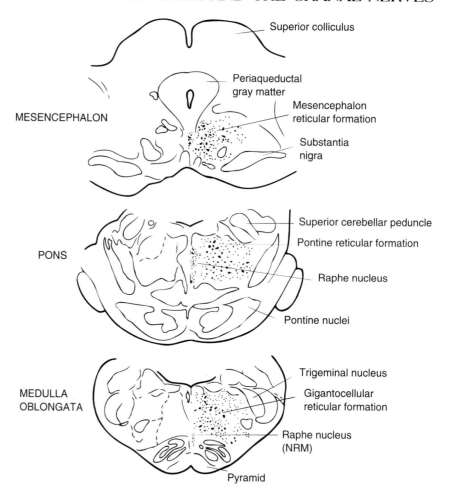

the brain and the spinal cord. Another special feature is that they send fibers directly to the cerebral cortex—that is, without synaptic interruption in the thalamus, as is typical of most cortical afferent pathways from lower levels.

STRUCTURE AND CONNECTIONS OF THE RETICULAR FORMATION

Structure and Subdivisions

The reticular formation received its name from the early anatomists because of its networklike appearance in microscopic sections (Figs. 15.2 and 15.4). It is built of cells of various forms and sizes that appear to be rather randomly mixed. Between the cells, there is a wickerwork of fibers passing in many directions. These fibers are partly axons and dendrites of the neurons of the reticular formation, partly afferent axons from other parts of the central nervous system. The reticular neurons have typically very long and straight dendrites, so that they cover a large volume of neuropil (Fig. 15.4). This distinguishes the reticular neurons from those found in specific nuclei of the brain stem, such as the cranial nerve nuclei (see the nucleus labeled XII in Fig. 15.4).

Figure 15.2 *The reticular formation.* Photomicrograph of section of the medulla, stained to show fibers (myelin) and cell bodies. Note how the perikarya—some of them very large—are distributed diffusely without clear nuclear borders, and with small fiber bundles coursing in various directions. The section is from the so-called gigantocellular subdivision of the reticular formation (see Fig. 15.1). Magnification, ×300.

A more detailed analysis of the reticular formation makes clear, however, that it consists of several subdivisions, among which the cells differ in shape, size, and arrangement even though the borders between such subdivisions are not sharp (Fig. 15.1). It is especially important that such cytoarchitectonically defined subdivisions also differ with regard to fiber connections and content of neurotransmitters. Not surprisingly, therefore, they differ functionally as well. In the pons and the medulla, approximately the medial two-thirds of the reticular formation consists of many large cells, in part so-called giant cells (Figs. 15.1 and 15.2). The lateral one-third contains almost exclusively small cells. Tract-tracing methods have shown that the medial part sends out many long, ascending and descending fibers, whereas the lateral small-celled part receives most of the afferents coming to the reticular formation. In general, therefore, we may say that *the lateral part is receiving, whereas the medial part is efferent and conveys the influence of the reticular formation to higher parts, such as the thalamus, and lower parts, such as the spinal cord.*

Studies with the Golgi method (and recently with intracellular tracers) give evidence of how complexly the reticular formation is organized. The long ascending and descending efferent fibers give off numerous collaterals on their way through the brain stem (Fig. 15.3). As can be seen in Figure 15.4, the collaterals run primarily in the transverse plane. Most dendrites of reticular cells have the same preferential orientation, so the reticular formation may be described as consisting of numerous transversely oriented disks (Fig. 15.4). The numerous collaterals of the axons from the cells in the medial parts ensure that signals from each reticular cell may reach many functionally diverse cell groups (such as other parts

Figure 15.3 *Neurons in the medial part of the reticular formation with long ascending and descending axons.* To the **right** is an example of a neuron with a bifurcating axon, with one ascending and one descending branch. Both branches give off collaterals as they course through the reticular formation. To the **left** are shown two neurons with ascending and descending axons, respectively. In this way, neurons with ascending axons can influence the activity of neurons with descending axons.

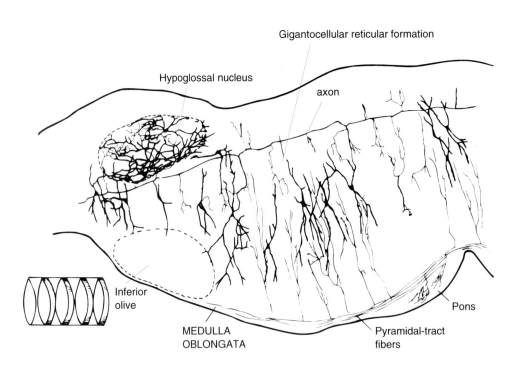

Figure 15.4 *Orientation of dendrites in the reticular formation.* Sagittal section through the medulla (rat). Note the long, straight dendrites, which are typical of the neurons of the reticular formation, in contrast to the neurons of a cranial nerve nucleus (the hypoglossal) and other specific brain stem nuclei. A long axon with numerous collaterals extending ventrally in the transverse plane is also shown. Collaterals of the pyramidal tract fibers also enter the reticular formation. From Scheibel and Scheibel (1958).

of the reticular formation, cranial nerve nuclei, the dorsal column nuclei, the colliculi, the spinal cord, certain thalamic nuclei, and the hypothalamus).

The Raphe Nuclei

The raphe nuclei (raphe = seam) together form a narrow, sagittally oriented plate of neurons in the midline of the medulla, pons, and mesencephalon (Figs. 15.1 and 15.5). In many ways, these nuclei have similarities with the reticular formation proper and are often considered part of it. On the basis of cytoarchitectonic and connectional differences, several raphe nuclei have been identified (Fig. 15.5) even though their borders are far from sharp. Together, the raphe nuclei receive *afferents* from many sources, such as the cerebral cortex, the hypothalamus, and the reticular formation. The *efferent* connections are special because *each axon ramifies extensively and reaches large parts of the central nervous system* with little topographic arrangement. Some topography is nevertheless present since the caudal raphe nuclei send their efferents to the spinal cord, whereas the rostral nuclei send fibers upstream to the cerebral cortex, among other places (Fig. 15.5).

Their *direct projections to the cerebral cortex* place the raphe nuclei among other nuclei with this same characteristic: dopaminergic cell groups in the mesencephalon, the locus coeruleus and adjoining scattered cell groups, and the basal nucleus. Another characteristic feature of the raphe nuclei is that most of the neurons contain *serotonin*. The actions of serotonin appear to be multifarious, depending on the kinds of receptor that are present postsynaptically. Most neurons in addition contain one or more *neuropeptides*, which presumably contribute to the synaptic effects of efferent fibers from the raphe nuclei.

The functions of the raphe nuclei are only incompletely known. In Chapter 7, we discussed the inhibitory actions of raphespinal fibers on the central transmission of signals from nociceptors. Later in this chapter we will briefly discuss the nuclei's relation to sleep. Lesions of the raphe nuclei have also been reported to evoke various kinds of behavioral changes, such as aggression and increased motor activity (to destroy the raphe nuclei in isolation however, is, virtually impossible).

A final peculiarity of the raphe nuclei is that they send fibers ending in close relation to the ependymal cells (which cover the interior aspect of the brain ventricles). The function of these fibers is unknown but may perhaps be related to regulation of transport processes through the ependyma.

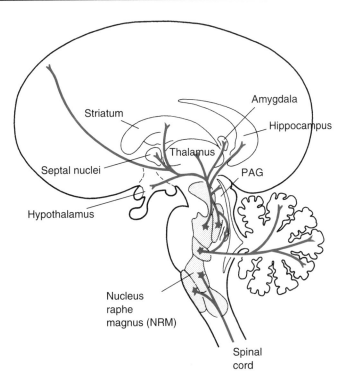

Figure 15.5 *The raphe nuclei.* Schematic midsagittal section through the brain, showing the various subdivisions of the raphe nuclei and some main connections. The most rostral nuclei send their fibers rostrally to the thalamus, cortex, and other cell groups, whereas the caudal nuclei project to the spinal cord.

The Locus Coeruleus

This nucleus consists of a small group of strongly pigmented cells located under the floor of the fourth ventricle (Fig. 15.6). It appears to be present in all mammalian species. After it was shown in the 1960s that the cells contain *norepinephrine*, the nucleus attracted considerable interest. The locus coeruleus has clear borders except ventrally, where it merges gradually with the adjoining reticular formation—which also contains many noradrenergic neurons. This is one reason why the locus coeruleus is often considered a part of the reticular formation.

The *efferent* fibers from the locus coeruleus are highly branched and *reach virtually all parts of the central nervous system*. It sends direct fibers to the cerebral cortex, the hypothalamus, the hippocampus, and other limbic structures. Direct fibers also reach the spinal cord but only parts of the brain stem (especially sensory nuclei). The dense noradrenergic innervation of the reticular formation and the motor nuclei must therefore originate in cell groups outside the locus coeruleus.

The *afferent* connections of the locus coeruleus have been traced with the HRP method from the hypothalamus, the amygdala, PAG, the solitary nucleus, the reticular formation, the spinal cord, and other areas. More recent and detailed studies show, however, that most of these sources send only few fibers to the locus coeruleus. Anatomic and physiological studies agree that the *main input arises in two cell groups in the medullary reticular formation*. One group, with an excitatory action on the locus coeruleus, is located ventrolaterally. The other group is found dorsomedially and has an inhibitory action.

Neurons in the locus coeruleus respond preferentially to novel, "exciting" sensory stimuli. Since norepinephrine increases the response to specific stimuli and improves the signal-to-noise ratio of postsynaptic neurons, the locus coeruleus is believed to play a particular role in mediating arousal in response to sensory stimuli. The highly branched and widespread organization of its fibers and the lack of topographic organization would enable such effects on many parts of the brain. One example is the facilitatory effect of norepenephrine on spinal motoneurons, discussed in Chapter 12 (*Monoaminergic Pathway from the Brain Stem to the Spinal Cord*). We return to the role of locus coeruleus in control of wakefulness when discussing sleep below.

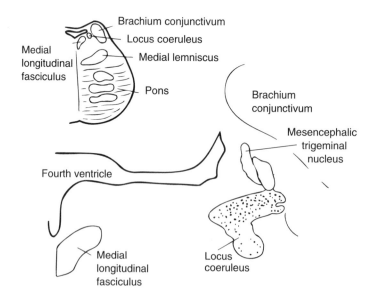

Figure 15.6 *The locus coeruleus*. Its position just below the floor of the fourth ventricle is shown in a transverse section of the pons. This nucleus and other noradrenergic cell groups in the vicinity have neurons with highly branched axons ending rather diffusely in most parts of the central nervous system.

*The Efferent Connections of
the Reticular Formation*

The reticular formation sends fibers to (and thereby acts on) four main regions: the *thalamus*, the *spinal cord*, *brain stem nuclei*, and the *cerebellum*. The influence on brain stem nuclei, such as the cranial nerve nuclei, is mediated in large part by collaterals of the long ascending and descending fibers destined for the thalamus and the cord. The reticular cell groups sending fibers to the thalamus overlap with cell groups sending fibers to the cord. The overlap is only partial, however, so that areas can be distinguished which send either ascending or descending efferent fibers (Fig. 15.9).

The *descending reticular fibers* to the cord run in the ventral part of the lateral funiculus and in the ventral funiculus (Fig. 15.7). Such *reticulospinal fibers* end primarily on interneurons, which in turn can influence motoneurons. The *ventral reticulospinal tract*[2] is discussed in Chapter 12 in relation to motor control (*More About Reticulospinal Pathways*). This is in reality not one tract but several that differ with regard to both anatomic organization and functional properties. The ventral reticulospinal tracts are both crossed and uncrossed and mediate both inhibitory and excitatory effects on spinal motoneurons. The reticulospinal neurons are further characterized by their axonal branching pattern, with collaterals given off at several levels of the spinal cord. Thus, muscles in different parts of the body can be influenced by each neuron. As discussed in Chapter 12, the *ventral reticulospinal tracts are of particular importance for postural mechanisms, for the orientation of the head and body toward external stimuli, and for voluntary movements of proximal body parts.* Connections from the *superior colliculus*—mediating sensory information to the reticular formation—are crucial for orienting movements toward novel stimuli. Combined anatomic and physiological studies of single cells have shown the importance of a tecto-reticulo-spinal pathway for such movements.

The *ascending fibers* from the reticular formation end in the *intralaminar thalamic nuclei* (Figs. 3.23, 7.19, and 15.8) unlike the specific sensory tracts ending in the lateral thalamic nucleus. Some fibers also end in the *hypothalamus*. We will discuss the functional significance of the ascending reticular connections later in this chapter; suffice it to say here that they are of particular importance for the general level of activity of the cerebral cortex, which in turn is related to consciousness and attention.

Figure 12.9 shows that the cell groups giving off ascending axons are located somewhat more caudally than those emitting descending axons. By means of the numerous collaterals of both the ascending and descending fibers in the reticular formation (Figs. 15.3 and 15.4), the two kinds of cell groups can influence each other. Furthermore, there are also many interneurons connecting different parts of the reticular formation. Thus a close cooperation is possible between the parts of the reticular formation acting on the cerebral cortex and those acting on the spinal cord.

Figure 15.7 *The descending connections of the reticular formation and afferents from higher levels.* Note that descending fibers from the cerebral cortex end on reticulospinal neurons. Most of the long connections are both crossed and uncrossed, although this is not shown in the figure. Numerous shorter fibers interconnecting subdivisions of the reticular formation are not shown.

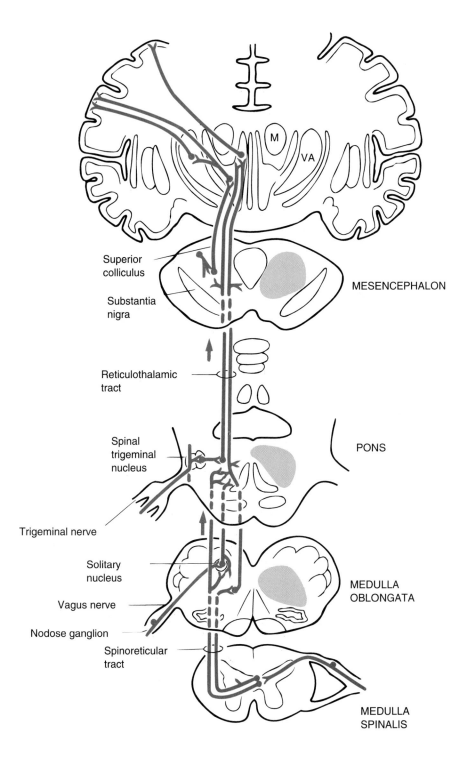

Superior
colliculus

Substantia
nigra

Reticulothalamic
tract

Spinal
trigeminal
nucleus

Trigeminal nerve

Solitary
nucleus

Vagus nerve

Nodose ganglion

Spinoreticular
tract

M

VA

MESENCEPHALON

PONS

MEDULLA
OBLONGATA

MEDULLA
SPINALIS

Figure 15.8 *The ascending connections of the reticular formation and afferents from lower levels.* The afferents from lower levels arise in the
cord (spinoreticular neurons) and in
the cranial nerve nuclei. The ascending
fibers from the reticular formation end
in the intralaminar thalamic nuclei. In
addition, there are direct connections
to the cerebral cortex from the raphe
nuclei and the locus coeruleus, not
shown in this figure (Figs. 15.5 and
15.6).

Connections from the Reticular Formation to the Cerebellum

Three distinct cell groups within the reticular formation send most of their efferent fibers to the cerebellum. They are therefore regarded as being among the *precerebellar nuclei*. The first of these is the *reticulotegmental nucleus* (nucleus reticularis tegmenti pontis), situated immediately dorsal to the pontine nuclei. It receives afferent connections from the pretectal nuclei and the superior colliculus among other cell groups, and sends fibers in particular to regions of the cerebellum known to participate in the *control of eye movements*. The second cell group, the *lateral reticular nucleus*, lies in the medulla, lateral to the inferior olive. It receives its main afferent input from the spinal cord and is therefore a link in one of the indirect spinocerebellar pathways (see Chapter 12). It also receives vestibular inputs (from the vestibular nuclei), however, and may therefore serve to *integrate information about the activity in motor-related spinal interneurons with information about the position of the body* (head). The smallest of the precerebellar reticular nuclei is the *paramedian reticular nucleus*, located medially in the medulla. It receives afferents from the spinal cord and some other sources. Its functional role is not known.

The Afferent Connections of the Reticular Formation

Various cell groups send fibers to the reticular formation (Figs. 15.7 and 15.8). *Spinoreticular fibers* are discussed in Chapter 7 (*Additional Pathways for Somatosensory Information*). They ascend in the ventral part of the lateral funiculus together with the spinothalamic tract,[3] but diverge in the lower medulla. Among other destinations, the fibers end in the parts of the reticular formation giving off long ascending axons to the thalamus. This provides a spinoreticulothalamic pathway that is anatomically and functionally different from the major sensory pathways discussed in Chapter 7. Some of the spinoreticular fibers end in areas where neurons send axons back to the spinal cord, thus establishing feedback loops between the reticular formation and the cord.

Corticoreticular fibers arise mainly in the cortical areas that give origin to the pyramidal tract. They end mainly in the regions of the reticular formation sending axons to the spinal cord. Therefore, a corticoreticulospinal pathway exists. It is known to be of importance for the control of voluntary and automatic movements, as discussed in Chapter 12.

The *superior colliculus* sends fibers to parts of the reticular formation, as mentioned above. These connections make it possible for visual signals to influence the reticular formation, since the superior colliculus receives visual information directly from the retina and from the visual cortex. In addition, the superior colliculus receives somatosensory information from the cortex, thus enabling integration of visual and somatosensory stimuli that are used for orientation toward external stimuli.

In addition to spinal neurons that send their axons only to the reticular formation, many *secondary sensory neurons send collaterals to the reticular formation*. This concerns many of the fibers of the spinothalamic tract, which, presumably, mediate *nociceptive and thermoceptive signals* to the reticular formation. The same kind of information from the face is provided by collaterals of ascending axons from the sensory (spinal) trigeminal nucleus. *Visceral sensory* impulses reach the reticular formation by collaterals of ascending fibers from the solitary nucleus (which receives afferents from the vagus nerve, for example). *Auditory signals* reach the reticular formation by collaterals of ascending fibers in the auditory pathways. *Vestibular signals* come from the vestibular nuclei.

We discuss in Chapter 13 that the *basal ganglia* (the substantia nigra) send efferents to the mesencephalic reticular formation (the locomotor region, PPN). Fibers from the *hypothalamus* ending in parts of the reticular formation serve to coordinate the activity of diffferent peripheral parts of the autonomic system. *Limbic structures*, notably the amygdala, also send fibers to the reticular formation. Such connections probably mediate emotional effects on autonomic and somatic motor functions. The *PAG* is discussed in Chapter 7 in relation to suppression of nociceptive signals. This mesencephalic complex of smaller nuclei have a wider specter of functions, however. Thus, it helps to initiate defensive reactions to external threats or other kinds of stress. This happens by way of its efferent connections to premotor networks in the reticular formation.

Finally, the reticular formation receives afferents from the cerebellum (primarily the fastigial nucleus, Fig. 14.4). This is an important pathway for the cerebellar influence on α and γ motoneurons.

The Reticular Formation Integrates Various Kinds of Information

The above description of afferents indicates that *signals from virtually all kinds of receptors can influence neurons of the reticular formation.* This is also shown by physiological experiments. Electrodes placed in the reticular formation can record potentials evoked by stimulation of receptors for light, sound, smell, and taste. Furthermore, stimulation of peripheral nerves carrying signals from cutaneous receptors and proprioceptors and of visceral nerves evokes activity. Whenever a receptor is stimulated, the signals reach not only the cortical areas of importance for the perception of the stimulus but also the reticular formation. Finally, stimulation of *the cerebral cortex, the hypothalamus, and limbic structures can produce changes in the activity of the reticular formation.* Thus, under normal conditions, there are always signals coming into the reticular formation, keeping it in a state of tonic activity. The extent of the tonic activity depends on how strongly the reticular formation is "bombarded" by receptors and by other parts of the brain. We return to this below when discussing control of wakefulness.

Anatomic and physiological data indicate that large parts of the reticular formation are characterized by *integration* of various kinds of information. The efferent signals from the reticular formation do not provide specific information about features such as stimulus modality. The very long dendrites and numerous interneurons with widely branching axons form a structural basis for integration. Such findings, together with physiological data showing that electrical stimulation of the reticular formation typically produces widespread and unspecific effects, led to the assumption that the reticular formation functions as a unity (without regional specialization). More recent investigations with more refined methods have shown, however, that the reticular formation is heterogeneous both anatomically and functionally, even though the borders between different subregions are not sharp.

FUNCTIONS OF THE RETICULAR FORMATION

It follows from the above discussion of its efferent connections that the reticular formation can act on virtually all other parts of the central nervous system. We have previously considered its effects on the spinal cord (Chapters 7 and 12), and we will add more below on this point. In addition, we will discuss the effects on the cerebral cortex, which are of particular importance. Parts of the reticular formation that are involved in the control of eye movements are discussed in Chapter 16, whereas the parts involved in the control of autonomic functions are described briefly in Chapter 17.

The Activating System

It is striking that the efferent connections of the reticular formation can *activate* both lower and higher levels of the central nervous system. Electrical stimulation alters several functions mediated by the spinal cord, such as muscle tone, respiration, and blood pressure. Also, the general activity of the cerebral cortex—which is closely related to the level of consciousness—can be altered by stimulation of the reticular formation. *The activating system of the brain stem* was therefore introduced as another name for the reticular formation. Stimulation of the reticular formation, however, can also produce inhibitory effects on several processes.

As mentioned above, we believe that there is a tonic activity of the reticular formation maintained by a constant inflow of impulses from various sources. The level of tonic activity is reflected by the level of consciousness, among other things. *The activity of the reticular formation is essential for the conscious awareness of specific sensory stimuli and for adequate behavioral responses to them.* When our attention is caught by a novel stimulus, this is mediated by the reticular formation. At the same time, the reticular formation produces the motor responses that ensure automatic orientation of the head and the body toward the source of the stimulus. The motor apparatus is mobilized, together with alterations of respiration and circulation.

Actions on Skeletal Muscles

Animal experiments during the 1940s led to the identification of two regions within the reticular formation that influence the *tone of the skeletal muscles*. Stimulation of a region in the medulla that sends particularly strong connections to the spinal cord (Figs. 15.9 and 15.10) could inhibit stretch reflexes and also movements induced by stimulation of the motor cortex. This region was therefore called the *inhibitory region*. A region with opposite effects, the *facilitatory region*, was found rostral to the in-

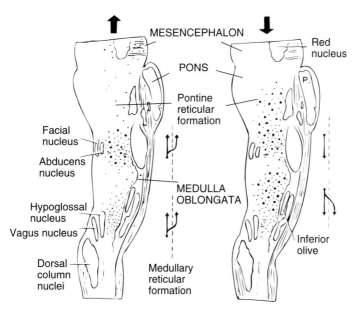

Figure 15.9 *Position of efferent reticular cell groups.* Drawing of sagittal section through the brain stem (cat). To the **left**, the areas with neurons sending axons to higher levels (the thalamus) are indicated with dots, whereas areas sending fibers to the spinal cord are shown in the **right** drawing. Note that the cell groups sending descending fibers are located somewhat more rostrally than the regions sending ascending fibers, providing opportunity for mutual influences by collaterals (as shown in Fig. 15.3).

hibitory one. It extends rostrally into the mesencephalon and is located somewhat more laterally than the inhibitory region.[4] The actions in the cord concern not only α but also γ motoneurons, so that the reticular formation can control the sensitivity of the muscle spindles. The activity of the γ motoneurons is increased by stimulation of the facilitatory region and inhibited by the inhibitory region. The muscle tone can therefore be up- and down-regulated by changes in the balance between the influences from the two regions. Since the cerebral cortex, the cerebellum, the basal ganglia, and other regions send fibers to the reticular formation, it is not unexpected that muscle tone can be influenced from these parts as well. It should be recalled, however, that cell groups other than the reticular formation also have direct access to the motoneurons, notably the vestibular nuclei with their strong facilitatory effects on the tone of muscles main-

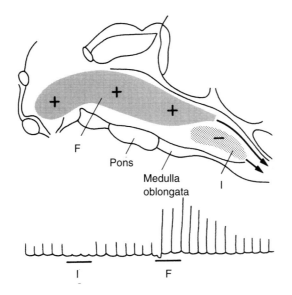

Figure 15.10 *Facilitatory (F) and inhibitory (I) regions of the reticular formation.* Schematic sagittal section through the brain stem (cat). The diagram **below** shows the amplitude of the patellar reflex (measured with EMG). In the period marked I, the inhibitory region was stimulated electrically, and the reflex response is almost abolished. In the F period, the facilitatory region was stimulated, and the patellar reflex response is markedly enhanced. From Kaada (1950).

taining the upright position (the concept of muscle tone is discussed in Chapter 11).

In addition to the rather diffuse effects on muscle tone obtained by electrical stimulation of the reticular formation, its role in the control of certain kinds of voluntary and reflex movements is discussed in Chapter 12. There is, however, no principal difference between the influence of motoneurons in eliciting a movement and in maintaining a (static) posture. On the basis of the present state of knowledge of the organization of the reticular formation, *the emphasis is more on its control of fairly specific motor tasks than on its diffuse effects on the muscle system as a whole.* Certain subregions have, for example, a particular role in control of the rhythmic *locomotor movements* (Chapter 12), whereas other regions are devoted to the control of *eye movements* (Chapter 16), and some are concerned primarily with *orienting movements of the head and the body* in response to optic and vestibular stimuli. In such cases, parts of the reticular formation—often consisting of fairly extensive networks—collect the relevant information about, for example, the position of the head and body, and ensure through their output signals the coordinated activity of all the muscles that are necessary to produce a proper response. Such reticular cell groups are, as mentioned, called *premotor networks (centers).* Common to premotor networks is their control of the activity of large groups of muscles.

Effects on Respiration and Circulation

The early investigations with stimulation of the reticular formation indicated that inspiratory movements are evoked from a region that coincides roughly with the inhibitory region (Fig. 15.10). Expiratory movements were produced by stimulation within the facilitatory region in the medulla. Later studies with microelectrodes have shown, however, that neurons with respiratory movement-related activity are found in several regions of the reticular formation, and not only in the medulla. Furthermore, a clear-cut separation of an inspiratory and an expiratory region appears not to be tenable. The current view is that *respiration is controlled by a network formed by several cell groups in the reticular formation of the ventrolateral medulla.* The neurons of the network change their activity in relation to specific phases of the breathing rhythm, and are collectively responsible for the production of rhythmic breathing. This network has properties in common with other *rhythm generators*, for example those producing locomotor movements. The respiratory rhythm generator is unstable shortly after birth in rats (but not in pigs and cats). A theory proposes that similar immaturity—so that the breathing rhythm is easily disturbed or abolished—lies behind sudden infant death.

Several kinds of information reaching reticular neurons are relevant for the *control of the respiratory rhythm generator*, such as signals from receptors within the lung tissue and from receptors in the walls of the large arteries, which monitor the blood concentration of oxygen and carbon dioxide.

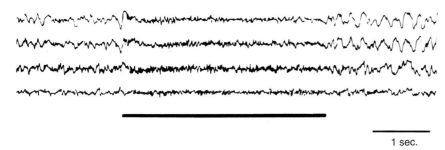

1 sec.

Figure 15.11 *EEG recordings from the classic studies of Moruzzi and Magoun of the activating system of the brain stem.* The four tracings are recorded over different parts of the cerebral cortex of a cat. The thick line shows the period of electrical stimulation of the reticular formation. The stimulation produces desynchronization of the EEG (activation), which returns to a synchronized pattern when the stimulation stops.

The reticular formation also receives all information necessary *to control blood pressure, the distribution of the blood volume among the organs, the stroke volume, and the heart rate* (see Chapter 17). To some extent, a distinction can be made between inhibitory and facilitatory regions for circulatory control, too. A "pressor" region producing increased blood pressure on stimulation and a "depressor" region with the opposite effect were originally identified in the medulla. Conditions have turned out to be more complex, however. As with respiratory control, rather extensive parts of the reticular formation participate in the coordination of the proper adjustments of the work of the heart and the diameter of the vessels. The effects are mediated chiefly by reticulospinal fibers that act on preganglionic sympathetic neurons and by reticular efferents to the dorsal motor nucleus of the vagus.

Effects of the Reticular Formation on the Cerebral Cortex

The ascending effect of the reticular formation was brought into focus by a paper published by the neurophysiologists Moruzzi (Italian) and Magoun (American) in 1949. Suddenly, new perspectives were opened on important aspects of brain functioning, especially consciousness, sleep, and wakefulness. On the basis of their animal experiments, Moruzzi and Magoun formulated a new concept: *the ascending activating system of the brain stem.*

Electrical stimulation of the reticular formation in anesthetized animals produces certain changes of the electrical activity in the cortex, as recorded by EEG. This method samples the collective activity of neurons in large parts of the cerebral cortex. Depending on how coordinated, or *synchronized*, the neuronal activity is, different kinds of waves are seen in the encephalogram. Under anesthesia (without stimulation), relatively slow waves dominate (Fig. 15.11). On stimulation of the reticular formation, the slow waves of the EEG are replaced by waves with a faster and more irregular rate and with a lower amplitude. We say that the EEG changes from *synchronization* to *desynchronization*. Together with desynchronization or activation of the EEG occur signs of increased attention and alertness—that is, an *arousal* is produced. Such an arousal can be produced also in unanesthetized animals with implanted electrodes. For example, a cat lying still with no obvious interest in its surroundings becomes suddenly alert and attentive when the reticular formation is stimulated with a high-frequency train of impulses. Various kinds of experiments confirmed the hypothesis of Moruzzi and Magoun that *the reticular formation is necessary for the maintenance of normal wakeful consciousness*. The reticular formation determines the level of wakefulness, with its many variations from tense alertness to drowsiness and sleep. Marked reduction of the activity of the reticular formation is associated with unconsciousness, as shown experimentally in animals with selective lesions. In humans with prolonged periods of unconsciousness after head injuries, there is often damage of the mesencephalic reticular formation. The lesion can be surprisingly small and yet produce deep unconsciousness.

As mentioned above, the reticular formation can have either activating or inhibiting effects on functions mediated by the spinal cord, depending on which region is stimulated (Fig. 15.10). Similar findings were made with regard to the ascending effects on the cerebral cortex, even though we so far have discussed only the activating effects. It ap-

Electroencephalography

Direct recording from the surface of the cerebral cortex of animals shows that the patterns of electrical waves differ among parts of the hemispheres. In humans, too, direct recordings from the exposed cortex can be done during brain surgery (electrocorticography). The electrical waves are conducted through the skull and the soft tissues of the scalp and can therefore be recorded with electrodes placed on the skin of the head. With this method, *EEG*, the electrical signals are dispersed and attenuated on their way through the skull and soft tissues, so that the origin of the signals within the hemisphere can only be roughly determined. Nevertheless, the method has been of great importance both for research and diagnostically since its introduction around 1930.

The electroencephalogram or EEG varies considerably with age; most marked are the changes during the first couple of years. There are also individual variations. Furthermore, the EEG pattern changes during sleep and during general anesthesia. Hyperventilation, which leads to a reduced carbon dioxide concentration in the blood, changes the excitability of cortical neurons, and this is reflected in the EEG. Finally, several drugs affect the EEG.

When analyzing the EEG, one can discern various wave forms and patterns. The α waves are relatively slow, with a frequency of 8–12/sec (Fig. 15.12). They occur typically in an awake person who is relaxed and resting with her eyes closed. When the person opens her eyes or starts to think about a mental task (Fig. 15.12), the EEG immediately changes to a pattern with more irregular waves with a higher frequency and lower amplitude. These are called β *waves*. The change of wave pattern from α to β waves is called *desynchronization* or *activation* of the EEG. During *sleep*, other wave forms and patterns occur that are typical of specific stages of sleep. Various neurological diseases can be diagnosed because they are associated with characteristic changes of the EEG. To some extent, the EEG can also help to localize the disease process. EEG is particularly important in the *diagnosis of epilepsy*.

It is not fully understood how the various wave forms in the normal EEG arise, but it is clear that they depend in large measure on different activity states in thalamocortical neurons. *Thalamocortical neurons* (functioning as relay cells for transmission of sensory and other signals to the cortex) have unique membrane properties owing to the presence of a special kind of Ca^{2+} channel that opens only when the cell is hyperpolarized to a certain level. Thalamocortical neurons generate action potential in two different patterns or modes: They may fire in *bursts* (that is, they fire 2–8 action potentials with a high frequency followed by a pause), or they fire *single spikes* with a varying overall frequency. The bursting pattern is associated with synchronization of the EEG (in states of drowsiness and so-called slow-wave sleep), whereas the single-spike firing occurs together with desynchronization (during attentiveness and during rapid-eye-movement sleep). It appears that these different functional states of the thalamocortical (relay) neurons determine whether they transmit signals to the cortex; Only in the single-spike mode do the cells transmit to the cortex the information they receive from, for example, peripheral receptors.

Figure 15.12 *EEG (electroencephalography)*. Three traces are shown, all of them recorded over the occipital lobes. **A.** The person is in a relaxed state, with his eyes closed. There are α waves typical of synchronization. **B.** At the arrow, the person opens his eyes and the α waves are replaced by faster, irregular waves with smaller amplitude, called β waves. The EEG is desynchronized. **C.** Desynchronization produced by solving a mental task. The person is asked to make a calculation (13 × 9). After the calculation is completed (117), the slower waves return.

pears that inhibition—that is, synchronization of the EEG—is evoked most easily from the caudal parts, whereas activation or desynchronization is evoked from the rostral parts (corresponding to the effects on skeletal muscles). We return to this below when discussing sleep.

Impulse Pathways and Transmitters for the Activation of the Cerebral Cortex

What are the pathways used by the reticular formation to influence consciousness, attention, and sleep? All of the major specific sensory pathways (the spinothalamic tract, the medial lemniscus, and the visual and auditory pathways) can be interrupted without affecting consciousness or the activation of the EEG produced by stimulation of the reticular formation. On the other hand, when these sensory pathways are left intact but the ascending connections of the reticular formation are interrupted by a cut in the mesencephalon, the animal becomes unconscious. Electrical stimulation of the reticular formation can no longer activate the EEG, even though stimulation of peripheral receptors evokes potentials in the cortical sensory regions. Thus, the sensory signals reach the cortex, but they are restricted to the sensory regions, and, most importantly, they are unable to arouse the animal.

Pathways other than the major sensory ones must therefore be responsible when the reticular formation activates the EEG over major parts of the cerebral hemisphere and produces behavioral changes indicating increased attention. Connections from the reticular formation to the *intralaminar thalamic nuclei* are likely candidates. Thus, electrical stimulation of these nuclei can produce activation of the EEG similar to that seen after stimulation of the reticular formation itself. The intralaminar thalamic nuclei send widespread efferents to the cerebral cortex. Therefore, a reticulothalamocortical pathway probably is important for the actions of the reticular formation on the cerebral cortex. Many, but not all, of the reticulothalamic fibers to the intralaminar nuclei are *cholinergic*. In addition to this indirect reticulothalamocortical pathway, there are direct projections to the cerebral cortex from *monoaminergic cell groups* in the brain stem—usually considered parts of the reticular formation—such as the *raphe nuclei* and the *locus coeruleus*. These projections are also related to attentional mechanisms and the states of sleep and wakefulness, as indicated by physiological and pharmacological studies. For example, neurons in the locus coeruleus increase their firing frequency shortly be-

Can Consciousness Be Explained in Neurobiological Terms?

The term consciousness does not lend itself to precise definitions; yet we all "know" what it is. For clinical use, we do not need elaborate definitions: it is of value simply to distinguish between levels of consciousness (from attention to coma, as the extremes). Consciousness has been described and characterized in many ways, although a satisfactory *definition* may be impossible to give. The American philosopher John Searle gives this description: "By 'consciousness', I simply mean those subjective states of sentience or awareness that begin when one awakes in the morning from a dreamless sleep and continue through the day until one goes to sleep at night or falls into coma, or dies, or otherwise becomes, as one would say, 'unconscious'." One central feature is *unity* or *wholeness*. We perceive ourselves as a whole, and all the bits and pieces of information analyzed by different specialized neural systems are subordinated and incorporated into a unitary experience. (Certain brain lesions, however, can dramatically change this; for example a stroke patient can deny that his paralyzed leg is a part of his body.)

Most people would accept that consciousness is a product of neuronal activity, and as such a property of the brain. This in itself does not explain the phenomenon, and consciousness cannot be fully understood by a reductionistic approach, studying in ever more detail the constituent parts of the brain. The brain—consisting of billions of neurons— produces as a whole something that is more than the sum of its parts, and even the most detailed knowledge of synaptic couplings, transmitters, and receptors does not suffice to explain consciousness and other mental phenomenons. Perhaps we must limit ourselves to the simple fact that consciousness is a property that can arise in a neuronal network exceeding a certain size and complexity. Looking for the "consciousness center" or "module" somewhere in the brain is— judging from our present knowledge—based upon a false assumption of how the brain works. That unconsciousness follows interruption of the ascending activating system in the mesencephalon, does not imply that the locus of consciousness is somewhere in the mesencephalon (similarly, the fact that a car cannot run without a battery does not imply that the battery *is* the car). Consciousness cannot be separated from its content including subjective sensations, moods, motives, inner images, and thoughts. For such mental functions the cerebral cortex is essential (in Chapter 8 we discuss whether conscious visual experiences could be linked to specific parts of the cortex). However, it would be misleading to state that the cerebral cortex alone "owns" the property of consciousness. As discussed above it must communicate with several other parts of the brain to "produce" consciousness. Neither should we conclude that all mental processes of the cerebral cortex take place in "the searchlight of consciousness." A patient illustrating this was described in Chapter 8. Another patient, described by the American Michael Gazzaniga, also illustrates this point. She had a stroke affecting the mid-portion of the corpus callosum (linking, among other regions, the somatosensory areas). She was asked to identify objects with the left or the right hand without seeing them. Holding, for example, a rubber in her right hand she could easily name and describe it. This is as expected because sensory information would reach her left hemisphere that is responsible for speech in most people (see Chapter 20). She could afterwards pick out with her right hand similar objects among many others in a bag. However, when the rubber was placed in her left hand—sending sensory information to the "mute" right hemisphere—she said she did not know what it was, or that she did not feel anything. Nevertheless, she could pick out with her left hand the rubber among the many other objects in the bag. Thus, the right hemisphere can analyze the sensory information in the same way as the left. It can initiate a purposeful, voluntary response—is it then conscious or not? Notably, in this patient most of the corpus callosum was undamaged. Thus, the two hemispheres could communicate except regarding somatosensory information. The left hemisphere remained ignorant of the information reaching the right. Gazzaniga regards the left hemisphere as a kind of interpreter of what goes on in the specific systems for information processing—only when the information reaches the left hemisphere can it be subjected to conscious attention. On the other hand, this does not fit easily with the fact that neglect of bodily parts or extra personal space most often occurs after *right*-hemisphere lesions.

fore and during periods of activation and focused attention. The cerebral cortex also receives direct *dopaminergic* projections from the ventral tegmental area in the mesencephalon. *Histaminergic* projections to the thalamus (including the intralaminar nuclei) can bring thalamocortical neurons from a state of burst firing to single-spike firing. Histamine receptor antagonists (H_1) block this effect, and might explain why the histamine antagonists commonly used for allergy and motion sickness have sleepiness as a side effect.

To summarize: *Several cell groups, using many transmitters, cooperate in the control of consciousness and attention. The effects are exerted partly in the thalamus, partly in the cerebral cortex. Most likely, each of the cell groups and transmitters influence partly different aspects of the awake state.*

The Reticular Formation and the Control of Sensory Information

In Chapter 7, we discuss how the central transmission of sensory signals can be controlled from higher levels of the central nervous system. Descending connections to the spinal cord from the raphe nuclei and various (other) parts of the reticular formation have been shown to suppress the central conduction of signals from nociceptors. Furthermore, the central transmission of visual, auditory, and other sensory impulses is subjected to control by the reticular formation. Thus, even though it is not alone in this capacity, the reticular formation plays an important role in the elimination of sensory signals that are considered irrelevant, so that our attention can be focused on the relevant signals.

Together with other mechanisms, inhibition from the reticular formation can ensure that, for example, we do not notice that someone is talking to us while we are absorbed in a book. This role is closely related to the one played by the reticular formation in attention and consciousness. Thus, the reticular formation is perhaps more concerned with the *focusing of our attention* on certain stimuli or internal events—that is, restricting our awareness—than with a global control of consciousness.

Sleep

Sleep consists of several phases that can be distinguished on the basis of differences in the EEG. The transition from alertness to drowsiness changes the EEG in the direction of synchronization. When a subject is falling into a deep, quiet sleep, the α waves disappear altogether and are replaced by irregular slow waves with greater amplitude (*slow-wave sleep*). After an initial light *phase I*, the sleep becomes gradually deeper, until *phase IV*. To waken a person in sleep phase IV requires relatively strong stimuli, whereas only weak stimuli are necessary in phase I. *Phase V* is special because the EEG is desynchronized, and there are conjugated movements of the eyes, much like a person looking at moving objects.[5] Because of these rapid eye movements (REM), this phase is also called *REM sleep* or *paradoxical sleep*. Muscle tone is generally reduced, with occasional muscular twitches, and there are changes of blood pressure and heart rate. *Dreaming* occurs—at least mainly—during REM sleep. The various phases of sleep follow each other with the same order throughout the night. Usually, the first REM phase occurs after about 1Ω hours of sleep and lasts for about 10 minutes. Thereafter the REM phases return at intervals of 1–2 hours, and become gradually longer up to about 30 minutes. When waking up (or being wakened) just after a REM phase, a person remembers the content of the dream vividly.

The cerebral cortex is as active during REM sleep as when awake. It is, however, partly uncoupled from the thalamus, which in the awake state delivers a constant stream of information about the external world. The EEG pattern during sleep is produced by complex interactions between neuronal firing patterns in the thalamus and the cortex. Inhibitory interneurons in both places play important roles in this respect.

Why we dream, has been the subject of much speculation and many theories. REM sleep appears to occur in all mammals,[6] even in the earliest species that developed about 140 million years ago. This fact alone suggests that REM sleep has an important function. Further support for its biological significance comes from other observations. Thus, the proportion of REM sleep increases after a period with REM-sleep deprivation, and it is much more difficult to prevent the occurrence of REM sleep than the other phases of sleep.

Newborn infants have approximately 8 hours of REM sleep per day and a special sleep rhythm. It consists of periods of 50–60 minutes of sleep usually starting with REM sleep rather than slow-wave sleep. By the age of 2 REM sleep is reduced to about 3 hours, and the sleep pattern is essentially as it is in adults. The reason that REM sleep is so dominating during infancy (and also before birth) is unknown. One possibility is that REM sleep is necessary for neuronal growth and development of connections. The dominating view today is that *dreams contribute to the processing and consolidation of newly learnt material*, and the integration of new experiences with older ones. Animal experiments indicate that storage of new material is reduced by prevention of REM sleep a certain period after the learning situation. During REM sleep in certain animals, a particular pattern of electrical activity (theta rhythm) occurs in the hippocampus. Since the hippocampus plays a crucial role in learning (see Chapter 19), this has been taken to support the relationship between REM sleep and learning.

The view that dreams are psychologically meaningful, relating in a disguised form to inner conflicts and life events, is the basis for their central place in the psychoanalysis since Freud. Rather than emphasizing the role of dreams in learning, psychoanalytic tradition would stress their importance for the elaboration of inner conflicts that are not consciously accessible. These two possibilities are not mutually exclusive, however. Perhaps a common purpose for all dreams is to help the individual develop *coping strategies*, since this requires both the integration of new with old experiences and that inner conflicts do not block learning and appropriate behavior.

The neural basis of sleep and its various phases is still not fully clarified and has turned out to be very complex. Several brain regions and neurotransmitters are of importance. Lesions of the *hypothalamus*, for example, can lead to increased or reduced amounts of sleep, but it is clear that the neuronal groups directly involved in sleep control are located in the brain stem, especially in the *pons*. Initially, after the discovery of the activating system, it was assumed that sleep was simply the result of reduced activity of the activating system—that is, a purely passive process. Further studies showed, however, that sleep could be induced by electrical stimulation of the lower parts of the reticular formation and that lesions of the same region prevented sleep (insomnia).

For *induction* of sleep, activity in *cholinergic neurons in the dorsolateral pons* is crucial (the peribrachial region, the pedunculopontine nucleus, and some smaller cell groups). These neurons project to the thalamus to influence the activity of the large sensory relay nuclei (the geniculate nuclei, the VPL). In addition, they project to neurons in the nearby reticular formation, which in their turn project to cholinergic neurons in the hypothalamus and the basal nucleus (among other targets). The effects of acetylcholine in the thalamus are mediated by muscarinic receptors. The pontine cholinergic neurons fire in bursts (*bursting neurons*) ahead of the eye movements in REM sleep. Their close relation to REM sleep is further shown by the observation that micro injection of acetylcholine in the dorsolateral pons increases REM sleep for several days.

The roles of *serotonin* and *norepinephrine* in control of sleep are less clear, probably because they are difficult to study in isolation. Thus, cholinergic and monoaminergic neurons lie partly intermingled in the dorsolateral pons. It seems established, however, that the monoamines exert their main effect on sleep by *modulating the activity of the pontine cholinergic neurons*. Mostly the monoamines *inhibit* the cholinergic neurons, thus increasing wakefulness. This conclusion is based on, among other things, that the monoaminergic neurons fire during wakefulness and are "silent" during REM sleep. Furthermore, microinjection of serotonin hyperpolarizes the bursting neurons in the dorsolateral pons. Finally, drugs that enhance the synaptic effect of serotonin (such as re-uptake inhibitors) have been found to reduce REM sleep in humans.

Spinal motoneurons are strongly inhibited from the brain stem during REM sleep. This prevents the execution of movements that are part of the dream (small, "miniature" movements can nevertheless be observed during dreaming). The inhibition is partly initiated by the pontine cholinergic neurons, although the major control most likely is exerted by noradrenergic neurons close to the locus coeruleus (the subcoeruleus nucleus). Reticulospinal neurons in the medial medullary reticular formation mediate the effects on the motoneurons. After destruction of descending norepinephrine-containing fibers animals still have REM sleep, but behave as if they were acting out their dreams with orienting movements, more complex exploratory behavior, and attack or flight.

Other transmitters, *GABA, dopamine*, and several *neuropeptides*, are involved in control of sleep by influencing the activity of the pontine cholinergic neurons. In addition, *glutamate* and *glycine* act by way of more indirect pathways. Thus, many drugs acting on the brain would be expected to influence sleep and wakefulness.

Narcolepsy

Narcolepsy is a genetically linked disease with sudden, irresistible *attacks of REM sleep* (or components of REM sleep). Starting usually between the ages of ten and thirty, the disease affects equally often men and women. The patients experience increased sleepiness during daytime, whereas the night sleep is fragmented. The symptoms are most likely related to an increased concentration of *muscarinic receptors* within the brain stem (cf. the increased REM sleep caused by injection of acetyl choline in the dorsolateral pons, mentioned above). Furthermore, there is evidence that *monoamine metabolism* is deficient. Both drugs that block muscarinic receptors and drugs that increase synaptic concentration of monoamines (such as amphetamine and tricyclic antidepressants) are reported to reduce the narcoleptic attacks.

The Reticular Formation and the Relationship between Mental and Bodily Processes

Variations in the activity of the reticular formation are reflected in virtually all aspects of the nervous processes and also in the activity of the endocrine organs controlled by the hypothalamus. Knowledge of such interactions may help to explain how mental and bodily processes are so intimately correlated and often change in parallel. There is much evidence to suggest that *the activity of the reticular formation is influenced by our mental state*. The thought of a forthcoming, unpleasant event or the memory of an embarrassing or agonizing situation may suddenly make a drowsy person alert and tense (increased muscle tone), produce sweating, increase the heart rate, and so forth. Every doctor who routinely tests reflexes knows that apprehension and anxiousness is accompanied by increased reflex responses and increased muscular tone. An exaggerated patellar reflex at the start of a consultation becomes "normal" as the patient relaxes. Another everyday example is the difficulty in falling asleep when one is preoccupied with distressing thoughts.

All of the above effects are expressions of increased activity of the reticular formation produced by the *influence of psychic processes*—presumably closely linked with neuronal activity in the cerebral cortex, limbic structures, and the hypothalamus. Thus, stimulation of certain cortical areas can increase the activity of reticular neurons, and this is followed by desynchronization of the EEG. Nonanesthetized animals at the same time become attentive. These effects are mediated by direct and indirect connections from the cortex to the brain stem. There are also connections from the hypothalamus and limbic structures (such as the amygdala) to the reticular formation, which may be of particular importance because emotionally colored psychic phenomena are most effective in causing activation. That insomnia is related to increased activity in the reticular formation is suggested by the fact that most drugs used against insomnia reduce the activity of reticular neurons. General anesthesia abolishes the transmission through central parts of the reticular formation (resulting in lack of activation of the EEG and unconsciousness), whereas the transmission in the specific sensory pathways is less affected.

It is also well known that *bodily processes can influence our mental state*. For example, a treatment that leads to muscle relaxation usually also reduces mental tension. Again, the effects are probably mediated by a reduction of the activity of the reticular formation. At the same time there are alterations of respiration, blood pressure, heart rate, and other autonomic functions, such as sweat secretion, peristaltic movements of the bowel, and secretion of gastric juice. Most likely, some of the autonomic expressions of anxiety may by themselves serve to maintain and increase the anxiety.

We return to the interactions between the mind and the body in Chapters 18 and 19.

NOTES

1. Some authors include certain thalamic cell groups—especially the intralaminar nuclei—in the term "the reticular formation of the brain stem."

2. Reticulospinal fibers are located also in the dorsal part of the lateral funiculus (dorsal reticulospinal tract). Many of these fibers are monoaminergic and come from, among other places, the raphe nuclei and adjoining parts of the reticular formation, as discussed in Chapter 7. These dorsal pathways appear to be primarily concerned with control of sensory transmission from the dorsal roots to motoneurons (segmental reflex arcs) and to second-order sensory neurons, which are links in the ascending sensory pathways.

3. The medial lemniscus does not give off collaterals to the reticular formation. Information from low-threshold mechanoreceptors must therefore reach the reticular formation via spinoreticular neurons.

4. The distinction between inhibitory and facilitatory regions is less sharp than originally believed. In several places, single neurons with inhibitory or facilitatory actions on muscles are intermingled.

5. That the eye movements are related to the content of the dream, is suggested by patients suffering from neglect of the left visual hemifield (after damage to the right hemisphere). They have conjugated eye movements during REM sleep only to the right side; that is, the visual field they attend to when awake.

6. Whales (Cetacea) appear not to have REM sleep. In these mammals the two hemispheres alternate to exhibit slow-wave sleep. Perhaps constant vigilance is a necessity for adaptation and survival.

CHAPTER 16

CRANIAL NERVES

We usually count 12 cranial nerves, even though neither the first (the olfactory nerve) nor the second (the optic nerve) are true nerves. These two and, in addition, the cochlear nerve are dealt with in Chapters 8, 9, and 10. A brief survey of the anatomy of the cranial nerves is given in Chapter 3 (Figs. 3.13 and 3.14). The prenatal development of the cranial nerve nuclei is treated in Chapter 4.

GENERAL ORGANIZATION OF THE CRANIAL NERVES

Before dealing with specifics for each of the cranial nerves (Fig. 16.1), we will discuss some features that are common to them all. Like the spinal nerves that connect the spinal cord with the body, the cranial nerves connect the brain stem with the peripheral organs. Several structural features are shared by the spinal cord and the brain stem, and thus also by the spinal and cranial nerves. Nevertheless, the brain stem is less regularly built and more complex in its organization than the spinal cord, and the cranial nerves are not as schematic in their composition as the spinal nerves. Most of the cranial nerves, for example, lack a distinct ventral (motor) root and a dorsal (sensory) root. Some of the cranial nerves are purely sensory, others are purely motor, and others are mixed. Like the spinal nerves, several of the cranial nerves contain autonomic (preganglionic) fibers supplying smooth muscles and glands. Finally, some also contain afferent fibers from visceral organs.

The Cranial Nerves Can Contain Four Different Kinds of Nerve Fibers

The cranial nerves can contain the following kinds of fibers:

1. *somatic efferent* fibers innervating skeletal (striated) muscles;
2. *visceral efferent* fibers supplying smooth muscles and glands and belonging to the parasympathetic part of the autonomic nervous system;

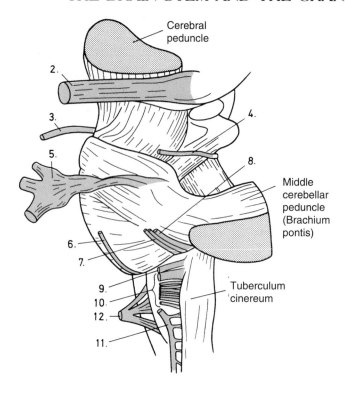

3. *somatic afferent* fibers with sensory impulses from the skin and mucous membranes of the face, from muscles and joints, and from the vestibular apparatus; and

4. *visceral afferent* fibers with sensory impulses from the visceral organs.

The *efferent fibers* of the cranial nerves have their perikarya in brain stem nuclei corresponding to the columns of spinal motoneurons (Fig. 11.2) and the intermediolateral cell column of the cord (Fig. 14.2). We use the terms *somatic efferent* and *visceral efferent* cranial nerve nuclei of these cell groups (Figs. 16.2 and 16.3). The *afferent fibers* have their perikarya in ganglia close to the brain stem, corresponding to the spinal ganglia. The central process of the ganglion cells enters the brain stem and ends on neurons in nuclei corresponding to the spinal dorsal horn and the dorsal column nuclei (Fig. 16.4). We use the terms *somatic afferent* and *visceral afferent* cranial nerve nuclei for such groups. From such afferent (sensory) nuclei, signals are conducted centrally to the thalamus and the cortex, and via brain stem interneurons to the somatic and visceral efferent (motor) cranial nerve nuclei (as links of brain stem reflex arcs; Fig. 16.4).

The Position of the Cranial Nerve Nuclei: An Overview

In early embryonic life, all neurons giving origin to a particular kind of fiber lie together in one longitudinal column in the brain stem. During further development, however, these columns break up into smaller

Visceral efferent
oculomotor nucleus

Oculomotor nucleus

Trochlear nucleus

Trigeminal motor
nucleus

Abducens nucleus

Facial nucleus

Superior salivatory nucleus

Inferior salivatory nucleus

Hypoglossal nucleus

Nucleus ambiguus

Dorsal motor vagus nucleus
(visceral efferent)

Accessory nucleus

Mesencephalic trigeminal
nucleus

Main trigeminal
nucleus
(somatic afferent)

Vestibular
nuclei

Cochlear
nucleus

Solitary nucleus
(visceral afferent)

Spinal
trigeminal
nucleus

Figure 16.2 *Position of the columns of the cranial nerve nuclei*. Schematic drawing of the brain stem seen from the dorsal aspect. The somatic efferent nuclei innervating myotome muscles are shown in dark red. The special somatic efferent nuclei innervating branchial arch muscles are marked with red dots. The visceral efferent nuclei are shown in red. In the **right** half, the sensory nuclei are shown.

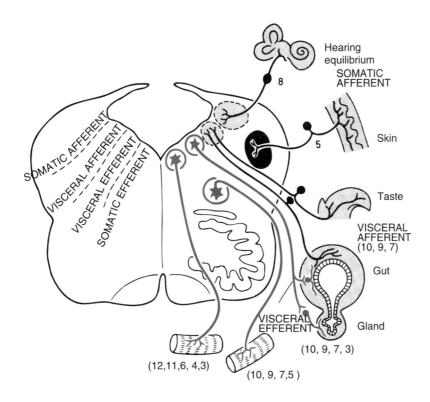

Hearing
equilibrium
SOMATIC
AFFERENT

Skin

Taste

VISCERAL
AFFERENT
(10, 9, 7)

Gut

VISCERAL
EFFERENT

Gland

SOMATIC AFFERENT

VISCERAL AFFERENT

VISCERAL EFFERENT

SOMATIC EFFERENT

(12,11,6, 4,3)

(10, 9, 7,5)

(10, 9, 7, 3)

Figure 16.3 *Position of the columns of the cranial nerve nuclei*. Schematic cross section of the medulla.

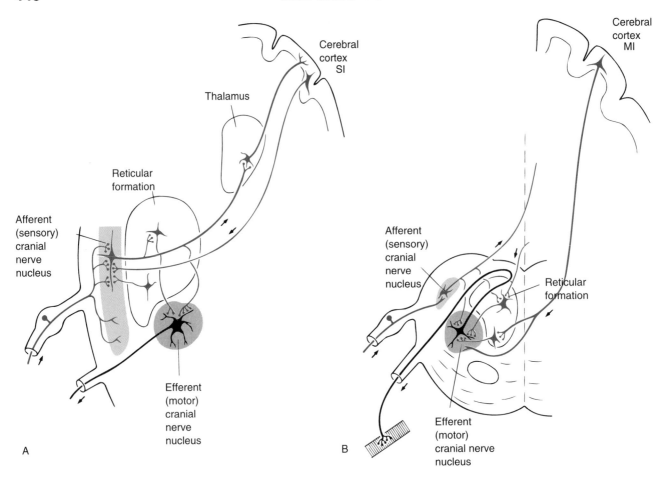

Figure 16.4 *Main features of the organization of the cranial nerve nuclei.* **A**. Sensory nucleus (for example, the trigeminal nucleus). The efferent fibers of the nucleus ascend to the thalamus of the opposite side, and from there the next neuron projects to the cerebral cortex. The fibers destined for the thalamus give off collaterals on their course through the reticular formation and the motor cranial nerve nuclei. Thus, a reflex arc with reflex center in the brain stem is established. The sensory nucleus is influenced by descending fibers from the cerebral cortex. **B**. Motor nucleus (for example, the facial nucleus) sending its efferent fibers out of the brain stem to striated muscles. The neurons of the nucleus are influenced by the cerebral cortex, by the reticular formation, and by collaterals of the ascending fibers from the sensory nuclei.

groups, and some of these groups move away from the original column. Nevertheless, the tendency for cranial nerve nuclei of the same category to form columns can be recognized also in the adult brain (Fig. 16.2). The demonstration of this regular pattern has been of value in understanding the functions of the cranial nerves. Furthermore, knowledge of this pattern aids us in learning about the cranial nerves and their nuclei.

It is helpful at the outset to remember the following general rule (evident from Figs. 16.2 and 16.3): *The efferent (motor) nerve nuclei lie medially in the brain stem, whereas the afferent (sensory) nuclei are located laterally.* Furthermore, in most cases the *nuclei are located at about the same rostrocaudal level as their nerves leave* the brain stem. In clinical neurology it is important to know the approximate rostrocaudal level of each nucleus (in the mesencephalon or pons, in the upper or lower part of the medulla).

The *somatic efferent nuclei* are in early embryonic life all arranged in a column close to the midline, but later some move away in a ventro-lateral direction (Fig. 16.3). Those remaining in the medialmost column are termed *general somatic efferent* and comprise (from caudal to rostral) the *nucleus of the accessory nerve* (11), the *nucleus of the hypoglossal nerve* (12), the *nucleus of the abducent nerve* (6), and the *nucleus of the oculomotor nerve* (3). (In the following we will for practical reasons use abbreviated names, such as the accessory nucleus and the hypoglossal nucleus.) All of these nuclei innervate *myotome muscles*—that is, muscles that are developed from the segmentally arranged somites of early embryonic life. The somatic efferent nuclei that have moved away from the medial column all innervate *branchial muscles*—that is, striated muscles developed from the branchial (visceral) arches (facial and masticatory muscles, and muscles of the pharynx and larynx). We call these nuclei *special somatic efferent* (although they most commonly are termed special visceral efferent).[1] This group comprises the *nucleus ambiguus* (9, 10), the *facial nucleus* (7), and the *motor trigeminal nucleus* (5).

The *visceral efferent* (parasympathetic) column of cranial nerve nuclei is located immediately lateral to the somatic efferent column (Fig. 16.3) and comprises the *dorsal motor nucleus of the vagus* (10), the small *inferior and superior salivatory nuclei* (9, 7), and the *parasympathetic oculomotor nucleus of Edinger-Westphal* (3). The *visceral afferent* fibers all end in one long nucleus, the *solitary nucleus* (solitary nucleus), which is located lateral to the visceral afferent column (Fig. 16.3).

Most laterally we find the *somatic afferent* nuclei. This group comprises the *sensory trigeminal nucleus* (5), the *vestibular nuclei* (8), and the *cochlear nuclei* (8). The sensory trigeminal nucleus consists of three functionally different parts (the spinal, the principal, and the mesencephalic nuclei). Together the three parts form one continuous column, however, which extends from the upper cervical segments of the cord into the mesencephalon (Fig. 16.2).

The fibers of the vestibulocochlear nerve are often classified as *special somatic afferent* because they originate from special sense organs; the trigeminal fibers are then termed *general somatic afferent*.

Figures 16.2 and 13.3, and the above account, show that *fibers of one kind all come from one of the columns of nuclei only, even though the fibers peripherally may follow several of the cranial nerves.* Thus, all (general) somatic afferent fibers end in the sensory trigeminal nucleus, whereas the fibers peripherally follow not only the trigeminal nerve but also the glossopharyngeal and the vagus nerves.

*The Cranial Nerves and Their Nuclei Are Links in
Reflex Arcs: Brain Stem Reflexes*

Like the spinal nerves that are links in spinal reflex arcs, the cranial nerves constitute afferent and efferent links of reflex arcs with reflex centers in the brain stem (Fig. 16.4). Often, such reflex centers are fairly complex, comprising neurons at several levels of the brain stem (for some, even at the cortical level). Thus, the afferent fibers may enter the brain stem at one level, whereas the efferent fibers leave at another. One example is the *corneal reflex* (touching of the cornea elicits an eye wink), in which the afferent fibers of the trigeminal nerve, entering at the midpontine level, descend in the brain stem and form synapses in the lower medulla (the spinal trigeminal nucleus). From the medulla, the impulses are conveyed by interneurons to the facial nucleus on both sides, located in the lower pons. The reflex center is in this case rather extensive, and as a consequence lesions at various levels of the brain stem may produce a weakened or abolished corneal reflex. However, depending on the location of the lesion, the change of the corneal reflex will be accompanied by various other symptoms, which helps in determining the exact site of the lesion.

Some brain stem reflexes are simple, such as the monosynaptic stretch reflex that can be elicited of the masticatory muscles.

The Cranial Nerve Nuclei Are Connected with Central Sensory and Motor Tracts

As mentioned, the cranial nerves and their nuclei are organized in accordance with the same general rules as the spinal nerves (with some exceptions). This means that the cranial nerves are the first links in sensory pathways corresponding to the *dorsal column–medial lemniscus system* and the *spinothalamic pathway* (Fig. 16.4). Furthermore, like the nuclei involved in the sensory pathways conducting from the spinal cord, those of the brain stem are subjected to descending control of the sensory transmission. This concerns influences from parts of the reticular formation and from the cerebral cortex.

Several of the somatic efferent (motor) cranial nerve nuclei are influenced by the *pyramidal tract*—that is, by fibers forming the *corticobulbar tract* (Fig. 16.4). An important difference between the corticospinal and corticobulbar fibers is that several of the cranial nerve nuclei receive both crossed and uncrossed fibers. Unilateral damage to the descending fibers (for example, in the internal capsule) produces clear-cut pareses only in some of the muscle groups innervated by the cranial nerves (most marked in the mimetic muscles).[2]

Examination of the cranial nerves is of great importance in clinical neurology because it can provide exact information about the site of a disease process. A prerequisite, however, is that the examiner has reasonably precise knowledge of where the cranial nerves exit from the brain stem (Figs. 3.16 and 16.1) and the position of their nuclei both rostrocaudally and mediolaterally (Figs. 16.2 and 16.3). Furthermore, the functions of the various nerves must be known in sufficient detail as a basis for the necessary tests.

Figures 3.15–3.17, 3.19, and 16.5 show the location of the cranial nerve nuclei in cross sections of the brain stem.

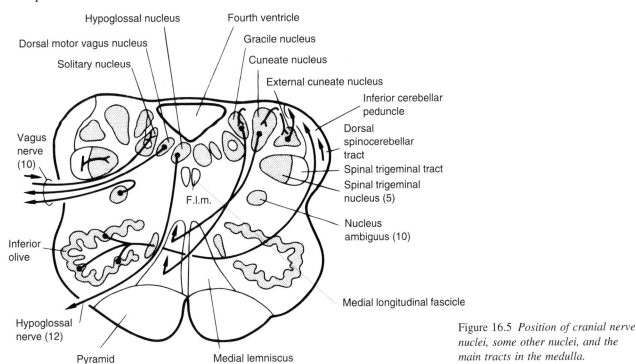

Figure 16.5 *Position of cranial nerve nuclei, some other nuclei, and the main tracts in the medulla.*

THE HYPOGLOSSAL NERVE

The twelfth cranial nerve, the hypoglossal nerve (Fig. 16.1), is the motor nerve of the tongue. It is composed of only *somatic efferent* fibers. The fibers come from the *hypoglossal nucleus*, which forms a slender, longitudinal column close to the midline in the medulla (Figs. 16.1 and 16.5). The nucleus produces an elongated elevation in the floor of the fourth ventricle (the hypoglossal trigone) (Fig. 3.18). The root fibers of the nerve pass ventrally and leave the medulla just lateral to the pyramid (Figs. 3.16, 16.1, and 16.5). Several small fiber bundles join to form the nerve, which leaves the skull through the *hypoglossal canal* in the occipital bone. The nerve then forms an arc as it courses downward and forward in the upper neck—external to the carotid artery—to the root of the tongue. The fibers innervate the striated muscle cells of the tongue.

The muscles of the tongue are used *voluntarily* during speech and eating. At such times the neurons of the hypoglossal nucleus are influenced by fibers of the pyramidal tract coming from the face region of the motor cortex of the opposite hemisphere. The descending fibers cross in the medulla just above the nucleus. A central motor lesion above the nucleus (for example, in the internal capsule) can produce pareses of the opposite half of the tongue, together with the more obvious pareses of the extremities. No clear-cut atrophy of the tongue occurs in cases of central motor lesions.

Reflex movements of the tongue occur in swallowing (and vomiting). The hypoglossal motoneurons are then activated from brain stem reflex centers, located in the reticular formation. Various kinds of stimuli can activate the reflex center for swallowing, notably touch and pressure receptors at the back of the tongue.

A unilateral lesion of the hypoglossal nerve or nucleus produces paralysis of the tongue on the same side. Since this is a peripheral paresis, a pronounced atrophy of the tongue muscles ensues. This is witnessed by a wrinkled surface of the tongue because the mucous membrane becomes too big for the reduced volume (Fig. 16.6). When the tongue is stretched out, it deviates to the paretic side, because of paresis of the genioglossus muscle. This muscle passes backward and laterally into the tongue from its origin at the inside of the mandible; its normal action when acting unilaterally is to draw the tongue forward and to the opposite side.

The Ansa Cervicalis

Some of the motor fibers from the first cervical spinal segment join the hypoglossal nerve and follow it for some distance before leaving it and descending in the neck. The descending fibers join other motor fibers from the second and third cervical segments and thereafter form a (fairly obvious) arc external to the internal jugular vein, called the *ansa cervicalis* (*ansa* means handle). The fibers of the ansa cervicalis innervate the infrahyoid muscles and have no relation to the hypoglossal nucleus or the muscles of the tongue. Damage to the hypoglossal nucleus or the proximal part of the nerve (before the fibers from C_1 join it) therefore produces no pareses of the infrahyoid muscles.

THE ACCESSORY NERVE

The eleventh cranial nerve, the accessory nerve, brings *somatic efferent fibers* to two muscles in the neck, the sternocleidomastoid and the trapezius. The accessory nucleus is located in a column in the upper part of the cervical cord (Fig. 16.2) and contains neurons that are of the ordinary motoneuron type. The root fibers leave the cord and ascend to enter the posterior fossa through the foramen magnum. The nerve then leaves the skull through the jugular foramen together with the vagus and the glossopharyngeal nerves (Fig. 16.7). Outside the skull, the nerve passes internal to the sternocleidomastoid muscle and superficially through the upper part of the lateral triangle of the neck before continuing under the upper part of the trapezius muscle.

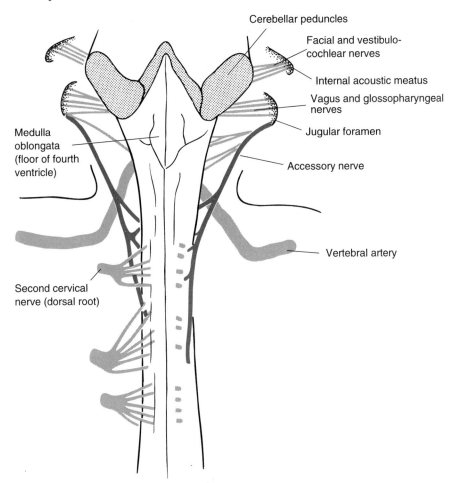

Cerebellar peduncles

Facial and vestibulo-cochlear nerves

Internal acoustic meatus

Vagus and glossopharyngeal nerves

Jugular foramen

Medulla oblongata (floor of fourth ventricle)

Accessory nerve

Vertebral artery

Second cervical nerve (dorsal root)

Figure 16.7 *The accessory nerve.* The lower part of the brain stem and the upper cervical cord seen from behind. The cerebellum is removed. The fibers of the accessory nerve proper emerge from the three upper cervical segments. They leave the cord between the ventral and dorsal roots (the ventral roots are not visible in the figure). Compare with the emergence of the vagus fibers in Figure 16.1.

The accessory nerve is joined for a short distance intracranially by some fibers from the nucleus ambiguus. These fibers leave the nerve just outside the jugular foramen and follow the vagus nerve in their further course. They should therefore be considered a part of the vagus with a somewhat aberrant course rather than a part of the accessory nerve.

In *central motor lesions* (of the corticobulbar component of the pyramidal tract), pareses of the contralateral sternocleidomastoid and the trapezius are usually observed. Because of its superficial position, the nerve may be damaged in the lateral triangle, producing a peripheral paresis. In such a case only the trapezius is paretic, since the fibers innervating the sternocleidomastoid leave the nerve higher up. Furthermore, the upper part of the trapezius muscle is usually most seriously affected, the lower part being supplied also from the cervical plexus. Paresis of the trapezius muscle makes it difficult to elevate the arm, because the trapezius is necessary for the rotation of the shoulder blade around its anteroposterior axis.

THE VAGUS NERVE

The vagus nerve is the tenth cranial nerve and is characterized by containing *fibers of all four kinds described above*.[3] Correspondingly, it is

Figure 16.8 *The course and distribution of the vagus nerve.*

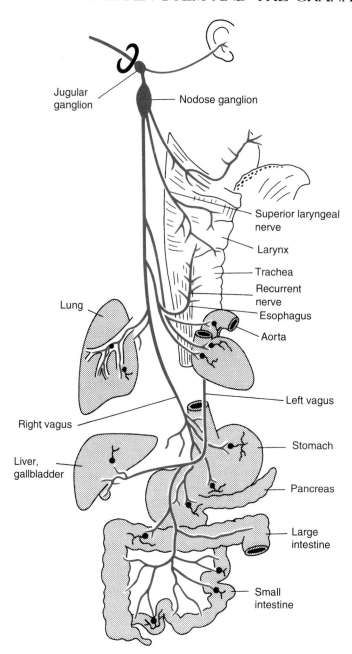

Jugular ganglion

Nodose ganglion

Superior laryngeal nerve

Larynx

Trachea

Recurrent nerve

Esophagus

Aorta

Lung

Left vagus

Right vagus

Stomach

Liver, gallbladder

Pancreas

Large intestine

Small intestine

connected with four different nuclei in the medulla. The root fibers emerge in a row at the lateral aspect of the medulla (Figs. 16.1 and 16.5) and join to form one nerve, which leaves the skull through the jugular foramen (Fig. 16.7).

In the jugular foramen and immediately below, the nerve has two swellings, the *jugular* and the *nodose ganglia* (Fig. 16.8), which contain the pseudounipolar perikarya of the sensory vagus fibers.

As implied by the name (Latin: vagus = wandering), the vagus nerve sends branches to widespread regions of the body. After leaving the skull, the nerve passes as a fairly thick cord downward in the neck together with the common carotid artery, further through the thorax, and into the abdomen through the diaphragm. It gives off branches in the neck, in the thorax, and in the abdomen.

Visceral Efferent (Parasympathetic) Vagus Fibers

The visceral efferent neurons belong to the parasympathetic part of the autonomic nervous system. The perikarya are found in the *dorsal motor nucleus of the vagus* (Figs. 3.16, 13.2, and 16.5).[4] The fibers do not pass directly to the organs, but end on a second set of neurons in parasympathetic ganglia close to or in the wall of the organs (Fig. 16.8)—as is the case for all parasympathetic nerves (Fig. 17.1). The neurons leading from the central nervous system to the ganglia are called *preganglionic*, and those leading from the ganglion to the organ are called *postganglionic*.

In the neck, the vagus gives off visceral efferent fibers to the *heart* (Fig. 16.8). The perikarya of the postganglionic neurons are located in the wall of the heart and around the great vessels in the vicinity of the heart, and the postganglionic fibers end among the muscle cells of the heart, especially those of the sinus node, which determines the heart rate.

Other branches from the vagus supply the *esophagus* and the *trachea* and, further down in the thorax, the *bronchi* of the lung. The postganglionic fibers innervate smooth muscles and glands in these structures.

In the *abdomen*, the vagus sends fibers to the *stomach*, the *small intestine*, and the *first half of the large intestine*. The vagus also supplies the *liver*, the *gallbladder*, and the *pancreas* with parasympathetic fibers. To reach the various organs, the fibers follow the arteries and form plexuses around them together with sympathetic fibers.

Impulses in the vagus nerve *reduce the heart rate, constrict the bronchi, and increase bronchial secretion, whereas the peristaltic movements and secretion are increased in the stomach and intestine. The secretion of the pancreas is also increased.*

Visceral Afferent Vagus Fibers

All branches of the vagus with visceral efferent fibers also contain afferent (sensory) fibers. These neurons have their pseudounipolar perikarya in the large *nodose ganglion* (Fig. 16.8). When the fibers enter the brain stem, they form a small bundle that passes caudally: the *solitary tract* (this is not a true tract, however, but the central course of a nerve). The fibers establish synapses in the solitary nucleus (Figs. 3.16, 16.2, and 16.5). The efferent fibers from this nucleus pass to the reticular formation and other cranial nerve nuclei in the vicinity and to higher levels such as the thalamus and the hypothalamus (Figs. 10.4 and 16.4).

All of the sensory fibers from the larynx and some from the pharynx follow the vagus.[5] The sensory fibers from the larynx follow the *superior laryngeal nerve* (from the part above the vocal cords) and the *recurrent laryngeal nerve* (from the lower part of the larynx).

Visceral Reflexes

The visceral afferent impulses in the vagus nerve do not reach consciousness, apart from perhaps feelings of hunger or satiety and more vague sensations. The visceral afferents are, however, links in *reflex arcs* that *control secretion and peristaltic movements of the gastrointestinal tract* (and vomiting). Such reflexes also mediate alterations of airway secretion and of the airway resistance by changing the tone of the bronchial smooth muscles. The *reflex centers* of all these reflexes are located in the medulla, and the efferent links are visceral efferent fibers coming from the dorsal motor nucleus of the vagus.

Visceral afferents from *baroreceptors* in the wall of the large vessels provide information about the blood pressure in the aorta. Increased blood pressure gives rise to increased firing frequency of the afferent fibers. This in turn produces increased firing of visceral efferent vagus fibers, which reduces the heart rate. The reflex center must involve connections from the solitary nucleus to the dorsal motor nucleus of the vagus (these two nuclei are close neighbors, as can be seen in Fig. 16.2).

The dorsal motor nucleus of the vagus can be influenced also by impulses other than those coming from the viscera. For example, the sight, the smell, or even the thought of food can produce increased secretion of gastric juice. These are examples of conditioned responses, whereas the stimulation of taste receptors produces an unconditioned (true reflex) response.

Other examples of visceral reflexes are discussed in Chapter 17.

The Vomiting Reflex

Vomiting is usually caused by marked dilatation of the stomach or irritation of its mucosa. The biologic significance of the reflex is presumably to rid the stomach of potentially harmful contents. As we all know, however, vomiting can also be provoked by irritation of the pharynx (putting a finger in the throat), by foul odors, strong emotions, and by travel sickness. Finally, vomiting can be produced by certain substances in the blood stream (such as apomorphine). Several different afferent links to the reflex center must therefore exist. The emptying of the stomach is caused by coordinated contractions of the smooth muscles in the stomach wall and striated muscles in the diaphragm and the abdominal wall. In addition, laryngeal muscles (closing the airways), and muscles of the pharynx, the soft palate and the tongue also participate. Thus, the reflex center must activate in a specific sequence visceral efferent neurons (motor vagus nucleus) and motoneurons at several levels of the brain stem and the spinal cord. The *reflex center* is actually quite widespread, but usually matters are simplified by restricting it to the medulla, including the *solitary nucleus*. This receives the visceral afferent fibers from the stomach, forming the afferent link when the reflex is elicited from the stomach itself. From the reflex center in the medulla impulses are coupled to the motor nuclei via synaptic interruption in the reticular formation and reticulospinal fibers. In addition, there are also direct spinal projections from the solitary nucleus to the motoneurons of the diaphragm and abdominal wall.

Substances in the bloodstream cause vomiting by direct action at the *area postrema* of the medulla (this is one among several regions of the brain lacking a blood–brain barrier; see Chapter 3, *Some Parts of the Brain Lack a Blood–Brain Barrier*). Neurons in the area postrema project to the solitary nucleus. Apomorphine and other alkaloids are given orally or subcutaneously to provoke vomiting.

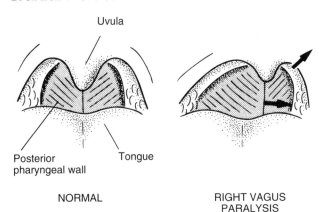

Uvula

Posterior pharyngeal wall   Tongue

NORMAL   RIGHT VAGUS PARALYSIS

Figure 16.9 *Paralysis of the right vagus nerve.* The uvula and the posterior pharyngeal wall are pulled toward the normal side when the patient says "aah." Redrawn from Mumenthaler (1979).

Somatic Efferent Vagus Fibers

The somatic efferent vagus fibers come from the *nucleus ambiguus* (Figs. 16.2 and 16.5), which belongs to the special somatic efferent nuclei. The fibers supply all striated muscles of the *larynx* and parts of the muscles of the *pharynx*. The fibers to the pharynx take off from the vagus as several small branches, whereas most of the fibers to the larynx are collected in the *recurrent laryngeal nerve*. This nerve takes off from the main vagus trunk at the level of the aortic arch on the left side and the subclavian artery on the right. It then arches behind the vessels and ascends in the furrow between the trachea and the esophagus, to reach the larynx. One of the laryngeal muscles located on the outside, the *cricothyroid muscle*, receives motor fibers in the *superior laryngeal nerve* (which is a predominantly sensory nerve, as mentioned above). The vagus also innervates one of the muscles of the soft palate (the *levator veli palatini muscle*).

A *lesion of the vagus nerve* above the exit of the motor branches to the pharynx and the soft palate produces deviation of the uvula and the posterior pharyngeal wall to the normal side (as can be seen, for example, when a patient is asked to say "aah") (Fig. 16.9). Pareses of the soft palate and the pharynx cause fluid and food to enter the nasal cavity when swallowing (owing to inadequate closure of the nasopharynx). Furthermore, the voice becomes hoarse because the vocal cords cannot be properly adducted. Such a symptom will obviously also occur after a lesion of the recurrent laryngeal nerve anywhere along its course. In case of a unilateral lesion, the voice hoarseness will gradually disappear, because the muscles of the normal side adapt to the changed conditions.

The neurons of the nucleus ambiguus are influenced by, among other sources, the *pyramidal tract* during speech. They can also be activated reflexly, however, by irritating stimuli of the respiratory tract (cough reflex).

Somatic Afferent Vagus Fibers

This is the smallest contingent of fibers in the vagus nerve. They have their perikarya in the small *jugular ganglion*, and come from a small region of the *skin of the external ear* (the auricular ramus). The fibers terminate in the *trigeminal sensory nucleus*. Touching the innervated area may evoke a cough reflex, and in some individuals stimulation of the external meatus (for example, by an otoscope) can cause a vomiting reflex. The causes of these phenomena are unknown. They might be due to connections from the trigeminal nucleus to the solitary nucleus, or by abnormal impulse transmission between sensory fibers of the vagus nerve (ephaptic transmission).

THE GLOSSOPHARYNGEAL NERVE

The ninth cranial nerve, the glossopharyngeal, resembles the vagus but is smaller and innervates a more restricted region. The root fibers leave the medulla immediately rostral to the vagus fibers (Fig. 16.1). The root fibers fuse to form one trunk that leaves the cranial cavity through the jugular foramen (together with the vagus and the accessory nerves). The nerve follows an arched course (ventrally) lateral to the pharynx, which it penetrates to reach the base of the tongue. Close to the jugular foramen, the nerve contains two small sensory ganglia with pseudounipolar ganglion cells (the superior and petrous ganglia).

Of the peripheral branches, some innervate the *muscles and the mucous membrane of the pharynx* (together with the vagus, which appears to be the most important quantitatively); other sensory fibers reach the *posterior part of the tongue, to innervate taste buds, and the mucous membrane* (and also the mucous membrane of the soft palate and the tonsillar region). The glossopharyngeal nerve also contains *visceral efferent* (parasympathetic) fibers to the *parotid gland* (and to the salivary glands in the posterior part of the tongue).

The Sinus Nerve and Baroreceptors

A special contingent of visceral afferent fibers in the glossopharyngeal nerve come from the wall of the *carotid sinus* (the thin-walled, dilated part of the internal carotid artery). The fibers conduct impulses from

The Nuclei of the Glossopharyngeal Nerve

The somatic efferent fibers to the striated pharynx muscles come from the *nucleus ambiguus*, whereas the visceral efferent fibers have their perikarya in the small *inferior salivatory nucleus* (Fig. 16.2). The impulses from this nucleus follow a somewhat complicated course to reach the parotid gland (as is the case for several of the parasympathetic fiber components of the cranial nerves). The preganglionic parasympathetic (visceral efferent) fibers from the inferior salivatory nucleus end in the small *otic ganglion* just outside the cranial cavity. The axons from the ganglion cells (postganglionic) join one of the trigeminal branches—*the auriculotemporal nerve*, which passes close to the ganglion—to the gland.

The visceral afferent fibers carrying impulses from the taste buds in the posterior third of the tongue end in the solitary nucleus. From there, the impulses are sent to the thalamus and further on to the cerebral cortex. The sensory fibers from the posterior part of the tongue, the tonsils, the soft palate, and the pharynx end in the *sensory trigeminal nucleus*.

mechanoreceptors recording the tension of the arterial wall; that is, the receptors monitor the blood pressure and are therefore called *barorecep-tors*. The afferent fibers end in the solitary nucleus, and from there the impulses are conveyed to the dorsal motor nucleus of the vagus. Increased impulse frequency of the cardiac vagus fibers reduces the heart rate, and the blood pressure thereby is reduced. When the blood pressure falls, there will be reduced firing of the cardiac vagus fibers, with increased heart rate and blood pressure. This is one of several mechanisms to ensure that the blood pressure is maintained within certain limits and that the cere-bral blood flow is sufficient at all times.

THE VESTIBULOCOCHLEAR NERVE: THE SENSE OF EQUILIBRIUM

The eighth cranial nerve, although consisting of only one trunk, is in re-ality two functionally different nerves, the *cochlear nerve* (dealt with in Chapter 9) and the *vestibular nerve*, which we will describe here. The nerves fuse after leaving the labyrinth (the cochlea and the vestibular ap-paratus) and follow the internal acoustic meatus. At the lower end of the pons, in the *cerebellopontine angle* (Figs. 16.1 and 16.7), the nerve en-ters the brain stem. Most of the fibers in the vestibular nerve end in the *vestibular nuclei*. The perikarya of the primary (afferent) vestibular fibers are located at the bottom of the internal meatus, forming the *vestibular ganglion*.[6] The main structural features of the labyrinth are described in Chapter 9 (Figs. 9.1 and 9.2) and will not be repeated here.

The Vestibular Apparatus

The vestibular apparatus, together with the cochlea, constitute the labyrinth. Unlike the cochlea, however, it does not depend on the exter-nal ear and the tympanic cavity to function. Like the cochlear duct with the organ of Corti (Figs. 6.3 and 6.7), the membranous labyrinth con-taining the vestibular receptors is embedded in the temporal bone and sur-rounded by a space containing perilymph (Figs. 16.10 and 16.12). The membranous labyrinth is filled with endolymph.

The vestibular part of the labyrinth consists of two small vesicles, the *utricle* and the *saccule*, and three circular tubes connected to the utricle, the *semicircular ducts* (Fig. 16.11). Each of the semicircular ducts has a swelling, the *ampulla*, in the end close to the utriculus. The ducts are ori-ented in three planes perpendicular to each other. In the erect position and with the head in a neutral position, the *lateral semicircular duct* lies ap-proximately in the horizontal plane, whereas the posterior and the ante-rior ducts are oriented vertically (Fig. 16.11).

Sensory epithelium with hair cells (Fig. 16.13) is found at five places in the vestibular labyrinth. The hair cells are similar to those in the cochlea. In each of the ampullae of the semicircular ducts, there is a transversely oriented elevation, the *ampullar crista* (Fig. 16.12). Hair cells with long cilia are present between the epithelial cells forming the crista. The cilia

Figure 16.10 *The sacculus*. Photomicrograph through the region of the saccular macula. Compare Figure 16.12.

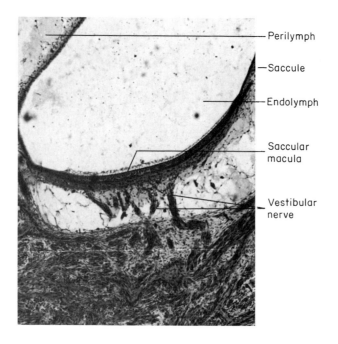

Perilymph

Saccule

Endolymph

Saccular macula

Vestibular nerve

Figure 16.11 *The position in the skull of the vestibular apparatus*. Note the orientation of the semicircular ducts in relation to the conventional planes of the body. The **lower** figure shows the base of the skull seen from above with the vestibular apparatus projected to the surface of the pyramid of the temporal bone.

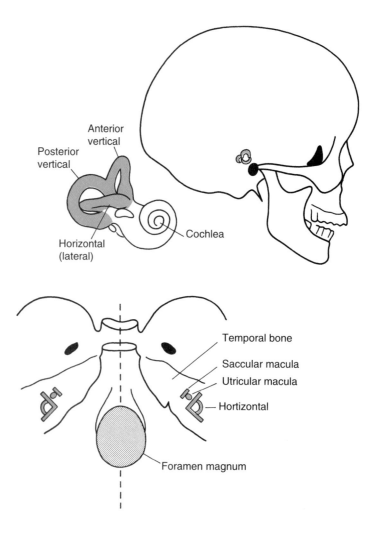

Anterior vertical

Posterior vertical

Horizontal (lateral)

Cochlea

Temporal bone

Saccular macula

Utricular macula

Hortizontal

Foramen magnum

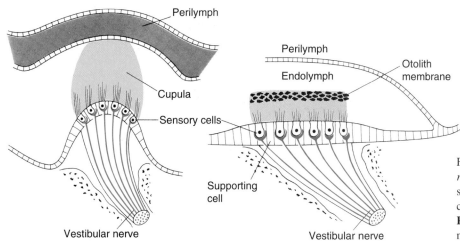

Figure 16.12 *The vestibular receptor regions.* Schematic. **Left**. Longitudinal section through the ampulla of a semicircular duct with the ampullar crista. **Right**. Section through the saccular macula. Compare Figure 16.10.

Figure 16.13 *Sensory (hair) cells of the utricular macula.* Scanning electron micrograph. The apical surface of one sensory cell is indicated. Magnification, ×10,000. Compare Figures 16.12 and 16.15. Courtesy of Prof. H. Lindeman.

Figure 16.14 *Otoliths from the utricular macula* (cat). Scanning electron micrograph. Magnification, ×2100. Courtesy of Prof. H. Lindeman, The National Hospital of Norway, Oslo.

461

project into a jellylike mass, the *cupula*. In the utricle and the saccule there are small patches of hair cells like those in the ampullae, the *utricular and saccular maculae* (Figs. 16.10 and 16.12). The macular hair cells are also covered by a jellylike mass, which is special because of its content of small "stones," the *otoliths* (Figs. 16.12 and 16.14). The otoliths are crystals of calcium salts. The utricular macula lies in approximately the same plane as the lateral semicircular duct (that is, horizontally in the neutral position), whereas the saccular macula is oriented almost vertically (Fig. 16.11).

The Adequate Stimulus for the Semicircular Ducts Is Rotation of the Head

Flow of the fluid (the endolymph) inside the semicircular ducts displaces the cupula, thereby bending the cilia. This activates or inhibits the sensory cells, depending on the direction of bending. *Flow of the endolymph in the semicircular ducts is produced by rotational movements of the head.* This is explained by the inertia of the fluid: When the head starts to rotate, the fluid "lags behind." When the rotation stops, the fluid continues to flow for a moment (like the water in a bowl that is rotated rapidly for a couple of turns). If the head rotation continues at even velocity, the fluid and the head will after a short time move with the same speed and in the same direction, which means that the cilia are not bent. Thus, it is clear that not every rotational movement is recorded by the receptors of the semicircular ducts: *Alteration of the velocity of the rotational movement— that is, positive or negative angular acceleration—is the adequate stimulus for the semicircular duct receptors. Thus these receptors have dynamic sensitivity* (see Chapter 6, *Receptor Properties*). Linear acceleration does not affect (or affects only slightly) the semicircular ducts. By linear displacement of the head (a translatory movement) without concomitant rotation, there is no stimulation of the semicircular duct receptors. An example of linear acceleration is a car that starts or brakes on a flat, straight road. If the road goes up and down and is curved, rotational accelerations of the car (and the heads of its passengers) are superimposed on the linear ones.

The orientation of the semicircular ducts ensures that rotation of the head in any conceivable plane produces change of activity of the receptors in one or more of the ducts. The pattern of activity produced by all the receptors is used by the brain to monitor the rotational movements of the head at all times. The semicircular ducts of both sides must function normally to supply the brain with the necessary information. A pair of ducts (for example, the right and left lateral ones) gives *complementary signals* to a given rotation—that is, increased impulse frequency from the one and reduced from the other.

Sacculus and Utriculus Signal the Position of the Head and Linear Acceleration

The small otoliths have higher specific weight than the endolymph and the substance in which they are embedded and are therefore more strongly influenced by gravitational forces. Taking as an example the utricular macula, which in the neutral head position is oriented horizontally (Fig. 16.11), a change of head position tilts the macula, and the otoliths pull the cilia in that direction. Different angles of tilt produce different patterns of activity of the macular hair cells. Owing to their different orientations in space, *the utricular and saccular hair cells together provide information about all possible head positions.*[7] Its ability to provide information about the position of the head at any one time (in the absence of movement) shows that the vestibular apparatus has *static sensitivity.* This property depends on the presence of receptors that adapt slowly or not at all (as discussed in Chapters 6 and 7), so that the receptors give a constant signal as long as a certain position is maintained. The static sensitivity of the vestibular apparatus depends, as we have seen, on the force of gravity and disappears in a state of weightlessness (such as in space travel).

Since the static sensitivity is a property of the utricle and the saccule, these parts of the vestibular apparatus are called the *static labyrinth.* We will see, however, that this part of the labyrinth also has dynamic properties.

The *dynamic sensitivity* of the utricle and the saccule is seen when their activity is recorded during linear acceleration. The response increases

More About the Vestibular Receptor Cells

Electron microscopic studies have shown that there are two kinds of vestibular receptor cells, which are found both in the cristae of the semicircular ducts and in the maculae of the saccule and utricle (Fig. 16.15). One kind, the *type 1* cell, is bottle-shaped, whereas the *type 2* cell is slender. The sensory fibers (the peripheral process of the vestibular ganglion cells) end differently on the two cell types (Fig. 16.15A). On the apical end of the cells there are numerous (50–110) *stereocilia* and one longer and thicker *kinocilium.* The stereocilia are unusually long microvilli and contain actin filaments like other microvilli. The kinocilium contains microtubuli (like cilia of the respiratory epithelial cells), indicating that the kinocilium is capable of active movements. The stereocilia are arranged regularly in accordance with their height (Figs. 16.13 and 16.15). This structural *polarization* of the receptor cells corresponds with the functional polarization mentioned above. Thus, bending of the stereocilia *toward* the kinocilium increases the firing frequency of the sensory fibers in contact with the cell, whereas bending in the opposite direction reduces the firing frequency. This is because the receptor cell is *depolarized* or *hyperpolarized* by bending of the cilia. The transmission of the signal from the receptor to the afferent nerve fiber is chemical, but the substance involved is not known. The alteration of the membrane potential of the receptor cell is believed to be caused by mechanical deformation of various parts of the so-called basal plate to which the cilia are anchored. The deformation changes the permeability of cation channels. Even a displacement of 0.2 μm at the tip of a cilium—corresponding to a displacement in the apical membrane of only 10 nm—elicits a robust response from the receptor!

Displacement of the cilia perpendicular to the direction of the polarization produces no response, whereas oblique displacements give a reduced response compared with a stimulus that is properly aligned with the polarization. This means that a given firing frequency of an afferent fiber is ambiguous—it can, for example, be caused by a weak stimulus in the direction of the polarization or a stronger obliquely oriented one. This may be the reason why the hair cells in the maculae are arranged differently with regard to the orientation of the polarization axes, so that all the cells together cover 360° (Fig. 16.15C). This ensures that the information received by the brain about head position in space is unambiguous. This requires, of course, that the brain be able to compare the magnitude of the signals from various parts of the maculae to reach a conclusion.

Figure 16.15 *Sensory cells of the vestibular apparatus.* **A** and **B**. Note the polarization of the cilia. **C**. The utricular macula seen from above. The **arrows** indicate the direction of polarization of the sensory cells in the various parts, which altogether cover all directions of deflection of the sensory hairs. From Brodal (1981).

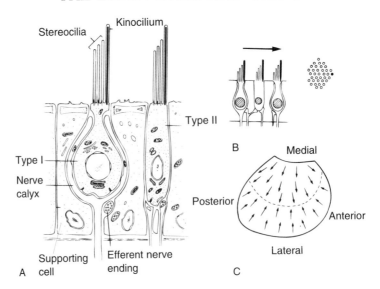

(that is, the firing frequency of the afferent fibers) with increasing acceleration. This is again explained by the inertia of the otoliths. On linear displacement of the head with changing velocity, as in a car that is accelerating, the otoliths lag behind and thereby bend the cilia backward (in relation to the direction of the movement). The opposite happens when the car slows down; the otoliths continue to move for a moment and bend the cilia forward (compare with the forces acting on a loose object in a car when the car speeds up or slows down).

The Primary Afferent Vestibular Fibers and the Vestibular Nuclei

The primary afferent fibers end in various parts of the vestibular nuclei. The collection of large and small vestibular nuclei is collectively called the *vestibular complex*. It covers a large area in the floor of the fourth ventricle and consists of four large nuclei and several small cell groups. (Not all cell groups within the vestibular complex receive primary vestibular fibers, however, and are therefore not vestibular, strictly speaking.) Figure 16.16 shows the location of the four major nuclei: the *superior*,

The Vestibular Nuclei Receive Afferents from Regions Other Than the Labyrinth

The physiological properties of neurons in the vestibular nuclei are not copies of those of the primary afferent fibers. This is explained by convergence on the cells of various kinds of afferents (such as fibers from the semicircular ducts and the utricle) and by interconnections between the nuclei (for example, commissural fibers linking the two sides). Furthermore, the vestibular complex receives afferents from other parts of the central nervous system, especially the spinal cord, the reticular formation, certain mesencephalic nuclei, and the cerebellum. Afferents from the mesencephalon arise, for example, in the superior colliculus, and the cerebellar fibers come from both the flocculonodular lobe and the anterior lobe (Figs. 14.3 and 16.28).

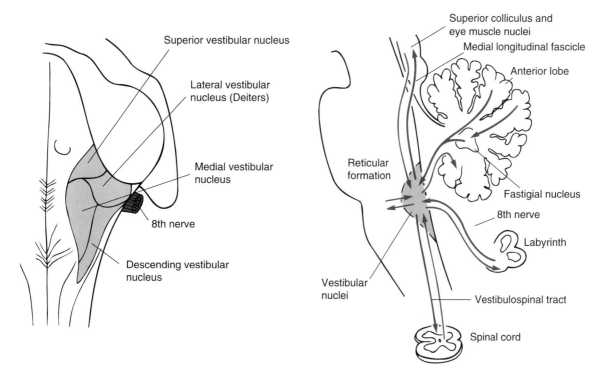

the *lateral* (or nucleus of Deiters), the *medial*, and the *descending* (or in-ferior).

Most of the afferent fibers from the *semicircular ducts* end in the su-perior nucleus and the rostral part of the medial nucleus, whereas the fibers from the *utricular macula* end primarily in the lateral nucleus. In agreement with the distribution of primary afferents, neurons in the su-perior nucleus are found to respond best to rotational head movements (angular acceleration), whereas the cells in the lateral nucleus are partic-ularly sensitive to static head position.

Efferent Connections of the Vestibular Nuclei

Schematically, the vestibular nuclei (and therefore also the vestibular re-ceptors) act on three main regions (Fig. 16.16):

1. *the spinal cord*, and especially the motoneurons, as discussed in Chap-ter 12;
2. *the cranial nerve nuclei of the extraocular muscles*; and
3. *the cerebellum.*

Information from the vestibular apparatus is used primarily to influence muscles that contribute to the equilibrium and to eye movements that en-sure that the retinal image is kept stationary when the head moves.

Most of the *fibers to the spinal cord* come from the lateral vestibular nucleus and form the *(lateral) vestibulospinal tract*. The fibers descend in the ventral funiculus on the same side as the nuclei from which they come. In the ventral horn they end—in part monosynaptically—on α and γ motoneurons (Fig. 16.17). The tract is *somatotopically organized*, so that various body parts can be selectively controlled. The vestibulospinal

Figure 16.16 *The vestibular nuclei*. To the **left**, the location of the nuclei is shown in a dorsal view of the brain stem. To the **right**, the main afferent and efferent connections are shown. Note reciprocal connections with the spinal cord, the cerebellum, the reticu-lar formation, and the nuclei of the ex-traocular muscles and other visually related nuclei of the mesencephalon.

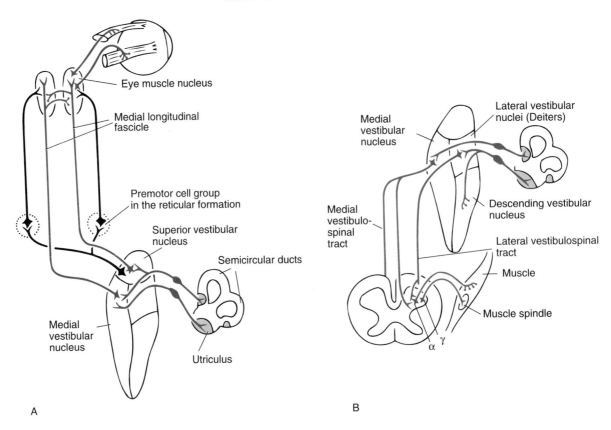

A

B

Figure 16.17 *The connections of the vestibular nuclei* with the nuclei of the extraocular muscles (**A**) and spinal cord (**B**).

tract has strong effects on muscles contributing to equilibrium and posture (see Chapter 12, *Vestibulospinal Tracts*). As mentioned, the lateral nucleus receives afferents from the utricular macula; these provide information about the static position of the head in space and thereby indirectly about the position of the body. Change of body position also changes its center of gravity, with a resulting need to adjust muscle tone to maintain equilibrium.

A smaller *(medial) vestibulospinal tract* arises in the medial nucleus. It also descends in the ventral funiculus and acts on motoneurons. The fibers do not reach below the upper thoracic segments, however, and are thought to be of importance primarily for head movements elicited by the vestibular receptors.

Fibers to the *nuclei of the extraocular muscles* arise mainly in the superior and medial nuclei, which receive many primary afferent fibers from the semicircular ducts (Fig. 16.17). The fibers leave the nuclei medially and join to form a distinct fiber bundle, the *medial longitudinal fasciculus*, located close to the midline below the floor of the fourth ventricle (Figs. 3.17, 16.16, and 16.29). Some of the fibers cross to the other side as they ascend, to end in the abducent, the trochlear, and the oculomotor nuclei. The connections are precisely organized so that the vestibular nuclei can select the combinations of muscles to be influenced. In addition to the direct connections in the medial longitudinal fasciculus, there are *indirect pathways* from the vestibular nuclei to the eye muscle nuclei via the reticular formation (Fig. 16.17). We will return to this below when discussing vestibular reflexes.

Vestibular fibers to the *cerebellum* are described in Chapter 14. They end primarily in the vestibulocerebellum and arise in the medial and descending nuclei (in restricted parts of these nuclei that do not appear to receive primary vestibular afferents). Fibers from the vestibulocerebellum to the vestibular nuclei can adjust the sensitivity (the gain) of the vestibulo-ocular reflex, as will be discussed below (see also Fig. 16.28).

Connections to the *thalamus* (to the VPL and the nearby VPI nucleus) from the vestibular nuclei have been demonstrated anatomically, and there is physiological evidence that impulses from the vestibular apparatus can reach the *cerebral cortex*.

Central Processing of Vestibular Signals

Vestibular impulses reach several small areas in the cortex, among them one close to the *face area of SI* (Fig. 7.21). An area at the junction between the parietal lobe and the insula contains neurons that are activated by signals from both the semicircular canals (head rotation) and from proprioceptors around the upper cervical joints. Since, in addition, the neurons are influenced by visual signals it seems likely that they integrate all kinds of movement-related information. Impulses from the labyrinth would thus contribute to the *awareness of bodily posture and movements in space*. In addition, signals from the labyrinth may mediate the signals producing a feeling of *dizziness (vertigo)* during certain kinds of vestibular stimulation. Furthermore, whereas the maintenance of body balance is caused by reflex control of muscle tone, the conscious awareness of how the body is oriented in space presumably depends on signals from the utricular and saccular maculae transmitted to the cerebral cortex.

Impulses from the utricle and the saccule are indeed necessary for the proper orientation of the body in space when visual information is prevented, as can be shown in animals whose otoliths have been removed and in persons with loss of vestibular function. Whereas such persons manage well as long as they can see, they have serious problems in maintaining the body's equilibrium in the dark.

Vestibular Reflexes

The anatomic basis and the physiological mechanisms underlying reflexes elicited from the vestibular apparatus have been investigated intensively recently. This interest is in part caused by the special problems encountered in space journeys. As with other parts of the brain being comprehensively investigated, conditions turn out to be more complex than initially thought. We will discuss only a few salient points.

Tonic and *phasic labyrinthine reflexes*, mediated by the vestibulospinal tracts, are described in Chapter 12. Here we will primarily address reflex actions on movements of the eye, *vestibulo-ocular reflexes*. This topic is also discussed toward the end of this chapter, when dealing with the cranial nerves supplying the extraocular muscles.

In general, *tonic* vestibular reflex effects are produced by impulses from the utricle and the saccule, whereas *phasic* reflex responses are caused by signals from the semicircular ducts when the stimulus is rotation of the head (angular acceleration) and from the utricle or saccule when the stimulus is linear acceleration.

There are several vestibulo-ocular reflexes, mediated by reflex arcs of various complexities. The simplest one consists of *three neurons* (Fig. 16.28):

1. *primary afferent fibers* from the cristae of the semicircular ducts;
2. *neurons in the vestibular nuclei* that send their axons to the *nuclei of the extraocular* muscles (passing in the medial longitudinal fasciculus); and
3. *motoneurons* in these nuclei, which send their axons to the *extraocular muscles*.

There are, furthermore, other impulse pathways with additional synapses, interrupted in the reticular formation and some other brain stem nuclei. The vestibulo-ocular reflexes ensure, as mentioned, that *the image is kept stationary on the retina when the head moves (rotates)*. A movement of the head in any direction is accompanied by a compensatory movement of the eyes in the opposite direction and with exactly the same velocity as the head movement. Rotation of the head produces movement of the endolymph inside the semicircular ducts. Taking a rotation in the horizontal plane (turning the head from one side to the other) as an example, mainly the lateral semicircular duct records the movement and elicits a compensatory eye movement in the horizontal plane.

When the head movement is relatively small, the eyes move with exactly the same velocity as and in the opposite direction of the head, and the image is kept in the same position on the retina all the time. This kind of movement, in which the eyes track an object accurately, is called the *smooth pursuit movement*. When the head movement becomes larger, so that it becomes impossible to keep the image stationary even with maximal excursion of the eyes, a fast *saccadic movement* occurs in the same direction as the head movement. Then the gaze is fixed again on the object and another smooth-pursuit phase follows (as long as the head continues to move in the same direction). Such an alternation between smooth-pursuit and saccadic eye movements is called *nystagmus*. In this case, the nystagmus was produced by stimulation of the semicircular ducts (rotation of the head) and is therefore called *vestibular nystagmus*. Nystagmus can, however, also be elicited by movement of the surroundings when the head is stationary. This *optokinetic nystagmus* occurs, for example in a train passenger watching the landscape pass by (we return to this below when discussing control of eye movements).

As mentioned, the vestibular nuclei receive afferents from sources other than the labyrinth, such as nuclei in the mesencephalon, the reticular formation, and the cerebellum. Some of these sources mediate visual information that can modify the vestibular reflex responses. This convergence of various inputs seems logical. Thus, to achieve optimal control of the eye movements, *the responsible neural cell groups must receive and integrate vestibular information about movements of the head, visual signals about movements of the image on the retina, and proprioceptive signals about movements of the eyes relative to the head.*

The Cerebellum Can Adjust the Vestibulo-Ocular Reflex to Changing External Conditions

The magnitude of the reflex response (not the response itself) to a certain rotational stimulus depends on signals to the vestibular nuclei from the cerebellum (Fig. 16.28). The Purkinje cells of the vestibulocerebellum receive primary vestibular fibers (ending as mossy fibers) that provide information about direction and velocity of the head movement. In addition, the same Purkinje cells receive information, via the inferior olive and climbing fibers, about whether the image is stationary or slips on the retina. A retinal slip indicates that the velocity of the compensatory head movement is too high or too low. The cerebellum is then capable of adjusting the excitability of the neurons in the vestibular nuclei—that is, in

Nystagmus and Falling Tendency Can Be Caused by Vestibular Stimulation

When an upright person rotates fairly rapidly a few times around his axis and then stops, the eyes can be seen to move rapidly one way (saccade) and slowly the other (slow pursuit) for some seconds afterwards. Obviously, the rotation has induced nystagmus. By using special instruments, it can be seen that there is nystagmus also at the start of the rotation, but in the opposite direction of that occurring after the rotation has stopped. When the person rotates to the right, the saccade movement is to the right and the slow pursuit movement is to the left—as if the person fixes her gaze on a stationary point and then moves the eyes rapidly when this point is slipping out of the visual field. The eyes then move to a new fixation point, and the same sequence of events is repeated. When the rotation of the body continues for some time, the nystagmus disappears and the person gets dizzy (compare with ballet dancers who deliberately ensure that the head does not move with even velocity during pirouettes; this way they have sufficient time for fixation so that the brain gets information to determine the orientation of the body in space).

The nystagmus is caused by stimulation of the receptors in the semicircular ducts. As mentioned, at the start of the movement the inertia of the endolymph makes it lag behind, thereby bending the cilia of the receptor cells, whereas the endolymph continues to flow for a moment after the rotation has stopped. The person who had just stopped rotating feels as if he were still rotating, but now in the opposite direction. The direction of the nystagmus corresponds to the illusion of such a rotation—that is, with the saccade phase to the left after a rotation to the right.

After stopping the rotation, the person is also unsteady and tends to fall to one side, especially if he is asked to keep his eyes closed. Furthermore, the arm deviates to the right if the person is asked to point straight ahead (with his eyes closed). This is called *postrotational past pointing*. After the rotation stops, the illusion of the opposite movement (that is, the person feels he is turning to the left) causes the past pointing to the right: The person feels that the room is moving to the right.

The postrotational effects on postural muscles are mediated via the vestibulospinal tracts (Fig. 16.17) and show that the receptors of the semicircular ducts also influence the spinal cord and the postural muscles, and not only the cranial nerve nuclei and the extraocular muscles.

Nystagmus, falling tendency, and past pointing can also be produced by irrigation of the external auditory meatus with hot or cold water. The change of temperature makes the endolymph flow in the semicircular ducts and thus produces stimulation of the receptors. Such a *caloric test* is used clinically to examine the function of the vestibular labyrinth and the conduction of impulses to the brain stem.

Various *diseases* affecting the vestibular receptors or the impulse pathways to the motoneurons of the extraocular muscles (the vestibular nerve, the vestibular nuclei, and the medial longitudinal fasciculus) can produce nystagmus in the absence of vestibular or visual stimulation. This is called *spontaneous nystagmus*. In certain cases, the nystagmus may be present only in certain positions of the head (positional nystagmus).

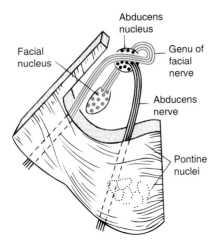

Figure 16.18 *The course of the facial nerve and its relation to the abducent nucleus.* Schematic cross section through the lower pons.

the reflex center of the vestibulo-ocular reflex. We also say that the cerebellum can change the gain of the reflex. Such adaptive change of gain of the reflex is presumably needed continuously during growth and also in situations of muscular fatigue. How much the gain can be altered is shown by experiments in which animals wear optic prisms that deflect the light so that it appears to come from another direction than it really does.

THE FACIAL AND INTERMEDIATE NERVES

The seventh cranial nerve belongs to the second visceral (branchial) arch and innervates structures developed from this. The facial nerve is the motor nerve of the facial (mimetic) muscles, supplying them with *special somatic efferent* fibers. The small *intermediate nerve* follows the facial nerve and is usually considered to belong to it. Thus, parts of the intermediate nerve can be said to represent a sensory root of the facial nerve with its *visceral afferent* fibers. The intermediate nerve also contains *visceral efferent* (parasympathetic) fibers, however.

The facial nerve (together with the intermediate nerve) leaves the brain stem laterally at the lower border of the pons, just ventral to the eighth nerve (Figs. 3.14 and 16.1). It then follows the eighth nerve to the bottom of the internal auditory meatus. The *facial nerve proper* (with the special somatic efferent fibers) then arches first posterolaterally and thereafter downward in a canal in the temporal bone. It leaves the skull through the *stylomastoid foramen* immediately medial and anterior to the mastoid process. The nerve then passes forward through the parotid gland and divides into several branches, spreading out like a fan to all the facial muscles.

The fibers of the *intermediate nerve* leave the facial nerve in the bottom of the internal meatus and in the facial canal. The *visceral efferent* (parasympathetic preganglionic) fibers bring secretory impulses to the *lacrimal gland* and two of the large *salivary glands* (the submandibular and the sublingual glands). See Figure 16.9 for details of the complicated route followed by the parasympathetic fibers. We also return to the intermediate nerve in some detail below. The *visceral afferent* fibers of the intermediate nerve innervate *taste buds in the anterior two-thirds of the tongue.*

The Facial Nerve

The motor fibers of the facial nerve have their perikarya in the *facial nucleus,* located in the lower pons. It belongs to the column of special somatic efferent nuclei (Figs. 16.2 and 16.3). The nucleus consists of several subdivisions, each supplying small groups of muscles. The root fibers of the facial nerve have a peculiar course before they leave the brain stem (Fig. 16.18). First, the fibers pass medially and lie dorsal to the abducent nucleus, forming the genu of the facial nerve, before they bend in the lateral and ventral direction. The facial fibers pass just beneath the floor of the fourth ventricle and form a small elevation, the facial colliculus (Fig. 3.18). Owing to the course of the nerve, symptoms of a peripheral facial paresis may occur in lesions located considerably more medial and dorsal than the nucleus itself. Figure 16.18 shows that damage to the abducent nucleus (affecting the lateral rectus muscle of the eye) is also likely to be accompanied by signs of pareses of the facial muscles of the same side.

Central and Peripheral Facial Pareses

Impulses from the facial nucleus evoke contractions of the mimetic muscles and are therefore responsible for our facial expressions. These muscles are used also in conjunction with speech, eating, blinking, and so forth. Impulses for voluntary movements of the facial muscles are conveyed through the *pyramidal tract* (corticobulbar fibers). The fibers arise from the face region of the MI in the precentral gyrus.

The part of the facial nucleus supplying the muscles in the forehead and around the eyes receive both uncrossed and crossed pyramidal tract fibers, whereas the muscles in the lower part of the face receive purely crossed fibers. *A lesion of the pyramidal tract (for example, in the internal capsule) therefore produces clear-cut pareses only in the lower part of the face on the opposite side of the lesion.* Most obvious is the sagging corner of the mouth. The patient can still wrinkle the forehead and close the eyes voluntarily. A *peripheral lesion* (of the facial nucleus or the nerve), however, produces pareses of all the facial muscles on the same side as the lesion (Fig. 16.19). For example, the eye cannot be closed, so there is danger of drying and ulceration of the cornea (and permanent loss of vision).

Peripheral lesions of the facial nerve may be caused by hemorrhage, infarctions, or tumors in the pons, by infections of the middle ear (to which the nerve passes in close proximity), or damage to the branches in the face. Most often, however, the cause of peripheral facial paresis is unknown. In such cases the muscle power usually returns after some time.

Figure 16.19 *Peripheral facial paralysis* (right side). The patient is asked to close her eyes and to retract the corners of the mouth. Based on Monrad-Krohn (1954).

The Mimetic Muscles

The facial or mimetic muscles originate from the facial skeleton and insert with elastic tendons in the dermis. There is a large number of small muscles, with the majority located around the mouth and the eyes. Of particular practical value are the muscles responsible for blinking and closure of the eye (the orbicularis oculi muscle) and the muscles around the mouth (the orbicularis oris and several other muscles), which move the lips. The buccinator muscle prevents the cheeks from being pressed out when the intraoral pressure is increased and, perhaps more importantly, prevents the cheeks from being sucked in between the teeth.

Facial Expressions of Emotion Do Not Depend on the Integrity of the Pyramidal Tract

Whereas impulses mediated by the pyramidal tract activate the motoneurons of the facial nucleus in voluntary movements (such as speech and eating), other descending pathways are responsible for facial expressions of emotions, such as sorrow and pleasure. As most of us know from personal experience, a genuine smile cannot be produced on command but arises independent of any conscious will. In contrast, our facial expressions often reveal emotions we would rather have concealed. A voluntary effort is required to suppress our spontaneous facial expressions, which most likely are controlled by descending connections from the hypothalamus and possibly the basal ganglia. Thus, lesions of the pyramidal tract do not abolish spontaneous facial expressions. The patient smiles and laughs when told a good joke but is unable to present a polite social smile. In contrast, in central pareses (such as capsular hemiplegia) emotional facial expressions are often exaggerated, and the patient cannot suppress a smile or prevent crying. Diseases of the basal ganglia, such as Parkinson's disease, present the opposite picture: The emotional, spontaneous expressions are lacking, whereas a voluntary, social smile is possible.

The Facial Nerve and Reflexes

The facial nucleus is also a link in some important reflex arcs. One is the *corneal* or *blink reflex*. It is elicited by touch or irritation of the cornea, and the sensory impulses are conducted centrally in the trigeminal nerve to the spinal trigeminal nucleus (Fig. 16.2). From there the impulses are transferred via interneurons in the reticular formation to the facial nucleus of both sides, and a contraction of the muscles of the eyelid is produced. The corneal reflex can be weakened or abolished by a lesion anywhere along the course of the afferent and efferent links or in the rather extensive reflex center.

Another reflex mediated by the facial nerve is the *stapedius reflex*, in which the response is contraction of the tiny stapedius muscle in the middle ear. The stimulus is an intense sound conducted centrally in the cochlear (acoustic) nerve to the cochlear nuclei. Most likely, interneurons in the reticular formation transfer the signals to the facial nucleus. The stapedius muscle pulls the stapes a little out of the oval window (Fig. 9.7)

The Intermediate Nerve

Where the facial nerve bends posteriorly in the temporal bone, there is a small ganglion (the *geniculate ganglion*) containing the perikarya of the sensory fibers of the intermediate nerve. Here a branch of the intermediate nerve, the *greater petrosal nerve*, leaves the main trunk of the facial nerve. It leaves the skull behind the orbit and contains visceral efferent (parasympathetic) fibers. These preganglionic fibers end in the small parasympathetic *pterygopalatine ganglion* located behind the orbit. From there postganglionic fibers follow trigeminal branches to the *lacrimal gland* and *glands in the nasal cavity* (Fig. 17.9). The rest of the intermediate nerve fibers leave the facial nerve as it passes downward posterior to the middle ear. This branch is called the *chorda tympani* because it passes through the middle ear (tympanic cavity) on its way forward to join the lingual nerve (a trigeminal branch) outside the skull. The chorda tympani contains *visceral afferent* fibers from taste buds in the anterior two-thirds of the tongue. These fibers have their perikarya in the geniculate ganglion. In addition, the chorda tympani carries *visceral efferent* (parasympathetic) fibers that end in the small *submandibular ganglion*. From this ganglion, postganglionic parasympathetic fibers pass to the *submandibular* and the *sublingual (salivary) glands*.

and thereby dampens the transmission of sound waves to the cochlear duct. Accordingly, peripheral facial paresis can produce hypersensitivity to sounds (*hyperacusis*).

Secretion of Tears and Saliva

The preganglionic parasympathetic fibers of the intermediate nerve—acting on the lacrimal, the submandibular, and sublingual glands—have their perikarya in the small *superior salivatory nucleus*. This nucleus belongs to the column of visceral efferent nuclei (Fig. 16.2). As mentioned, preganglionic parasympathetic fibers acting on the parotid gland have their perikarya in the *inferior salivatory nucleus* and follow the glossopharyngeal nerve.

The secretion of saliva is brought about primarily by stimulation of the taste receptors but also by impulses from higher levels of the brain (such as the thought of tasty food; it is especially effective to imagine that one is eating a lemon).

The secretion of tears, even more than the salivary secretion, is an example of how visceral functions can be influenced from higher levels of the brain. The continuous secretion of tears is of course primarily a physiological protection of the eyes and is increased in response to any irritation of the cornea or the conjunctiva; nevertheless, the most profuse tear production occurs when we express strong emotions by crying. The impulses to the superior salivatory nucleus producing the flow of tears when crying are not mediated by the pyramidal tract or other efferent cortical fibers descending in the internal capsule—in correspondence with the fact that tears cannot be produced voluntarily nor can the secretion of tears be suppressed. Most likely, fibers from the hypothalamus are responsible for the activation of the visceral efferent neurons during crying. But the hypothalamus is under the influence of higher levels, such as parts of the cerebral cortex and the limbic structures. Thus, it is the conscious experience of the emotions (such as sorrow or pity) that starts the train of neural events leading to tear secretion.

THE TRIGEMINAL NERVE

The fifth cranial nerve is first and foremost the sensory nerve of the face, with mainly *somatic afferent fibers*. In addition, it contains a small portion with *special somatic efferent* fibers to the masticatory muscles. The trigeminal nerve is the nerve of the first visceral (branchial) arch and innervates structures that are developed from this arch.

The nerve leaves the brain stem laterally on the pons (Figs. 3.14 and 16.1) with a small (medial) motor root and a large (lateral) sensory root. Shortly after leaving the pons, the nerve expands to form the large *semilunar ganglion*, which contains the perikarya of the pseudounipolar (sensory) ganglion cells (Fig. 16.20). Three large branches continue anteriorly from the ganglion: the *ophthalmic*, the *maxillar*, and the *mandibular nerves* (Figs. 16.20 and 16.24).

Figure 16.20 *The positions of the trigeminal nuclei.*

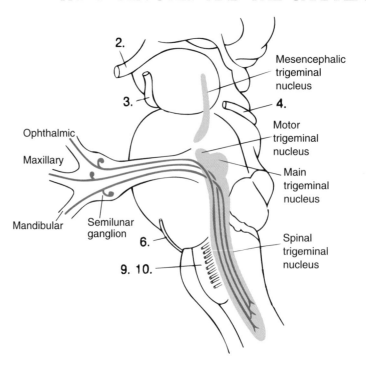

The *ophthalmic nerve* enters the orbit and supplies the eye bulb (including the cornea), the upper eyelid, the back of the nose, and the skin of the forehead with sensory fibers (Fig. 16.21). It also sends fibers to the mucous membranes of the anterior part of the nasal cavity. The *maxillary nerve* runs forward in a sulcus in the bottom of the orbit and sends fibers to the lower eyelid, the skin above the mouth, the upper teeth and the gingiva, and, finally, the hard palate and the posterior (major) part of the nasal cavity. The *mandibular nerve* innervates the lower teeth and gingiva, the tongue, and the skin of the lower jaw and upward, well into the temporal region (Fig. 16.21). The branch of the mandibular nerve supplying the tongue with somatic sensory afferent fibers is called the *lin-

Figure 16.21 *Distribution in the facial skin of the three main trigeminal branches*. The location of some further branches is indicated. The segmental origins of sensory fibers to the rest of the head and the neck are also indicated.

gual nerve. This nerve receives visceral afferent (taste) fibers from the chorda tympani, destined for the anterior two-thirds of the tongue.

The *motor fibers* of the trigeminal nerve follow the mandibular nerve but leave this in several smaller twigs to the masticatory muscles (and some other muscles with relation to the lower jaw and the soft palate).

The Sensory Trigeminal Nucleus

With regard to function and fiber composition, the sensory part of the trigeminal nerve corresponds to the spinal dorsal roots. The trigeminal nerve, therefore, belongs to the somatosensory system and conducts impulses from *low-threshold mechanoreceptors, thermoreceptors, and nociceptors* in the face and in the mucous membranes of the face. As with other spinal nerves, fibers leading from different kinds of receptors are intermingled in the nerve but have become arranged by receptor type when entering the central nervous system. Then the fibers are distributed to three subdivisions of the long sensory trigeminal nucleus (Figs. 3.15–3.17, 16.2, and 16.20). Fibers from *proprioceptors* (muscle spindles, joint re-

More About the Subdivisions of the Sensory Trigeminal Nucleus

The *thinnest fibers* of the trigeminal nerve (Aδ and C fibers), conducting primarily from nociceptors and thermoreceptors, bend caudally after entering the pons (Fig. 16.20). They continue as a small bundle, the *spinal tract of the trigeminal nerve*, located just beneath the medullary surface. It is joined by somatic afferent fibers, which have followed the glossopharyngeal and the vagus nerves peripherally. Just like the solitary tract, the spinal tract, strictly speaking, is not a tract, since it consists of the central process of the pseudounipolar ganglion cells. The spinal tract continues down into the upper cervical segments and corresponds to the bundle of Lissauer in the cord (Fig. 3.10). The fibers enter the *spinal trigeminal nucleus* (or nucleus of the spinal trigeminal tract), which corresponds largely to the dorsalmost laminae of the cord. For example, a layer very similar to the substantia gelatinosa is present. The spinal trigeminal nucleus can be further subdivided in a rostrocaudal sequence. The caudal part or subnucleus appears to be especially involved in pain mechanisms and corresponds most closely with the dorsal laminae of the cord. It also receives dorsal root fibers from the upper cervical segments. This may perhaps explain why a certain condition with paroxysms of facial pain of unknown origin *(trigeminal neuralgia)* may sometimes irradiate outside the area innervated by the trigeminal nerve (see the explanation of referred pain in Chapter 7, *Spinothalamic Cells Receive Impulses from Both Somatic and Visceral Structures: Referred Pain*). The spinal tract of the trigeminal nerve is sometimes surgically transected to alleviate severe, chronic facial pain *(medullary trigeminal tractotomy)*. This abolishes pain and temperature sensitivity in the face on the same side.

Thick myelinated fibers (Aβ) in the trigeminal nerve from the skin end mostly in the *main (principal) sensory trigeminal nucleus* (Fig. 16.20) with a precise somatotopic pattern. This part of the trigeminal nucleus corresponds functionally to the dorsal column nuclei.

The *mesencephalic trigeminal nucleus* stretches as a slender column from the upper part of the pons and into the mesencephalon. This is a very unusual nucleus, since its neurons look like pseudounipolar ganglion cells and indeed send one process peripherally into the trigeminal nerve. Afferent fibers from the *muscle spindles* of the masticatory muscles follow the mandibular nerve, whereas those from the extraocular muscles follow the ophthalmic and perhaps the oculomotor nerve. Impulses from mechanoreceptors in the root sheaths of the teeth end in the mesencephalic nucleus.

The trigeminal nucleus, especially the spinal subdivision, has numerous connections with the *reticular formation*. This is partly by means of reflex arcs involving the trigeminal nerve as the afferent link but also as links in ascending pathways to the thalamus with signals from nociceptors.

Figure 16.22 *Deviation of the jaw as a sign of peripheral trigeminal pareses.* Paresis of the right trigeminal nerve. Normally, the two lateral pterygoid muscles pull the jaw forward when opening the mouth. When unopposed by the paretic right pterygoid, the left (normal one) deviates the jaw to the right when the patient opens her mouth.

ceptors) end in the *mesencephalic nucleus*, fibers from *low-threshold mechanoreceptors* end in the *main* or *principal nucleus*, whereas impulses from *nociceptors* end in the *spinal trigeminal nucleus*.[8]

Central Transmission of Signals from the Trigeminal Nucleus

Functionally, the spinal trigeminal nucleus (especially its caudal part) corresponds to the dorsalmost laminae of the cord, whereas the main sensory nucleus corresponds to the dorsal column nuclei. These similarities are evident also in the central pathways. The secondary sensory fibers from the cells in the spinal nucleus join the spinothalamic tract and end in the thalamus. Fibers from the main nucleus join the medial lemniscus. The somatotopic pattern within the thalamic terminal region is such that the fibers from the trigeminal nucleus—carrying impulses from the face— end most medially, in the *VPM* (Fig. 7.20). The ascending fibers from the trigeminal nucleus cross to the opposite side before they join the large sensory tracts. A *lesion affecting lateral parts of the medulla* is likely to interrupt the spinothalamic tract and the spinal trigeminal nucleus. This will cause reduced or abolished pain and temperature sensation in the opposite body half but on the same side of the face (Fig. 7.15 and 7.17). From the thalamus, the signals are transmitted to the face region of the SI in the postcentral gyrus (Figs. 7.21 and 7.22).

Reflexes Involving the Trigeminal Nerve

Like the spinal dorsal root fibers, the trigeminal nerve constitutes the afferent link of several reflex arcs. We have described the *corneal reflex* (the blink reflex) above, in conjunction with the facial nerve that constitutes the efferent link of this reflex. Other reflexes are the *sneeze reflex*, elicited from the mucous membrane of the nasal cavity, and the *sucking reflex*, elicited in the newborn from mechanoreceptors of the lips. A stretch reflex can be produced by a brief tap downward on the chin, stretching the masticatory muscles (among them, the masseter muscle). This *masseter reflex* is monosynaptic and involves the mesencephalic trigeminal nucleus. The peripheral processes of the neurons of this nucleus innervate the muscle spindles, and the central processes reach the motor trigeminal nucleus in the pons. This reflex, with its reflex center in the mesencephalon and pons, is one of those routinely tested in clinical neurology.

The Motor Trigeminal Nucleus

The *special somatic efferent* fibers in the trigeminal nerve come from the motor trigeminal nucleus, located in the pons at the level of the main sensory nucleus (Figs. 3.17 and 16.20). All of the motor fibers follow the mandibular nerve. A *peripheral paresis* of the motor fibers of the trigeminal nerve (or the nucleus) leads to atrophy of the masticatory muscles and reduced force of biting on the side of the lesion. A unilateral paresis of the masticatory muscles is most easily detected by asking the patient to open his mouth widely; the lower jaw then deviates toward the side of the paretic muscles (Fig. 16.22). This is caused by paresis of the lateral pterygoid muscle, which normally pulls the mandible forward in conjunction with opening of the mouth.

Voluntary movements of the jaws during speech and chewing depend on the pyramidal tract (corticobulbar fibers). The fibers from the MI to the motor trigeminal nucleus are often both crossed and uncrossed (bilateral), but in some persons they appear to be purely crossed. Only in the latter case will there be clear-cut signs of pareses of the masticatory muscles after a lesion of the internal capsule (capsular hemiplegia). There may also be other signs of a central paresis, such as an increased masseter reflex on the paretic side.

Reflex movements of the masticatory muscles occur during swallowing, sucking, and vomiting. The afferent fibers of such reflexes are partly sensory trigeminal fibers from the oral cavity and partly sensory fibers passing in the vagus and the glossopharyngeal nerves.

Brain Stem Infarctions Can Produce Symptoms from Several Cranial Nerves and Long Tracts

Infarctions of the brain stem are caused by closure of the arterial branches supplying it (Fig. 3. 41). Any branch can be affected (although some more often than others), and the resulting symptoms depend on which structures are supplied by the occluded branch. There are large variations, however, both regarding the area supplied by a particular artery in different individuals, and between the right and left side in the same individual. Thus, symptoms will vary after occlusion of a particular artery. Rather than memorizing detailed lists of symptoms for each arterial branch, one should therefore combine the findings of a thorough clinical examination with knowledge of the functional anatomy of the brain stem. This will usually enable a fairly precise localization of the lesion.

We use as an example infarction in the *lateral part of the pons*. This part of the brain stem is usually supplied by the *inferior anterior cerebellar artery*, which leaves the basilar artery in the lower third of the pons. Besides the pons, the artery often supplies the brachium pontis, the flocculus, and middle parts of the cerebellar hemispheres. The most common symptoms are due to damage of the root fibers and the nuclei of the trigeminal, the facial, and the vestibulocochlear nerves (see Figs. 3.17 and 16.1). Cerebellar symptoms and symptoms due to damage to the long ascending and descending tracts are more variable, presumably due to individual variations in the area supplied by the artery. Thus, a lateral pontine infarction will usually produce ipsilateral peripheral facial paresis (the root fibers leave laterally in the lower pons), ipsilateral sensory loss in the face (all sensory qualities due to interruption of trigeminal root fibers), deafness and dizziness (the vestibulocochlear nerve, vestibular nuclei), and in some gaze paralysis to the side (ascending connections from the vestibular nuclei, see Fig. 16.17). In addition, there is usually ipsilateral ataxia (the cerebellar hemispheres), and sometimes contralateral weakness and an inverted plantar reflex (pyramidal tract), and contralateral reduced pain and temperature sensibility (the spinothalamic tract).

THE ABDUCENT, TROCHLEAR, AND OCULOMOTOR NERVES

These three cranial nerves (the sixth, fourth, and third) supply the extraocular muscles with *somatic efferent* fibers. In addition, the oculomotor nerve contains *visceral efferent* (parasympathetic) fibers to the smooth, intrinsic eye muscles. Simplified, we may say that by moving the eye in the orbit, the *extraocular muscles ensure that the images we look at fall on the central part of the retina (the macula), whereas the intrinsic muscles control the amount of light that reaches the retina and adjust the curvature of the lens so that the retinal image is always in focus.* Most of these tasks are performed reflexly, and usually eye position, light access, and lens curvature are all controlled simultaneously.

Before describing the nerves to the eye muscles and their nuclei, we will discuss a few salient features of eye movements in general. The central connections of the eye muscle nuclei are best treated collectively in a discussion of central control of eye movements.

Horizontal, Vertical, and Rotatory Movements of the Eye

The eye is a sphere, lying in the orbit, surrounded by fat. The eye can rotate freely in any direction around its center, whereas translatory movements are prevented. To describe the rotatory movements of a sphere, we define three axes, all passing through the center, oriented perpendicular to each other. For convenience, we describe the movements as taking place in three planes: a frontal, sagittal, and a transverse or horizontal plane. A movement in the horizontal plane takes place around a vertical axis, and the anterior part of the eye—and therefore the gaze—moves from side to side. Such *horizontal eye movements* are performed when we look to one side; when looking to the left, the left eye rotates laterally and the right eye rotates medially. A movement in the sagittal plane takes place around a transverse axis, and the anterior part of the eye moves up and down. Such movements, directing the gaze up and down, are called *vertical eye movements.* Movements in the frontal plane take place around a sagittal axis, and the eye rotates without any horizontal or vertical movement. For practical reasons only, such movements around a sagittal axis are called *rotatory eye movements* (even though, strictly speaking, all eye movements are rotations around the center of the eyeball).

The *six extraocular (extrinsic) muscles* ensure that the visual axes of the eyes (Fig. 8.3) can be directed precisely toward any point in the visual field. The scheme in Figure 16.25 shows the main movements produced by each of the extraocular muscles when acting alone. It can be seen that most of the muscles produce vertical, horizontal, and rotatory movements. We can nevertheless simplify matters by stating that *two muscles produce predominantly horizontal movements* (the medial and lateral rectus muscles), *two produce predominantly vertical movements* (the superior and inferior rectus muscles), whereas *two muscles produce mainly rotatory movements* (the superior and inferior oblique muscles).

The Extraocular Muscles

The small extraocular muscles (Figs. 16.23 and 16.24) all attach to the sclera and originate from the wall of the orbit (a brief account of the structure of the eye bulb is given in Chapter 8).

We analyze the actions of the extraocular muscles in relation to the above-defined three axes through the center of the eyeball. We then need to know the direction of the force exerted by the muscles in relation to

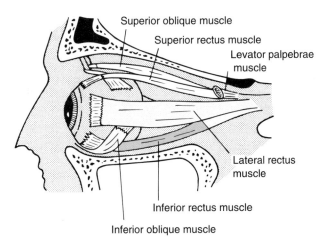

Figure 16.23 *The extraocular muscles seen from the lateral aspect.* The lateral wall of the orbit is removed. Note that the straight muscles insert in front of the equatorial plane of the eye, whereas the oblique muscles insert behind.

the axis. We must furthermore know whether the muscle insertion in the sclera is anterior or posterior to the *equatorial plane of the eye*, a frontal plane dividing the eye in an anterior and a posterior half.

There are *four straight* and *two oblique* extraocular muscles (Figs. 16.24 and 13.25). The straight ones (the rectus muscles) come from the posterior end of the orbit and run forward to insert in front of the equatorial plane. This means that the *lateral rectus* muscle pulls the eye (the cornea) laterally, whereas the *medial rectus* muscle pulls it medially. These two muscles thus produce *pure horizontal movements*. Correspondingly, the *superior rectus* muscle pulls the eye (the cornea) upward, whereas the *inferior rectus* muscle pulls it downward. These two therefore produce *vertical movements*. Because the superior and inferior rectus muscles run anteriorly in a lateral direction, however, they do not pro-

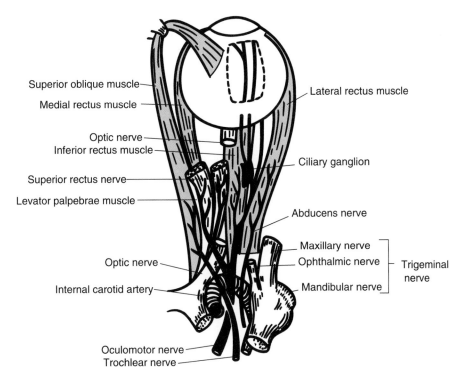

Figure 16.24 *The right eye with muscles and nerves seen from above.* Note the three cranial nerves innervating the muscles of the eye. Some of the extraocular muscles and the optic nerve have been cut. The external layers of the eye bulb have been partly removed to expose the postganglionic fibers from the ciliary ganglion on their way to the intrinsic eye muscles. Note also the position of the trigeminal ganglion and the internal carotid artery.

Figure 16.25 *The actions of the extraocular muscles*. The **arrows** indicate the direction of the action (but not the force). Note that all muscles except the medial and lateral recti rotate the eye, in addition to their other actions. The actions shown are, strictly speaking, true only when the eye is in the neutral position. Movements away from the neutral postion may alter the actions of the muscles. For example, the superior rectus is a pure elevator when the eye is 23 degrees abducted.

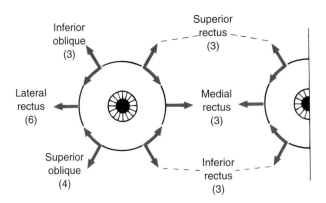

duce purely vertical movements but also some horizontal movement (in the medial direction). Thus, when the superior rectus muscle acts alone, it produces an upward movement combined with a (smaller) medial—that is, an oblique movement (Fig. 16.25). In addition, the muscle produces a small medial rotation of the eye (around the sagittal axis).

The *superior oblique muscle* has a rather complicated course (Figs. 16.23 and 16.24). It originates posteriorly in the orbit and runs forward medially. Just behind the anterior margin of the orbit, it bends sharply around a small hook of connective tissue and continues in a posterolateral direction to insert posterior to the equatorial plane. The muscle has actions around all three axes: It rotates the eye so that the upper part moves medially and directs the gaze downward and laterally. The *inferior oblique*

The Eye Muscles Are Built for Precise Control

The structure of the extraocular muscles reflects their use in extremely delicate and precisely controlled movements. The muscle fibers are very thin compared with ordinary skeletal muscle fibers, and the motor units are among the smallest in the body (only 5–10 muscle fibers per motoneuron). Consequently, the nerves to the extraocular muscles contain many nerve fibers: The abducent nerve in humans (supplying only one muscle) contains around 6000 axons. The extraocular muscles are composed of a mixture of fibers with fast and with slow twitch contractions. The muscles are required both to hold a certain tension for a long time (static position holding) and to produce extremely fast movements. The maximal speed of contraction is, accordingly, high compared with other skeletal muscle fibers. Furthermore, the maximal firing frequency of the motoneurons innervating the extraocular muscles is unusually high and occurs during saccadic movements. EMG recordings in awake human subjects with their eyes open show that there is some activity in virtually all of the extraocular muscles. The tension produced by each muscle varies, of course, with the position of the eyes.

There is a high density of *muscle spindles* in the extraocular muscles. Apart from the general rule that muscles subject to precise control have a high density of muscle spindles, their functional role in the extraocular muscles is not clear. Thus, signals from extraocular muscle spindles are apparently not consciously perceived—that is, they do not contribute to the awareness of eye position and movements (in this respect differing from muscle spindles elsewhere, as discussed in Chapter 7). Nor do signals from extraocular muscle spindles evoke stretch reflexes. In general, it seems highly likely that muscle spindle signals, providing information about the length and the change of length of the extraocular muscles, are integrated with signals providing information about movements of the head from the labyrinth and with signals from the retina. The latter signals can, for example, supply information about whether the image is stationary or is slipping on the retina. Experiments with transection of the ophthalmic nerve (assumed to contain most of the muscle spindle afferents from the extraocular muscles) produce pronounced instability of the eyes and slow pendular movements in darkness.

muscle originates from the bottom of the orbit in its anteromedial part and runs, like the superior oblique, posterolaterally to insert behind the equator. It directs the gaze laterally and upward and rotates the eye with its upper part laterally. The main action of the oblique muscles is to rotate the eyes (in the opposite direction around the sagittal axis).

It should be emphasized that the above considerations concern movements starting from a neutral position of the eye. Changing the position of the eye in the orbita also changes the action of the muscles (for some muscles the change is small, for others quite marked). For example, the superior rectus is a pure elevator when the eye is 23° abducted.

The Eye Movements Are Conjugated

Virtually all natural eye movements are combinations of the various movement directions described above. By combining proper amounts of vertical and horizontal movements, any oblique movement can be produced. Furthermore, all natural eye movements are *conjugated*—that is, the two eyes move together to ensure that the image always falls on *corresponding points* of the two retinae (Fig. 8.3). Double vision (*diplopia*) results if the eye movements do not occur in conjugation. This is a typical symptom of pareses of the extraocular muscles (caused, most frequently, by lesions of one of the nerves to the muscles). Other typical symptoms are strabismus (squint), vertigo (dizziness), and an altered position of the head (the latter to avoid diplopia).

Almost all eye movements require a complicated cooperation of numerous muscles, with activation of synergists and inhibition of antagonists. When, for example, we look to the left, the left lateral rectus is activated and the left medial rectus is inhibited, whereas the right medial rectus is activated and the right lateral rectus is inhibited. This is the simplest possible example, with a purely horizontal movement. In most other situations the cooperation between various muscles becomes much more complicated and requires an extensive, sophisticated neural network for control. We return to this below.

The Abducent Nerve

The abducent nerve leaves the brain stem close to the midline at the junction of the medulla and the pons (Figs. 3.14 and 16.1). Figure 16.18 shows the location of the *abducent nucleus* and its relation to the facial nerve. The abducent nerve runs forward intracranially and passes through the *cavernous sinus* before entering the orbit through the superior orbital fissure (Fig. 16.24). It supplies only one muscle, the *lateral rectus*. The muscle pulls the eye so the cornea faces laterally (abducts the eye) (Fig. 16.25). Even though other muscles can abduct the eye somewhat (the superior and the inferior oblique muscles), the lateral rectus is necessary for more than a slight lateral movement. A person with a unilateral lesion of the abducent nerve usually keeps the head turned somewhat to the side of the lesion to compensate for the loss of lateral motion of the eye.

The Trochlear Nerve

This is the only one of the cranial nerves to leave the brain stem on the dorsal side (just below the inferior colliculus) (Figs. 3.18 and 16.1).[9] The *trochlear nucleus* is situated a little ventrally to the aqueduct in the mesencephalon (Figs. 3.19 and 16.29). Like the abducent nerve, the trochlear traverses the cavernous sinus and enters the orbit through the superior orbital fissure. It innervates the *superior oblique muscle* (Figs. 16.24 and 16.25), which directs the gaze downward and laterally.

The Oculomotor Nerve

The nerve emerges from the ventral aspect of the mesencephalon, in the interpeduncular fossa (Figs. 3.14 and 3.19). This is the largest of the three nerves supplying the extraocular muscles and, as mentioned, contains somatic efferent and visceral efferent fibers. The *somatic efferent* fibers come from the large *oculomotor nucleus* (or nucleus of the oculomotor nerve) situated close to the midline in the mesencephalon, ventral to the aqueduct (Figs. 3.19 and 16.29). The medial longitudinal fasciculus, with ascending fibers from the vestibular nuclei, lies close to the oculomotor nucleus (and to the abducent and trochlear nuclei as well). The *visceral efferent* (parasympathetic) fibers come from the small *nucleus of Edinger-Westphal* located in the vicinity of the oculomotor nucleus. Often the term *oculomotor complex* is used for the somatic efferent and visceral efferent nuclei together.

The oculomotor nerve passes forward to the orbit through the cavernous sinus together with the other nerves to the eye (entering through the superior orbital fissure). The somatic efferent and parasympathetic fibers part in the orbit (Fig. 16.24). The somatic efferent fibers innervate the following extraocular muscles: the *superior and inferior rectus*, the *medial rectus*, and the *inferior oblique*. These muscles can move the eye medially, upward, and downward and rotate it around the sagittal axis (Fig. 16.25). In addition, the oculomotor nerve supplies the *levator palpebrae superioris* muscle, which serves to lift the upper eyelid.

The *visceral efferent* (preganglionic parasympathetic) oculomotor fibers end in the small ciliary ganglion situated behind the eye (Fig. 16.24). Here the fibers establish synapses with the postganglionic neurons, which send their axons anteriorly in the wall of the eye to innervate the intrinsic (smooth) muscles of the eye: the sphincter pupillae and the ciliary muscle (Fig. 8.2). Contraction of the *ciliary muscle* increases the lens curvature when looking at near objects (see Chapter 8, *The Lens and the Far and Near Points of the Eye: Accommodation*). The *sphincter pupillae* constricts the pupil to reduce the amount of light reaching the retina.

A *lesion of the oculomotor nerve* produces, among other symptoms, an abnormal position of the eye, which is directed laterally (due to the unopposed pull of the lateral rectus) and downward (due to the superior oblique muscle). As in lesions of the abducent or the trochlear nerves, the patient will have double vision. In addition, the upper eyelid droops (*ptosis*) because of paralysis of the levator palpebrae (Fig. 16.27). The inter-

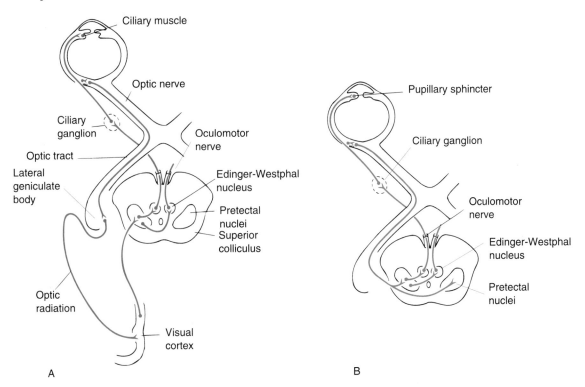

Figure 16.26 *Visual reflexes*. The reflex arcs for (**A**) the accommodation reflex and (**B**) the light reflex.

ruption of the parasympathetic fibers makes the pupil larger (due to loss of action of the sphincter pupillae), and the light reflex is absent (in an incomplete lesion of the nerve, the pupil may be slightly larger and the reaction to light more sluggish than on the normal side). The ability to accommodate the lens is abolished, making it impossible to see near objects sharply. The intracranial course of the oculomotor nerve makes it especially vulnerable in cases of temporal herniation caused by increased intracranial pressure (see Chapter 3). *Thus, examination of the size of the pupils, and their reaction to light, is of great practical value in patients who are unconscious after head trauma.*

The Light Reflex and the Accommodation Reflex

The oculomotor nerve is the efferent link of both of these reflexes, even though they are quite different in other respects. The *light reflex* is relatively simple, with its reflex center in the brain stem (Fig. 16.26). An increase in the amount of light reaching the retina elicits a contraction of the sphincter pupillae muscle. Both pupils constrict even when the light hits only one eye. The afferent link consists of fibers of the optic nerve that leave the optic tract before it reaches the lateral geniculate body. The fibers end in the *pretectal nuclei* on both sides (Fig. 16.26). From these nuclei, the impulses are conveyed to the Edinger-Westphal nuclei on both sides, and via the ciliary ganglion the impulses reach the sphincter pupillae. The bilaterality of the connections explains why a unilateral stimulus produces a bilateral response.

Interruption of the oculomotor nerve abolishes the light reflex in the eye on the side of the lesion, but the reflex is present in the other eye. In

Figure 16.27 *Paresis of the oculomotor nerve* (right side). **Top**. The upper eyelid droops (ptosis) due to paresis of the the levator palpebra muscle. **Bottom**. The examiner lifts the eyelid and reveals that the right eye is abducted and lowered due to the unopposed actions of the lateral rectus and the superior oblique muscles.

case of interruption of the afferent link on one side (damage to the retina or the optic nerve), the light reflex is absent in both eyes when light is shone into the eye on the lesioned side but is present in both sides when the other eye is illuminated. Thus, examination of the light reflex can provide valuable information with regard to the site of a lesion.

The *accommodation reflex* is a cortical reflex: The reflex arc passes via the cerebral cortex. The afferent link is fibers passing in the optic nerve from the retina, and the efferent link consists of parasympathetic fibers in the oculomotor nerve to the ciliary ganglion (Fig. 16.26). From there the postganglionic fibers pass to the ciliary muscle. The *reflex center* is not known in detail, but recent studies indicate that the cortical fibers pass to the superior colliculus (not the pretectal nuclei as shown in Fig. 16.26) and from there to the nearby reticular formation. Neurons in the reticular formation mediate the impulses to the parasympathetic oculomotor nucleus. The accommodation reflex is elicited only when we fix the gaze on an object that is moving toward us. Together with the accommodation, a *pupillary constriction* occurs as the object comes closer.

CONTROL OF EYE MOVEMENTS

All ocular movements are produced by impulses to the extraocular muscles from the nuclei of the sixth, fourth, and third cranial nerves. The activity of the motoneurons in these three nuclei must be precisely coordinated and is indeed controlled by a highly complex set of interconnected neuronal groups. Studies of such "preoculomotor" nuclei and networks have provided a wealth of interesting data. Best known are the networks involved in control of the saccadic (fast) eye movements, whereas the anatomic basis of the control of smooth-pursuit movements is less well understood. Before going into some main features of these oculomotor networks, we will discuss briefly the kinds of eye movement we are dealing with.

Classification of Eye Movements

In general, the control system for eye movements must ensure that the gaze can be moved quickly from one point of fixation to another—that is, by *saccadic movements*, or *saccades*—but also that the gaze can be kept stationary on an object even when the object or the head moves: by *slow-pursuit movements*. Rhythmic alternation between saccades and pursuit movements is called *nystagmus* (see "Vestibular Reflexes" above). The eye movements may be *voluntary*, as when we follow a moving object with the eyes, or *reflex*, when the head moves (the vestibulo-ocular reflex) or the surroundings move (optokinetic reflex). Nystagmus can be produced by vestibular stimulation or optokinetically.

More About Classification of Ocular Movements

A schematic classification of eye movements is given below. Several of the points have been discussed previously in this chapter, but a collective treatment and more details are given here.

1. *Saccades* are conjugated movements that change the optical axis of the eyes from one point of fixation to another with maximal speed. Saccades can (at least in a certain sense) be *voluntary*, as when we look at a stationary landscape and fix the gaze at one point for a moment, and then move on (with a saccade) to another point of fixation. Saccades can also be *reflex*, as with vestibular or optokinetic nystagmus. When awake, we perform saccades all the time, often several per second.
2. *Smooth-pursuit movements* are performed when we follow a small moving object to keep the image stationary on the central part of the retina. As a rule, we use pursuit movements both of the eyes and of the head when looking at a moving object. One might think that the movements of the head would elicit conjugated eye movements in the opposite direction of the head (the vestibulo-ocular reflex). Since this does not occur, the vestibulo-ocular reflex must be suppressed during such smooth-pursuit movements.
3. *Optokinetic-response* movements are saccadic or smooth-pursuit movements intended to stabilize the retinal image when the whole visual field moves relative to the head.
4. *Vestibulo-ocular reflex* movements are smooth-pursuit movements and saccades elicited by movements of the head (Fig. 16.28).
5. *Vergence* movements change the visual axes of the eyes in relation to each other when the point of fixation moves away from or toward the eyes. This is necessary to keep the image on corresponding points of the retina. Vergence movements are a prerequisite for fusion of the two images and for stereoscopic vision. Convergence of the optic axes, which takes place when an object is approaching the eyes, depends primarily on the activity of the medial rectus muscles, with some contribution also from the superior and inferior recti (Fig. 16.25). Convergence movements are accompanied by accommodation and pupillary constriction.

Each of the above movement types is controlled at least partly by different central neural structures, finally focusing on the motoneurons of the eye muscle nuclei.

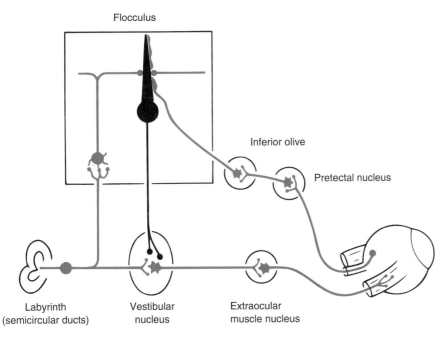

Flocculus

Inferior olive

Pretectal nucleus

Labyrinth
(semicircular ducts)

Vestibular
nucleus

Extraocular
muscle nucleus

Figure 16.28 *Main structural elements of the vestibulo-ocular reflex.* Only excitatory connections are shown (even though there are inhibitory neurons in the vestibular nuclei that influence the motoneurons of the antagonists). The reflex arc consists of three neurons from the semicircular duct to the extraocular muscles. The cerebellar flocculus receives signals from the labyrinth and from the retina, and the output of the Purkinje cells can adjust the sensitivity of the vestibular neurons, if necessary, to avoid retinal slip. Based on Ito (1984).

Figure 16.29 *Centers for vertical and horizontal eye movements.* Sagittal section through the monkey brain stem. Redrawn from Büttner-Ennever (1988).

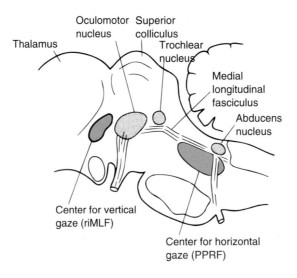

Pathways and Cell Groups Involved in Control of Eye Movements: An Overview

For control of *horizontal* eye movements (especially saccades), the most important premotor area, paramedian pontine reticular formation (*PPRF*), lies close to the abducent nucleus on each side (Fig. 16.29). The PPRF sends fibers to the abducent and oculomotor nuclei and coordinates their activities (Fig. 16.30). Unilateral damage in the region of the PPRF abolishes (or makes smaller and more sluggish) saccades to the side of the lesion (*horizontal gaze paralysis*). A corresponding premotor area for *vertical* eye movements is found in the mesencephalic reticular formation close to the oculomotor nucleus (Fig. 16.29). Lesions in this region can abolish vertical eye movements (*vertical gaze paralysis*).

The premotor "gaze centers" are supplied from the vestibular nuclei, the superior colliculus, the cerebral cortex, and other sources with relevant information about movements of the head and the eyes, about reti-

Figure 16.30 *Control of horizontal conjugate eye movements.* Highly simplified scheme to show some of the connections responsible. Only excitatory connections are included. The figure also shows how interruption of the medial longitudinal fascicle produces a paralysis of the gaze in the medial direction (internuclear ophthalmoplegia).

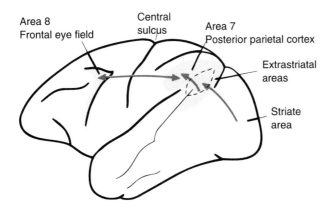

Area 8
Frontal eye field

Central
sulcus

Area 7
Posterior parietal cortex

Extrastriatal
areas

Striate
area

Figure 16.31 *Cortical areas involved
in control of eye movements* (monkey).
The arrows show some association
connections of these areas. The dashed
line indicates that some of the area is
hidden in a sulcus.

nal slip, and the desired gaze direction. In addition, various cell groups
besides the "gaze centers" send fibers directly to the eye muscle nuclei
(for example, the vestibular nuclei).

We know less about the subcortical nuclei and tracts that control pursuit than saccadic movements. Recent studies, however, suggest that the
pontine nuclei and the *cerebellar flocculus* are necessary for their generation. The relevant parts of the pontine nuclei receive projections from
the cortical regions involved in control of pursuit movements.

At least two regions of the *cerebral cortex* are closely involved in the
control of eye movements (Fig. 16.31): The *frontal eye field* is primarily
related to initiation of saccadic movements, whereas several smaller areas in the *parieto-temporal region* are mainly involved in the control of
pursuit movements. Unilateral lesions of the frontal eye field reduce or
abolish voluntary saccades to the opposite side of the lesion. (Pursuit
movements to follow a moving object are still possible, however.)

Afferent Connections to the Extraocular Motor Nuclei

Many kinds of information must be integrated and translated into commands to the eye muscle motoneurons to achieve the extremely precise
control of eye movements necessary for the normal functioning of the visual system. We will review some of the most important cell groups and
connections controlling the eye muscle nuclei.

We have previously mentioned connections from the *vestibular nuclei*, which, via the *medial longitudinal fasciculus*, reach all the cranial
nerve nuclei of the eye muscles (Fig. 16.17). These connections are both
crossed and uncrossed. Some of the vestibular neurons sending their axons into the medial longitudinal fasciculus are excitatory; other neurons
are inhibitory (GABA). The connections are precisely organized, enabling
the activation of specific synergists and the inhibition of their antagonists
(with regard to the intended eye movement). Other efferent fibers from
the vestibular nuclei end in cell groups situated in the vicinity of the eye
muscle nuclei, which send their axons to the latter. The *perihypoglossal
nuclei* are examples of such preoculomotor cell groups. These nuclei (the
most prominent one is the *prepositus nucleus*) are situated around the hypoglossal nucleus in the medulla. In addition to afferents from the vestibu-

More About Brain-Stem and Cortical Centers for Control of Eye Movements

Brain Stem Centers

By combining anatomic data on the fiber connections with physiological results (obtained by single-cell recordings, electrical stimulation, and lesions), we have identified brain stem cell groups of particular importance for eye movements. As metioned above, a *center for horizontal eye movements* has been identified in the PPRF. This center is situated close to, and sends fibers to, the abducent nucleus. It also sends fibers to the parts of the oculomotor nucleus containing the motoneurons of the medial rectus muscle. Together with the lateral rectus (innervated by the abducent nucleus), the medial rectus participates in horizontal movements. In addition, there are so-called *internuclear neurons* in the abducent nucleus that send axons to the medial rectus motoneurons of the opposite side (Fig. 16.30). This premotor network ensures simultaneous activation of the lateral rectus on one side and the medial rectus on the other, and inhibition of the antagonists.

A *lesion in the region of the PPRF* reduces horizontal conjugate movements to the side of the lesion. Especially marked is the reduction in saccadic movements. A unilateral lesion of the *medial longitudinal fasciculus* between the abducent and the oculomotor nucleus produces so-called *internuclear ophthalmoplegia* with abolished ability to adduct the eye on the same side (the medial rectus muscle). This may be understood on the basis of the diagram in Figure 16.30. However, vergence movements are possible even though the medial rectus is responsible also in that case. Thus, pathways other than the medial longitudinal fasciculus are responsible for the activation of the medial rectus muscle during vergence movements.

As mentioned, the PPRF receives impulses directly and indirectly from the vestibular nuclei, the superior colliculus, and the frontal eye field. It appears to function as the last premotor station for the initiation of conjugate horizontal saccadic movements. In agreement with this, there are neurons in the PPRF that are active immediately before and during a saccade to the same side, whereas they are inactive during slow-pursuit movements and fixation. These so-called *excitatory burst neurons* are believed to establish excitatory connections with the motoneurons responsible for the saccade. There are also *inhibitory burst neurons*, located close to the PPRF, with a pattern of activity similar to the excitatory burst neurons. They inhibit monosynaptically the motoneurons in the abducent nucleus of the opposite side. The activity of both kinds of burst neurons appears to be controlled by a third kind of neuron in the PPRF, which is tonically active. Such *omnipause neurons* probably inhibit the burst neurons tonically, except in relation to saccades. Thus, the omnipause neurons are silent immediately before and during saccades, regardless of the direction and amplitude of the movement. Recent studies indicate that the omnipause neurons receive direct connections from both the superior colliculus and the frontal eye field (they must also presumably receive impulses from the vestibular nuclei, since saccades can be elicited by vestibular signals as well).

A *center for vertical and rotatory eye movements* has been identified in the reticular formation close to the oculomotor nucleus. This region includes a nucleus called the rostral interstitial nucleus of the medial longitudinal fasciculus (*riMLF*) and probably also another small cell group (the *interstitial nucleus of Cajal*). This region receives, most likely, afferents from the vestibular nuclei, the pretectum (and thereby indirectly from the superior colliculus), and frontal eye field. Physiological studies indicate that there are monosynaptic connections from the region of the riMLF to the trochlear nucleus and motoneuron groups within the oculomotor nucleus that produce vertical eye movements.

The PPRF and the region of the riMLF are interconnected, indicating that they do not operate independently of each other. The fact that many natural eye movements are neither purely horizontal not purely vertical but combinations of both strongly suggests that the centers for horizontal and vertical movements must coordinate their activity.

Recent studies strongly suggest that lateral parts of the *pontine nuclei* (sending efferents to the cerebellum) are necessary for *pursuit movements* and for the slow phase of optokinetic nystagmus. This is based on recordings of single-cell activity and lesion experiments in monkeys, as well as a few patients with small brain-stem infarctions. Among cerebellar regions, the *flocculus* appears to be the most important for pursuit movements. Clinical observations support the role of the cerebellum in control of pursuit movements also in humans. The deficits observed in patients with cerebellar lesions resemble the dose-dependent effects of alcohol on pursuit movements.

Cortical Centers

The *frontal eye field* (area 8 of Brodmann, Figs. 16.31 and 20.3) is located immediately frontal to the premotor area. It is of particular importance for *voluntary saccades* (regions in the parieto-occipital region also contribute to control of saccades). Electrical stimulation of the frontal eye field elicits conjugated eye movements to the opposite side. The effect is mediated by fibers descending in the internal capsule to brain stem premotor cell groups, such as the superior colliculus, the pretectal nuclei, and the PPRF, which in their turn activate motoneurons in the eye muscle nuclei. A unilateral lesion of the frontal eye field makes the patient unable to move the gaze voluntarily to the side opposite the lesion (for example, when asked by the examiner to move the gaze). The ability to move the gaze laterally is not completely lost, however. Thus, smooth-pursuit movements occur when an object is brought into the visual field and then moved slowly laterally—that is, the patient is able to follow the object with her gaze.

With regard to *cortical control of smooth-pursuit movements*, a region in the parietotemporal region seems to be of particular importance. This notion is based on, among other things, observations of the activity of single cells in relation to eye movements. The subcortical cell groups intercalated between these cortical regions and the eye muscle nuclei are, however, not identified with certainty.

The ability to *fix the gaze* is a prerequisite for slow-pursuit movements. A *fixation center* is assumed to be localized within the cortical region responsible for the initiation of slow-pursuit movements. The term fixation reflex implies that the tendency to fix the gaze on an object is not really voluntary, at least not in the strict sense of that word (even though fixation is dependent on the person being conscious). *Optokinetic nystagmus* is an expression of the fixation tendency or reflex. When a screen with alternating black and white vertical stripes is moved horizontally in front of a person, nystagmus occurs. The gaze is fixed automatically on one of the stripes and follows it until it leaves the visual field. Then the eyes move rapidly back to the starting position and the gaze is fixed again on another stripe. This sequence repeats itself as long as the screen moves.

lar nuclei, the perihypoglossal nuclei receive afferents from other structures involved in eye movement control, such as parts of the reticular formation and the cerebellum.

The direct and indirect impulse pathways from the vestibular nuclei to the eye muscle nuclei mediate the *vestibulo-ocular reflexes* (Fig. 16.28) and are probably also involved in *optokinetic reflexes*. In the latter case, signals from the retina reaching the vestibular nuclei (synaptically interrupted in several nuclei) must be involved rather than signals from the labyrinth.

Proprioceptive impulses from muscle spindles of the extraocular muscles reach the eye muscle nuclei from the mesencephalic trigeminal nucleus. Proprioceptive signals have been shown to be necessary for the long-term correction and adaptation of the mutual position of the eyes in fixation and saccades. Especially in childhood with continously changing proportions, proprioceptive information is presumably necessary to ensure fusion of the retinal images (avoid strabismus with double vision).

Optic impulses do not pass directly from the retina to the eye muscle nuclei but are mediated by several brain stem nuclei, which also receive impulses other than visual information. This concerns the *superior colliculus* and the *pretectal nuclei* (situated rostral and ventral to the superior colliculus; Fig. 16.26). These nuclei receive afferents from the retina and from parts of the cerebral cortex involved in control of eye movements (the frontal eye field, the posterior parietal cortex, and parts of the extrastriatal visual areas; Fig. 16.31). Many neurons in the superior colliculus are active immediately before a saccade, and play most likely an important role in the organization of conjugated saccades.

There are no direct connections from the *cerebral cortex* to the eye muscle nuclei. Activation of the extraocular muscles from the cortex in conjunction with voluntary eye movements is mediated via other brain stem cell groups, among them the premotor "gaze centers" mentioned above (Fig. 16.30).

NOTES

1. As mentioned above, the fibers to the striated muscles of the visceral (branchial) arches are usually termed special visceral efferent. Both anatomically and functionally, however, they are more similar to the somatic efferents. First, visceral arch striated muscles are among those subject to the most precise voluntary control (the mimetic muscles of the face and the muscles of the larynx) and should therefore not be mixed up with visceral (smooth) muscles. Secondly, the neurons are structurally like α motoneurons; that is, they are larger than the preganglionic, parasympathetic neurons. In addition, the visceral arch neurons contain the neuropeptide CGRP that is found in spinal motoneurons but not in preganglionic parasympathetic neurons. Therefore, for didactic reasons we find it preferable to use the term *special somatic efferent*. Otherwise it is of no great importance which terms are used to group the neurons of the cranial nerves; the important thing is to know where the cell bodies of the various cranial nerves are located, the course of their fibers, and their functions.
2. The accessory, the hypoglossal, and the part of the facial nucleus supplying the lower part of the face—and often also the motor trigeminal nucleus—receive only crossed fibers, as judged from clinical observations (Monrad-Krohn).
3. Embryologically, the vagus nerve belongs to the fourth, fifth, and sixth branchial arches, and this explains the peculiar course of some of its branches.
4. Experiments with modern tracing techniques show that the neurons supplying the heart (and probably also the lungs) have their perikarya in an external, distinct part of the nucleus ambiguus. The perikarya are morphologically like those of the dorsal motor vagus nucleus, and differ from the larger motoneurons in the main nucleus ambiguus, which innervate striated muscles (of the pharynx and larynx).
5. On an embryological basis, all sensory fibers from the pharynx (and the posterior part of the tongue) should be classified as visceral afferent. There is evidence, however, that such fibers end in the somatic afferent trigeminal nucleus and not in the visceral afferent nucleus. Functionally, they may therefore be considered somatic afferent rather than visceral afferent.
6. There are also efferent cholinergic fibers in the vestibular nerve, ending in contact with the vestibular receptors. Their actions are not known in man. In lower mammals, they have been shown to have an inhibitory action, whereas the action in monkeys appears to be excitatory. The efferent fibers come from a small cell group in the lower pons close to the vestibular nuclei.
7. The utricle records especially head positions that vary around a sagittal axis (that is, a lateral tilt), whereas the saccule probably records positions mainly around a transverse axis (that is, flexion–extension in the cervical joints).
8. The separation of fibers of different kinds is not quite as sharp as this account may indicate, however. Thus, many trigeminal fibers divide after entering the brain stem into an ascending and a descending branch (just like the sensory fibers entering the cord). In this manner, single ganglion cells may end in more than one nuclear subdivision.
9. Another peculiarity of the trochlear nerve is that it crosses the midline before leaving the brain stem, so that the left trochlear nucleus innervates the right superior oblique muscle and vice versa. Some of the fibers of the oculomotor nerve also cross before leaving the brain stem.

PART V

THE AUTONOMIC NERVOUS SYSTEM

The *autonomic nervous system* (or visceral system) is not a term that can be defined precisely, either anatomically or functionally. The old belief that the somatic and the autonomic parts of the nervous system are completely independent is not tenable. The more we have learned about the structure and function of the nervous system, the clearer it has become that simplistic divisions like this are rather arbitrary. The somatic and visceral processes are so intimately interrelated that any subdivision becomes by necessity artificial. For practical reasons, it is nevertheless helpful to use the term autonomic nervous system and to define it very broadly as *the neuronal groups and fiber connections that control the activity of visceral organs, vessels, and glands* (also the vessels and glands that are not parts of visceral organs). Visceral organs contain smooth-muscle cells and glands. We can therefore also define the autonomic system as *the parts of the nervous system that control the activity of smooth muscles and glands*, regardless of their location in the body (in contrast to the somatic or cerebrospinal system, which controls striated skeletal muscles). Mostly, we are not aware of the processes going on in the organs controlled by the autonomic nervous system, and their activities are not subject to voluntary, conscious control. The autonomic nervous system cooperates with the endocrine system, as we will see in this section.

The autonomic system can be subdivided in different ways. As with the somatic system, we distinguish *peripheral* and *central* parts. Whereas the peripheral parts of the autonomic and somatic systems can be separated fairly well, the division becomes much less clear within the central nervous system. The peripheral parts of the autonomic system are described in Chapter 17, whereas the central parts, notably the hypothalamus, are discussed in Chapter 18.

The autonomic system can also be divided into a *sympathetic* and a *parasympathetic* part, differing anatomically and functionally (again, the separation is most obvious in the peripheral nervous system). The actions of the two parts of the autonomic system are often antagonistic: Where the sympathetic system activates, the parasympathetic reduces the activity, and vice versa. In addition, the *enteric nervous system* is now regarded as a distinct part of the autonomic nervous system. It consists of some million neurons and an extensive network in the wall of the digestive tract. The enteric system is influenced by both the sympathetic and the parasympathetic systems but functions independently as well.

In a broad perspective, a major function of the autonomic system is to contribute to bodily *homeostasis*, that is, the maintenance of a relatively constant internal milieu.[1] The autonomic nervous system is not the only means by which the central nervous system can control homeostasis, however. In addition, the *endocrine system*—which is controlled from the central nervous system via the *pituitary gland*— serves this purpose. Furthermore, homeostasis requires appropriate somatic motor activity to secure, for example, the supply of water and nutrients.

The role of the *hypothalamus* is to organize the autonomic, endocrine, and somatic-motor processes into behavior that is appropriate for the immediate and long-term needs of the organism.

NOTES

1. Definition of homeostasis (The New Shorter Oxford): maintenance of a dynamically stable state within a system by means of internal regulatory processes that counteract external disturbances of the equilibrium.

CHAPTER 17

PERIPHERAL AUTONOMIC NERVOUS SYSTEM

Although the nerves to visceral organs contain both efferent (motor) and afferent (sensory) fibers, the structural and functional differences between the autonomic and the somatic systems concern primarily the efferent side. Therefore, this chapter deals mainly with the visceral efferent neurons, briefly describing special features of visceral afferent neurons and visceral sensibility.

In general, the actions of the *sympathetic system* suggest that it is of special importance in *situations of stress, requiring mobilization of bodily resources*. The parasympathetic system, on the other hand, contributes primarily to *processes of maintenance*, such as digestion and reproductive behavior. The actions of the two systems, however, are much more varied than this, and such generalized statements should be taken only as useful rules of thumb.

Figure 17.1 *Basic organization of the peripheral part of the autonomic system.* Two consecutive neurons conduct the impulses from the central nervous system to the effectors. Note the difference in length between the pre- and postganglionic fibers in the sympathetic and the parasympathetic systems. Effectors may be glandular cells and not only smooth-muscle cells, as shown here.

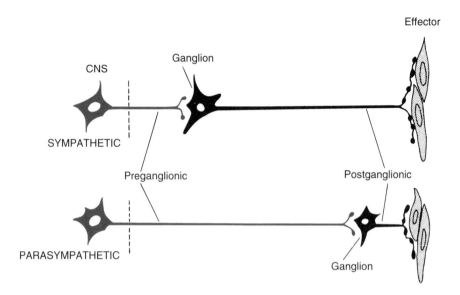

GENERAL ORGANIZATION OF THE AUTONOMIC SYSTEM

Two Succeeding Neurons Constitute the Efferent Pathway

Despite their different actions, the sympathetic and the parasympathetic systems have certain features of peripheral organization in common. These should be known before discussing the differences between them.

In contrast to the somatic efferent fibers (leading from motoneurons to skeletal muscles), the visceral efferent fibers do not pass nonstop to the organs. The transmission of signals is interrupted by *autonomic ganglia* (Figs. 17.1 and 17.2). The multipolar cells in the ganglia send their axons to the effectors (smooth-muscle cells and glands) in visceral organs. The neurons conducting impulses to the ganglia are called *preganglionic*, whereas the ganglion cells and their axons are called *postganglionic*. The *perikarya of the preganglionic neurons* are located in the spinal cord and the brain stem. The *preganglionic neurons*, both the sympathetic and the parasympathetic ones, use *acetylcholine* as a neurotransmitter.

Figure 17.2 *Autonomic ganglion.* Microphotograph of thionine-stained section. To the **right**, a nerve is seen to enter the ganglion with preganglionic fibers.

Another typical feature of the autonomic nervous system is that the postganglionic fibers as a rule form extensive *plexuses* around the organs they innervate.

Postganglionic Fibers Do Not Establish Typical Synapses

The thin, unmyelinated postganglionic fibers do not form typical synapses with the effector cells, in contrast to the somatic efferent fibers innervating skeletal muscle cells (Fig. 11.4). When the postganglionic fibers reach the vicinity of the effector cells, they branch extensively, and there are small swellings—*varicosities*—along the branches (Fig. 17.1). In each varicosity there are vesicles with neurotransmitter. The varicosities do not form synapses but can be located fairly close to the effector cells. In some places the distance is only 50 nm, permitting very direct and precise control of the effector cell. Most often, however, the distance between the varicosities and the effectors is so great that the transmitter, after being released, must diffuse over fairly long distances to reach its target. This means that the neurotransmitter acts on several effector cells within a certain distance. When the diffusion distance is great, the transmitter acts slowly—that is, with a fairly long latency and a prolonged action (compared with the fast action at the neuromuscular junction). Often, only a few of the smooth-muscle cells in the wall of a hollow organ—such as a vessel—are close enough to the varicosities to be directly influenced by the transmitter. In such cases, the action potential elicited in some smooth-muscle cells is propagated from cell to cell via gap junctions between them (which couple the cells electrically). In general, therefore, *the actions of the autonomic nervous system are more diffusely distributed, both spatially and temporally, than is the case in the somatic system.* The properties of the smooth-muscle cells contribute to increase this difference, because their action potentials last much longer than those of skeletal muscles. Furthermore, smooth-muscle cells (for example, in the wall of the gastrointestinal tract) can be made to contract by stimuli other than nervous ones, such as by stretching and by the actions of hormones. The autonomic system therefore *contributes* to the regulation of the contraction of smooth-muscle cells in the gastrointestinal tract and in the walls of the vessels, but it is not alone in this capacity (again in contrast to the control of skeletal muscle cells by the motoneurons).

There are, nevertheless, *great differences between different organs with regard to the precision of their autonomic innervation.* Some visceral organs require much faster and more accurate control than others. The smooth muscles of the eye (the ciliary muscle and the sphincter pupillae, regulating the curvature of the lens and the diameter of the pupil) must be subject to very precise control. The same holds for the muscles of the ductus deferens, in which the propulsive contractions must be fast and well coordinated. Such demands are not made of the smooth muscles of the gastrointestinal tract and the vessels. Corresponding to different functional requirements, the pattern of autonomic innervation varies in different organs. The intrinsic eye muscles, for example, receive a large number of nerve fibers so that all muscle cells come in close contact with varicosities of nerve fibers. This arrangement is called *multiunit*, because it is similar to the conditions in the somatic system with many precisely controlled motor units. In places with few nerve fibers to supply a large number of smooth-muscle cells, so that only a few cells are close to nerve varicosities, we use the term *single-unit* arrangement. Thus, numerous muscle cells behave as a unit when one or a few are activated.

Autonomic Ganglia and Plexuses

The autonomic ganglia contain *multipolar neurons* of various sizes (Fig. 17.2) with long, branching dendrites. The axons are mostly unmyelinated and very thin. The perikarya of the ganglion cells are embedded in a meshwork of fibers consisting of afferent fibers, ganglion cell dendrites, and axons of the ganglion cells. At least some of the ganglia receive *sensory fibers* from visceral organs. There are also *interneurons* in the autonomic ganglia. Such features, and other data, indicate that the ganglia are not just simple synaptic interruptions of purely motor (efferent) pathways but can serve as *reflex centers* for some visceral reflexes.

When an organ is innervated by both sympathetic and parasympathetic fibers, these two components intermingle and form *autonomic plexuses* just outside or in the wall of the organs. At many places cell bodies of postganglionic cells form small clumps intermingled with the fibers of the plexuses. Thus, ganglia and plexuses often coexist, and the ganglia then have the same prefix as the plexuses. For example, the *cardiac plexus* on the outside of the heart contains both kinds of fibers and, in addition, the perikarya of the postganglionic parasympathetic neurons. Especially well-developed plexuses are found around the large vessels in the upper abdomen, where vagus fibers intermingle with sympathetic fibers from (mainly) the splanchnic nerves. These *prevertebral plexuses* get their names from the arteries they surround and follow peripherally: the *celiac plexus*, the *superior and inferior mesenteric plexus*, and the *renal plexus*. The prevertebral plexuses continue into the pelvis as the *hypogastric plexus*.

Differences between the Sympathetic and the Parasympathetic Systems

The two systems differ in several respects. The *preganglionic neurons* are situated in different parts of the central nervous system: The *sympathetic* ones are found in the T_1–L_2 spinal segments, whereas the *parasympathetic* preganglionic neurons lie in the brain stem and the $(S_2)S_3$–S_4 spinal segments (Figs. 17.6 and 17.9). Furthermore, the *ganglia* are located differently: *Sympathetic* ones lie close to the central nervous system, whereas the *parasympathetic* ganglia are located close to the target organs. Thus, the sympathetic preganglionic fibers are short, and the parasympathetic ones are long (Fig. 17.1).

Another difference between the two systems is the *neurotransmitters* utilized by the postganglionic fibers: The sympathetic fibers release *norepinephrine*, whereas the parasympathetic fibers release *acetylcholine* from their varicosities.

Finally, the distribution of postganglionic fibers is different. Thus, *virtually all parts of the body receive sympathetic fibers, whereas the*

TABLE 17.1 Summary of Some Main Actions of the Autonomic System*

Organ	Sympathetic System	Parasympathetic System
Skin	Vasoconstriction; sweat secretion; goose skin	No innervation
Skeletal muscles	Vasoconstriction	No innervation
Heart	Increased rate and stroke volume	Reduced heart rate
Airways	Dilatation of bronchi (reduced airway resistance)	Bronchial constriction; secretion from mucosal glands
Gastrointestinal tract	Reduced blood flow and peristaltic movements	Increased peristaltic movements; secretion of gastric juice, bile, and pancreatic juice
Urinary bladder	Relaxation of muscle for emptying (detrusor); contraction of urethral sphincter	Contraction of detrusor muscle; relaxation of urethral sphincter
Rectum	Relaxation of muscle of emptying; closure of the internal sphincter (smooth muscle)	Contraction of muscle for emptying; relaxation of internal sphincter
Genital organs	Contraction of the ductus deferens (ejaculation)	Erection (penis, clitoris)
Eye	Pupillary dilatation	Pupillary constriction; accommodation; secretion of tears

*See Table 17.2 for more details.

parasympathetic fibers are mostly restricted to the true visceral organs. The body wall and the extremities (skin, muscles, joints) do not receive parasympathetic fibers.

The functions of the two systems will be treated later in this chapter. Table 17.1 gives a broad overview.

The Parasympathetic Innervation Is Usually More Precise Than the Sympathetic

As a general rule (with notable exceptions), the sympathetic system is more diffusely organized than the parasympathetic. This is shown, for example, in the relation between the number of preganglionic and postganglionic fibers. In the parasympathetic ciliary ganglion (Figs. 16.24 and 16.26), two postganglionic fibers leave the ganglion for each preganglionic fiber reaching it—that is, a 2:1 relationship (in the cat). For the sympathetic superior cervical ganglion (Fig. 17.6), the relationship is 30:1 in the cat and 60–190:1 in humans (this ganglion contains more than 1 million neurons in man). Furthermore, the parasympathetic innervation is in several places arranged with *multiunits*—that is, small "motor units" and the possibility of precise control. This concerns, for example, the innervation of the intrinsic eye muscles. The sympathetic innervation is often (but not always) arranged with *single units*—that is, a large number of smooth muscle cells are activated from one postganglionic fiber and behave as a functional unit.

Another difference concerns the topographic arrangement of the preganglionic neurons. Whereas the sympathetic neurons show only a fairly rough topography within the intermediolateral column in relation to the location of the target (Fig. 17.6; Table 17.2), the parasympathetic neurons are as a rule collected in distinct nuclei (Fig. 17.9) or subdivisions of a nucleus (like the dorsal motor nucleus of the vagus), each related to one target organ.

The difference in innervation precision between the sympathetic and the parasympathetic systems mentioned above have several *exceptions*, however. One example is the ductus deferens, in which the rhythmic contractions are elicited by sympathetic fibers. A multiunit arrangement is required to ensure the necessary precision and speed of the contractile wave moving the sperm during ejaculation. On the other hand, the parasympathetic innervation of the gastrointestinal tract, eliciting contractile activity, is rather diffuse (single-unit arrangement).

TABLE 17.2 The Principal Features of the Autonomic Innervation of Some Organs

	The Sympathetic System		
Organ	Preganglionic Neuron	Postganglionic Neuron	Action
Eye	Th$_{1-2}$	Superior cervical ganglion	Pupillary dilatation
Lacrimal gland	Th$_{1-2}$	Superior cervical ganglion	?
Submandibular and sublingual glands	Th$_{1-2}$	Superior cervical ganglion	Vasoconstriction
Parotid gland	Th$_{1-2}$	Superior cervical ganglion	Vasoconstriction
Heart	Th$_{1-4(5)}$	Superior, middle, inferior cervical and upper thoracic ganglia	Increased heart rate and stroke volume, dilation of coronary arteries
Bronchi, lungs	Th$_{2-7(2-4?)}$	Inferior cervical and upper thoracic ganglia	Vasodilation, bronchial dilation
Stomach	Th$_{6-10}$ Greater splanchnic nerve	Celiac ganglion	Inhibition of peristaltic movement and secretion, vasoconstriction
Pancreas	Th$_{6-10}$ Greater splanchnic nerve	Celiac ganglion	Vasoconstriction
Small intestine ascending and transverse large intestine	Th$_{6-10}$ Greater splanchnic nerve	Celiac, superior and inferior mesenteric ganglia	Inhibition of peristaltic movement and secretion
Descending large intestine, sigmoid, rectum	Th$_{11}$–L$_2$	Inferior mesentery hypogastric and pelvic plexus (ganglia)	Inhibition of peristaltic movement and secretion
Ureter, bladder	Th$_{11}$–L$_2$	Hypogastr. and pelvic plexus (ganglia)	Relaxation of detrusor muscle and contraction of internal sphincter
Head, neck (skin and skeletal muscles)	Th$_{1-4}$	Superior and middle cervical ganglia	
Upper extremity	Th$_{3-6}$	Stellate and upper thoracic ganglia	Sweat secretion, vasoconstriction, pilo-erection
Lower extremity	Th$_{10}$–L$_2$	Lower lumbar and upper sacral ganglia	
	The Parasympathetic System		
Organ	Preganglionic Neuron	Postganglionic Neuron	Action
Eye	Edinger-Westphal nucleus	Ciliary ganglion	Pupillary constriction accommodation
Lacrimal gland	Superior salivatory nucleus	Pterygopalatine ganglion	Secretion of tears
Submandibular and sublingual glands	Superior salivatory nucleus	Submandibular ganglion	Secretion of saliva, vasodilation

TABLE 17.2 Continued

Organ	The Parasympathetic System		Action
	Preganglionic Neuron	Postganglionic Neuron	
Parotid gland	Inferior salivatory nucleus	Otic ganglion	Secretion of saliva, vasodilation
Heart	Dorsal motor nucleus, vagus nerve	Cardiac plexus	Reduced heart rate (bradycardia)
Bronchi, lungs	"	Pulmonary plexus	Bronchial constriction and secretion
Stomach	"	Myenteric and submucosal plexus (ganglia)	Peristaltic movement and secretion
Pancreas	"	Periarterial plexus	Secretion
Small intestine ascending and transverse large intestine	"	Myenteric and submucosal plexus (ganglia)	Peristaltic movement and secretion
Descending large intestine, sigmoid, rectum	S_{3-4}	Myenteric and submucosal plexus (ganglia)	Peristaltic movement and secretion
Ureter, bladder	S_{3-4}	Pelvic plexus (ganglion)	Contraction of detrusorand and inhibition of internal sphincter
Head, neck (skin and skeletal muscles)			
Upper extremity		No parasympathetic innervation	
Lower extremity			

PERIPHERAL PARTS OF THE SYMPATHETIC SYSTEM

Preganglionic Fibers and the Sympathetic Trunk

The peripheral parts of the sympathetic system consist of neurons conveying impulses to visceral organs, and sensory fibers leading in the opposite direction. The efferent, *preganglionic sympathetic fibers* belong to neurons with perikarya in the *intermediolateral column* in the spinal cord (Fig. 17.3). The fibers leave the cord (like other efferent fibers) through the ventral roots, but because the intermediolateral column is present only in the T_1–L_2 segments (Fig. 17.6), only the ventral roots of these segments contain preganglionic sympathetic fibers (the sympathetic system is also called the *thoracolumbar* system). The sympathetic fibers follow the somatic ones only for a short distance, however. Just after the ventral and the dorsal roots fuse, the sympathetic preganglionic fibers leave the spinal nerve to end in a sympathetic ganglion (Fig. 17.4). In early embryonic life, one ganglion is produced on each side for every spinal segment, but during further development some ganglia fuse, so the final num-

Figure 17.3 *The intermediolateral cell column* contains the perikarya of the preganglionic sympathetic neurons. Cross section of the thoracic cord.

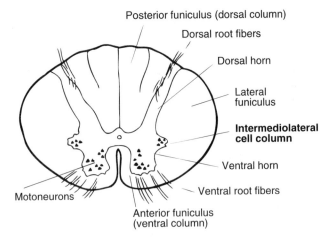

ber is smaller than the number of segments. This reduction is most marked in the cervical region.

The ganglia are located just outside the intervertebral foramen, laterally on the vertebral column (Fig. 17.5). The row of such *paravertebral ganglia* extends from the base of the skull to the coccygeal bone in the pelvis minor. Since the ganglia are interconnected by fiber bundles, a continuous string called the *sympathetic trunk* is formed (Figs. 17.5 and 17.6). The ganglia form small swellings along the trunk. There is usually one ganglion for each pair of spinal nerves, except in the cervical region, where there are only three: the *superior, middle,* and *inferior cervical ganglia.* The middle ganglion can be missing, and the inferior cervical ganglion is usually fused with the uppermost thoracic ganglion to form the

Figure 17.4 *The sympathetic system.* Postganglionic neurons are located in the ganglia of the sympathetic trunk and in the prevertebral ganglia. Sympathetic fibers to the trunk and the extremities follow the spinal nerves, whereas fibers to the visceral organs form separate nerves and follow the main vessels to the organs.

Middle cervical ganglion

Cardiac nerves

Common carotid artery

Stellate ganglion

Subclavian artery

Brachial plexus

Pulmonary branch

Thoracic nerves

Sympathetic trunk

Communicating rami

Ribs

Greater splanchnic nerve

Lesser splanchnic nerve

Diaphragm

Figure 17.5 *The sympathetic trunk.* A part of the thoracic vertebral column and the ribs seen from the right. Note the communicating rami and the splanchnic nerves. Redrawn from Spalteholz (1929).

large *stellate ganglion* (Fig. 17.5). In the lumbar and sacral parts of the sympathetic trunks, some cross connections are present.

The preganglionic sympathetic fibers leave the spinal nerve as a small bundle called the *white communicating ramus,* which connects the nerve with the sympathetic trunk (Figs. 17.4 and 17.5). Since many of the preganglionic fibers are myelinated, this communicating ramus is whitish. Because of the restricted extension of the intermediolateral column, *only the thoracic and the upper two lumbar spinal nerves give off white communicating rami.*

When reaching the ganglia of the sympathetic trunk, some preganglionic fibers establish synapses with postganglionic neurons in that ganglion, whereas others continue uninterrupted through the ganglion (Fig. 17.4). In the upper part of the trunk, the fibers continue rostrally, in the lower part caudally, to establish synapses with ganglion cells in ganglia at levels above and below the intermediolateral column (Figs. 17.6, 17.7, and 17.8). This arrangement ensures that *preganglionic fibers reach all the ganglia of the sympathetic trunk (the paravertebral ganglia).*

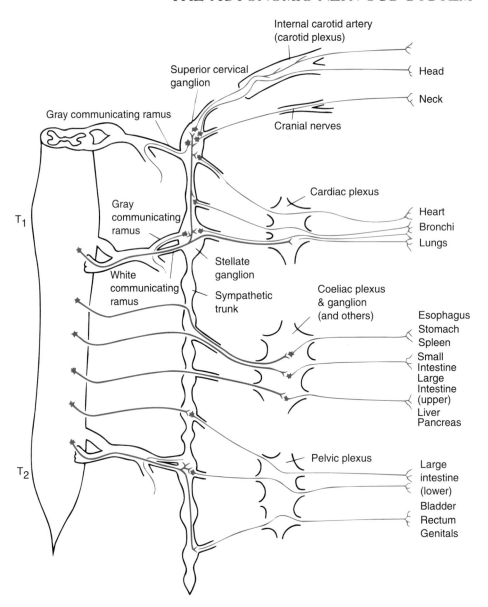

Figure 17.6 *The sympathetic system, highly schematized.*

Some of the preganglionic fibers pass directly through the ganglia and form separate nerves destined for prevertebral sympathetic ganglia (Figs. 17.4–17.6). We will return to this point later in this chapter.

Postganglionic Sympathetic Fibers

The postganglionic fibers from the ganglia of the sympathetic trunk take different routes. From all of the ganglia, some fibers pass back to the spinal nerve as the thin gray *communicating ramus* (Figs. 17.4 and 17.5). This ramus is more grayish than the white ramus because most of the postganglionic fibers are unmyelinated.[1] *All of the spinal nerves are supplied with postganglionic fibers through the communicating rami* (Fig. 17.6). The postganglionic fibers follow the spinal nerves out into all their branches.

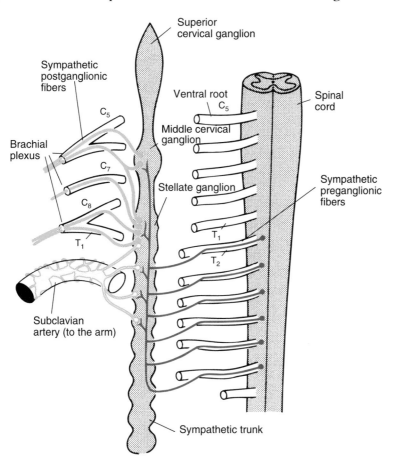

Superior
cervical ganglion

Sympathetic
postganglionic
fibers

Ventral root
C₅

Spinal
cord

C₅

Brachial
plexus

Middle cervical
ganglion

C₇

Stellate ganglion

Sympathetic
preganglionic
fibers

C₈

T₁

T₁

T₂

Subclavian
artery (to the arm)

Sympathetic trunk

Figure 17.7 *Sympathetic innervation of the upper extremity.* The preganglionic fibers come from the upper thoracic segments of the cord and synapse in the ganglia of the sympathetic trunk up to the middle cervical ganglion. The postganglionic fibers follow partly the spinal nerves and partly the subclavian artery to the arm. Redrawn from Haymaker and Woodhall (1945).

Other postganglionic fibers leave the trunk and *pass to larger arteries in the vicinity* and follow them peripherally (such as the subclavian artery to the arm, the common iliac artery with branches to pelvic organs and the lower extremity) (Figs. 17.7 and 17.8). Some of these fibers innervate the smooth-muscle cells of the artery. Many of the postganglionic sympathetic fibers that follow the spinal nerves leave them peripherally to innervate small vessels. Other fibers from the spinal nerves innervate sweat glands and smooth muscles attached to hair follicles (Fig. 17.4).

Sympathetic Innervation of the Head and Extremities

The *head, neck, and upper extremity* are supplied with preganglionic sympathetic fibers from the upper thoracic segments. The fibers enter the sympathetic trunk through the communicating rami. Some establish synaptic contacts with postganglionic neurons in the upper thoracic ganglia, whereas other fibers pass through these ganglia to end in the cervical ganglia (Figs. 17.6 and 17.8). From these ganglia, postganglionic fibers enter the spinal nerves to the neck (C₁–C₄) and the upper extremity (C₅–T₁).

Figure 17.8 *Sympathetic innervation of the lower extremity.* In the **right** side of the figure, pre- and postganglionic parasympathetic fibers from the sacral cord are also shown. Redrawn from Haymaker and Woodhall (1945).

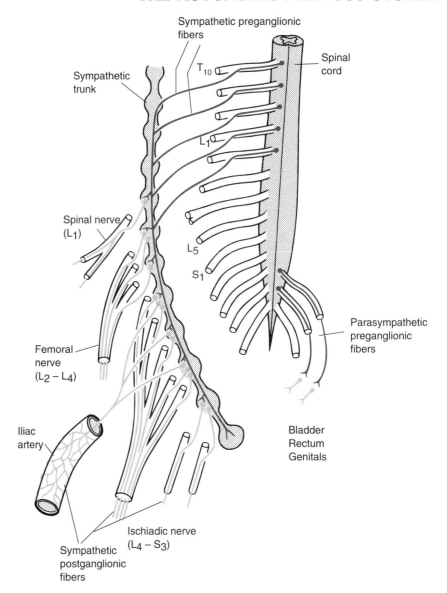

Interruption of the Sympathetic Innervation of the Head. Horner's Syndrome

Sympathetic denervation of the head is usually caused by lesions of the sympathetic trunk in the neck. Because all preganglionic fibers enter the trunk below the inferior cervical ganglion (Fig. 17.6), a lesion anywhere above the level of the thoracic outlet can interrupt the sympathetic innervation of the head. It may be caused, for example, by a tumor in the apex of the lung, in the thyroid gland, or in any of the numerous lymph nodes in the neck. The ensuing symptoms can be understood on the basis of the effects of sympathetic fibers on the skin and the eye (Table 17.1). In the case of a unilateral lesion, the *facial skin* on the side of the lesion becomes redder (warmer) and drier than that on the other side (caused by vasodilatation and lack of sweat secretion). The *pupil* is smaller (*miosis*) on the side of the lesion (paralysis of the sphincter pupillae), and the eyelid usually droops a little (*ptosis*) owing to paralysis of the tarsal muscle. This constellation of symptoms (red and dry skin, miosis, and ptosis) affecting half of the face is called *Horner's syndrome*.

Horner's syndrome can also be caused by lesions in the brain stem (for example, in the lateral part of the pons), interrupting the descending fibers to the intermediolateral column.

The *head* receives postganglionic fibers from the *superior cervical ganglion*. From the ganglion, the fibers follow arteries and cranial nerves to the skin, the eye, the lacrimal gland, and the salivary glands.

With regard to the *lower extremities*, the arrangement corresponds to that described for the upper extremity, with postganglionic fibers following partly the spinal nerves and partly the large arteries (Fig. 17.8).

Sympathetic Innervation of the Viscera

As mentioned above, the postganglionic sympathetic fibers to the extremities and the body wall follow to a great extent the spinal nerves. The visceral organs of the thorax and the abdomen do not receive branches from the spinal nerves, however. Therefore, the sympathetic fibers destined for these organs have to form separate nerves. Such *splanchnic nerves* are fairly thin twigs that leave the sympathetic trunk at various levels.

The sympathetic fibers to the *heart* follow the superior, middle, and inferior cardiac nerves leaving the corresponding cervical ganglia. The perikarya of the postganglionic neurons are found in the cervical ganglia (Fig. 17.6). In addition, some smaller branches to the heart take off from the upper thoracic sympathetic ganglia.

Most sympathetic fibers to the *abdominal viscera* form the *greater* and *lesser splanchnic nerves* (Fig. 17.5). These nerves consist mainly of preganglionic fibers from spinal segments T_6–T_{11}, which pass uninterrupted through the ganglia of the sympathetic trunk (Figs. 17.4 and 17.6). The nerves penetrate the diaphragm and end in ganglia located on the ventral side of the abdominal aorta in the upper abdomen. These are called *prevertebral ganglia*, to distinguish them from the paravertebral ganglia of the sympathetic trunk.

The largest among the prevertebral ganglia is the *celiac ganglion*, located where the celiac artery emerges from the aorta. Smaller prevertebral ganglia are found where the superior and inferior mesenteric arteries emerge. The postganglionic fibers follow the arteries to the various organs.

The *greater and lesser splanchnic nerves* and the corresponding prevertebral ganglia supply the visceral organs in the *upper and middle part of the abdomen*, such as the stomach, pancreas, gallbladder, small intestine, and the large intestine to the descending part. The *adrenal medulla*, which also receives preganglionic fibers from the splanchnic nerves, is special. The medullary endocrine cells (chromaffin cells)—which are transformed postganglionic neurons—release *epinephrine* (and small amounts of norepinephrine) into the bloodstream on sympathetic stimulation.

The visceral organs of the *lower abdomen* receive their sympathetic innervation from the intermediolateral column in the lower thoracic and upper two lumbar segments. These fibers also leave the sympathetic trunk as separate nerves (*lumbar splanchnic nerves*) to reach prevertebral ganglia. The postganglionic fibers follow the arteries to the organs (Fig. 17.6).

The prevertebral ganglia are embedded in a meshwork of fibers, forming prevertebral plexuses, with names corresponding to those of the ganglia (Fig. 17.6). The plexuses formed mainly by sympathetic fibers continue from the lower part of the abdominal aorta into the pelvis minor as the *hypogastric plexus*. In the pelvis, the hypogastric plexus mixes with parasympathetic fibers from the pelvic nerves and forms the *pelvic plexus* around the pelvic organs, as mentioned above.

PERIPHERAL PARTS OF THE PARASYMPATHETIC SYSTEM

As mentioned above, the preganglionic parasympathetic (visceral efferent) neurons have their perikarya in the brain stem and in the sacral cord. The cells are morphologically similar to the sympathetic preganglionic neurons of the intermediolateral column.

The Cranial Nerves Contain Preganglionic Parasympathetic Fibers

The preganglionic fibers of the cranial part of the parasympathetic system follow the *oculomotor*, the *facial* (intermediate), the *glossopharyngeal*, and the *vagus nerves*. The fibers come from the visceral efferent column of cranial nerve nuclei (Figs. 16.2 and 16.3). The preganglionic fibers of the cranial nerves supplying structures in the head end in several parasympathetic ganglia, located outside the skull close to large cranial nerve trunks (Fig. 17.9). These are the *ciliary*, the *pterygopalatine*, the *otic*, and the *submandibular ganglia*. From these ganglia, the postganglionic fibers pass to the effector organs (the intrinsic muscles of the eye, the lacrimal gland, and the salivary glands).

The preganglionic fibers of the *vagus nerve* do not end in well-defined ganglia but in more diffusely distributed collections of postganglionic neurons in the walls of (or just outside) the organs. These postganglionic neurons have short axons running in the wall of the organ and innervate smooth-muscle cells and glands. As mentioned in Chapter 16, the vagus nerve sends parasympathetic fibers to the heart, the lungs, the gastrointestinal tract down to the descending colon, the gallbladder, the liver, and the pancreas (Fig. 16.8). With postganglionic sympathetic fibers the vagus form the *cardiac plexus*, which lies around the aortal arch and extends down onto the heart. The cardiac plexus also contains scattered groups of postganglionic parasympathetic perikarya; the largest group being just underneath the aorta. The *sinus node* and the *atrioventricular node* receive the densest innervation of parasympathetic postganglionic (vagus) fibers, whereas the ventricles receive few such fibers (they receive a dense sympathetic postganglionic innervation, however). In the *airways* the vagus participates in plexuses around the trachea and the bronchi (the *tracheobronchial plexus*), containing scattered postganglionic neurons.

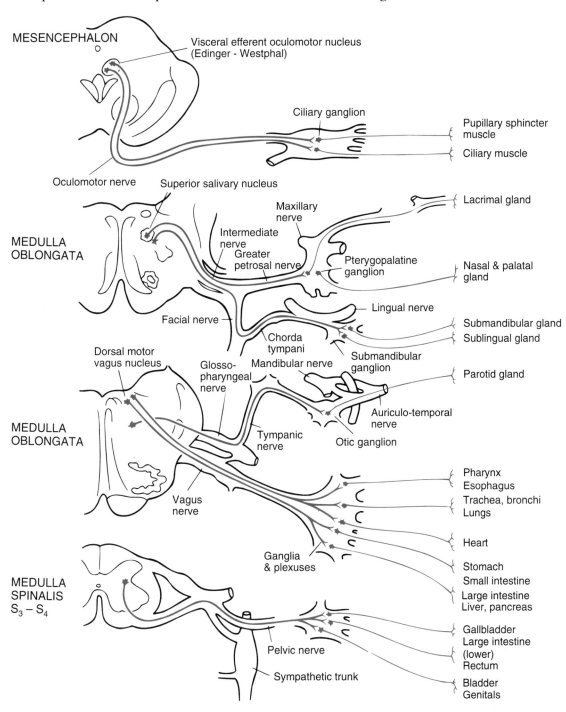

MESENCEPHALON

Visceral efferent oculomotor nucleus
(Edinger - Westphal)

Ciliary ganglion

Pupillary sphincter muscle

Ciliary muscle

Oculomotor nerve

Superior salivary nucleus

MEDULLA OBLONGATA

Maxillary nerve

Intermediate nerve

Greater petrosal nerve

Pterygopalatine ganglion

Lacrimal gland

Nasal & palatal gland

Facial nerve

Lingual nerve

Chorda tympani

Mandibular nerve

Submandibular ganglion

Submandibular gland

Sublingual gland

Parotid gland

Dorsal motor vagus nucleus

Glosso-pharyngeal nerve

Auriculo-temporal nerve

MEDULLA OBLONGATA

Tympanic nerve

Otic ganglion

Vagus nerve

Pharynx
Esophagus

Trachea, bronchi
Lungs

Heart

Stomach
Small intestine
Large intestine
Liver, pancreas

Ganglia & plexuses

MEDULLA SPINALIS
S₃ – S₄

Pelvic nerve

Sympathetic trunk

Gallbladder
Large intestine (lower)
Rectum

Bladder
Genitals

The Sacral Part of the Parasympathetic System Supplies the Genitals, Bladder, and Rectum

Figure 17.9 *The parasympathetic system.* Note the location of the perikarya of the preganglionic neurons in the brain stem and in the sacral cord.

The perikarya of the preganglionic neurons in the sacral cord are located in the $(S_2)S_3$–S_4 segments, with a position corresponding to the intermediolateral column of the sympathetic system (Figs. 17.9 and 17.10). The parasympathetic preganglionic fibers leave the cord through the ventral roots and follow the spinal nerves for a short distance. Then they leave

Figure 17.10 *Innervation of the bladder.* To the **left** is the parasympathetic innervation of the smooth muscles responsible for emptying the bladder. The preganglionic neurons are located in the spinal segments S_3–S_4, whereas the postganglionic perikarya are found just outside or in the wall of the bladder. To the **right** is the course of the sensory fibers from the bladder. From the lower part, the sensory fibers follow the efferent parasympathetic fibers, whereas the sensory fibers from the upper part (the fundus) follow the sympathetic fibers (via the sympathetic trunk). The striated, external sphincter muscle is innervated by motoneurons in the sacral segments S_3–S_4 (not shown).

the spinal nerves as separate, small *pelvic nerves*. In contrast to the sympathetic preganglionic fibers, the parasympathetic ones do not pass to the sympathetic trunk but join postganglionic sympathetic fibers in the *pelvic plexus*, located immediately lateral to the rectum, the bladder, the prostate gland (in the male), and the cervix (in the female). Many of the postganglionic parasympathetic neurons are located in the pelvic plexus (the *pelvic ganglion*).

Postganglionic parasympathetic fibers innervate *all the organs of the pelvis* and, in addition, the *corpora cavernosa* (erectile tissue) of the penis and the clitoris. The *descending* and *sigmoid colon* and the *rectum* are innervated from the sacral parasympathetic division. Of particular practical importance is the parasympathetic innervation of the rectum and the bladder, which is responsible for emptying these organs (Fig. 17.10). We treat the emptying reflex of the bladder later in this chapter.

THE ENTERIC NERVOUS SYSTEM

As mentioned above, the digestive tract contain millions of neurons embedded in two plexuses in the wall. Largest is the *myenteric plexus*—located between the circular and the longitudinal external smooth-muscle layers, whereas the smaller *submucous plexus* is situated below the mucous membrane. The plexuses are formed by the axons of the enteric neurons, together with postganglionic sympathetic fibers (with their cell bodies in the prevertebral ganglia). The neurons of the enteric system monitor the tension in the intestinal wall and the chemical milieu of the mucosa, and control the peristaltic movements of the bowel, moving the content toward the anus. In addition, they influence blood flow, the secretion from mucosal glands, and the absorbtion of nutritients.

It was formerly believed that the enteric neurons were parasympathetic postganglionic. Only a minority contain acetylcholine, the classic transmitter of postganglionic parasympathetic neurons, however. It has become increasingly clear, that these plexuses and ganglia represent a part of the peripheral nervous system that is to a large extent independent of the rest of the nervous system. Some even use the term "the mini-brain of the gut." Thus, the neurons in the myenteric and submucous ganglia are able to function even after the sympathetic and parasympathetic nerves to the gastrointestinal have been cut. The number of neurons in the enteric system is large, and only a few of these are under direct control from the central nervous system (by means of parasympathetic preganglionic fibers).

Broadly speaking, the *enteric system integrates information about the local conditions with central commands through sympathetic and parasympathetic postganglionic fibers.*

Neurons and Neurotransmitters of the Enteric System

The enteric plexuses contain not only motor neurons—innervating smooth muscle cells and glands—but also interneurons and most likely sensory cells. Numerous neurotransmitters, in particular many *neuropeptides*, have been found in the enteric ganglion cells. With few exceptions, however, they are not yet functionally characterized. Different kinds of neurons contain different combinations of neuropeptides and classic transmitters (acetyl choline, GABA, and serotonin). *Excitatory neurons*, sending their axons upward (toward the mouth), ensure constriction of the bowel above a bolus of intestinal contents. Such neurons typically contain *acetylcholine* and *SP*. Inhibitory neurons send their axons downward (toward the anus) and inhibit the circular muscle layer in front of a bolus, thus easing its propulsion. Such neurons may contain ATP, VIP, or NO. Neurons acting on *epithelial cells* to increase the *transport of water and electrolytes*, may contain either VIP or acetylcholine (with a variety of peptides, such as galanin, neuropeptide Y, CCK, or CGRP).

A special kind of neuron contains the *gastrin-releasing peptide* (GRP). A group of such neurons are found in the wall of the stomach and send processes to the gastrin-producing cells in its distal part (the antrum). Stimulation of the vagus causes release of GRP, which then induces release of gastrin to the bloodstream. It affects acid producing cells (parietal cells) in the upper part of the stomach.

Finally, some enteric neurons are most likely sensory and send their central process to prevertebral ganglia. Thus, local reflex arcs not involving the central nervous system are established.

FUNCTIONAL ASPECTS OF THE AUTONOMIC NERVOUS SYSTEM

When the autonomic system is considered as a whole, certain main functional features are clear (Table 17.1). The *parasympathetic system* controls primarily processes that are necessary for the maintenance of the organism over the long term. The parasympathetic system thus activates the digestive processes, ensures that waste products are expelled by contraction of the bladder and rectum, protects the eye against strong light, ensures focused vision, reduces the activity of the heart, reduces the diameter of the airways, and increases bronchial secretion. The *sympathetic system* as a whole is more concerned with mobilizing the resources of the body when an extra effort is required. In situations of fear and anger, there are usually signs indicating increased sympathetic activity, such as increased blood pressure, increased heart rate, and dilatation of the pupils. At the same time, stored energy is mobilized by *epinephrine* secreted into the bloodstream from the *adrenal medulla* (increased blood level of glucose and fatty acids). Epinephrine also activates the heart and dilates the bronchi (relaxation of smooth-muscle cells). The activity of the gastrointestinal tract is inhibited. In general, such responses are adequate in flight-or-fight situations.

The above simple dichotomy disregards, however, that in addition the sympathetic system takes part in "daily maintenance" and is active not only in stressful situations. For example, the sympathetic system is crucial for the temperature-regulating functions of the skin, and sympathetic activity is required every time we rise from the sitting position to avoid fall in blood pressure and fainting. Furthermore, the sympathetic system cooperates with the parasympathetic system in control of reproductive functions. We should also realize that the sympathetic and parasympathetic influences on an organ can be regulated up and down independently. Finally, both systems may send impulses at the same time to an organ (the heart, for example, receives both kinds of impulses at the same time). The traditional scheme with reciprocal autonomic innervation—with autonomic "tone" determined by a point on a continuum from sympathetic to parasympathetic—is therefore not tenable.

Actions of Sympathetic Fibers on the Circulatory and Respiratory Organs

The postganglionic sympathetic fibers innervate *vessels in all parts of the body*. Because the vascular smooth-muscle cells are arranged circularly, contraction reduces the diameter and increases the vascular resistance. Such *vasoconstriction* is most marked in the smallest arteries, the *arterioles*, which are especially concerned with the regulation of blood flow to the organs. Action potentials in the sympathetic fibers ending in the vessel walls produce vasoconstriction and, thus, reduced blood flow. By varying the impulse frequency of the sympathetic nerves, they can vary the diameter of the vessels.[2] When there are no impulses in the sympathetic fibers innervating the vessel (and no other substances act to produce contraction), the arterioles are maximally widened by the internal blood pressure. This is called *vasodilation.*

In many situations the task of the sympathetic system is to ensure that there is a sufficient blood flow through "high-priority" organs, primarily the brain and the heart. When the blood flow through these organs diminishes, sympathetic neurons to vessels in other parts of the body increase their firing rate. Thus, the blood flow through skeletal muscles and the visceral organs is reduced. Sudden vasodilation in large parts of the body leads to a fall in blood pressure and fainting, because the cerebral blood flow is reduced.[3]

Sympathetic innervation of the *large veins* is also of importance for the maintenance of adequate blood pressure. Constriction of such capacity vessels distributes more of the blood volume to the arterial side—that is, the *effective blood volume* increases. This mechanism is of importance in case of reduced blood volume (on bleeding or dehydration).

Impulses in sympathetic fibers to arterioles in *skeletal muscles* produce vasoconstriction. Epinephrine—released from the adrenal medulla on sympathetic stimulation—may, however, inhibit the vascular smooth-muscle cells and thereby produce vasodilation.

The *heart* receives sympathetic fibers partly through separate nerves from the cervical sympathetic ganglia (Figs. 17.5 and 17.6) and partly through direct branches from the upper thoracic ganglia. Sympathetic impulses produce increased heart rate (by action on the pacemaker cells in the sinus node), increased stroke volume, and dilation of the coronary arteries.

In general, the *sympathetic innervation of the circulatory system ensures that the cardiac output can be increased, that the blood pressure can be maintained, and that the blood flow is directed to the organs needing it the most.*

Cardiac Muscle Cells and Impulse Conduction in the Heart

The heart is built of a special kind of striated muscle cell but does not receive somatic nerve fibers. The cardiac muscle cells differ from skeletal muscle cells by, for example, being electrically coupled by gap junctions (nexus). Thus the action potential spreads from cell to cell. In this respect, the cardiac muscles resemble smooth musculature. Another difference is that the cardiac muscles do not require nerve impulses to produce action potentials. The heart muscle cells have pacemaker properties—the cells depolarize spontaneously and produce regular action potentials. The speed of depolarization and thus the frequency of spontaneous action potentials vary considerably, however, among muscle cells in different parts of the heart. The highest frequency is found among the cells in a small bundle of specialized muscle cells, the *sinus node*, located in the upper part of the right atrium. Normally the impulse that triggers contraction of the whole heart starts in the sinus node. From there it spreads outward to the rest of the atria and further on to the ventricles through a bundle of specialized muscle cells. Cardiac muscle cells with a lower spontaneous firing frequency than the cells of the sinus node are activated by spread of the impulse from the sinus node before the spontaneous depolarization has reached the threshold for an action potential.

The sympathetic and parasympathetic fibers to the heart end partly in the sinus node, whereby the heart rate can be regulated either up or down. At rest, the heart is under a certain dominance of the parasympathetic system (the vagus nerve), which "restrains" the cardiac activity. Actions on the stroke volume by the autonomic system are mediated by fibers ending near the muscle cells of the ventricles.

The vessels of the *lungs* receive sympathetic fibers producing vasodilatation. It is doubtful whether postganglionic sympathetic fibers act on the bronchial smooth musculature in humans[4] (even though such innervation is present in several animal species). Epinephrine, however, has a powerful inhibitory effect on the bronchial musculature; that is, it produces bronchial dilation. Thus the sympathetic system, by its stimulation of the adrenal medulla, acts indirectly on the resistance of the airways.

Effects of Sympathetic Fibers in Other Organs

The *sweat glands* of the skin are innervated by sympathetic fibers, producing sweat secretion. Sweat secretion normally occurs together with dilatation of cutaneous vessels when there is a need for increased loss of heat. Sweat secretion may, however, also occur in extreme situations with a large drop in blood pressure or with strong pain. In such situations, the skin vessels are maximally constricted and the skin is, consequently, pale and cold (cold sweat). A special feature of the innervation of sweat glands is that the neurotransmitter released from the postganglionic fibers is acetylcholine (and not norepinephrine).

Impulses in sympathetic fibers also activate the small smooth muscles attached to the hair roots, which make the hairs stand up. This is called *piloerection*. At the same time, the muscles compress the sebaceous glands, so that they empty their product into the hair follicle. In humans, the sympathetic control of hair position is of minor importance, whereas in animals it is of great significance for control of body temperature.

In the *abdominal viscera*, impulses in sympathetic fibers produce vasoconstriction and reduced contractile activity of the smooth muscles of the walls of hollow organs (that is, reducing the amplitude and frequency of the peristaltic movements). At the same time, the secretion of the glands of the digestive tract is reduced. In sum, these effects result in a marked reduction of the digestive processes. The sympathetic system also inhibits the emptying of the rectum, both by inhibition of the smooth muscles of the wall and by activating the smooth muscles of the internal anal sphincter. In addition, the smooth muscles of the *bladder* wall are inhibited.

The sympathetic innervation of the *genital organs* concerns vessels and the smooth musculature. The innervation of the *ductus deferens* is of particular importance because impulses in sympathetic fibers are responsible for the rhythmic contractions during ejaculation. The *uterus* receives sympathetic fibers, even though their functional role is not clear. Even after complete denervation the uterus may function normally in pregnancy and in parturition.

The sympathetic fibers to the *eye* have their perikarya in the superior cervical ganglion. They produce dilation of the pupil by activating the *dilatator pupillae* muscle and by causing contraction of the radially oriented vessels of the iris (the latter effect is probably most important for pupillary dilation). A small smooth muscle attached to the upper eyelid, the *tarsal muscle*, is also innervated by sympathetic fibers. The tonic activity of this muscle helps to keep the eyelid up while we are awake.

Irritation of Peripheral Nerves Can Produce Changes in the Skin

The effects of sympathetic fibers to the skin—that is, sweat secretion, vasoconstriction, and piloerection—can be reproduced by electrical stimulation of the ventral roots or the peripheral branches of the spinal nerves. Under abnormal conditions, the sympathetic fibers can be irritated by infections or by compression or traction of the nerves. In such cases there is abnormal sweat secretion from areas of the skin that are pale and cold. Destruction of the sympathetic fibers (by, for example, prolonged compression) leads to abolished sweat secretion and vasodilation, resulting in areas of the skin that are abnormally warm and red and at the same time dry. Observations of such local changes of the skin can be helpful in the diagnosis of diseases affecting the peripheral nerves.

Control of Blood Pressure and Blood-Flow Distribution

Normally, the sympathetic neurons are activated reflexly, and many of them are links in arcs for so-called vasomotor reflexes—that is, reflexes in which the response is a change of vascular diameter (and thus resistance). The superior aim of the control of *blood pressure* is to ensure that the brain (and the heart) always has a sufficient blood flow. *Baroreceptors* in the large arteries in the neck and the aortal arch record the slightest fall in blood pressure and produce an automatic increase of the impulse frequency of sympathetic fibers. This is most marked for the sympathetic fibers to skeletal muscles but if necessary, fibers to the heart are also activated. In this manner, vasoconstriction of the skeletal muscle arterioles is produced. This increases the vascular resistance and the blood pressure is elevated, with the end result that the blood flow to the brain is increased to an adequate level.

Such vasomotor reflexes have been studied with the *microneurographic technique*, enabling the recording of the activity of small groups of postganglionic sympathetic fibers in humans. This makes it possible to study the relationship between the sympathetic impulse frequency and, for example, blood pressure. The postganglionic sympathetic fibers to *muscle arterioles* fire in bursts in pace with the pulse. The bursts are evoked by baroreceptor activation during the diastole of the heart. The overall firing frequency changes in association with changes of blood pressure. Considering the enormous blood flow that can pass through working muscles, we must obviously have central control of this part of the vascular system. Only if the heart increases its output and other vascular beds are constricted (for example, in the abdominal organs) can the sympathetic "throttling" of the muscles be relieved without serious fall in the blood pressure.

The activity of the postganglionic sympathetic fibers to the *skin* appears not to be clearly related to the blood pressure, in contrast to the activity of fibers supplying vessels in skeletal muscles. On the other hand, skin sympathetic fiber activity is closely correlated with the *ambient temperature*; the sympathetic innervation of the skin serves first and foremost the control of body temperature. Increased activity of fibers innervating the sweat glands occurs together with reduced activity of fibers to the small vessels. This produces vasodilation and sweat secretion with increased loss of heat.

The activity of sympathetic fibers to the skin is, however, also strongly influenced by *emotions*—as witnessed by blushing when "having made a fool of oneself" and paleness when frightened. In case of very strong emotions or extreme physical stress (shock, intense visceral pain), simultaneous sympathetic activation of vascular smooth muscles and sweat glands can occur (*cold sweat*).

There are striking *differences between various persons* with regard to the level of activity of sympathetic fibers under identical circumstances, as shown with the microneurographic technique. Postganglionic fibers to skeletal muscles—which constitute a large fraction of all postganglionic fibers in peripheral nerves—have been studied in particular. As mentioned, the activity of these fibers changes in close correlation with changes of the central blood pressure. Comparison of persons with normal blood pressure shows that the resting activity of sympathetic fibers varies by a factor of ten from person to person. Thus, each person appears to have his own characteristic pattern, which is unchanged over a long time. From this "baseline" value, the impulse frequency is up- or down-regulated in response to alterations in blood pressure caused by, for example, the change of body position from sitting to standing. No clear correlation has been found in the level of activity between sympathetic fibers to muscles and elevated blood pressure (*hypertension*).

Function-Specific Sympathetic Control

The above shows that various categories of sympathetic fibers can be controlled independently. There is not a uniform "sympathetic tonus" for all parts of the sympathetic system. High activity in some parts must coexist with low activity in others if the sympathetic system is to fulfill its tasks in controlling blood pressure and body temperature, in reproduction, and so forth. Accordingly, recent *anatomic* studies show that sympathetic neurons innervating different targets are more clearly segregated than formerly believed. Double labeling with retrograde tracers show, for example, that in the intermediolateral column neurons supplying the upper cervical ganglion and the stellate ganglion are largely segregated (although they are found mainly in the same spinal segments, with 90% in T_1–T_6). Thus, higher levels of the central nervous system (such as the hypothalamus) can selectively control subdivisions of the sympathetic system.

Microneurographic observations further support that selective control takes place. Recording from muscle sympathetic fibers during rest show that the firing frequency is uniform to different muscles. Thus, in this situation all sympathetic neurons controlling muscle blood flow receive a common command signal (probably from the brain stem). As soon as a muscle starts working, however, the sympathetic impulse frequency drops in the nerve to this muscle, although it remains unaltered to the resting muscles. Thus, in this situation the sympathetic system exerts a differential control of the muscles; that is, the impulse frequencies depend on their individual needs.

The *specificity of sympathetic control* of muscle blood flow can presumably arise in two ways. One possibility is lowered central drive (from the brain stem) to preganglionic neurons controlling specific muscles. This may in turn be due to sensory signals from the working muscle (ergoreceptors), or that the motor cortex informs higher levels of the autonomic system about which muscles are being selected for a motor task. The other possibility is that a purely spinal reflex inhibits the preganglionic neurons controlling blood flow to the working muscles.

The Effects of Parasympathetic Fibers

As mentioned above, the sympathetic and the parasympathetic systems have mostly antagonistic effects (on the organs innervated by both; Tables 17.1 and 17.2). Because the postganglionic fibers usually contain neuropeptides in addition to acetylcholine, however, their actions may be more complex than either stimulation or inhibition of the organ.

The parasympathetic postganglionic fibers produce *glandular secretion* (for example, from the lacrimal gland, salivary glands, and glands of the respiratory and gastrointestinal tracts). Parasympathetic fibers are furthermore responsible for increased strength and frequency of *peristaltic contractions in the gastrointestinal tract and the bladder.* The parasympathetic innervation is particularly important for the emptying of the bladder (Fig. 17.10) and the rectum (control of micturition is treated below in connection with visceral reflexes).

As mentioned above, the *heart* receives parasympathetic preganglionic fibers through the vagus nerve. The sinus node and the atrioventricular node receive particularly dense innervation of postganglionic (cholinergic) fibers. Lowering of the heart rate—by affecting the sinus node—is the most marked effect of vagus stimulation. In addition, the vagus exerts more complex effects on the ventricles. Most likely, this happens by presynaptic inhibition of sympathetic postganglionic fibers, thus reducing the contractile force of the heart muscle. Some effects of vagus stimulation are not mediated by acetylcholine but, most likely, by *neuropeptides* such as somatostatin and VIP. In the resting situation the heart receives parasympathetic impulses with a low frequency (higher in endurance-trained than in untrained persons). During work the influence of the vagus diminishes with the need for increased cardiac output. The effect of the vagus on the *coronary arteries* in humans is believed to be constrictor. In the *airways* the vagus produces bronchial constriction and secretion.

Most of the vessels of the body do not receive parasympathetic innervation. Exceptions are vessels of glands and of the external genitals, in which parasympathetic impulses cause vasodilation (that is, they inhibit the smooth-muscle cells). Increased activity of the parasympathetic fibers to the penis (and the clitoris) produces erection (see *Control of the Erection and Ejaculation Reflexes,* later in this Chapter).

In the *eye* parasympathetic fibers of the oculomotor nerve reduce the diameter of the pupil and produce accommodation of the lens.

NEUROTRANSMITTERS IN THE AUTONOMIC NERVOUS SYSTEM

An Overview

The impulse transmission between neurons of the autonomic system is mediated by neurotransmitters, as elsewhere in the nervous system. The preganglionic fibers end with typical synapses on the dendrites of the postganglionic neurons. As mentioned above, all (or the vast majority of) *preganglionic neurons* use *acetylcholine*; that is, they are cholinergic. Many (perhaps all) preganglionic neurons contain in addition *neuropeptides* (enkephalin, somatostatin, neurotensin, and others), as demonstrated with immunocytochemical techniques. The various neuropeptides appear to be expressed differentially in subgroups of autonomic ganglion cells. The functional significance of these neuropeptides, which coexist with acetylcholine in preganglionic neurons, is so far not clear, but the two substances are most likely released together. The released acetylcholine binds to *nicotinic receptors* in the membrane of the postganglionic neurons (in the autonomic ganglia).

Most *postganglionic parasympathetic neurons* release *acetylcholine.* In the peripheral organs, acetylcholine binds to *muscarinic receptors* in the membrane of cardiac, smooth-muscle, and glandular cells.

Most *postganglionic sympathetic neurons* release *norepinephrine* and are noradrenergic. The effects on the effector cells are mediated by two kinds of receptors, the α- and the β-adrenergic receptors, which are distributed differently and have different effects on the postsynaptic cells. In the heart, norepinephrine produces increased heart rate by its binding to β receptors. By binding to α receptors, norepinephrine produces contraction of smooth-muscle cells in most blood vessels, in the ductus deferens, and in the dilatator pupillae muscle of the eye. Binding to β-receptors elicits relaxation of smooth-muscle cells in the wall of the bladder, the uterus, and the airways.

Epinephrine, which is released from the chromaffin cells of the adrenal medulla by sympathetic stimulation, has largely the same effects as norepinephrine. Thus, epinephrine binds to α- and β-adrenergic receptors of the heart, vessels, and the respiratory tract. In addition, epinephrine stimulates the release of free fatty acids from adipose tissue and the breakdown of glycogen to glucose. These metabolic effects are mediated by β-receptors in fat and liver cells.

Besides the cholinergic and noradrenergic postganglionic neurons, some use neither of these transmitters (*noncholinergic and nonadrenergic transmission*; see below). This fact, with the ubiquitous coexistence of the classical transmitters with neuropeptides or other neuroactive substances (ATP, NO) explains why the effects of stimulation of autonomic nerve fibers turn out to be so varied and complex (in contrast to what was believed earlier).

Subgroups of Adrenergic Receptors

Each of the two main kinds—α- *and* β-adrenergic receptors—has several subtypes with different distributions and actions. When norepinephrine binds to the α_1-*receptor*, this produces opening of Ca^{2+} channels, which leads to depolarization, and in turn elicits contraction or secretion. The action of the α1-receptor is not directly on the Ca^{2+} channel but indirectly via intracellular second messengers (diacylglycerol and activation of protein kinase C). The α_2-receptor is mostly localized presynaptically and modulates the transmitter release. The β_1-*receptor* is mostly localized postsynaptically in the heart, on adipose cells, and in the central nervous system. It acts via cAMP as a second messenger. The β_2-*receptor* has a different distribution than the β_1-receptor, being primarily found in smooth- muscle cells of the respiratory tract. Binding of epinephrine (or drugs with similar action) to β_2-receptors causes relaxation of the smooth-muscle cells, notably in the walls of the bronchi. This produces dilation of the bronchi and reduces airway resistance.

Noncholinergic and Nonadrenergic Transmission in the Autonomic System

In addition to the classical neurotransmitters acetylcholine and norepinephrine, several other neuroactive substances have been demonstrated in the autonomic nervous system. The majority of pre- and postganglionic neurons probably contain neuropeptides in addition to acetylcholine or norepinephrine. Furthermore, some autonomic neurons—notably in the enteric system—contain neither acetylcholine nor norepinephrine. Such *noncholinergic and nonadrenergic* (NANC) autonomic fibers are also found in the respiratory tract, the gastrointestinal tract, the bladder, and the external genitals. Some of these release ATP or NO as neurotransmitter; others contain neuropeptides such as somatostatin, SP, VIP, and CCK.

The coexistence of norepinephrine and other transmitters was first suggested by the observation that blocking the receptors for norepinephrine did not prevent all effects of sympathetic nerve stimulation. In the *ductus deferens*—which receives a very dense sympathetic innervation—stimulation of the nerves produces first a fast contraction caused by release of ATP and subsequently a slow contraction produced by norepinephrine. In the *salivary glands*, the parasympathetic postganglionic fibers release both acetylcholine and VIP. The acetylcholine produces secretion from the glandular cells, whereas the VIP produces vasodilatation. Another example concerns the *arteries of the penis*, which dilate to cause erection. This vasodilatation is caused by parasympathetic postganglionic fibers that release VIP (and not acetylcholine).

Some parasympathetic postganglionic fibers in the *heart* release somatostatin and probably VIP (increasing the heart rate). In the *stomach* vagus stimulation can produce release of VIP in addition to acetylcholine. Stimulation of nerves to the human airways can produce bronchial dilatation, although not by release of norepinephrine or acetylcholine. The effect appears to be mediated by release of VIP from postganglionic nerve varicosities.

A final example of exceptions to the general rules about neurotransmitters and the autonomic system concerns the *sweat glands*. As mentioned, these are innervated by sympathetic fibers that use acetylcholine instead of norepinephrine.

Presynaptic Receptors Modulate the Transmitter Release from Postganglionic Nerve Terminals

Neurotransmitters released from the postganglionic neurons bind not only to postsynaptic receptors in the membrane of smooth-muscle and glandular cells but also to presynaptic receptors in the membrane of the varicosities along the fibers. Thus, for example, norepinephrine that is released from sympathetic fibers can bind presynaptically and inhibit further release of norepinephrine or bind to parasympathetic cholinergic terminals in the vicinity. In the heart, sympathetic fibers inhibit the release of acetylcholine in this manner. The sympathetic inhibiting effect on the peristaltic contractions of the gastrointestinal tract is mediated, at least partly, by binding of norepinephrine to α-receptors on the parasympathetic, cholinergic terminals—that is, the release of acetylcholine is inhibited.

Sensitization

When the postganglionic autonomic fibers to an organ are interrupted, the sensitivity of the organ to the transmitter (which is no longer released) is increased. Epinephrine and norepinephrine in the bloodstream, for example, have a more powerful action after an organ has lost its sympathetic innervation, and the same holds for adrenergic drugs. This phenomenon, called *sensitization*, is not restricted to the autonomic system, however.

Drugs with Actions on the Autonomic Nervous System

Several drugs influence the synaptic transmission in the autonomic nervous system. *Atropine* blocks the action of acetylcholine (released from postganglionic parasympathetic fibers) on muscarinic receptors. Other drugs have similar *anticholinergic* effects, often as a side effect. This is the case for several psychopharmaceuticals. The peripheral actions of the parasympathetic system are inhibited, causing symptoms such as dilated pupils (mydriasis) and reduced accommodation of the lens (causing difficulties in seeing close objects clearly). The heart rate increases, and the secretory activity is reduced in several glands. Atropine, for example, is used to reduce secretion of glands in the respiratory tract during surgical anesthesia. The reduced salivary secretion causes dryness of the mouth, a very bothersome side effect of anticholinergic drugs. The peristaltic contractions of the bowel are reduced, causing constipation. The bladder contractility is reduced, with danger of incomplete emptying (especially in cases of prostatic enlargement causing increased urethral resistance, the danger of urinary retention should be kept in mind). Because the sweat glands receive a cholinergic innervation, their secretion may also be reduced (most antiperspirants contain substances with an anticholinergic action).

Pilocarpine is an example of a drug with a *parasympathicomimetic* action: that is, a cholinergic drug. Administration of pilocarpine causes increased salivation, tear flow, reduced heart rate, and increased secretion from, and peristaltic movements of, the gastrointestinal tract. The pupil is small (miotic), causing reduced vision in dim light.

Many drugs activate adrenergic receptors—that is, they have *sympathicomimetic* effects. Some act on both α- and β-receptors, others act preferentially on one or the other receptor type (or on subtypes). *Isoprenaline* (isoproterenol) acts selectively on β-receptors. It thus produces increased heart rate and bronchial dilatation. *Metaraminol* acts preferentially on α-receptors and causes peripheral vasoconstriction and, thereby, increased blood pressure.

Drugs that block α-receptors (such as *phentolamine*) produce peripheral vasodilatation and a fall in blood pressure, whereas drugs that block β-receptors mainly cause reduced heart rate and stroke volume and bronchial constriction. The development of more *selective β-blockers*, acting selectively on β_1-receptors present in the heart, has made it possible to treat hypertension without unwanted bronchial constriction (β_2-receptors are found primarily in the lungs). On the other hand, the development of adrenergic drugs acting selectively on β_2-receptors (and not on β_1-receptors) has made it possible to treat patients with bronchial obstruction (as asthmatics) without such side effects as increased cardiac activity and hypertension.

The impulse *transmission in the autonomic ganglia* can also be influenced by drugs. As mentioned above, acetylcholine is the main transmitter in both sympathetic and parasympathetic ganglia. The nicotinic receptors in the ganglia are nevertheless somewhat different from those present at the neuromuscular junction. This makes it possible to influence one of these targets without affecting the other.

All neurotransmitters present in the peripheral parts of the autonomic system are also found in the central nervous system, together with adrenergic and cholinergic receptors. Thus, drugs designed to act on peripheral parts of the autonomic nervous system may produce side effects through actions on central neurons—that is, in case they pass the blood–brain barrier. β-blockers for example, which are used extensively to treat hypertension, can give central side effects, such as dizzines, disturbed sleep, and depression.

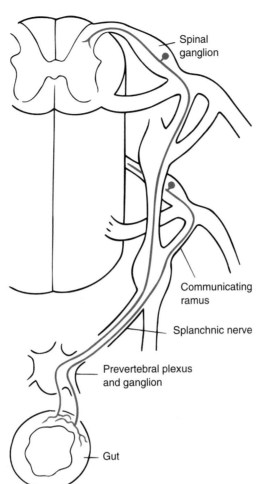

Figure 17.11 *Sensory fibers of sympathetic nerves to the visceral organs.* Note that the fibers pass through the prevertebral plexuses and ganglia before entering the spinal nerves via the communicating rami.

Labels in figure: Spinal ganglion; Communicating ramus; Splanchnic nerve; Prevertebral plexus and ganglion; Gut

It occurs, presumably, after denervation of any neuron. For example, skeletal muscle cells have increased sensitivity to acetylcholine after having lost their nerve supply. The underlying mechanism is probably increased postsynaptic density of receptors, as though the neuron attempts to maintain normal synaptic activity.

SENSORY INNERVATION OF VISCERAL ORGANS

Together with the visceral efferent (sympathetic and parasympathetic) fibers in the nerves to the internal organs, there are afferent fibers conveying sensory information from the viscera to the central nervous system (Fig. 17.11). Sensory fibers follow the sympathetic splanchnic nerves leaving the sympathetic trunk at various levels (Fig. 17.6), the parasympathetic cranial nerves (the oculomotor, the intermediate, the glossopharyngeal, and the vagus nerves; Fig. 17.9), and, finally, the parasympathetic pelvic nerves leaving the sacral spinal nerves to innervate pelvic organs (Figs. 17.9 and 17.10).

The visceral afferent neurons are structurally indistinguishable from the somatic afferent ones—that is, they have their pseudounipolar perikarya in ganglia of the spinal and cranial nerves (Fig. 17.11). The peripheral process follows the sympathetic or parasympathetic nerves to the organs, whereas the central process enters the dorsal horn or the brain stem sensory nuclei (the solitary nucleus). The vast majority of the visceral afferent fibers are thin (Aδ and C fibers).

With some exceptions, such as taste and fairly diffuse sensations of hunger, fullness, and so forth, the sensory signals from the viscera are not consciously perceived. Under abnormal conditions, sensory signals from the viscera can, of course, produce the sensations of intense pain and nausea. The normal function of the sensory innervation of the internal organs is probably related to their mediation of *visceral reflexes*, such as coughing, vomiting, swallowing, circulatory and respiratory reflexes, emptying of the rectum and bladder, and so forth. Many of these reflexes have their reflex centers in the reticular formation. In addition, "silent nociceptors" (see Chapter 7) may mediate information about the local mileu of the internal organs, contributing to homeostasis.

As a general rule, *fibers conducting impulses from visceral nociceptors (producing sensations of pain) follow sympathetic nerves*, whereas the parasympathetic nerves contain fibers conducting from other kinds of receptors. Thus, there is no evidence of fibers leading from nociceptors in the vagus nerve. The above conclusions are based primarily on the clinical results of cutting various nerves in attempts to alleviate visceral pain.

Visceral Receptors

Morphologically, most of the visceral receptors are free nerve endings (Fig. 7.1).[5] They respond to various kinds of stimuli, even though they are structurally identical. A large group consists of *mechanoreceptors* recording the tension of the tissue in which they are located. Such receptors are found, for example, in the heart, lungs, and in the walls of hollow abdominal organs. They provide information about the degree of filling of hollow organs and can elicit reflex contractions aimed at emptying the organ or moving the content. Some stretch receptors may give rise to sensations of pain by responding to strong dilatation of a hollow organ and to forceful contractions of the smooth musculature. Most *visceral nociceptors* are, however, believed to be sensitive to substances in the tissue produced by inflammation or ischemia (chemoreceptors).

Other *chemoreceptors*, strategically placed in the vascular system (at the aortic arch and at the bifurcation of the common carotid artery), react to the carbon dioxide and oxygen concentration in the blood.

Central Pathways and Visceral Reflexes

The sensory impulses from the visceral organs pass through the dorsal roots and end in the *dorsalmost parts of the dorsal horn* (Fig. 7.11). The sensory fibers following the cranial nerves end in the *solitary nucleus* in the medulla (Fig. 16.2). From these receiving cell groups in the cord and in the brain stem, the signals are transmitted to motor nuclei (especially those consisting of preganglionic autonomic neurons), to the reticular formation, and to the hypothalamus and the thalamus. Visceral afferent signals arriving through the dorsal roots are transmitted centrally, at least for the most part, through the *spinothalamic and spinoreticular tracts* (Fig. 7.15). Details are not known, however, with regard to the central transmission of visceral afferent impulses.

Many of the *visceral reflexes* elicited by signals from visceral receptors and receptors in the walls of vessels have their reflex centers in the spinal cord. The more complex reflexes, however, requiring coordination of activity in several parts of the body, have reflex centers in the brain stem or in the hypothalamus. We return to this in Chapter 18.

Vasomotor reflexes were discussed earlier in this chapter. Other important visceral reflexes are produced by stimulation of receptors in the *lungs* and the *airways*, such as coughing and respiratory adjustments. The *vomiting reflex* can be elicited by irritation of the mucosa of the stomach but also in various other ways. It is discussed in Chapter 16, *The Vomiting Reflex*. The *emptying reflexes of the rectum and the bladder* are elicited by stimulation of stretch receptors in their walls and have reflex centers partly in spinal segments $(S_2)S_3$–S_4 and partly in the brain stem. These visceral reflexes are unusual because they can be suppressed voluntarily. The emptying reflex of the bladder is discussed further below.

Reflexes Elicited from Receptors of the Lungs

Signals from stretch receptors in the bronchial walls contribute to *inhibition of inspiratory movements* when the lungs have been inflated to a certain extent (the *Hering-Breuer reflex*). Receptors producing coughing are probably free endings between the epithelial cells of the airways, in part located very close to the epithelial surface (irritation receptors). Such free nerve endings contain SP (as do many other sensory neurons).

A special kind of receptor—the *J- or juxtapulmonary receptor*—is located close to the lung alveoles. It responds to increased pulmonary capillary pressure. Increased pressure in the left atrium (which receives the blood from the lungs) immediately leads to increased pulmonary capillary pressure, with the danger of developing lung edema. Thus, it seems reasonable that the capillary pressure must be monitored closely. Stimulation of the J-receptors produces increased heart rate but may also cause bronchial constriction (this is known to occur in patients with heart failure and increased pulmonary capillary pressure). It is furthermore believed that signals from the J-receptors can reach consciousness and cause a feeling of dyspnea.

The Emptying Reflex of the Bladder and the Control of Micturition

As mentioned above, this reflex is evoked by stimulation of stretch receptors in the wall of the bladder, which record filling. The impulses are conducted in myelinated afferent fibers to the lumbosacral cord (Fig. 17.10). Many sensory units leading from the bladder are slowly adapting with dynamic sensitivity—that is, they respond more to rapid than slow distension of the bladder. No signals are sent when the bladder is empty but when urine starts to accumulate the sensory units start firing. The pressure in the human bladder during filling is typically between five and 15 mm Hg, whereas emptying is normally elicited at 25–30 mm Hg. Urine does not leak out in the filling phase because the intraurethral pressure is kept higher than the intravesical pressure. The intra-urethral pressure is maintained by several factors, among them smooth muscles and elastic tissue in the urethral wall. In the filling phase the smooth muscle of the bladder wall (the *detrusor muscle*) is relaxed, whereas smooth muscles around the urethral outlet are most likely contracted due to sympathetic impulses. When the intravesical pressure reaches the critical level, brisk activity of parasympathetic neurons makes the detrusor muscle contract, while sympathetic influence in the outlet area is reduced. In addition, the striated sphincter muscle in the pelvic floor must relax. *Normal emptying of the bladder thus requires coordinated control of parasympathetic preganglionic neurons in the S_3–S_4 segments, sympathetic preganglionic neurons in the T_{11}–L_2 segments (Table 17.2)*, and α motoneurons in the S_1–S_3 segments.

The parasympathetic control of the detrusor muscle is mediated by *acetylcholine*, whereas *norepinephrine* mediates the sympathetic effect on the urethral outlet area. In addition, *VIP* released from parasympathetic fibers is probably responsible for inhibition of the smooth muscles surrounding the urethra, and sympathetic fibers inhibit the detrusor muscle in the filling phase. Few sympathetic fibers are found in this part of the bladder wall, however. Since many are found in the pelvic plexus and associated small parasympathetic ganglia, the sympathetic inhibition of the detrusor muscle is most likely due to inhibition of the postganglionic parasympathetic neurons.

Normal emptying of the bladder requires more than intact spinal-reflex arches, however. This is evident in patients with *transections of the cord* above the sacral level. If the lesion is complete, all descending connections acting on the sacral reflex centers are interrupted. The patients experience great difficulties with emptying the bladder because the activities of the detrusor muscle and the internal sphincter are incoordinate (*dyssynergia*). Patients with lesions of the brain stem above the pons do not have dyssynergia. Further observations show that the dorsolateral pons (near the locus coeruleus) contains a neuronal network coordinating the spinal reflexes involved in micturition (the *pontine micturition center*). Ascending spinoreticular fibers—informing about the filling pressure—join the spinothalamic tract in the cord. The descending reticulospinal fibers from the pontine micturition center lie dispersed in the lateral funiculus, although the majority are found in its dorsal part.

Although *lesions above the pons* do not disturb the normal emptying of the bladder, patients with such lesions may have problems with the control of the *initiation of micturition* (inhibition in particular). The cell groups responsible for the voluntary control of micturition are not known in detail, although medial parts of the frontal lobe and the hypothalamus appear to be involved.

The Erection and Ejaculation Reflexes

As mentioned above, *erection* depends on parasympathetic impulses to the vessels of the penis or the clitoris, whereas *ejaculation* is due mainly to sympathetic impulses to the smooth muscles of the ductus deferens and the prostate. The preganglionic neurons of these functions have their cell bodies in the lumbosacral cord (Figs. 17.6 and 16.9). In addition, successful expulsion of the semen requires coordination of smooth muscles closing the upper urethra (preventing the semen from entering the bladder) and striated muscles of the pelvic floor (sphincter muscles and muscles around the penile cavernous bodies, especially the bulbocavernosus muscle). The α motoneurons of the latter muscles are found in the sacral cord. In male rats these groups of motoneurons are three times larger than in female rats. This *sexual dimorphism* arises early in the prenatal development and depends on the presence of minute amounts of androgens.

Evidently, erection and ejaculation require *precise temporal coordination of several muscles*. The coordination is carried out in the spinal cord by a complex network of interneurons. For example, the activity of sympathetic preganglionic neurons in the lower thoracic-upper lumbar cord must be coordinated with the activity of parasympathetic preganglionic neurons and α motoneurons in the sacral cord. Both erection and expulsion of the semen can occur after *transection of the cord* in humans, provided the lesion is above the mid-thoracic level. In such patients, erection is evoked by sensory stimuli from the penis. The patient has no conscious sensations, however, since the ascending sensory tracts are interrupted.

Supraspinal control of the reflex centers for erection and ejaculation is carried out by various cell groups in the *reticular formation* (close to those controlling micturition) and the *hypothalamus*. The hypothalamic cell groups are influenced, among other areas, from the cerebral cortex and the amygdala. Normally, of course, descending connections from these higher levels are involved in the induction of erection—more or less independently of sensory impulses acting via the spinal reflex arch. Inhibitory impulses reach the spinal reflex centers of erection and ejaculation from an area in the ventral part of the upper medulla (that is, there are descending connections acting on parasympathetic and sympathetic preganglionic neurons and α motoneurons). The lack of such inhibitory connections may explain why some patients with transection of the cord above the sacral level suffer from a hyperactive erection reflex (*priapism*). Thus, the reflex arch is intact and may be activated by irrelevant sensory stimuli.

Visceral Pain

As mentioned above, visceral afferent signals do not usually reach consciousness. Under abnormal conditions, one may experience sensations from the visceral organs and vessels. Pain is of special interest in this connection. Most fibers carrying signals from visceral nociceptors follow the sympathetic nerves of the organs.[6] Fibers conveying signals from nociceptors in the walls of the arteries of the extremities follow the peripheral (spinal) nerves, just like the efferent sympathetic fibers.

Surgery of visceral organs (for example, of the abdomen) can be performed without the patient feeling pain as long as the abdominal wall is anesthetized. Pain is felt only when the mesenteries or the peritoneum is pulled. Cutting with a sharp knife, for example, is not painful. That the abdominal viscera are not insensitive, however, is witnessed by the intense pain accompanying certain diseases, such as stones blocking the ureter or the gall ducts, or intestinal obstruction. In other diseases, pain can be completely lacking for a long period, such as in many cases of cancer of the lungs, the kidneys, or the gastrointestinal tract. The adequate stimuli for visceral nociceptors are obviously different from those of somatic nociceptors in the skin. This is perhaps not surprising since the visceral organs are not normally exposed to harmful stimuli that the organism has to respond to with a certain behavior.

As mentioned, visceral pain can be provoked by *stretching* the tissues. When the wall of a hollow organ is distended above an obstruction, forceful contractions of the smooth musculature are produced in an attempt to overcome the obstruction. Such spasmic contractions usually occur with regular intervals, explaining the typical bouts of pain experienced when, for example, a stone is stuck in the ureter.

Another cause of visceral pain is *ischemia*, which can occur when an artery is thrombosed. The commonest example is the pain felt when a coronary artery is narrowed (angina pectoris) or occluded (heart infarction).

Pain is also felt when irritating substances come in contact with the peritoneum, as in cases of perforation of a gastric ulcer or an inflamed gallbladder. The spread of bile, gastric content, or blood to the peritoneal cavity causes extreme pain and shock. Inflammation of the mucosa of the bladder changes the behavior of the sensory units leading from the bladder. First, mechanoreceptors recording stretching of the wall become more sensitive (lowered thresholds), and secondly many "silent nociceptors" (see Chapter 7, *Not all Nociceptors May Signal Tissue Damage*) start firing. Under normal conditions even marked stretching of the wall does not activate such receptors, whereas in inflammation they respond to even moderate distension of the bladder. This may explain the frequent voiding in patients with cystitis, and the urge to void even when the bladder is almost empty. The *arteries* are also sensitive to painful stimuli. An arterial puncture (for example, to draw a blood sample) is painful. Furthermore, spasmic contractions or strong dilatation of arteries is also painful.

Special Features of Visceral Sensation: Referred Pain

Visceral pain differs in many respects from pain originating in somatic structures. Visceral pain is usually more *diffuse*, *less precisely graded*, and of a *different quality* than pain arising in the skin. Furthermore, visceral pain is accompanied typically by slowing of the heart, lowered blood pressure, cold sweat, nausea, and a tendency to keep still. Many of these effects are probably orchestrated by the *PAG*. The PAG receives nociceptive impulses, and coordinates a varied specter of autonomic and somatic reactions to stressfull stimuli (see Chapter 7, *The Functional Role of the Pain-Suppressing Systems*). Several factors might contribute to the diffuseness of visceral pain. The density of sensory innervation is generally low in visceral organs with consequently very large receptive fields of the sensory units. In addition, the central branches of the visceral spinal ganglion cells run for a long distance both rostrally and caudally in the cord. Thus, signals entering in one dorsal root can activate spinothalamic cells at many segmental levels.

Often the pain is not felt where the organ is located but in some other place, often in the body wall or the extremities. The pain is referred to another site than where it originates, and this phenomenon is called *referred pain* (See Chapter 7, *Spinothalamic Cells Receive Impulses from Both Somatic and Visceral Structures: Referred Pain*). This pain (for example, in the left arm in the case of angina, and under the right scapula in the case of a gallstone) can be localized fairly precisely by the patient. At the site of the diseased organ, however, there is usually only a diffuse pain, difficult both to localize and to describe.

Referred pain is most likely caused by the convergence on nociceptive neurons in the cord and the thalamus of signals from somatic structures (especially the skin) and viscera innervated from the same spinal segments. The signals coming from the visceral organs are interpreted as arising in the skin and not in the visceral organ, presumably because impulses from the visceral organs are never consciously perceived under normal circumstances (for example, nociceptors of the heart are not normally stimulated). This explanation fits with the observation that the *pain is regularly referred to areas of the skin (dermatomes) innervated from the same spinal segments as the visceral organ.*

Pain Can Be Relieved by Sympathectomy

Knowledge of the special features of visceral pain and of the segmental innervation of visceral organs is of importance for surgical interventions of the autonomic nervous system. Such operations are performed occasionally, especially on the sympathetic system, to interrupt the pathways for pain impulses and sometimes to increase the blood flow of the extremities (to interrupt vasoconstrictor fibers). For example, interruption of the lumbar sympathetic trunk interrupts the sympathetic outflow to the lower extremities (Fig. 17.8). In some patients with intractable pain arising in the upper abdomen (usually because of terminal cancer of the pancreas or the stomach) the transmission of sensory signals can be blocked by alcohol injections in the celiac plexus. Because this procedure also blocks the efferent sympathetic impulses, the patients experience orthostatic hypotension due to vasodilatation in the abdominal organs (this side effect is usually only transitory, however).

There is also evidence that abnormal activity of sympathetic efferent neurons can contribute to a certain kind of painful condition that occurs especially after trauma to the extremities (*causalgia, reflex dystrophy*). The pain in such cases has an intense, burning character and can be provoked by trivial, normally innocuous stimuli (such as light touch). Often the pain is accompanied by signs of abnormal efferent sympathetic activity, such as pale, cold skin. If the condition lasts, the skin becomes thin and glossy with loss of hairs. There may also be atrophy of muscles and osteoporosis of the skeleton. The cause of the pain is unknown, but interruption of the sympathetic outflow to the painful extremity can often reduce or completely remove the pain—for example, by blocking the stellate ganglion in case of pain in the arm (Fig. 17.7). In the latter case there has been no interference with the sensory innervation of the arm, since this passes in the spinal nerves.

The pain arising in the *heart* is usually referred to the ulnar aspect of the left arm or the upper part of the chest because these regions of the skin and the heart both receive sensory innervation from the upper thoracic segments of the cord. The *gallbladder* and the skin in the region of the lower end of the scapula are both innervated from the eighth thoracic segment. The shoulder pain on *irritation of the diaphragm* is explained by the common innervation from the fourth and fifth cervical segments. Pain from the urinary bladder can be referred to two areas of the skin, one innervated by the spinal segments S_2–S_3 and another area higher up on the back innervated by the lower thoracic and upper lumbar segments (Figs. 7.12 and 7.13). This fits with the segments of the cord innervating the bladder (Fig. 17.10).

The phenomenon of *cutaneous hyperesthesia* in cases of visceral diseases is also explained in Chapter 7. In *appendicitis*, for example, there is often a band-like area of hyperesthesia on the right side of the lower abdomen (usually within the dermatomes T_{10}–T_{11}).

The Axonal Reflex

It has been known for a long time that electrical stimulation of dorsal roots can produce vasodilatation in the dermatome of the root concerned. Originally, this was interpreted as evidence of the existence of efferent fibers in the dorsal root, but this has not been verified by modern methods. The phenomenon is undoubtedly caused by impulses conducted in the peripheral direction by the sensory fibers. Such impulses, conducted in the direction opposite the normal direction, are called *antidromic*. The action potentials are of course exactly the same as those conducted in the normal direction (orthodromically). Antidromic impulses in C fibers appear to release *SP* from the peripheral branches. SP probably causes the release of *histamine* (presumably from mast cells). Histamine causes vasodilatation, especially of the capillaries, and at the same time the capillaries become leaky. Thus, a local edema is produced.

Various phenomena can probably be explained by this phenomenon. When the skin is stroked with a fairly sharp object, it reddens (vasodilatation) after a few seconds on both sides of the stripe. This can be explained as follows: The stroking of the skin stimulates C fiber nociceptors, and action potentials are conducted to the central nervous system (and we experience a sharp pain). At the same time, however, the action potential is also conducted peripherally in the branches of the C fiber not innervating the stimulated skin stripe. These branches end in the skin outside the stripe, where they liberate SP and cause vasodilatation. The process is called a reflex, and since it utilizes only the peripheral process of a pseudounipolar ganglion cell, it is called an *axon reflex*. The reflex cannot be elicited in an area of the skin that has been deprived of its sensory innervation.

Under normal conditions, the antidromic impulses in sensory fibers hardly play any role. They may, however, help to explain certain pathological phenomena. An example from the airways can be mentioned. In disposed individuals, irritating gases can produce a marked edema of the mucous membranes. The edema is caused apparently by histamine release, which in turn is caused by SP released by an axon reflex from sensory fibers innervating the mucous membrane (partly coming close to the surface of the epithelium).

NOTES

1. White and gray rami are often fused into one, so that even at the levels T_1–L_2 there may be only one communicating ramus on each side. This contains, as will be understood, both the pre- and postganglionic fibers. In the case of two rami, the color difference between them is not very marked.

2. The degree of vasoconstriction is influenced not only by the nervous system but also by circulating hormones, in particular epinephrine. Furthermore, substances produced by

the local metabolism in the tissue influence the degree of contraction of the vascular smooth-muscle cells.

3. Some people have poor control of the blood-flow distribution in such situations (*orthostatic hypotension*). This is believed to be due to a failure of the sympathetic system. Such persons also often feel limp and uncomfortable after a meal, because of a fall in the blood pressure (*postprandial hypotension*). Microneurographic studies show that this is caused by a lack of sympathetic activity. Normally after a meal, the sympathetic impulse activity increases in nerves to the lower extremities, whereas in the patients with postprandial hypotension no such increase occurs (to upheld the blood pressure the blood flow to the lower part of the body must be reduced when that to the digestive tract increases).

4. Studies in humans with histofluorescence techniques, which visualize catecholaminergic nerve fibers in tissue sections, have shown the presence of such fibers around the vessels but not around the bronchi.

5. There are some encapsulated nerve endings in the visceral organs. Thus, Pacinian corpuscles are present in the pancreas, the mesenteries, and the vessel walls. Their functional role at these sites is unknown.

6. An exception to this rule is the transmission of signals from nociceptors in the neck of the bladder, the prostate, the cervix uteri, and the rectum. "Pain fibers" from these organs follow the parasympathetic pelvic nerves to the sacral spinal nerves (Fig. 17.10). Signals from nociceptors in the fundus of the uterus and of the bladder, however, follow the sympathetic nerves of the hypogastric plexus ending in segments T_{11}–L_2.

CHAPTER 18

CENTRAL AUTONOMIC SYSTEM: HYPOTHALAMUS

Sympathetic and parasympathetic parts cannot be clearly separated in the higher centers that control autonomic functions. Thus, the cell groups at higher levels are centers for coordination of reflex responses involving various autonomic processes that require cooperation of sympathetic and parasympathetic neuronal groups at the lower levels. This chapter will be concerned mainly with the hypothalamus, which is the most important higher center for control of autonomic (visceral) functions. The control exerted by the hypothalamus is mediated by the peripheral parts of the autonomic system and by the endocrine system. In addition, the *hypothalamus serves to coordinate endocrine, autonomic, and somatic motor responses to behavior that is appropriate for the immediate needs of the body, such as feeding, drinking, and reproduction.* The overall aim is to maintain bodily *homeostasis* in a wide sense. The hypothalamus is, however, also connected with higher parts of the central nervous system, such as the cerebral cortex and the amygdala. These connections are important links in the interactions between bodily and mental processes *(psychosomatic interrelations)*, which play a role in both health and disease.

AUTONOMIC CENTERS IN THE BRAIN STEM

Physiological experiments have localized several regions of the brain stem involved in the control of autonomic processes, as mentioned in Chapter 15. Electrical stimulation and lesions of restricted parts of the reticular formation of the pons and medulla produce changes in *blood pressure, cardiac activity, respiration, sweat secretion, gastrointestinal activity*, and other processes. Such higher-level centers exert control of the lower autonomic reflex centers of the spinal cord and coordinate their activities. The anatomic substrates of the brain stem centers are groups of neurons in the medullary and pontine reticular formation. It should be noticed, however, that the centers as a rule are not well-defined nuclei but are formed by extensive networks of interconnected neurons. The brain stem centers ensure, for example, that the segmental vasomotor *reflexes operate together to serve the needs of the whole organism*, and not only its individual parts. We discussed in Chapter 16 how the blood supply of other organs is subordinate to the needs of the brain, and how the micturition center in the pons coordinates the activity of several smooth and striated muscles. Furthermore, cell groups in the reticular formation initiate movements and postural adjustments as parts of complex behaviors in response to thirst, hunger, external dangers, sexual arousal, and so forth. Several such behaviors are coordinated from the *superior colliculus* and the *PAG* in the mesencephalon by way of their connections to the reticular formation.

A perfect coordination cannot be performed by the brain stem autonomic centers, however. This is witnessed by the poor control of autonomic functions such as blood pressure and body temperature in decerebrate animals. Optimal autonomic control, and coordination of autonomic with endocrine and somatic processes, requires that the brain stem and spinal centers be supplied with afferent fibers from higher centers, especially in the hypothalamus.

STRUCTURE AND CONNECTIONS OF THE HYPOTHALAMUS

This small part of the brain, weighing only 4–5 g in humans, is a mosaic of minor nuclei that can be distinguished on the basis of their cytoarchitectonics, connections, cytochemistry, and physiological properties. Only the main features will be discussed here.

Hypothalamic Nuclei

In the wall of the third ventricle, below the hypothalamic sulcus, some identifiable nuclei are embedded in a more diffuse mass of neurons (Figs. 3.22 and 2.23); together these constitute the hypothalamus. The borders between the hypothalamic nuclei and the neighboring regions are not sharply demarcated. This explains why the borders have been drawn differently by different authors. Figure 18.1 shows the classic subdivisions of the British neuroanatomist Le Gros Clark. It is now common to distinguish a *medial part of the hypothalamus*, containing several fairly distinct nuclei, and a *lateral hypothalamic area* (or nucleus) with a diffuse structure. The latter is traversed by numerous fibers running mainly longitudinally. Collectively they are usually termed the *medial forebrain bundle*, though this is not a single tract anatomically or functionally and has

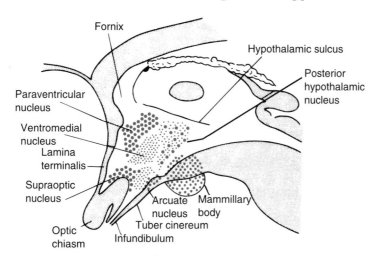

Figure 18.1 *The hypothalamus.* Median section through the third ventricle. Some of the major hypothalamic nuclei are shown with red dots. The size of the dots indicates the relative size of the neurons of the various nuclei. Redrawn after Le Gros Clark et al. (1936)

no sharp borders (see Chapter 19, *The Medial Forebrain Bundle*). Within the *medial part*, one can distinguish *anterior, middle (tuberal)*, and *posterior (mammillary) nuclear groups*. Particularly well defined are two anterior large nuclei, the *paraventricular nucleus* and the *supraoptic nucleus*. The first is located close to the wall of the third ventricle, the latter just above the optic chiasm (Fig. 18.1). In the same region lies the SCN that functions as a biologic clock (see below *Circadian Rhythms*).[1] In the *middle or tuberal nuclear group* we find the *ventromedial*, the *dorsomedial*, and the *arcuate (infundibular)* nuclei. The latter nucleus is located in the bottom of the third ventricle (Fig. 3.23), below the ventromedial nucleus. In the *posterior part* of the hypothalamus we find the *posterior nucleus* close to the ventricular wall, whereas the characteristic *mammillary nucleus* (consisting of several subnuclei) is located in the bottom of the ventricle (Figs. 18.1 and 20.8) The term *mammillary body* is used for the macroscopically visible part of the mammillary nuclei (Figs. 3.12, 3.22, and 18.1). In general, there is a high degree of cooperation among the hypothalamic nuclei, mediated by short intrahypothalamic fibers. Notably, there are numerous reciprocal connections between the medial nuclei and the lateral area (nucleus) of the hypothalamus.

The Connections and Functions of the Hypothalamic Nuclei Have Been Hard to Clarify

Determining the exact connections and functional roles of the various nuclei has proved more difficult in the hypothalamus than in most other parts of the brain. This is partly because the nuclei are so small and are located in a part of the brain that is difficult to reach with experimental manipulations and partly because most of the afferent and efferent fibers are unmyelinated and mixed with fibers destined for other parts of the brain. In particular, lesions or stimulations of the lateral hypothalamic area are bound to affect the medial forebrain bundle and thereby fibers destined for other regions than the hypothalamus. The hypothalamic nuclei furthermore have a rich network of mutual connections, so that, for example, a lesion of one nucleus will interfere with the functioning of several others as well. Modern methods utilizing toxic agents that destroy the cell bodies without affecting fibers of passage have helped to settle some controversies, however. Finally, there are notable species differences regarding both connections and neurotransmitters, and most experimental data have been obtained in rats or cats.

Figure 18.2 *Main afferent connections of the hypothalamus.* Arrows indicate the direction of impulse conduction.

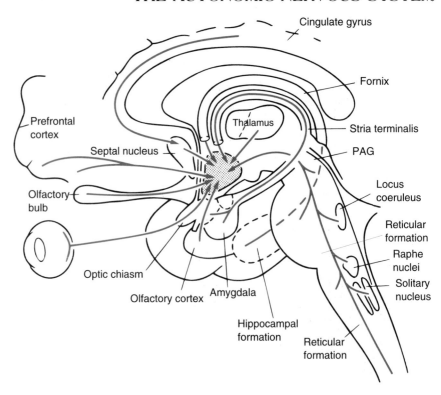

The Hypothalamus Contains Many Neurotransmitters

Numerous neurotransmitter candidates are present in the hypothalamus, as demonstrated with immunocytochemical and biochemical methods. *Acetylcholine, norepinephrine, dopamine, serotonin, histamine*, and many *neuropeptides* are found with a differential distribution among the hypothalamic nuclei. Norepinephrine is among the neurotransmitters found in highest concentration (some of the norepinephrine is related to terminals of fibers from the locus coeruleus). Some of the neuropeptides are involved in the hypothalamic control of the pituitary gland or released to the bloodstream in the pituitary (see below, *The Hypothalamus and the Endocrine System*). The functional role of the various neurotransmitters in the hypothalamus is still incompletely known (as is, indeed, why so many different neurotransmitters are needed in the brain). Several neurotransmitters and neuropeptides are discussed later in this chapter.

Afferent Connections and Other Kinds of Input to the Hypothalamus

Figure 18.2 shows diagrammatically the main afferent connections of the hypothalamus. It is immediately clear that many—perhaps most—parts of the brain are able to influence the hypothalamus! (The mammillary nucleus is in several aspects different from the other hypothalamic nuclei and will be treated separately below.) In addition, the hypothalamus is special since it receives information by *hormones* acting on specific receptors, and *special sensory neurons* that record blood temperature (*ther-

moreceptors) and salt concentration (*osmoreceptors*). These features reflect the functions of the hypothalamus in homeostatic control.

Hypothalamic afferent nerve fibers bring signals from *most kinds of receptors* and also from *higher levels of the brain*, such as the cerebral cortex and the limbic structures. Thus, hypothalamus receives information about olfactory and taste stimuli, the conditions in the gastrointestinal tract, the blood pressure, nociceptor activation, skin temperature, and the intensity of ambient light. The afferent fibers from limbic structures inform about emotional and motivational aspects.

The many groups of *afferents end in at least partially different parts of the hypothalamus*, which fits with physiological evidence that the hypothalamus consists of many functionally different parts (some of these will be discussed later in this chapter). Nevertheless, both the many intrinsic connections and the properties of single cells show that the *various afferent signals are considerably processed and integrated before command signals are sent to the pituitary, autonomic preganglionic neurons, somatic efferent cell groups, and higher levels of the brain.*

More About Afferent Connections

We will treat in some more detail the various afferent hypothalamic connections and the information they may supply.

The *retina* supplies the hypothalamus with visual information (probably unspecific information concerning the total amount of light rather than patterned vision). This information is used to control bodily functions with daily variations (see below, *The Hypothalamus and Circadian Rhythms*). *Olfactory* information reaches the hypothalamus indirectly from regions receiving fibers from the olfactory bulb, such as the amygdala and the olfactory cortex (Fig. 10.1), which send fibers to parts of the hypothalamus (Fig. 18.2). This information is important for sexual behavior (shown in rats) and for autonomic control of digestion. Physiological studies show that *auditory* information can reach the hypothalamus, and the same holds for signals from *cutaneous receptors*. Anatomically, direct fibers have been traced from the *spinal cord* to the hypothalamus. Many such direct fibers arise in lamina I and convey *nociceptive* information, and may contribute to autonomic and endocrine responses to painful stimuli. Most information from the cord reaches the hypothalamus indirectly via the *reticular formation*, however. In that case, the sensory information is presumably highly integrated—that is, not providing specific information about stimulus features. Impulses from visceral organs reach the hypothalamus after synaptic interruption in the solitary nucleus and most likely a further synaptic relay in the reticular formation. Such signals may, for example, inform about the filling of the stomach, which influences the feeling of fullness.

Fibers from the *amygdala* may, as mentioned, convey olfactory information but also signals related to emotions and motivation. The *hippocampal formation* in the medial part of the temporal lobe (another of the limbic structures) sends many fibers in the fornix to end in the hypothalamus. We do not know what information these fibers transmit. Presumably, it is a synthesis of several sensory modalities. The *ventral striatum* sends fibers to the lateral hypothalamus, and the *cingulate gyrus* can act via the septal nuclei. Part of the *orbitofrontal cortex* has direct connections to the hypothalamus, presumably mediating processed information about taste and smell; that is, information that has been interpreted regarding its significance. Sensory signals linked to motivation may also be conveyed to the hypothalamus from the orbitofrontal cortex.

Hormones Act on Hypothalamic Neurons

In addition to receptors for the endogenous neurotransmitters, many hypothalamic cells also contain *receptors for various hormones*, such as for the steroid sex hormones, the thyroid hormones, and for hormones released from the anterior pituitary. Often the hormones act on the brain as part of feedback loops regulating the production of hormones from the pituitary. Hormones also influence other functions of the brain, however.

The sex and thyroid hormones pass the blood–brain barrier easily. The steroid sex hormones bind to intracellular receptors, and thereby influence the activity of hypothalamic cells (and cells in other parts of the brain, particularly in certain limbic structures). Glucocorticoids (from the adrenal cortex) bind to specific receptors in the paraventricular nucleus, among other places. Binding of clucocorticoids elicits behavior with the aim to increase carbohydrate intake in experimental animals.

Some hormones that do not pass the blood–brain barrier easily can nevertheless act on the hypothalamus and certain other brain regions. This is possible because certain regions of the brain close to the ventricles lack a blood–brain barrier (see Chapter 3, *Some Parts of the Brain Lack a Blood–Brain Barrier*), and the neurons in such regions send axons to other parts of the brain. One example is the *subfornical organ*, located below the fornix close to the wall of the third ventricle. The hormone *angiotensin II*, the production of which is increased by a reduction of the blood volume, binds to specific receptors in the subfornical organ. The latter sends axons to the supraoptic and paraventricular hypothalamic nuclei (which produce the antidiuretic hormone). This exemplifies that hormones acting on the hypothalamus (directly or indirectly) provide feedback information of importance for the hypothalamic control of the pituitary gland. Other hormonal actions on the brain are discussed briefly later in this chapter.

Efferent Connections

The efferent connections of the hypothalamus are widespread, enabling this tiny part of the brain to influence the activity of many cell groups at lower as well as higher levels (Fig. 18.3). By its characteristic projection to the *pituitary* the hypothalamus control the production of several hormones (this is discussed in more detail below). In addition, the hypothalamus sends fibers to most of the cell groups from which it receives afferents, such as the *amygdala*, the *septal nuclei*, nuclei of the *reticular formation*, the *PAG*, some of the *cranial nerve nuclei*, and the *spinal cord*. The hypothalamus can also influence the *cerebral cortex*.

Hypothalamic influences on *autonomic processes* such as blood pressure, heart rate, temperature regulation, and digestion are mediated by direct and indirect *descending connections to the preganglionic sympathetic and parasympathetic neurons*. Many hypothalamic neurons send axons to parasympathetic cell groups of the brain stem (such as the dorsal motor nucleus of the vagus) and to the sympathetic neurons of the intermediolateral column of the cord. In addition, effects on these cell groups are mediated via the reticular formation, which receives many afferents from the hypothalamus.

Hypothalamic effects on the *cerebral cortex* occur via direct projections and via the thalamus (this concerns especially the mamillary nucleus, see below). Whereas the mediodorsal thalamic nucleus is unlikely

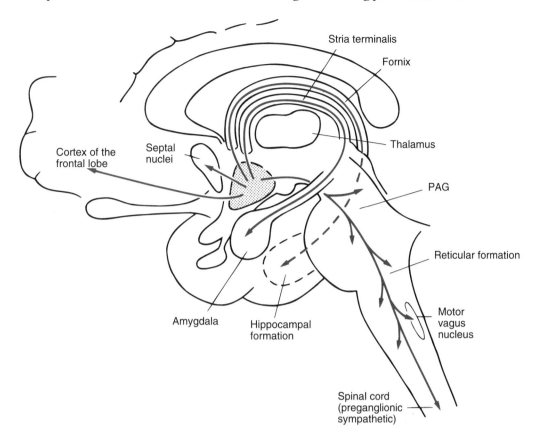

to receive direct hypothalamic afferents, several nuclei mentioned above that receive fibers from the hypothalamus project to the mediodorsal nucleus (such as the amygdala and the septal nuclei). The MD projects to the prefrontal cortex (Fig. 20.7) Direct connections from the hypothalamus pass to the orbitofrontal cortex and temporal associations areas (some

Figure 18.3 *Main efferent connections of the hypothalamus.* The connections to the pituitary gland are not included, nor are the efferent connections of the mammillary nucleus.

The Mammillary Nucleus

Situated most posteriorly in the hypothalamus, the mammillary nucleus differs in several respects from the other nuclei. It consists of several subnuclei and forms the characteristically shaped mammillary bodies (one on each side) at the ventral aspect of the diencephalon (Figs. 3.12, 3.22, 18.1, and 18.4). The subnuclei differ to some extent with regard to connections, although we will disregard such differences here.

Among the *efferent* mammillary connections (Fig. 18.4), the *mammillothalamic tract* is most conspicuous. The fibers, forming a thick bundle, run anteriorly and upward in the wall of the third ventricle to end in the *anterior thalamic nucleus* (Figs. 3.23, 20.7, and 20.8). This nucleus projects to the *cingulate gyrus* (Fig. 18.7). Thus, a major target of the mammillary nucleus is the cerebral cortex. Another large efferent fiber tract descends in the brain stem as the *mammillotegmental tract*. These fibers end primarily in certain nuclei of the mesencephalic and pontine reticular formation.

Most of the *afferent* fibers to the mammillary nucleus originate in the *hippocampal formation* and pass in the *fornix* (Figs. 3.22, 18.4, and 19.2). In humans, the fornix contains more than 1 million axons. In addition, the mammillary nucleus receives afferents from the septal nuclei and some brain stem nuclei.

The mammillary nucleus appears to be an important *link in the signal transmission from structures in the temporal lobe to the cingulate gyrus.* These connections, and thus the mammillary nucleus, may be related to *spatial memory* and orientation in space (see Chapter 19, *Clinical Examples of Amnesia*).

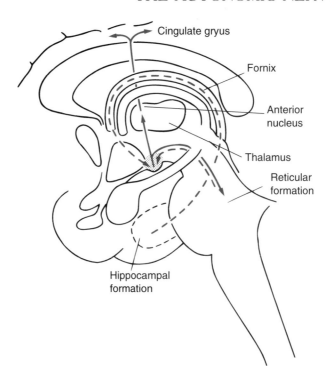

Figure 18.4 *Main connections of the mammillary nucleus.*

of these direct hypothalamic fibers are GABAergic). In addition, a diffusely organized *histaminergic* projection to large parts of the cortex arises in the small *tuberomammillar nucleus*. This projection may be involved with other ascending connections in cortical activation (see Chapter 14 for a discussion of the ascending activating system).

THE HYPOTHALAMUS AND THE ENDOCRINE SYSTEM

The effects of the hypothalamus on organs innervated by the autonomic nervous system can be explained by direct and indirect connections to the preganglionic sympathetic and parasympathetic neurons of the brain stem and the spinal cord. Diseases or lesions affecting the hypothalamus can, however, disturb *functions controlled by the endocrine system*, too, such as sexual functions, growth, and metabolism. Of the endocrine organs, only the adrenal medulla receives an important autonomic innervation. The effects of the hypothalamus on the endocrine organs are explained by the hypothalamic control of the superior endocrine organ, the pituitary. This control concerns both the anterior and posterior parts of the pituitary (Fig. 18.5). Two different pathways are used for the hypothalamo-pituitary interactions. The *posterior pituitary* is reached by a direct neural tract (often referred to as the supraopticohypophysial or the hypothalamohypophysial tract), whereas the *anterior pituitary* is reached by the so-called tuberoinfundibular tract and a special portal vascular system (Fig. 18.5C). We will return to this below.

The *pituitary gland* (the hypophysis) consists of an anterior lobe, the *adenohypophysis*, that is developed from the epithelium of the primitive

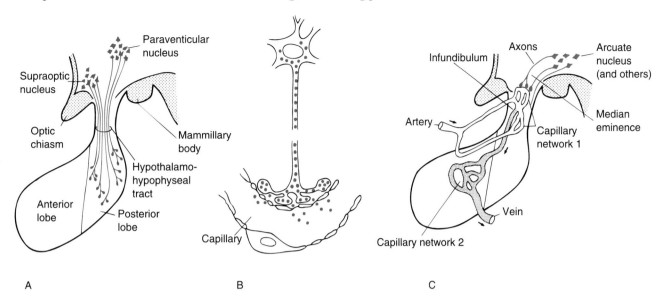

foregut and is built up of clusters of epithelial cells with a rich supply of wide capillaries (sinusoids). The posterior lobe of the pituitary, the *neurohypophysis*, is developed from the neural tube and consists of nerve terminals of fibers from the hypothalamus and a special kind of glial cell, the *pituicytes*.

Figure 18.5 *The relationship between the hypothalamus and the pituitary gland.* **A.** Connections from the hypothalamus to the posterior lobe. **B.** Axonal transport of peptide hormones (neuropeptides) from the hypothalamus to the pituitary. **C.** The portal vessels of the pituitary stalk ensure that releasing hormones (factors) are transported from the median eminence in the upper part of the stalk to the epithelial cells of the anterior lobe.

The Anterior Pituitary Produces Several Hormones

The following hormones are produced and secreted by the epithelial cells of the adenohypophysis:

1. *Growth hormone* (GH) or somatotrophic hormone, which stimulates body growth, particularly growth of long bones;
2. *Thyroid-stimulating hormone* (TSH);
3. *Adrenocorticotrophic hormone* (ACTH), which stimulates the production of steroid hormones, such as cortisol, in the adrenal cortex;[2]
4. Two *gonadotrophic hormones*—one follicle-stimulating hormone (FSH) that promotes the growth of the oocyte and its surrounding follicle cells and one luteinizing hormone (LH) that is necessary for the ovulation and formation of the corpus luteum from the follicle cells; and
5. *Prolactin* (or lactogenic hormone), which stimulates growth of the mammary gland during pregnancy and maintains the milk production during the nursing period.

Various observations indicate that as a rule each hormone is produced by a specific cell type. The cells are named for the hormone they produce, and are called *somatotrophs* (GH), *thyrotrophs* (TSH), *mammotrophs* (prolactin), and so forth. In routine histological sections, however, only three kinds of epithelial cells can be recognized in the anterior pituitary: *acidophils, basophils*, and *chromophobes*. The acidophils produce GH and prolactin, whereas the basophils probably produce the rest. The chromophobes may represent precursors to the acidophils and basophils. It follows that the basophils and the acidophils both are heterogeneous groups, as indeed has been shown with immunocytochemical techniques with antibodies raised against the various hormones.

The Relation between the Hypothalamus and the Posterior Pituitary

Two peptide hormones are released to the bloodstream in the posterior pituitary: *vasopressin* or *antidiuretic hormone* (ADH) and *oxytocin*. Both hormones are synthesized in the hypothalamus and are brought to the pituitary by axonal transport. The thin, unmyelinated axons reaching the posterior lobe (in man, about 100,000) come from two hypothalamic nuclei in the anterior part of the hypothalamus: the *supraoptic nucleus* and the *paraventricular nucleus* (Figs. 18.1 and 18.5A). These two nuclei are quite similar and the hormones are produced in both nuclei, although by different neurons. Most of the hormone-producing cells are large, with large vesicles in their cytoplasm containing precursor molecules of the final hormones. The neurons are collectively termed the *magnocellular neuroendocrine system* (to distinguish them from the parvocellular neuroendocrine system that is discussed below). Even though both ADH and oxytocin are produced in both cell groups, ADH is produced predominantly in the supraoptic nucleus and oxytocin mainly in the paraventricular nucleus. The hormones can also be demonstrated within the axons. The axons end with large boutons in close contact with the fenestrated capillaries of the posterior lobe (Fig. 18.5B). Action potentials reaching the boutons constitute the signal for release of the hormone (just as for the release of neurotransmitter in ordinary nerve cells). The cells of the supraoptic and the paraventricular nucleus are called neurosecretory because they have all the characteristic features of neurons but at the same time release their product to the bloodstream.

The antidiuretic hormone was extracted from the posterior lobe quite early, before the neural connection between the hypothalamus and the posterior lobe had been ascertained. The hormone acts by increasing the water reabsorption in the kidneys—that is, it reduces the urine secretion (the hormone also elicits contraction of vascular smooth-muscle cells, which explains why it is also called vasopressin). It was known that destruction of the posterior lobe leads to a condition called *diabetes insipidus*, which is characterized by daily urine volume of 10–15 liters. Later it was discovered that the disease could be produced also by cutting the pituitary stalk. This was the beginning of a full understanding of the nature of the relationship between the hypothalamus and the pituitary.

The production of ADH varies in accordance with the osmalarity of the blood. Most likely, the cells of the supraoptic nucleus (and in some other nuclei) function as *osmoreceptors*.[3] When the osmotic pressure of the blood increases because of extraordinary loss or reduced intake of fluid (for example, by heavy sweating, diarrhea, or vomiting), the cells of the supraoptic nucleus are excited and increase the frequency of their action potentials, thus releasing more ADH into the bloodstream. This results in reduced urine volume (the urine becomes more concentrated). At the same time the synthesis of the hormone is increased. Even a salty meal is enough to stimulate the osmoreceptors. The hypothalamus is thus a control center for the body's "housekeeping" of water. Diabetes insipidus, mentioned above, also occurs as an inherited disease. Such patients have pronounced cell loss in the supraoptic and paraventricular nuclei.

Oxytocin elicits contraction of the smooth-muscle cells in the wall of the *uterus* and thus plays a role during delivery. It also produces contraction of the smooth-muscle cells (myoepithelial cells) of the *mammary gland*, thereby assisting in emptying the breast. When the infant suckles, sensory impulses travel from the nipple (through the spinal nerves) to the cord and further to the hypothalamus, where the neurons of the paraventricular nucleus are influenced. Increased firing frequency leads to increased secretion of oxytocin to the bloodstream, and the hormone reaches the mammary gland in seconds. This is called the *milk ejection reflex.* It is special in that only the afferent link is neural, the efferent link being humoral. Although oxytocin is present in males, its function is so far unknown.

The Influence of the Hypothalamus on the Anterior Pituitary: The Hypophyseal Portal System

It has long been known that diseases affecting the hypothalamus can be accompanied by altered growth, metabolism, and sexual functions—processes that are controlled by hormones produced in the anterior pituitary (adenohypophysis). There are, however, no axonal connections from the hypothalamus to the anterior lobe. Thus, mechanisms other than those concerning the posterior lobe must be responsible for the influence of the hypothalamus on the anterior lobe. The discovery of a *special vascular arrangement in the infundibulum* (stalk) of the pituitary—the *hypophyseal portal system*—was a breakthrough in this respect (Fig. 18.5C). Most of the arteries reaching the anterior pituitary do not branch into capillaries among the epithelial cells but continue upward in the stalk (some arteries enter this directly). In the upper part of the stalk, they form wide capillaries (sinusoids) that finally collect into large veins. These *hypophyseal portal veins* course back to the anterior lobe, where they form a new set of sinusoids among the epithelial cells. From these sinusoids the blood is collected in veins that leave the pituitary. *The blood in the sinusoids of the anterior lobe has first been through a capillary net in the stalk of the pituitary.* Thus, substances can be transported from the stalk to the anterior lobe. Numerous thin axons from the hypothalamus end in the uppermost part of the hypophyseal stalk. This region is called the *median eminence* (Fig. 18.5). The fibers of the tuberoinfundibular tract end in contact with the capillaries in the median eminence. These fibers transport peptides from their parent cell bodies (axonal transport) and release them into the hypophyseal portal system. From the capillaries in the median eminence, the peptides are brought by the blood to the second capillary network among the epithelial cells of the anterior lobe.

The neurons sending axons to the median eminence lie mainly close to the wall of the the third ventricle (periventricularly). The neurons are relatively small and they are therefore collectively termed the *parvocellular neuroendocrine system* (to distinguish them from the magnocellular system). Many of the neurons are found in the *arcuate nucleus* (Fig. 18.1).

Most of the peptides transported by the portal system cause hormonal secretion from the epithelial cells of the anterior lobe and are therefore called *releasing factors or hormones*. One releasing hormone acts preferentially (but not only) on one kind of cells in the anterior pituitary and thus produces secretion of mainly one hormone. Some peptides transported in the tuberoinfundibular tract have an inhibitory effect on the secretion of anterior lobe hormones and are called *inhibitory factors or hormones*. Most of the neurons of the parvocellular system release more than one peptide, however. The neurons may therefore have several different actions on the anterior pituitary. Although thus *peptides are colocalized* in the neurons, hormones in the bloodstream from the anterior pituitary and neurons in other parts of the nervous system can influence which peptide is preferentially secreted. Thus, the interplay between the hypothalamus and the endocrine system is indeed complex.

Several of the peptides involved in the control of the pituitary are found also in neurons in other parts of the brain, where they are released at conventional synapses. Examples are somatostatin (inhibits the release of GH), thyrotropin-releasing hormone (TRH), and corticotropin-releasing hormone (CRH). Thus, these peptides function as releasing hormones at one site and as neurotransmitters at another. This serves to emphasize the futility of assigning one function to each peptide.

More About Some Releasing Hormones

As mentioned above, the hormone that stimulates the synthesis and secretion of ACTH is called *CRH* or CRF (corticotrophin-releasing hormone or factor). In humans, neurons producing CRH are mainly found in a particular small-celled subdivision of the *paraventricular nucleus*. ACTH stimulates the secretion of *glucocorticoids* from the adrenal cortex, and such secretion is an important response to stress (see below). Besides multifarious metabolic effects, the glucocorticoids act on the anterior pituitary and the hypothalamus to inhibit the synthesis and release of ACTH and CRH (negative feedback). The neurons containing CRH have been shown immunocytochemically to contain several other peptides (among them vasopressin and enkephalin). Thus, the CRH neurons may have functions besides the control of ACTH.

Growth hormone-releasing hormone (GRH) is found mainly in the arcuate nucleus, which sends it efferents to the median eminence. The peptide *somatostatin*, which inhibits the release of the growth hormone, is present in neurons of the arcuate nucleus but in addition in many other cell groups that do not project to the median eminence. *Prolactin* is also controlled by two hypothalamic peptides, the stimulating prolactin-releasing hormone (PRH) and *dopamine* (also called prolactin release-inhibiting hormone, PIF). Hypothalamic neurons containing dopamine are mainly in two small paraventricular cell groups and in the supraoptic nucleus.

We do not know why some pituitary hormones are controlled by two hypothalamic peptides with opposite effects, while others are controlled by only one.

FUNCTIONAL ASPECTS

The above account of its connections suggests that the hypothalamus functions as a coordinator of information of many different kinds, particularly pertaining to homeostasis and "bodily maintenance." The hypothalamus contains cell groups that serve as control centers for several autonomic functions, such as blood pressure, body temperature, water balance, metabolism, digestion, and reproduction. Furthermore, the rhythmic variations of several bodily processes are governed by the hypothalamus. For each of the mentioned broad functional categories, the hypothalamus *serves to coordinate endocrine, autonomic, and somatic motor responses into appropriate behavior.*

Hypothalamic "Centers"

Even though the hypothalamus contains some well-defined nuclei, it is not possible to localize any of the functional centers mentioned above to one specific nucleus. The centers must be imagined as rather extensive networks of mutually interconnected hypothalamic cell groups. This agrees with the observation that many of the autonomic processes influenced by the hypothalamus are not controlled independently. Some factors, such as the diameter of the vessels, are of importance in several different processes, such as temperature regulation and control of blood pressure. Complex behavior, such as that necessary for feeding and drinking, depends on the integrity of both medial and lateral hypothalamic areas, even though subregions play different roles. Early studies with fairly crude methods—often destroying passing fibers from other nuclei in addition to parts of the hypothalamus—lead to incorrect identification of hypothalamic centers, and misconceptions regarding the independence of hypothalamic control functions. The altered view on hypothalamic "centers" parallels the change of view during the last 20–30 years on the existence of functional centers of the brain in general. Rather than focusing on individual cell groups as responsible (centers) for complex functions, we now emphasize how many cell groups contribute to execution of most tasks. When we nevertheless sometimes use the term center for convenience, the reader should realize its limited explanatory value. We have, for example, not explained how the central nervous system controls micturition by placing a "micturition center" in the pons.

Before discussing more specifically some main functions of the hypothalamus, we mention a rough functional subdivision based on early lesion experiments: the anterior parts of the hypothalamus are concerned with predominantly parasympathetic effects, whereas the posterior parts are more involved in functions carried out by the sympathetic system.

Control of Body Temperature

The hypothalamus receives information about ambient temperature from *thermoreceptors* in the skin. It initiates in response measures to increase heat production or heat loss. This is not suffcient, however, since the superior goal is to keep the *core temperature* constant (that is, in deep parts of the body)—not the skin temperature that may vary considerably, as we know from everyday experience. To be able to control the core temperature, the hypothalamus must also be informed about the blood temperature in central parts of the body. As mentioned above, some neurons in the anterior hypothalamus are temperature-sensitive. Accordingly, when the blood flowing through the anterior part of the hypothalamus is warmed, an experimental animal shows signs of increased heat loss. Cats, for example, pant and sweat through the paws. In humans skin vasodilatation (redness and warmth) and sweating occurs. If these parts of the hypothalamus are destroyed (on both sides), the animal no longer reacts to a rise in ambient temperature. The body temperature therefore rises. When, on the other hand, the posterior parts of the hypothalamus are destroyed, the animal no longer reacts with shivering and vasoconstriction to a fall in ambient temperature. Therefore, the body temperature drops (the vasoconstriction reduces heat loss, and the shivering increases heat production). This exemplifies how the hypothalamus coordinates autonomic (vasoconstriction) and somatic (shivering) responses. These and

Fever

Fever arises when the set point of the hypothalamic thermostat is altered. If the set point is changed to, for example, 39° C the normal body temperature is judged to be too low and measures to conserve and produce heat are started (skin vasoconstriction, shivering, curling up, putting on more clothes). The person feels cold while the temperature is below the new set point. Fever has most likely evolved as a defensive response, improving survival from infections (although fever is sometimes harmful).

Fever can be caused (indirectly) by lipopolysaccarides, called *pyrogens* from bacterial membranes, or by simple tissue injury leading to inflammation (for example, fever after severe sunburn). In any case, cytokines (interleukin-1β, interleukin-6, and probably others), which are mediators of immune cells, appear to be crucial for altering the set point of the hypothalamic thermostat. Thus, cytokines have been found in tissue fluid from the anterior hypothalamus in experimental animals with fever, and preventing their accumulation prevents fever. It is not clear, however, how these substances reach the hypothalamus. Thus, contrary to earlier beliefs, they most likely do not enter the hypothalamus from the blood stream. One possibility is that cytokines in the blood bind specifically in regions lacking a blood–brain barrier, such as the subfornical organ, and stimulate glial cells there to produce cytokines and *prostaglandins*. The latter substance is shown to increase the activity of cold-sensitive neurons and inhibit warm-sensitive ones. Furthermore, drugs that reduce fever (antipyretics), such as aspirin, inhibit the synthesis of prostaglandins. In addition, experimental evidence suggests that local hypothalamic production of cytokines can be induced by sensory *impulses in peripheral nerves*. Thus, circulating pyrogens from bacteria can induce production of cytokines in visceral organs (for example, in the liver), thereby activating the vagus nerve. The afferent signals arriving in the vagus are then transmitted to the hypothalamus (presumably via the solitary nucleus) and induce production of cytokines. These two mechanisms may not be mutually exclusive. It seems likely that several mechanisms may operate in concert to produce fever, although the overall picture is not yet clear.

Local adaptations in the hypothalamus ensure that the fever does not reach dangerous levels (*antipyresis*). Thus, cytokines activate neurons in the paraventricular nucleus producing CRH and vasopressin. As discussed above, CRH release leads to increased blood level of cortisol. This would reduce the peripheral production of cytokines and by that reduce the fever. Furthermore, fibers from the paraventricular nucleus release vasopressin in the septal nuclei. Experimental infusion of vasopressin in the septal nuclei suppresses almost completely the febrile response to intravenous injection of pyrogens. It appears most likely that the septal nuclei act back via septohypothalamic fibers to cancel the effect of cytokines on the thermostat.

other observations suggest that *neuronal groups in the anterior part of the hypothalamus are necessary for the coordination of the processes ensuring that the body temperature does not rise above normal levels (increasing heat loss), whereas the posterior parts contain neurons necessary for heat conservation.* Together, these parts function as a thermostat that tries to keep the body temperature as close as possible to a *set point* of 37° C. If the temperature drops below the set point, the "heater" is turned on, that is, measures are started to conserve heat (skin vasoconstriction, putting on more clothes) and if necessary increase heat production (shivering, or voluntary muscular activity).

In humans, abnormal rise in the body temperature, *hyperthermia*, can be produced by diseases affecting the hypothalamus or by an inadvertent lesion during surgery. Occasionally, hyperthermia occurs during general anesthesia.

Digestion and Feeding

Various metabolic processes are controlled by the hypothalamus. For example, lesions of certain parts can produce *abnormal fat deposition*, both in experimental animals and in humans. The gastrointestinal tract is influenced by the hypothalamus. Lesions can produce *ulcers of the mucous membranes* and bleeding in the stomach and the small intestine. Stimulation of the hypothalamus can elicit increased secretion of gastric juice and strengthening of peristaltic movements. Even though the intestinal changes are not identical after hypothalamic lesions in experimental animals and in humans with gastric and duodenal ulcers, it seems likely that the hypothalamus may be involved in the development of the latter.

Not only the digestive processes but also *feeding behavior* is controlled from the hypothalamus. Early stimulation and lesion experiments indicated that the lateral hypothalamic area can induce increased eating (or behavior directed at acquiring food), whereas the medial parts (especially the *ventromedial nucleus*) reduce eating (induce satiety). Further studies have shown that, although essentially correct, this scheme is too simple. The inputs to the hypothalamic "feeding" centers are multifarious, as witnessed by data from animal experiments, and by everyday experiences of the numerous factors that influence human feeding behavior. It is nevertheless remarkable how most people maintain their body weight over many years, although even the smallest daily surplus of food would cause a steady weight gain. The hypothalamic centers governing food intake are thought to operate as a homeostat.[4] Feedback loops ensure that the food intake oscillates around a set point. Overeating is automatically followed by reduced consumption. Of course, psychological factors—or occasionally, hypothalamic disease—may disturb this finely tuned control mechanism. The many connections between the hypothalamus and the cerebral cortex, the amygdala, and other limbic structures tell us that the hypothalamus does not function as an independent center. Rather, it is an organizer for motivated behavior related to digestion and feeding. Whether such behavior occurs is determined by other regions than the hypothalamus.

Neuropeptide Y and Energy Metabolism

Several transmitters are involved in the hypothalamic control of feeding behavior, although much remains before their mutual roles are clarified. One interesting neurotransmitter is NPY that is found in high concentration in nerve terminals in the paraventricular nucleus. Most of the NPY-containing terminals come from the arcuate nucleus. Injection of NPY near the paraventricular nucleus increases food intake in experimental animals. Furthermore, it decreases the metabolism in brown fat and increases fat storage in ordinary, fat tissue. This leads to a larger weight gain than expected from the food intake. The NPY-containing connections to the paraventricular nucleus might therefore regulate the energy balance of the body by controlling both appetite and metabolism. How NPY release in the hypothalamus produces this is not known, although some effects may be mediated by projections from the paraventricular nucleus to sympathetic preganglionic cell groups. The hormone *insulin* may act as one of several feedback signals to the arcuate nucleus from the periphery, informing about the energy status of the body. Thus, hypothalamic injection of insulin reduces the food intake in normal rats (but not in rats with genetically determined obesity). In addition, glucose-sensitive hypothalamic neurons are likely to be involved in the control of appetite (cf. the feeling of hunger when the blood glucose is low). Experiments suggest, however, that other feedback signals must be involved as well. One interesting candidate is called *leptin*. This is a small protein poduced by fat cells. It inhibits NPY release in the hypothalamus—probably by acting in the arcuate nucleus—and might thus serve as a feedback signal to reduce feeding. Mice with mutation in the gene coding for leptin (the *ob* gene) become obese, whereas normal mice reduce eating when given leptin. One study comparing serum concentrations of leptin in normal and obese people suggests that most obese people are insensitive to endogenous leptin production.

NPY is involved in other hypothalamic tasks, such as control of *circadian rhythms* (see below), and secretion of *releasing hormones*. It is often colocalized with cathecolamines, GABA, or somatostatin. Finally, NPY is also found in the amygdala where it is involved in stress reactions (having an anxiolytic effect). Obviously, each of the numerous transmitters present in the hypothalamus may be expected to participate in quite diverse functions.

The Hypothalamus and Sleep

Lesions of the hypothalamus in experimental animals and in humans are often accompanied by sleep disturbances, sometimes as an abnormal amount of sleep and sometimes as insomnia or disturbed sleep rhythm. Experimental evidence has led to the assumption that a "sleep center" exists in the anterior part of the hypothalamus and a "waking center" in the posterior part. Conditions are probably much less schematic, however. Our knowledge of the role of the reticular formation in sleep mechanisms (see Chapter 15, *Sleep*) has altered the interpretation of the experiments mentioned above. Thus, the "waking center" in the posterior hypothalamus coincides with regions known to produce an activating effect on the cortex and may not be a part of the hypothalamus. Stimulation of this region produces changes in the EEG and in behaviors that are characteristic for the awake state.

The Hypothalamus and Circadian Rhythms

The hypothalamus plays a role as a pacemaker for several functions showing a cyclic variation. Light stimuli from the retina (varying with length of the light/dark cycle) (Fig. 18.2) appear to be of particular importance for the set of such *circadian* rhythms. The pacemaker capacity appears to be inborn, however. Thus, in rats, rhythmic activity occurs in some hypothalamic cell groups in late embryonic life.

The retinohypothalamic fibers end in the SCN. Lesions of this nucleus disturb (but do not necessarily abolish) the cyclic variations of body temperature, blood level of steroid hormones from the adrenal cortex, and sexual functions. The SCN has connections with several other parts of the hypothalamus, which enable it to *synchronize* the various functions mentioned above (and other functions as well). *GABA* (colocalized with VIP and vasopressin) is most likely the transmitter used by most SCN neurons.

The *biologic significance* of the cyclic variations of bodily functions is to adapt the level of activity to the most stable and predictable variations in the environment. For example, in humans it seems appropriate that most bodily functions are at their lowest level during the night, whereas animals hunting at night would need a different activity profile. Persons staying in environments without any information about the time of the day develop a rhythm with cycles slightly longer than 24 hours.

Not all data fit with the SCN being the *only* synchronizer of biologic rhythms, however. For example, sleep rhythm and body temperature variations are desynchronized in persons deprived of time information.

See Chapter 3, *The Epithalamus and the Pineal Gland* where the effects of the SCN on the pineal gland, and the hormone melatonin are discussed.

Hypothalamus, Sexual Functions, and Sex Differences

The efferent connections of the hypothalamus also enable it to influence sexual behavior—that is, to start and coordinate the autonomic, endocrine, and somatic motor components. This is verified by many animal experiments. For example, injection of the female sex hormone estradiol in the ventromedial hypothalamic nucleus in castrated male rats elicits copulatory behavior. Lesions of the ventromedial hypothalamic nucleus in female rats reduce their sexual activity.

We have little precise knowledge of *how* the hypothalamus controls sexual functions, however. One among many relevant pathways passes from the paraventricular nucleus directly to spinal motoneurons innervating the bulbocavernosus muscle. This muscle, which is important during ejaculation, is large in male rats but tiny in females. Correspondingly, the descending pathway mentioned above is absent in female rats.

A nucleus called the *intermediate nucleus of the anterior hypothalamus* (INHA-1) is about twice as large in men as in women (the nucleus is found between the supraoptic and the paraventricular nuclei). This example of *sexual dimorphism* arises at the age of four by a neuronal loss in girls, whereas the cell number remains constant in boys.

As discussed above, the hypothalamus controls sexual functions also by its actions on the pituitary and its secretion of *gonadotrophic hormones*. The gonadal sex hormones act on the hypothalamus and other parts of the brain and can therefore influence sexual behavior. As shown in rats and monkeys, transient exposure to small amounts of sex hormones during early development determines later sexual identity and behavior.

THE HYPOTHALAMUS AND THE IMMUNE SYSTEM

Effects of the Nervous System on the Immune System

The relationship between the nervous system and the immune system has attracted increasing attention recently. This topic is important in several respects, for example, regarding the interactions between mental and bodily processes. Besides many anecdotal reports of somatic diseases that start at times of mental stress and imbalance, there is growing experimental evidence of hypothalamic influence on the immune system. This concerns, for example, the activity of *natural-killer cells* and *lymphocytes*. Furthermore, antigen stimulation appears to increase activity among certain hypothalamic cell groups. This also suggests that the hypothalamus be in some way involved in the defense against infections. Other studies show altered T-lymphocyte numbers in deeply depressed patients. How these interactions come about is not fully understood, and findings in this field are partly contradictory.

The nervous system can influence the immune system in two ways: one via the *endocrine system*, the other via *sympathetic innervation* of the lymphoid organs. The endocrine influence is primarily mediated by ACTH and secretion of clucocorticoids from the adrenal cortex. The inhibiting effects of the clucocorticoids on inflammation and resistance to infections are well known. Long-lasting stress with increased ACTH secretion might cause increased vulnerability to infections, allergy, autoimmunity, and other diseases.

The bone marrow, thymus, spleen, lymph nodes, and gut-associated lymphoid tissue all receive innervation by sympathetic postganglionic fibers. The innervation density is highest in T-lymphocyte areas. Lymphocytes express β-adrenergic receptors, and varicosities of sympathetic fibers are found close to lymphocytes. Chemical denervation of lymphoid organs causes, among other effects, reduced T-lymphocyte activity. Although we know little of the functional significance, the autonomic system is thus able to modulate the properties of the immune system.

Effects of the Immune System on the Nervous System

We deal with immune reactions *in* the central nervous system in Chapter 1, as part of defense mechanisms. However, the immune system can also influence normal nervous processes. One example is that cytokines from leukocytes cause *fever*, as discussed above. Furthermore, it seems highly likely that typical symptoms in infectious diseases like *drowsiness* and *loss of appetite* (anorexia) are caused by indirect action of cytokines on the hypothalamus.

Cytokines can also cause ACTH secretion from the anterior pituitary via the hypothalamus. Although the exact chain of events is unknown, we know that interleukin 1 (a cytokin) affects neurons in the solitary nucleus (Fig. 16.2), which project to the paraventricular nucleus in the hypothalamus (Fig. 18.1). There the release of CRH may be increased, with subsequent secretion of ACTH and clucocorticoids.

THE HYPOTHALAMUS AND MENTAL FUNCTIONS

Psychosomatic Interrelations

The relationship between the hypothalamus and the pituitary discussed above helps explain why diseases affecting the hypothalamus can produce alterations of hormonal secretion from the pituitary itself, the thyroid, the adrenal cortex, and the gonads. But it also helps in explaining the relationship between mental and bodily processes—what are called *psychosomatic interrelations*. Thus, the hypothalamus receives afferents from many parts of the brain, among them the cerebral cortex and the limbic structures, which are closely related to what we term mental or psychic functions. Furthermore, the hypothalamus has access to bodily processes through its connections with the peripheral parts of the autonomic nervous system. In short, *our mental state can produce alterations of endocrine organs and of autonomically innervated organs by acting on the hypothalamus*. Not all such effects are mediated via the hypothalamus, however. Thus, the autonomic and somatic cell groups of the reticular formation are accessed also by fibers from the cerebral cortex and limbic structures.

We will describe a few examples of psychosomatic interrelations. Women may lose their menstruation for some time after psychic stress (loss of a close person, dissatisfaction, depression, and so forth). The mechanism is apparently reduced secretion of gonadotrophic hormones from the pituitary. When subjected to bodily stress (such as infections, trauma, intoxications, and major surgery), the organism responds by, among other things, increasing the secretion of corticosteroids. The same response can also be produced by mental stress by causing increased secretion of releasing hormones from the hypothalamus, which in turn increases the secretion of ACTH from the anterior pituitary. In experimental animals, this hormonal response to mental stress is prevented by transection of the stalk of the pituitary. Functions controlled by the posterior pituitary (such as urinary volume) can be influenced by our mental state. A particularly striking example is that of a woman breast-feeding her baby, who can cause the milk to trickle from the nipples just by thinking of the child. The inner image of the child in some way influences the hypothalamus, with an increase of oxytocin secretion as the result. This reaches the mammary glands and makes the smooth muscles contract (milk ejection reflex).

Psychosomatic Disorders

A *psychosomatic disorder* (syndrome) can be defined as a condition in which psychological processes play a substantial role for the production of the somatic symptoms. Broadly speaking, it is thought that *endocrine and autonomic responses to psychic challenges that are adaptive when of short duration, may cause somatic disease if they persist for months and years.* From what we have discussed in this chapter, it seems likely that the hypothalamus is central in development of psychosomatic diseases, that is, as a link between psychic processes and altered bodily functions. As one might imagine, such causative relations are usually hard to establish with certainty, and there is probably no clear distinction between somatic diseases caused by psychological factors and diseases affecting primarily somatic structures. As discussed in relation to the placebo phenomenon (Chapter 7), all disease processes are more or less influenced by the mental attitude and expectations of the patient, while any somatic disease will lead to psychological reactions. In some conditions, such as irritable bowel syndrome, fibromyalgia, chronic fatigue syndrome, dyspepsia without an ulcer, and noncardiac chest pain, the influences of psychic factors are thought to be important and sometimes decisive, although we cannot explain the causative relationships. In other diseases, like gastric ulcers, coronary disease, asthma, and diabetes there is good evidence that psychic stress can increase the *vulnerability* (that is, the risk of developing the disease), without being a main causative factor. Furthermore, in such diseases, which are typically due to the interaction of many risk factors, individuals probably vary as to the importance of each risk factor.

Stress and Stress Reactions

Used in the present context, stress can be physical or psychological. A common definition is *something perceived by the individual as a threat to the homeostasis of the organism.* Besides in cases of extreme physical stress, the crucial point is *how* the challenge or extra demand is perceived—not the stress by itself. Although the word stress in common language denotes something that is bad for the health, extra demands on our physical or mental performance are inevitable and usually not harmful. On the contrary, without challenges to the *status quo*, there would be no development, no learning, and no improvement of adaptive behavior.

The coordinated sum of endocrine, autonomic, and somatic responses to stress is termed a *stress reaction*. Stress reactions are commonly assessed by measuring the blood level of *epinephrine* (activation of the sympathetic system) and of cortisol (activation of the hypothalamic-pituitary-adrenal axis). The function of the stress reaction is to maintain *homeostasis* in a wide sense, and it can be initiated by the stressful event itself or by the expectation of it. The hypothalamus obviously plays a central role in our ability to cope with stressful events; that is, the *stress reactions are largely expressed though the hypothalamic influences on the endocrine, autonomic, and somatic effector systems.*

The stress reaction should not be seen as an isolated phenomenon but rather as a part of bodily expressions of *arousal* (arousal was discussed in Chapter 15). In this perspective, *stress is a stimulus that increases arousal* (with changes of the EEG, attention, muscle tone, respiration, selective autonomic activation, and activation of the CRH-ACTH-glucocorticoid reaction chain).

The purposefulness of the stress reaction is most obvious with physical stress, such as situations demanding extreme endurance or force, or with injuries causing rapid blood loss. However, stress reactions are also adaptive and beneficial before and during extra mental demands such as examinations, performances, or novel situations. Overall, stress reactions are adaptive when they improve our ability to cope with the extra demands. Lack of corticosteroid hormones due to disease of the adrenals (Addison's disease), for example, greatly reduces our ability to tackle even minor challenges to homeostasis. The stress reaction becomes potentially disease-provoking only when it by far outlasts the actual stressful situation (with, among other things, persistently elevated level of "stress hormones").

When talking of stress causing disease, we usually mean psychic stress, and such that lasts for months or years. Whereas serious physical stress produces a stress reaction that is uniform among individuals, the individual variations are larger to psychic stress. Thus, the decisive factor is the *subjective perception and interpretation of the situation.* This depends on many conditions, such as prior experiences and how they were tackled (especially during early childhood). Among psychological stress factors (stressors), the *feeling of loss of control* is probably the most important. Closely related to this is *unpredictability* of a situation. Animal experiments show that stress reactions to painful stimuli are reduced if the stimulus is preceded by a warning signal. Perhaps this is because not knowing when the stimulus occurs requires constant arousal, whereas the warning enables the animal to relax (reduce arousal) between the stressful events.

The importance of the feeling of control is exemplified by the fact that humans with chronic pain reduce their consumption of analgetic drugs if they can decide themselves when to take the drug, rather than having to ask another person. Another important factor determining the level of psychic stress is the possibility of obtaining an *outlet for frustration*, for example with physical exercise. Finally, animal experiments support that *social attachments* reduce psychic stress.

Bodily Processes May Influence Psychic Ones

Such interactions are especially clear with regard to the *hormonal effects on the brain*. For example, increased production of *thyroid hormones* changes the mental state toward excitement, increased initiative, and lively associations, whereas reduced production leads to apathy, fatigue, and increased need of sleep. Many patients with a thyroid disease have been misdiagnosed as suffering from a mental disorder. Treatment with *corticosteroids* (as used, for example, with certain kinds of cancer) often elevates the mood (euphoria), making the patient appear unduly cheerful and unconcerned. The changes of mood often associated with the menstrual cycle in women (*premenstrual syndrome*) are probably caused, at least in part, by effects of female sex hormones on the brain. Thus, a high density of receptors for sex hormones has been demonstrated in various parts of the brain. This concerns in particular certain cell groups in the hypothalamus and the amygdala, but also neurons in other parts such as the cerebral cortex can bind sex hormones. It seems likely, therefore, that the excitability of many neuronal groups can be influenced by circulating hormones (steroid hormones pass the blood–brain barrier easily). In cats, heat behavior may be produced by implantation of female sex hormones in the posterior part of the hypothalamus. Many other experiments give further evidence that animal behavior can be influenced considerably by circulating hormones, presumably by their actions on the brain. The male sex hormone *testosterone* can produce male sexual identification and behavior when given to monkeys at an early stage of their development, regardless of the sex of the monkey. Thus, a female monkey may later behave like a male if given a small amount of testosterone for a period shortly after birth.

The Hypothalamus and Emotions

The hypothalamus is among the parts of the brain most directly involved in the expression of emotions or *emotional reactions* (in an experimental context, emotional reactions can be defined as behavior in response to stimuli producing sensations with an emotional coloring). This agrees well with the fact that the hypothalamus functions as a superior center for control of autonomic processes. Emotions are expressed, as we know from everyday experience, to a large extent through changes of the functions of autonomically innervated organs, such as palpitations, dryness of the mouth, fainting, blushing, paling, alterations of the digestive tract, sweating, frequent micturition, and so forth. In addition, emotions are witnessed by automatic movements, such as rapid, superficial breathing, facial expressions, and postures. Such movements, which are organized by brainstem premotor networks, are probably influenced from the hypothalamus (cf. the emotional smile and facial palsy, Chapter 16, *Facial Expressions of Emotion Do Not Depend on the Integrity of the Pyramidal Tract*).

So-called sham rage can be provoked in cats and dogs in which the whole cerebral cortex, the basal ganglia, and large parts of the thalamus have been removed. Since only the hypothalamus is connected with the brain stem in such animals, their expression of rage must depend on the hypothalamus. Such animals react much like normal animals to painful stimuli, with biting, scratching, snarling, and increased ventilation. Since the whole cortex is removed, it is unlikely that true emotions are experienced, however. It seems reasonable to conclude that the hypothalamus contains cell groups that coordinate and put into action the behavior expressing the rage. The rage of such "hypothalamic" animals is, in contrast to normal animals, not directed toward anything in particular; they seem to lack the ability to know the nature and the location of the stimulus provoking the pain (as one might expect in an animal lacking the cerebral cortex and most of the thalamus). Furthermore, the expression of the rage dies out very quickly after the stimulus is over, whereas the reactions continue for a while in normal animals (as in humans). This observation also suggests that other parts of the brain normally act on the hypothalamus when emotional reactions are produced, as we discuss in Chapter 19 (*The Amygdala Emotions, and Behavior*).

The above account indicates that to regard the hypothalamus as the locus of the emotions would be an impermissible oversimplification. Rather, the *hypothalamus is a superior center for the integration and coordination of emotional reactions*. This conclusion is supported by some observations in humans. During brain surgery with local anesthesia, pressure on or traction of the hypothalamic region can elicit reactions of panic, crying, laughter, or profuse talking. The patients sometimes, however, report a change of mood, such as depression or euphoria. It thus appears that the activity of the hypothalamus is not only of significance for emotional reactions but also in some way for the emotions themselves (perhaps mediated by connections back to the limbic structures and the cerebral cortex from the hypothalamus).

Emotions and Emotional Reactions

When discussing the relations between the hypothalamus and emotions, one must distinguish the emotions themselves from the emotional reactions—that is, the behavior expressing our emotions. We can experience the feelings or emotions only subjectively. Of course, we may learn that certain external stimuli or situations usually produce certain emotions in other people, but such correlations can only be tentative because so many psychological individual variations play a role. We cannot obtain information from animals about their emotions. The emotional reactions, however, can be directly observed and are often more reliable in animals than in humans. Factors such as upbringing, social conventions, and rational considerations determine to a large extent the emotional reactions in humans. That emotions in animals can only be inferred indirectly from their behavior explains why it is not quite clear how many basic emotions animals have. Commonly, however, only three basic emotions are identified (in cats, dogs, and monkeys): rage, fear, and pleasure (love). Even though the emotions of animals certainly are less schematic than this, there is no doubt that the emotions of humans have much more variation and nuances. This should be kept in mind when drawing conclusions with regard to emotions and psychosomatic interactions in humans on the basis of animal experiments. The anthropologist Paul Ekman identifies seven basic emotions in humans, based on their relation to culture-independent facial expressions: *happiness, sadness, anger, fear, disgust, surprise, and contempt.*

NOTES

1. The *suprachiasmatic nucleus* cannot be identified in ordinary Nissl-stained sections in contrast to the supraoptic and paraventricular nuclei. It is clearly visible, however, by use of immunocytochemical identification of several neuropeptides (vasopressin, VIP, neuropeptide Y, and neurotensin).

2. The hormone ACTH is synthesized from a large precursor protein called pro-opiomelanocortin or pro-ACTH/endorphin. This precursor molecule is cleaved into other peptides, notably β-lipotropin (β-LPH) with a yet-unsettled function, and β-endorphin, which is a potent opioid peptide with inhibitory actions on pain transmission. The functional role of the β-endorphin secreted from the pituitary is not clear, however. β-Endorphin is also found in a hypothalamic nucleus (the *arcuate nucleus*) with projections to brain stem nuclei of importance for pain transmission (see Chapter 7).

3. The ADH secretion is also influenced by other factors, although in primates these appear to be much less potent than changes of osmolarity. For example, reduced blood volume leads concentration of angiotensin II in the bloodstream, which in turn affects the supraoptic and paraventricular nuclei via the subfornical organ. Ethanol reduces the secretion of ADH, thereby increasing urine production.

4. *Homeostat*: a system maintaining a steady state by internal processes. A thermostat is thus a homeostat to keep a constant temperature.

PART VI

THE CEREBRAL CORTEX AND LIMBIC STRUCTURES

This part of the book deals with the cerebral cortex and parts of the forebrain closely associated with the cortex with regard to both development and connections. The cerebral cortex can be divided into two parts (without definite delimitations) on the basis of phylogenetic development: the *neocortex*, which is the most recent part and comprises most of the cortex in higher mammals, and the *allocortex*, which is the oldest part. The nomenclature used for the oldest part of the cortex varies, but usually the term allocortex is used for the parts of the cortical mantle with a simple, often only three-layered structure instead of the six layers that are typical of the neocortex. In reptiles the allocortex constitutes what little cortex there is. In humans the neocortex has completely outgrown the allocortex, which forms only a ring of varying thickness at the medial aspect of the hemispheres, encircling the corpus callosum and the brain stem (Fig. 19.1). In addition to the fact that the structure of the allocortex is simpler than that of the neocortex, there are other differences as well. The neocortex develops in parallel with the thalamus and receives most of its subcortical afferents from the thalamus, whereas the allocortex receives afferents from several other subcortical nuclei. Together, these nuclei and the allocortex are commonly said to comprise the so-called *limbic sys-*

tem. There are wide variations among authors, however, with regard to which cell groups are included in this term.

As a first rough indication of functional differences, one may say that *conscious thoughts and actions* depend primarily on the neocortex, whereas the allocortex and the other parts of the limbic system are more concerned with *emotions, motivation, and affective behavior.* As we will discuss in the following chapter, however, there are no sharp distinctions in such functional respects between the neocortex and the limbic structures. Nor do the cell groups comprising the limbic system represent a functionally homogeneous "system." It should finally be emphasized that higher mental functions—usually associated with the cerebral cortex—can only exceptionally be linked to specific nuclei or cortical areas. The most complex tasks of the nervous system are carried out by networks distributed between neurons in many parts of the cortex and in subcortical nuclei.

CHAPTER 19

LIMBIC STRUCTURES

Coordination of autonomic functions is a major task of the hypothalamus, as discussed in Chapter 18. We have also described how the hypothalamus influences processes such as metabolism, growth, and reproduction. Hypothalamic influences on bodily functions are mediated in part via peripheral regions of the autonomic nervous system and in part through the endocrine system. The afferent connections of the hypothalamus show that it can be influenced not only by the peripheral organs and tissues it controls but also by higher levels of the nervous system, primarily the frontal lobe, cingulate gyrus, hippocampal formation, septal nuclei, and the amygdala. It is therefore understandable that stimulation of most of these regions can produce effects like those from stimulation of the hypothalamus. In this chapter we will discuss some of these structures and their functions. Although mentioned several times in this chapter, the frontal lobes will be more systematically treated in Chapter 20.

The "Limbic System"

Several of the cell groups mentioned above (that is, the cingulate gyrus, the hippocampal formation, the septal nuclei, the amygdala, and sometimes also the mammillary nucleus and anterior thalamic nucleus[1]) are commonly embraced under the term "limbic system" (gyrus limbicus is another name for the cingulate gyrus). Sometimes terms like "the emotional brain" have been used to describe these regions. Whereas the amygdala is closely related to emotions, however, the hippocampus is primarily involved in cognitive tasks. The cell groups comprising the limbic system coincide in part with what was formerly called the *rhinencephalon*, although this term, strictly speaking, comprises only the parts of the brain receiving olfactory fibers. The value of such collective terms is questionable. Even though some of the effects of stimulation or ablation of several of the cell groups in the limbic system are similar, there are also clear-cut differences. Furthermore, the fact that many of the nuclei are interconnected does not imply that they constitute a system with a unified function. Studies with modern methods have served to strengthen this

Figure 19.1 *The limbic structures.* The right hemisphere seen from the medial aspect. The regions and cell groups indicated in red are usually included in the term "limbic system."

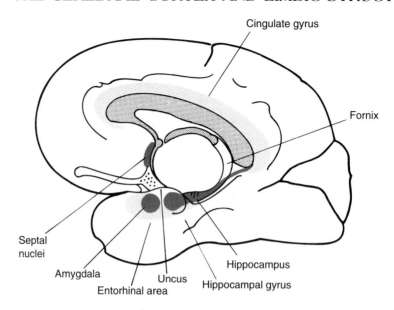

Cingulate gyrus

Fornix

Septal nuclei

Amygdala

Entorhinal area

Uncus

Hippocampus

Hippocampal gyrus

view by showing differences between the individual nuclei with regard to connections, neurotransmitters, properties of single cells, and effects of selective lesions. In fact, *it is not possible to define "the limbic system" with a reasonable degree of precision.* Thus, we will not treat the structures included under this term as a unit but rather will discuss each separately. We also prefer to use the neutral term *limbic structures* (Fig. 19.1) because it does not give a misleading impression of functional unity.

The Circuit of Papez

In 1937, Papez described what he considered a closed circuit of connections starting and ending in the hippocampus. From the hippocampus, the flow of signals was postulated to pass to the mammillary nucleus, from this nucleus to the anterior thalamic nucleus, from there to the cingulate gyrus, and then finally back to the hippocampus. This circuit of interconnected cell groups was hypothesized to form the anatomic basis of emotional reactions and expressions. These suggestions formed the basis for the concept of "the limbic system," which was introduced in the early 1950s. Even though the connectional scheme of Papez is basically correct, it has been modified on several important points. For example, the afferent fibers of the mammillary nucleus (passing in the fornix) do not come from the hippocampus itself but from adjacent regions in the parahippocampal gyrus (subiculum) (Figs. 19.2 and 19.3). Each of the cell groups of the circuit has other—and sometimes more important—connections than with each other. A unified functional role of the circuit in the expression of emotions has not been corroborated by later research.

THE CEREBRAL CORTEX AND "LIMBIC FUNCTIONS": THE CINGULATE GYRUS

Experimental and clinical data show that *autonomic functions* can be influenced by the cerebral cortex. From the cingulate gyrus in particular (Figs. 19.1 and 19.3), electrical stimulation elicits a combination of autonomic (visceral) and somatic effects.[2] Autonomic effects include, for

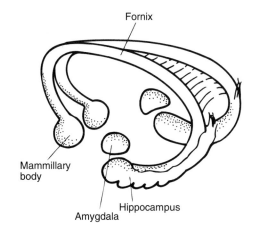

Figure 19.2 *The hippocampal forma-tion, fornix, mammillary nucleus, and the amygdala.* Above, they are seen obliquely from behind; below, from above.

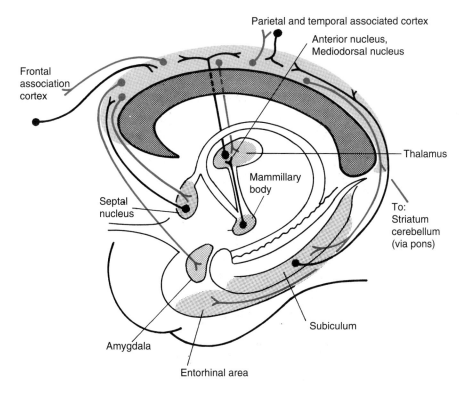

Figure 19.3 *Main connections of the cingulate gyrus.* The cingulate gyrus has connections with cortical associa-tion areas and with limbic structures and may act as a mediator between them.

example, alterations of *respiration* and *circulation* (reduced rate of breathing, heart rate, and blood pressure), of the *digestive tract* (altered peristaltic movements and secretory activity), and *pupillary dilatation*. Somatic effects are expressed mainly as changes of *muscle tone* and of ongoing *movements* (most often inhibition).

Behavioral changes can be elicited by stimulation of the anterior part of the cingulate gyrus in particular. Most attention has been paid to *aggressive reactions*. Bilateral removal of the cingulate gyrus in monkeys makes them tamer. They may also become socially indifferent—that is, they appear to have lost interest in other members of their group and do not try to make contact.

Surgical lesions of parts of the cingulate gyrus, *cingulotomy*, has been performed in some patients with intense, chronic pain that could not be alleviated by conventional means. Some of these patients were reported to experience their pain as less intense and disabling after the operation. Cingulotomy has also been reported to have beneficial effects when performed on some patients with chronic and severe depression. Several ethical objections have been raised to *psychosurgery* of this kind. Furthermore, the outcome for the individual person appears to be difficult to predict; the effect may in some cases be the opposite of that desired.

Alterations of functions controlled by the autonomic system can be produced by stimulation of parts of the cortex other than the cingulate gyrus. Stimulation of the underside (the orbital surface) of the *frontal lobes* and of the pole of the temporal lobe produces effects similar to those obtained from the cingulate gyrus. This may be explained by the known connections between the frontal and temporal lobes and the connections between these parts and the cingulate gyrus (Figs. 19.3 and 20.13). Also emotional changes are typical in patients with damage of the orbitofrontal cortex (most likely because this region is connected with the amygdala).

Stimulation of neocortical regions does not only produce effects on autonomic functions; somatic functions are altered as well. Thus, *no part of the cortex appears to serve autonomic functions only*. On the other hand, alterations of autonomic functions can occur after stimulation of cortical regions one might believe to be purely somatic, such as the *motor and the premotor cortical areas*. Thus, stimulation of the motor cortex produces vasomotor changes (that is, changes of the blood vessel diameter and, therefore, of blood flow) of the opposite body half. On damage to these cortical areas, as seen in patients with a cerebral *stroke*, vasomotor changes often occur in the paralyzed parts of the body. Even alterations of the heart rate and blood pressure and of the digestive tract can occur. As a final example of combined somatic and autonomic effects, stimulation of the *frontal eye field* (Fig. 16.31) produces pupillary dilatation in addition to the more obvious conjugated eye movements.

Pathways for Neocortical Influence on Autonomically Innervated Organs

How the neocortex influences the autonomic nervous system (and the endocrine organs) is not entirely clear. There are few direct connections from the cortex to the hypothalamus (even though cortical connections to

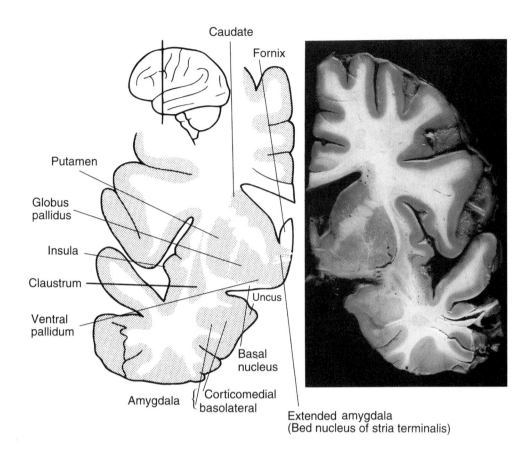

Caudate

Fornix

Putamen

Globus
pallidus

Insula

Claustrum

Ventral
pallidum

Uncus

Basal
nucleus

Amygdala { Corticomedial
basolateral

Extended amygdala
(Bed nucleus of stria terminalis)

Figure 19.4 The amygdala and parts of the basal forebrain. Photograph of a frontal section through the right hemisphere. Note the close relation between the amygdala and the cortex of the temporal lobe.

the reticular formation of the brain stem can explain some effects). The cingulate gyrus receives afferents from association areas of the parietal, frontal, and temporal lobes (Fig. 19.3), but it has no direct efferent connections to the hypothalamus. Indirect pathways are available, however. Thus, the cingulate gyrus projects to the hippocampal formation, to the septal nuclei, and to the amygdala, all of which have different connections to various parts of the hypothalamus. Furthermore, neocortical areas in the frontal and temporal lobes (Fig. 19.4) project to the amygdala and can therefore influence the hypothalamus indirectly.

Fairly large areas of the cerebral cortex can thus influence the hypothalamus and brain stem autonomic centers. To simplify, neocortical effects on autonomic functions appear to be mediated primarily by neocortical efferents to such limbic structures as the hippocampal formation, the amygdala, and the septal nuclei, which mediate the effects on hypothalamic nuclei (and to some extent directly on brain stem autonomic centers).

THE AMYGDALA
AND EMOTIONS

An Overview

The amygdala (the amygdaloid nucleus) is located in the temporal lobe, underneath the uncus (Figs. 19.1, 19.2, 19.4, and 19.6B). In humans, the amygdala is a complex of subnuclei, each with a distinctive internal structure, neurotransmitters, and connections. We will here mainly restrict ourselves to distinguish between a small *corticomedial* (including a central nucleus) and a large *basolateral* nuclear group. The basolateral group increases in size from lower to higher mammals and is particularly well developed in humans. The corticomedial nuclear group lies close to the olfactory cortex (Fig. 10.2). To simplify, we may say that *the corticomedial nuclei are connected primarily with the olfactory bulb, the hypothalamus, and the visceral nuclei of the brain stem, whereas the basolateral nuclei are mainly connected with the thalamus and prefrontal parts of the cerebral cortex.* In addition, the basolateral nuclei send fibers to the *ventral striatum.* This would suggest that the corticomedial part of the amygdala is concerned primarily with autonomic functions, whereas the basolateral parts are more involved in conscious processes related to the frontal and temporal lobes. The many intrinsic connections among the various nuclei show, however, that they must cooperate extensively.

The *functions of the amygdala* cannot be justly described in a few simple terms. Although partly due to insufficient knowledge, this mainly reflects that the amygdala participates in several higher mental functions, each of which are highly complex. Some main functional aspects can nevertheless be identified. Thus, no other part of the brain is found to be equally crucial for *emotions* and *emotionally conditioned behavior.* Furthermore, a central task of the amygdala is the establishment of *links between stimuli and their emotional value* (put very simply, whether something is good or bad). Most of our memories have some—often quite strong—emotional coloring, which is crucial for our ability to react appropriately to a stimulus. Think of the importance of being able to judge the facial expressions of other people, the emotional aspects of their speech, and so forth. As we will discuss below, damage to the amygdala in monkeys leads to, among other things, difficulties in social interactions.

Afferent Connections of the Amygdala

The *corticomedial nuclei* receive afferents from the *olfactory bulb*, the *hypothalamus*, the *intralaminar thalamic nuclei*, the *septal nuclei*, *dopaminergic* neurons in the mesencephalon, and the *parabrachial area* (in the dorsolateral pons). The latter projection may convey information about *taste* and, in addition, about *painful stimuli.* Thus, ascending fibers of spinal lamina I nociceptive neurons end in parts of the parabrachial area that project to the central amygdaloid nucleus (among other targets). The sensory units of this pathway have very large receptive fields and receive convergent inputs from the skin and viscera. It seems likely that this lamina I-parabrachial-amygdaloid pathway contributes to the emotional aspects of pain.

The *basolateral nuclei* receive fibers from the *thalamus*, the *neocortex of the frontal lobe* (prefrontal cortex), parts of the *temporal lobe*, and from the *cingulate gyrus* (Fig. 19.4). Together the basolateral nuclei (the lateral nucleus in particular) receive *all kinds of sensory information.* This may be both emotionally neutral information about sensory stimuli from

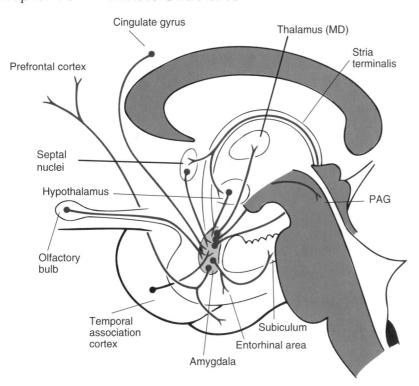

Figure 19.5 *Main connections of the amygdala.* Note the close connections with the hypothalamus and with association areas in the temporal and frontal lobes.

cortical association areas, and about unpleasant and threatening ones from the reticular formation, the intralaminar thalamic nuclei, and perhaps parts of the cortex (the insula). Thus, the amygdala receives, for example, information about fear-provoking stimuli and their context. Efferents from the lateral nucleus reach other amygdaloid nuclei that may influence the cortex (conscious experience of emotions) and brain-stem cell groups (behavioral reactions, including autonomic responses associated with emotions).

Efferent Connections of the Amygdala

The efferent connections of the amygdala are mostly reciprocal to the afferent ones. One major efferent pathway goes to the *hypothalamus*. Most of these fibers are collected in the macroscopically visible *stria terminalis*, which arches over the thalamus (Fig. 19.5). The fibers end primarily in the ventromedial hypothalamic nucleus (compare with the efferents from the hippocampal formation, which run in the fornix and end in the mammillary nucleus). Other efferents pass to the *thalamus* (especially to the mediodorsal nucleus, MD), enabling impulses from the amygdala to reach the *prefrontal cortex* (Fig. 20.7). As mentioned above, these connections may be important for the conscious experience of emotions, such as fear and anxiety. The amygdala also sends fibers to some parts of the cortex that do not project back, especially *visual areas* in the inferotemporal cortex (Fig. 20.10).

Parts of the allocortex receive fibers from the amygdala, especially the *hippocampal formation* (the entorhinal area and the subiculum) and the *septal nuclei*. Fibers to the *ventral striatum* (including the nucleus accumbens, Fig. 3.17) and the *basal nucleus* (Fig. 19.4) arise in the basolateral amygdaloid nuclei. The projection to the striatum may mediate emotional influences of movements. The projections to the basal nucleus can induce activation of the EEG (arousal and increased attention). There is experimental evidence that synaptic learning effects on neurons in the auditory cortex depend on inputs from the amygdala (and the basal nucleus) besides the specific auditory information via the medial geniculate body. It seems likely that this is related to the well-known effects of motivation on learning: We remember material better with emotional coloring.

Finally, there are connections from the amygdala to various brain stem nuclei, such as the *PAG*, parts of the *reticular formation*, and *parasympathetic cranial nerve nuclei*. These connections—with those to the hypothalamus—seem important for the autonomic and somatic expressions of emotions. The connections to the PAG are involved in eliciting conditioned fear behavior (the PAG sends fibers to various brain-stem premotor networks). In rats conditioned fear includes so-called *freezing*; that is, the animal becomes completely still. The freezing reaction, which includes suppressed pain transmission, occurs typically when a rat meets a predator, such as a cat.

Behavioral Effects after Damage or Stimulation of the Amygdala

Bilateral destruction of the amygdala in monkeys causes *tameness* (that is, loss of aggressive and defensive reactions) as the most marked behavioral change. All behavioral expressions of emotions are reduced, however. In contrast to normal monkeys, those without amygdala show no signs of fear when, for example, confronted with a snake. Furthermore, they do not seek contact with other animals in the group and therefore become socially isolated. Full explanations of these and other symptoms are not yet possible. Some can probably be explained, however, by the removal of amygdaloid effects on the hypothalamus and brain-stem autonomic and somatic motor centers (among them the PAG). Thus, sensory stimuli (such as the sight of a snake), although reaching consciousness, would not be able to elicit the normal behavioral reactions. In addition, the symptoms most likely depend on interruption of the amygdaloid connections to the cerebral cortex. Thus, the normal integration of the cognitive and emotional aspects of a stimulus would be disrupted. A patient with bilateral destruction of the amygdala (described by the British psychiatrist Jacobson) illustrates this point. She appeared calm and relaxed outwardly, and had normal heart rate in situations in which she experienced great anxiety and wanted to run away. Presumably, the coupling between the emotions and the emotional reactions was disrupted in this patient (cf. Chapter 18, *The Hypothalamus and Reactions*).

Many behavioral changes have been produced by electrical stimulation of the amygdala in animals with implanted electrodes. (In such experiments the electrodes have been inserted and fixed to the skull under general anesthesia. Afterward the electrodes cause the animal no pain or obvious discomfort.) Stimulation produces a *varied pattern of somatic and autonomic responses, which appear to be parts of more complex behavioral reactions.*

As would be expected from the anatomic data discussed above, stimulation of medial and lateral parts of the amygdaloid complex gives different responses. *Stimulation of the corticomedial nuclear group* produces smacking, salivation, and licking and chewing movements. Emptying of the rectum and the bladder may occur, together with inhibition of voluntary movements.

Stimulation of the basolateral nuclear group often produces arousal and signs of increased *attention*: The animal lifts its head, its pupils are dilated, and it looks around (especially toward the side opposite of the stimulating electrode). The attention of the animal appears to be directed toward something in the surroundings. As might be expected, together with these behavioral changes occurs *activation of the EEG*. Strong stimulation can produce more dramatic effects, such as signs of strong *fear or rage*. The animal (for example, a cat) might try to escape and show other signs of fear, or it may snarl and growl and perhaps attack the ex-

The Amygdala, Emotions, and Behavior

Conditioned Fear

As mentioned above, the amygdala plays a role in a variety of emotions and emotionally related behaviors. This, with its anatomic heterogeneity, strongly suggest that the amygdala is not a functional unit. In the search for the biologic substrate of specific behaviors, *conditioned fear* has been intensively studied. Crucial links in the pathways underlying this phenomenon have been "dissected" out in experimental animals. Such detailed data may help to understand how the amygdala participates in other kinds of tasks.

Situations with purely mental stress can produce a conditioned-fear reaction in rats as in humans. In rats the conditioning may be established by letting a tone be followed repeatedly by a painful stimulus (for example, an electric shock to the foot). After a while the tone alone elicits fear-related behavior, that is, behavior that normally occurs in threatening or dangerous situations (like the sight of a cat). As discussed earlier, the fear reaction of a rat includes autonomic, somatic, and endocrine responses, such as freezing and increased secretion of cortisol. When a tone is used as the conditioning stimulus, the necessary information about the sound is transmitted directly from the thalamus to the *lateral amygdaloid nucleus*. The auditory cortex is necessary for the occurrence of the fear reaction only if the animal has to discriminate two tones with different frequencies. The hippocampus is not necessary for the tone conditioning. It is necessary, however, for a weaker *contextual conditioning*; that is, the fear reaction can also be elicited by clues in the environment of the experimental situation (such as objects, sounds or odors). From the lateral nucleus signals are relayed (directly and indirectly) to the central nucleus. Efferents from the central nucleus to autonomic and somatic cell groups in the brain stem (among them the PAG) probably mediate main components of the fear reaction. Thus, destruction of the central nucleus abolishes both the freezing and autonomic responses in conditioned fear.

Anxiety and Neurotransmitters

The amygdala contains many neurotransmitters (among them most of the known neuropeptides). To sort out the functional role of each transmitter is a formidable task. For practical reasons, therefore, scientists concentrate upon studying one or a few at a time, with the danger of overlooking the contributions of other transmitters. We will restrict ourselves here to transmitters involved in conditioned fear and psychic stress.

As mentioned above, signals are transmitted from the lateral to the central nucleus via direct and indirect routes, and drugs that reduce anxiety (anxiolytics) may function by interfering at this level. Electrical stimulation of the lateral nucleus evokes primarily *GABA-mediated* inhibition in the central nucleus (acting at both GABA$_A$ and GABA$_B$ receptors). Some inhibition occurs presynaptically by reducing the release of glutamate. The *benzodiazepines* (Valium and others) bind to specific sites on the GABA receptor (benzodiazepine receptors) and potentiate the effect of GABA. Such drugs are used to reduce anxiety and as hypnotics. The density of benzodiazepine receptors is high in the amygdala and particularly high in the lateral nucleus (and one other subnucleus of the basolateral complex). Local infusion of benzodiazepines in these nuclei reduces expressions of conditioned fear in experimental animals.

The expectation of a painful stimulus evokes an *endocrine response*, as one part of a *stress reaction* (see Chapter 18, *Psychosomatic Disorders*). This may be mediated by fibers from the central nucleus to the paraventricular hypothalamic nucleus. This nucleus projects to the median eminence where *CRH* is released and reaches the anterior pituitary via the portal system (Fig. 18.5C). CRH increases the secretion of *ACTH*, thus increasing cortisol in the bloodstream.

CRH may be an important transmitter in the amygdala in relation to *anxiety and stress*. Besides containing CRH-positive cell bodies, the central nucleus receives many CRH-containing fibers (neurons several places contain CRH, for example, in the parabrachial area and the locus coeruleus). Injection of CRH into the cerebral ventricles increases stress reactions and fear-related behavior. This is probably caused by the action of CRH both in the amygdala and other cell groups. For example, noradrenergic neurons in the locus coeruleus are activated, which may contribute to arousal as part of a stress reaction. Acute and chronic stress increases CRH in the amygdala, and accordingly, microinjections of CRH-antagonists in the central nucleus abolish some stress reactions.

Several other than transmitters CRH show changes in relation to anxiety and stress. *NPY* has attracted much interest. Thus, microinjection of NPY in the amygdala evokes largely the opposite effects of CRH on stress and fear-related behavior. NPY is present in many neurons in the amygdala (colocalized with norepinephrine, GABA, or somatostatin) and in terminals of afferent axons. Animal experiments suggest that whereas CRH is crucial in setting off a stress reaction, NPY that is released *after* the reaction has started protects against overshooting.

The Amygdala and Depression

As mentioned above, CRH is one likely transmitter (among several) for evoking fear-related behavior and stress reactions and the amygdala is an important site of action.

CRH also appears to be related to mood. Thus, the concentration of CRH in the cerebrospinal fluid is increased in many deeply depressed patients and victims of suicide. In the latter group, lowered density of the CRH receptor was found in the frontal lobe (down regulation due to constantly increased CRH available?). A transgenic mouse-strain overproducing CRH has, as expected, increased levels of ACTH and cortisol in the blood. In addition, they show behavior indicative of anxiety (for example, the way they behave in novel situations). This behavioral pattern is normalized by supply of CRH-antagonists.

Measurement of regional cerebral blood flow supports that the function of the amygdala is altered in seriously depressed patients. Thus, compared with a control group, depressed patients had increased blood flow in the left prefrontal cortex and amygdala. We should realize, however, that this observation does not tell us how the amygdala is involved in depression—for example, whether the blood flow changes are secondary to a change of mood or whether changes in the amygdala come first.

Sexuality and Psychosurgery

Hypersexuality is one of the behavioral changes after bilateral destruction of the amygdala in animals. This may, however, be related to damage to allocortical areas in the vicinity of the amygdala rather than to the amygdala itself. Nevertheless, it is conspicuous that the amygdala is among the brain regions with the highest density of receptors for sex hormones. It therefore seems likely that the activity of neurons in parts of the amygdala is influenced by the level of sex hormones in the blood (the sex hormones are lipid-soluble and pass the blood–brain barrier easily).

Stereotactic destruction of the amygdala has been performed on some especially violent criminals to reduce their aggression. Bilateral destruction of the amygdala has even been performed in an attempt to cure hyperactive children. The ventromedial hypothalamic nucleus, receiving many fibers from the amygdala, has also been stereotactically lesioned in a small number of sex criminals. The ethical objections to all these psychosurgical interventions were so strong, however, that they were tried only for a short period of time. Furthermore, the results appear to be so unpredictable that psychosurgery of this kind would be difficult to defend even if there were no other objections.

aminer. Most likely, fear and rage are elicited from slightly different parts of the amygdala.

In *humans*, the amygdala has been stimulated in conjunction with brain surgery of the temporal lobe under local anesthesia. A wide spectrum of autonomic and emotional reactions have been produced in such cases, but most pronounced is a feeling of *anxiety*. Memory-like hallucinations and *déjà vu* experiences (the feeling of having experienced the same situation before) have also been reported. This is called a *dreamy state*, and can occur in epileptic seizures starting in the temporal lobe. Similar effects— that is, fear and various kinds of hallucinations—have been produced by stimulation of the anterior portion of the hippocampus and the lateral cortex of the temporal lobe (in the superior temporal gyrus). This can presumably be explained by the close connections between these regions and the amygdala, all being parts of a more widespread network for handling of emotions and memories.

The Amygdala and Learning

The conditioned-fear reaction discussed above requires a learning process. Thus, the rat learned to associate an innocuous stimulus with something painful. Destruction of the amygdala prevents establishing the conditioned response. Thus, experiments with monkeys after a lesion restricted as far as possible to the amygdala show that they have difficulties in learning the association between objects and their meanings. They can recognize objects but cannot relate them to other kinds of information, such as whether the object was associated with a reward or something unpleasant. Many other observations support that the amygdala is necessary for the *learning of associations between stimuli and their significance in terms of reward or punishment*. We may say that amygdala is crucial for the emotional coloring of experiences and sensations, and that it is remembered. Amygdala is not alone in this respect, however. Both the amygdala and parts of the *prefrontal cortex* are necessary in monkeys for the learning and later retrieval of associations between visual stimuli and food rewards. The connections involved are partly direct fibers from the amygdala to the ventromedial prefrontal cortex and partly a pathway interrupted in the mediodorsal thalamic nucleus (MD). Experiments in rats suggest that connections between the basolateral amygdala and the *ventral striatum* (including the nucleus accumbens) also are necessary for establishing stimulus-reward associations. (These experiments were different from the monkey experiments since they tested the association between the place of a stimulus and its reward value.)

NEURONAL GROUPS IN THE BASAL PARTS OF THE HEMISPHERES: THE BASAL FOREBRAIN

Below and medial to the well-defined basal ganglia many neurons are spread out rather diffusely. Unfortunately, the nomenclature for this region is not consistent among authors. Thus, different names are often applied to the region or parts of it without attempting to describe more precisely what is meant. The old anatomists named it the *substantia innominata* (the region without a name), presumably reflecting that nothing was known about its connections and functions. The *basal forebrain* (basal prosencephalon) is usually used synonymously with the substantia innominata. Only recently are its connections, cytochemistry, and functions being clarified, making it clear that the basal forebrain is no anatomical or functional unity. It is now commonly accepted to divide the basal forebrain into three overlapping regions, differing regarding neurotransmitters and connections: the *ventral striatopallidum*, the *extended amygdala*, and the *basal nucleus* (Figs. 4.17 and 19.4). The ventral striatopallidum was discussed in Chapter 13. We will here discuss only certain aspects of the basal forebrain, and start with a large group of cholinergic neurons that are found in the basal nucleus and some adjacent cell groups.

Cholinergic Neurons Projecting to the Cerebral Cortex

Cholinergic neurons of the basal forebrain form a thin disc close to the basal surface of the hemisphere—the *basal nucleus*—and are furthermore found in the *septal nuclei* and the *diagonal band of Broca* that extend dorsally close to the midline (Figs. 4.17 and 19.4). The septal nuclei form the most well-defined anatomic entity among these cell groups, and are found just in front of the anterior commissure[3] (Fig. 19.1). The diagonal band of Broca forms a transition between the basal nucleus and the septal nuclei.

The cholinergic neurons of the basal forebrain project to the *cerebral cortex* (both to the allocortex, including the hippocampus, and the neocortex).[4] The septal nuclei and the diagonal band send fibers mainly to the hippocampal formation (Fig. 19.9) whereas the basal nucleus projects to the neocortex with a rough topographic order.

Afferents to the cholinergic cell groups of the basal forebrain are still incompletely known. Important inputs arise in the brain stem, notably in the *locus coeruleus* and in *cholinergic cell groups in the dorsolateral pons* (such connections are involved in the ascending activating system discussed in Chapter 15). Furthermore, afferents come from the *hypothalamus*, the *gyrus cinguli*, and the *nucleus accumbens* of the ventral striatum.

Among the cholinergic cell groups, the *septal nuclei* first attracted much interest because early lesion and stimulation experiments showed that they influence autonomic functions, emotions, and behavioral reactions. For example, lesions of the septal nuclei in animals alter sexual and foraging behavior. Aggressive behavior appears to be reduced (as stimulation of the septal nuclei can produce aggression). The effects are similar to those produced by lesions of the amygdala and the anterior parts of the cingulate gyrus, and can be explained presumably by the connections of the septal nuclei with these parts and the hypothalamus. Symptoms specific to the septal nuclei, constituting the so-called septal syndrome, have not been proved convincingly.

Later studies turned to the role of the cholinergic neurons in *attention* and *memory* mechanisms. Particularly seminal in this respect was the discovery of cell loss in the basal nucleus in patients with Alzheimer's disease. Some studies in monkeys suggested that the septal nuclei, the diagonal band of Broca, and the basal nucleus all must be destroyed to produce memory impairments. On the other hand, more detailed experimental studies with injection of substances that destroy the cell bodies but not passing fibers suggest that the septal nuclei and the diagonal band of Broca are especially important for memory (presumably because of their connections with the hippocampus), whereas the basal nucleus is more concerned with maintaining and perhaps focusing attention. Furthermore, there are several reports of patients with small lesions in the anterior parts of the cholinergic cell groups who exhibited clear-cut memory loss (both for recent and past events). One such patient, for example, had a lesion affecting primarily the diagonal band of Broca, as judged with MRI. The difficulties with the exact localization of the damage in such patients warn against firm conclusions, however.

Other Components of the Basal Forebrain

The Ventral Striatopallidum and the Extended Amygdala

The ventral striatum (including the nucleus accumbens) is discussed in relation to the basal ganglia in Chapter 13. With a similar ventral extension of the pallidum it forms the *ventral striatopallidum*. These parts of the basal forebrain show similarities with the basal ganglia (dorsal striatum and dorsal pallidum) regarding cytoarchitectonics, cytochemistry, and connections (for example, a dense dopaminergic innervation from the mesencephalon). In contrast to the dorsal striatum (the caudate nucleus and the putamen), which receives the main afferent input from the neocortex, the ventral striatum receives main inputs from the allocortex and the amygdala. A further characteristic of the ventral striatum is that it projects to the hypothalamus and brain-stem nuclei, such as the PAG and the motor vagus nucleus. The ventral pallidum projects to the MD that sends fibers to the prefrontal cortex (cf. the projection of the dorsal pallidum to the VL/VA thalamic nuclei that project mainly to the premotor areas).

Another rather diffuse cell group in the basal forebrain—continuous with the ventral pallidum—is called the *extended amygdala*, because it forms a rostral extension of the medial amygdala (Fig. 19.4). Most of it is made up of the *bed nucleus of the stria terminalis* (the stria terminalis is a bundle of efferent fibers from the amygdala, Fig. 19.5). The bed nucleus is found medial to the pallidum at the same anteroposterior level and further anterior to the anterior commissure (that is, close to the septal nuclei). When lumping this part of the basal forebrain with the amygdala, it is because they share many transmitters and connections. The anatomic distinction between the extended amygdala and the nucleus accumbens is not sharp, however, and both receive, for example, dopaminergic fibers from the mesencephalon.

The Medial Forebrain Bundle

Many fibers interconnecting the various limbic structures are located in a diffusely delimited, parasagittal fiber mass in the basal part of the hemisphere. This ill-defined structure is called the *medial forebrain bundle* and is referred to in Chapter 18. It extends from the region of the anterior commissure anteriorly and posteriorly into the mesencephalon. Most of the fibers are short interconnecting nuclei found close to each other, such as the septal nuclei, other nuclei in the basal forebrain, various hypothalamic nuclei, and the PAG in the mesencephalon (Fig. 18.3). Fibers from the monoaminergic cell groups of the brain stem pass through the medial forebrain bundle on their way to forebrain structures, such as the cortex (including the hippocampal formation). Functionally, the medial forebrain bundle is heterogeneous, and lesions of it cannot be expected to reveal the function of any particular cell group or fiber tract.

Figure 19.6 *Magnetic resonance images* (MRIs) showing the hippocampus and the amygdala. **A.** Frontal plane. Note the position of the hippocampus medially in the temporal lobe (compare Figs. 3.26, 3.27 and 19.8). **B.** Parasagittal plane through the medial part of the temporal lobe, showing the amygdala and the uncus (compare Fig. 13.2). Courtesy of Dr. S.J. Bakke, The National Hospital, Oslo.

THE HIPPOCAMPAL FORMATION: LEARNING AND MEMORY

An Overview

The last among the limbic structures we will discuss are the *hippocampus* and nearby regions in the temporal lobe, the *dentate gyrus*, the *subiculum*, and the *entorhinal cortex* (the latter located in the hippocampal gyrus) (Figs. 19.1 and 19.2). Collectively, these structures form the *hippocampal formation* (unfortunately, what is included in this term varies among authors). Whereas the interest formerly was directed mainly to the hippocampus itself, recent studies have made us consider the function of the hippocampus in conjunction with the nearby structures in the hippocampal gyrus, which are interconnected with the hippocampus.

The *hippocampus* (Figs. 3.28, 3.32, 19.2, and 19.6–19.8) forms an elongated bulge medially in the temporal horn of the lateral ventricle, produced by invagination of the ventricular wall by the hippocampal sulcus (Fig. 19.7). Along the medial aspect of the hippocampus, the *dentate gyrus* forms a narrow, notched band (Figs. 3.32, 19.2, and 19.7). The hippocampus and the dentate gyrus belong to the allocortex and have a simplified laminar pattern compared with the neocortex. Nevertheless, they are far from simply built, with several different cell types and precisely organized, highly complex patterns of connections.

Two aspects of the connections of the hippocampal formation are, presumably, crucial for the understanding of its functional roles: First, *the extensive, two-way connections with various cortical association areas and, second, the direct and indirect connections with other limbic structures* such as the cingulate gyrus and the septal nuclei. As for neocortical connections, the hippocampus obviously processes large amounts of information. The parallel increase in the size of the hippocampus and the

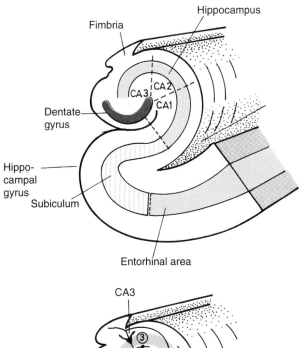

Figure 19.7 *The hippocampus.*
Schematized drawing of a frontal section through medial parts of the temporal lobe. Compare Figures 3.26, 19.6, and 19.8, which show corresponding sections. The section is oriented approximately perpendicular to the long axis of the lower, thickened part of the hippocampus (cf. Figs. 3.30 and 19.2). The **lower** drawing shows one (of several) impulse pathways through the hippocampus. 1 = Pyramidal cell in the entorhinal area; 2 = granule cell in the dentate gyrus; 3 = pyramidal cell in the CA3; 4 = pyramidal cell in the CA1; 5 = pyramidal cell in the subiculum projecting to the entorhinal area.

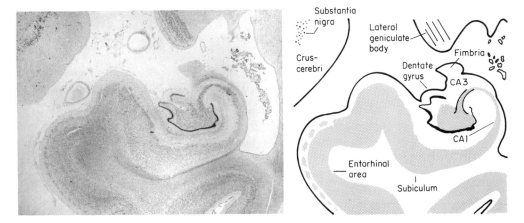

Figure 19.8 *The hippocampal formation.* Photomicrograph of thionine-stained frontal section through the human temporal lobe. The temporal horn of the lateral ventricle with some of the choroid plexus is seen above to the right of the hippocampus. The mesencephalon with the crus and the substantia nigra is seen to the left. The section corresponds to the drawing in Figure 3.26.

569

neocortex during evolution furthermore indicates that its main functions are related to the neocortex.

The quantitatively dominating *afferent inputs* to the dentate gyrus and the hippocampus arise in the *entorhinal area*. The neurons of the dentate gyrus send their efferents to the hippocampus, whereas the hippocampal projection neurons project to the subiculum (Figs. 19.7 and 19.8). The subiculum distributes fibers to several areas, notably back to the *entorhinal area* and to the *mammillary nucleus* (through the fornix). Thus, the *hippocampus acts largely back onto the areas from which it receives information*. The entorhinal area receives afferents both from nearby areas in the temporal lobe and more distant cortical areas. All are *association areas* (that is, not primary sensory or motor regions), which integrate various kinds of sensory information.

A large number of *commissural fibers* connect the hippocampus of the two sides, indicating a close cooperation between them.

There is now much evidence that the hippocampal formation plays a crucial role for certain kinds of *learning and memory*. These conclusions are based on many animal experiments and observations in humans with lesions in medial parts of the temporal lobe. Thus, bilateral damage of the hippocampal formation leads to *amnesia*, that is, impaired memory without intellectual reduction (cf. dementia, discussed in Chapter 4). Lesions restricted to the hippocampus proper produce amnesia, although much less severe than when the whole hippocampal formation has been damaged.

It should be emphasized that the hippocampal formation is not the only part of the brain important for memory, as we will discuss later in this chapter. Thus, *parts of the hippocampal gyrus outside the hippocampal formation* appear to play an independent role in memory formation and retrieval. Furthermore, amnesia has been reported also after lesions of the *medial thalamus*, and as discussed above, *cholinergic cell groups* of the basal forebrain also play a role (presumably by way of their connections with the hippocampus). Finally, the role of *amygdala* in learning of associations between stimuli and their emotional value was discussed above.

The hippocampal formation is important for memory only for a certain time after an event (probably about one year). Thus, isolated damage of the hippocampal formation does not abolish recall of older memories, although it prevents the learning of certain kinds of new material. This is probably because the memory traces after a certain time are stored in many parts of the cerebral cortex.

We can roughly distinguish two kinds of memory: One kind concerns the memory of events and facts, and is called *declarative* or *explicit memory*; the other concerns skills and habits and is called *nondeclarative* or *implicit memory*. Only the first kind depends critically upon the integrity of medial parts of the temporal lobe. For nondeclarative memory the basal ganglia, cerebellum, and parts of the neocortex appear to be most important.

Impulse Routes through the Hippocampus

Most of the neurons of the dentate gyrus are small so-called *granule cells*, whereas the only well-defined hippocampal cell layer consists of large *pyramidal cells* (Figs. 19.7 and 19.8). Above and below the pyramidal cell layer are layers containing the pyramidal cell dendrites and incoming axons. There are also various kinds of interneurons, notably the *GABAergic basket cells*, which inhibit the pyramidal cells. The hippocampus can be divided into three longitudinal zones, named *CA1 to CA3* (Fig. 19.7). The granule cell axons contact the pyramidal cell dendrites, and the pyramidal cells send axons out of the hippocampus.

Even though the internal architecture of the hippocampus is rather complicated, with several neuronal types with complex interconnections, a relatively simple main transmission route from input to output appears to exist, as first shown by the Norwegian neurophysiologist Per Andersen (Fig. 19.7). This pathway starts in the entorhinal area and has three synaptic interruptions. Neurons in the entorhinal area send their axons, forming the so-called *perforant path*, to the hippocampus, where many end in the dentate gyrus. The axons of the granule cells of the dentate gyrus, called *mossy fibers*, end primarily on the apical dendrites of the pyramidal cells of CA3 (Fig. 19.7). The CA3 pyramidal cells send so-called *Schaffer collaterals* to the apical dendrite of the CA1 pyramidal cells. From CA1 a significant part of the impulse traffic is directed to the *subiculum*, and from there to the *entorhinal area*—thus closing the circuit passing from the entorhinal area through the hippocampus and back to the entorhinal area. All links in this pathway are *excitatory* using glutamate as neurotransmitter.

Further anatomic and physiological studies show that conditions are more complex than the simple serial coupling illustrated in Figure 19.7. For example, the fibers of the perforant path not only contact granule cells of the dentate gyrus but also end directly on the hippocampal pyramidal cells. Thus, several parallel pathways enter the hippocampus. Furthermore, we do not know what kind of information processing takes place in the hippocampus before "answers" are issued to the entorhinal area and many other areas.

Has the Hippocampus a Lamellar Organization?

On the basis of primarily physiological data, it was postulated that the hippocampus is organized in thin lamellae oriented perpendicular to the long axis of the hippocampus, each lamella presumably representing a functional unit (Fig. 19.7 shows the circuitry in the plane of a lamella). This cannot be the whole story, however. Anatomic investigations performed in monkeys and in lower mammals show that the efferent fibers from a narrow transverse zone of the entorhinal area extend for a considerable distance longitudinally in the hippocampus. Thus, each entorhinal efferent neuron can presumably contact neurons in many hippocampal lamellae. Furthermore, the collaterals of the hippocampal pyramidal neurons extend not only in the plane of the lamellae (as shown in Fig. 19.7) but also longitudinally. In fact, it is still not clear what should be regarded as a functional unit within the hippocampus and the degree of functional localization present.

Afferent Connections of the Hippocampal Formation

As with other parts of the brain, improved methods for neural tracing have revealed that the hippocampal formation has connections with more areas than formerly believed. We will focus on those regarded as most important. As mentioned above, the main afferents to the dentate gyrus arise in the entorhinal cortex. Since the dentate gyrus sends its efferents to the hippocampus, *the entorhinal cortex is the quantitatively dominating deliverer of information to the hippocampus.* Therefore, to understand the nature of the information processed by the hippocampus, we must know the afferent connections of the entorhinal area. Recent studies with retrograde transport have shown that *most association areas of the neocortex* are likely to influence the entorhinal area, either directly or indirectly, by means of fibers to other areas in the hippocampal gyrus, which in turn project to the entorhinal area. Thus, the majority of direct entorhinal afferents arises in adjacent parts of the *hippocampal gyrus* and in the *perirhinal cortex* (located around the rhinal sulcus, see Fig. 10.2). These areas form a continuous cortical region, although different parts are not identical regarding connections. Together, the region receives *visual* information from extrastriate areas in the inferior part of the temporal lobe (Fig. 20.13), *auditory* information from the superior part of the temporal lobe, *somatosensory* information from posterior parietal cortex, and information from *polysensory association* areas—that is, areas that integrate several sensory modalities. Finally, afferents arrive from the cingulate gyrus, the insula, and the prefrontal cortex. Together, the entorhinal area receives highly processed sensory information. We assume, for example, that information about words comes to the hippocampus regardless of whether we see (read), hear, or read by touch (Braille writing).

We should realize, however, that the areas providing the entorhinal area (and thus the hippocampus) with its main inputs, project to other areas as well. For example, both the perirhinal cortex and the subiculum project to the mediodorsal thalamic nucleus (MD, which projects to the prefrontal cortex and parts of the cingulate gyrus). This might explain why the memory loss is more severe after damage of the perirhinal cortex and the areas neighboring the entorhinal area than after a lesion of the entorhinal cortex and the hippocampus (we will return to this point below).

Smaller but functionally important contingents to the hippocampal formation come from the *septal nuclei* and *monoaminergic cell groups in the brain stem.* The *septohippocampal* neurons release acetylcholine, which has a long-lasting depolarizing effect on the hippocampal neurons—that is, the pathway has a *modulatory* action. Electrical stimulation of the septal nuclei does not drive the hippocampal pyramidal cells to produce action potentials but increases their excitability for seconds or even longer. Other hippocampal afferents come from the *raphe nuclei* (serotonin) and the *locus coeruleus* (norepinephrine). These inputs, too, appear to have modulatory effects on the hippocampal cells. Thus, there is evidence that the long-term increase in synaptic effects that can be produced in the hippocampus by certain kinds of afferent stimulation (LTP; see below) is reduced after pharmacological removal of monoamines from the hippocampus. Thus, these *modulatory pathways appear not to provide the hippocampus with specific information but rather to control the firing rate of hippocampal cells in response to specific information from the entorhinal area* (and thus from many parts of the cortex). This may be related to degrees of attention and motivation, which we know have profound influence on both learning and memory.

Efferent Connections of the Hippocampal Formation

Until the mid-1970s it was believed that most efferents from the hippocampus were directed to the mammillary body, passing in the fornix (fibers destined for the mammillary nucleus comprise the majority of the fornix fibers, Fig. 18.4). This was based on the erroneous assumption that all axons in the fornix came from hippocampal pyramidal cells. This view on hippocampal efferents was presumably influenced by Papez and the postulated circuit interconnecting the limbic structures. Furthermore, the macroscopically visible fornix is such an impressive pathway that other possibilities were apparently not seriously considered. With the introduction of methods using axonal transport of radioactively labeled amino acids, it was shown, however, that the *fornix fibers originate in the subiculum*.[5] Furthermore, not all fibers in the fornix end in the mammillary body, some pass to the *ventral striatum* (nucleus accumbens) and the *ventromedial hypothalamus*. The subiculum also sends fibers to *amygdala*. It became furthermore clear that the *impulse flow from the hippocampus, via the subiculum, is directed as much (or more) towards association areas in the temporal and frontal lobes* (Fig. 19.7 and 19.9) *than towards the cingulate gyrus* (via the mammillary body and the anterior thalamic nucleus; Fig. 18.4). The parallel evolutionary increase of the hippocampus and the cerebral hemispheres also suggests that hippocampal functions are most closely related to the neocortex.

Comparison of the efferent connections with the afferent ones shows that the hippocampal formation is largely *reciprocally* connected with subcortical and cortical areas. Thus, we must assume that whatever the hippocampus is doing, it requires a constant *exchange of information* with many other areas.

Hippocampal Efferents are Topographically Organized

The connections from the hippocampus to the subiculum, and from there to other areas, are topographically organized. A longitudinal zone of the subiculum close to the dentate gyrus (Fig. 19.7), for example, sends fibers to parts of the allocortex and the nucleus accumbens, whereas a zone at the other extreme projects to the cingulate gyrus. This example serves to emphasize that the hippocampal formation cannot be understood as a unit. Thus, since different parts have different connections, symptoms after lesions may be expected to vary with their exact localization within the hippocampal formation. Some controversies among authors regarding the effects of hippocampal lesions on memory are probably due to disregard of such anatomic facts.

Different Kinds of Learning and Memory

Before discussing further the functions of the hippocampal formation some words about learning and memory may be useful. The following is a very superficial treatement of a large and important field in psychology. Other classifications than those used here exist, and the different forms of memory may not be as independent as this presentation may suggest.

Figure 19.9 *Some main connections of the hippocampus.*

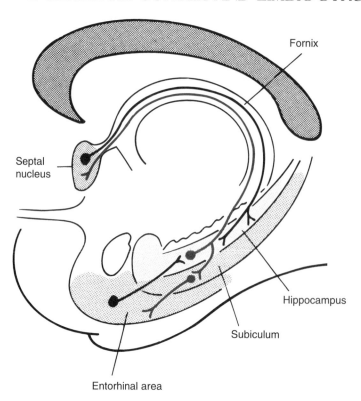

Learning in a wide sense is a prerequisite for memory—something new must be stored that can be recalled later. Problems with remembering may be due to either deficient *learning*, *long-term storage* of newly learnt material, or *retrieval* of the stored material. Thus, when destruction of a part of the brain causes amnesia, the part may not necessarily be the site of the memory traces—it may just be a link in a chain of events leading to retrieval.

Much of our learning is *associative*, that is, we learn from experience that two phenomena occur together. This holds for *classic conditioning* (learning of a conditioned response) when one stimulus always follows another, and for *operant conditioning* in which we learn that a certain behavior produces a certain response. An example of operant conditioning is a hungry rat learning by trial and error to press a lever to obtain food. In the same situation later the rat knows what the appropriate behavior is. Not learning is associative, however. With constant exposure to a stimulus the response is altered—for example, by ceasing to notice a loud sound we have heard many times (*habituation*). The response may also increase with repeated exposure, as with painful stimuli (*sensitization*). Other, more complex, kinds of learning are *non-associative*, such as learning by imitation elements of language and movement patterns. Often, however, learning includes several of these forms at the same time.

Another way to characterize learning and memory relates to *what* is learnt, rather than to how it takes place. One main category concerns episodes and events from ones own life ("Where did I put the scissors?," "What is the name of the person in that picture?") This is called *explicit*, *episodic*, or *declarative memory*. Afterwards we can recall the episode, often in the form of pictures, which may be described verbally (memory of *what*). Learning about the world we live in is of the same kind (the capital of Italy, the first president of the US, the location of the post office, and so forth). Common to such memories is that we must consciously "search our minds" to recall them. In contrast to such declarative memory is that necessary to learn and perform skills (riding a bicycle, dress, use knife and fork, and so forth). Habits and attitudes also largely fall in this category, which is called *implicit*, *procedural* or *nondeclarative memory*. The learning leads to altered behavior, but not necessarily so that the stored material can be subject to a conscious analysis. With skills like playing an instrument or arithmetic, the stored information becomes accessible only by performing the skill (memory of *how*). In ordinary teaching situations much of the learning is implicit—for example, the aquisition of attitudes of which both the teacher and the student are unaware.

As mentioned above, animal experiments and clinical observations suggest strongly that declarative and nondeclarative memory use at least partly different regions of the brain. One striking piece of evidence comes from patients with Alzheimer's disease who have markedly impaired de-

The Relation Between Memory and Long-Term Potentiation

Since the hippocampus is involved in learning and memory, it is of special interest that the synapses are *plastic* at several steps in the circuit shown in Figure 19.7. Thus, their efficacy can be increased for a long time after intensive stimulation (LTP; see Chapter 1, *Neurons Can "Remember" Previous Synaptic Influences* and *The NMDA Receptor: A Mediator of Both Learning and Neuronal Damage?*). Indeed, *LTP* was first discovered in the hippocampus, although it has later been found in many other areas of the brain, among them the cerebral cortex and the amygdala. LTP is produced whenever the pyramidal cells are subjected to excitatory inputs—for example, from the Schaffer collaterals—while they are in a depolarized state (caused by another excitatory input). Thus, simultaneous synaptic activation of the cell from two sources can make it "remember," in the sense that the next time the cell is activated by the same fibers, the postsynaptic effects are stronger than earlier. Binding of glutamate to the NMDA receptor opens a Ca^{2+} channel, but only when the membrane is in a depolarized state. The influx of Ca^{2+} acts as a signal to a long-lasting enhancement of the synaptic efficacy (or, in other words, LTP).

The *mechanism for LTP*, apart from being related to the NMDA receptor and calcium influx, is not yet fully understood. For example, it is not settled whether the increased synaptic effect of a single action potential in an afferent terminal is caused by increased transmitter release (that is, a presynaptic mechanism) or whether the changes occur postsynaptically.

To demonstrate a direct relation between LTP and learning is difficult, however. For example, only specific subsets of synapses are likely to show LTP in a natural learning situation. Nevertheless, much indirect evidence supports that hippocampal LTP is related to learning and memory. Increased synaptic efficacy has been found in the hippocampus in rats housed in an environment rich in stimuli and challenges (assuming that more learning takes place in this situation than in a standard cage). LTPlike phenomena have been observed in the hippocampus also after specific training situations. Another piece of evidence is that NMDA-receptor antagonists both prevent induction of LTP and reduce learning and memory in experimental animals. Gene-technological manipulations have produced strains of mice in which hippocampal LTP cannot be induced, and these animals also show reduced learning ability. Finally, structural synaptic changes have been observed in the hippocampus in conjunction with the induction of LTP. Even more compelling, structural synaptic changes (formation of new synapses and splitting of spines into two) have also been reported in the hippocampus in rats at the time they improve their performance in a learning situation.

There are, however, many pitfalls and problems with the interpretation of all of the above kinds of experiments, and not all studies point in the direction of a direct relationship between LTP and learning.

clarative memory but retain the ability to learn new skills. Also, observations of patients with memory deficits after lesions of the temporal lobe (without dementia) indicate that they learn and remember new movements better than new faces, words, places, and so forth.

The possible role of the *cerebellum* in motor learning was discussed in Chapter 14.

Medial Parts of the Temporal Lobe and Memory

The belief that the hippocampus is of importance for memory goes back to the end of the past century and was based on careful examination of patients with loss of memory as a result of brain damage. The degree and type of memory deficits were correlated with the site of the brain lesion, as determined histologically after the death of the patient. Patients with severe *amnesia* (loss of memory) that is not accompanied by intellectual reduction (dementia) typically have lesions affecting the medial parts of the temporal lobe (and often also the medial parts of the thalamus). The importance of the medial temporal lobe for *declarative or explicit memory* (see above) was strikingly demonstrated in the 1950s by observations of the patient H.M. with bilateral removal of the hippocampus and surrounding regions (see below, *Clinical Examples of Amnesia*). Such lesions include the hippocampal formation as the most constant finding. The amnesia is mainly *anterograde*—that is, the memory is lost for events taking place after the time of the brain damage. In case of *retrograde* amnesia, the patient is unable to recall events that took place before the damage. Retrograde amnesia virtually never occurs without anterograde amnesia. It should be stressed, however, that such lesions affect primarily *long-term memory*, whereas *short-term memory* may be virtually unimpaired (that is, the ability to remember, for example, numbers or words for up to a minute).

The interpretation of the data mentioned above is difficult, however, because the lesions were restricted very seldomly to the hippocampus or even the hippocampal formation. During the past few years, refined studies in monkeys with selective lesions, and observations with MRI and PET in humans, have clarified to a large extent the mutual roles of the hippocampus and other subregions of the medial temporal lobe. One such case was described recently, however (see below, *Can Destruction of CA1 Alone Produce Anterograde Amnesia?*), and it supports the notion that the hippocampus has a special role in certain kinds of memory. Furthermore, the perirhinal cortex appears to be critically involved in stimulus recognition memory.

It now seems established that the most severe memory loss occurs in monkeys after removal of not only the hippocampal formation but also the perirhinal cortex and the cortex surrounding the entorhinal area in the hippocampal gyrus. The former view that lesions of the amygdala also contribute to memory impairment was most likely based on inclusion of the perirhinal cortex in lesions of the amygdala. With refined techniques it was shown that isolated lesions of the amygdala does not reduce declarative memory (although the ability to remember associations between stimuli and emotions is reduced). Lesions comprising the hippocampus, the dentate gyrus, the subiculum, and parts of the entorhinal area produce clear-cut memory loss, but not as severely as when the perirhinal cortex is removed also. Thus, the perirhinal cortex and adjoining cortex of the hippocampal gyrus) appear to contribute to memory not only by their connections with the hippocampal formation but also by their connections to other parts of the brain. For example, perirhinal cortex projects to the thalamus (MD), amygdala, mammillary body, and parts of the prefrontal cortex.

Testing Memory in Monkeys

Various memory tests are used in experiments with monkeys to study the relation between brain structures and memory. Most common is the so-called *delayed nonmatching-to-sample test*. The monkey is briefly shown an object. After a certain time the same object is shown with a novel one. To receive a reward (for example, orange juice) the monkey must move the novel object, thus showing that it remembers which one was seen before. The experiment goes on with continually new pairs of items. With a brief interval between the first and second presentation, the performance is independent of the integrity of medial temporal structures. With intervals above 10 sec, however, the frequency of errors increases in monkeys with such lesions as a sign of failing memory. With more than two-minute intervals the performance is no better than chance, whereas normal monkeys reduce their performance to about 80% with intervals of three minutes.

What Is the Contribution of the Hippocampus to Learning and Memory?

Lesions restricted to the hippocampus are difficult to obtain. Nevertheless, recent experiments in monkeys with stereotaxic lesions, or with controlled global ischemia, come close to the ideal situation. Thus, global ischemia of limited duration may kill hippocampal pyramidal cells selectively. It now seems well documented that selective hippocampal lesions produce impaired memory in monkeys, although much less severe than when other parts of the hippocampal formation is included. The observations in the patient R.B., discussed below (*Clinical Examples of Amnesia*), strongly suggest that isolated hippocampal damage produce amnesia in humans also.

Possible unique contributions of the hippocampus to declarative memory—differing from those of the neighboring areas in the medial temporal lobe—are nevertheless not clear. Properties of single hippocampal cells, as described by O'Keefe and co-workers, are of particular interest in this connection. Thus, the firing of single hippocampal cells changes with the position of the animal in relation to its surroundings. The firing pattern changes, for example, with the location of the animal in different corners of the cage. On the basis of such experiments, it was proposed that the hippocampal neurons together form a *cognitive map* of our surroundings. This fits with the observation that monkeys with lesions of the hippocampal formation have difficulties with remembering *where* an object was located— the *association between objects and space*. We also know from cognitive psychology and from everyday experience that recall is strongly *context dependant*. For example, experiments with divers show that a series of numbers learned under water is better recalled under water than on dry land. Similarly, when unable to recall why we went into a room, it may help to go back to the place where we first got the idea to go into the room.

Clinical Examples of Amnesia

The Famous Case of H.M.

Patients with bilateral damage to medial aspects of the temporal lobe have pronounced anterograde (and often less severe retrograde) amnesia, as described above. The most famous case of this kind was described by Scoville and Milner. In 1953, this patient, called H.M. in the voluminous literature that deals with the results of tests to which he has been subjected, underwent surgery to remove bilaterally the medial aspects of his temporal lobes (the purpose was to cure his severe epilepsy). His lesion comprises most likely the hippocampal formation, additional parts of the parahippocampal gyrus, the uncus, and the amygdala. The epileptic fits became less frequent, but unfortunately he acquired a severe, permanent anterograde amnesia. Initially, he also had considerable retrograde amnesia that gradually improved to concern only 1 year before the operation. He remembered well the address of the place he lived before the operation, but he never learned the new address when moving afterward. He was furthermore unable to recall people he had met for the first time after the operation, even though he might have met them regularly for years. He could easily recall songs he had learned before the operation but not those he heard for the first time afterward. He never learned where the lawn mower was kept in his new house. Shortly after eating dinner, he could start on a new meal without remembering that he had just eaten. Nevertheless, his intelligence, as measured with various tests, was unaltered compared with before the operation, and his capacity for abstract reasoning was normal. Interestingly, his ability to learn new movements was much better than that for learning new faces, words, and so forth.

The memory deficits described above all concern events that took place some time previously—that is, long-term memory. His short-term memory was not correspondingly impaired, however. For example, he could recognize a word among nine presented to him 40 seconds earlier.

Once H.M. described his life as follows: "Every day is alone, regardless of the pleasures I have had or the sorrows I have had." Without long-term memory, we lose the continuity between the events of the present and the past.

Can Destruction of CA1 Alone Produce Anterograde Amnesia?

An interesting case was described recently by Zola-Morgan and co-workers, which supports the importance of the hippocampus proper for learning and memory. The patient, called R.B., had an episode of brain ischemia during cardiac surgery. Afterward, he had moderate anterograde amnesia that lasted until his death some years later. He was not appreciably reduced intellectually. Even though his amnesia was much less severe than that of H.M., he had grave problems remembering the events of the day before. During his visits to his doctor, he would repeat the same story at short intervals. Histological examination of the brain after his death showed that the most pronounced alterations were in the hippocampus and, interestingly, restricted to CA1 on both sides. Within the CA1 there was an almost total loss of pyramidal cells (Fig. 19.5). That the CA1 field of the hippocampus is particularly vulnerable (to ischemia) was suggested in the past century on the basis of observations of patients with epilepsy. The mechanism in such cases may be excessive release of glutamate that activates NMDA receptors (see Chapter 4, *Ischemic Cell Damage and the Glutamate Hypothesis*). This results in an uncontrolled influx of calcium, with subsequent cell damage.

As a possible explanation of the marked symptoms of R. B. caused by a seemingly minor damage to the hippocampus, Zola-Morgan and co-workers suggest that destruction of the CA1 field (in its entire length) effectively interrupts signal transmission through the hippocampus and thus isolates it from the rest of the brain (see Fig. 19.5).

Permanent Memory Traces Lie in Many Parts of the Brain

As mentioned above, the amnesia after lesions of the hippocampus and surrounding structures is predominantly or solely anterograde. This shows that information about events taking place some time before the lesion must be stored in other parts of the brain.

Other clinical observations of patients with damage in various parts of the brain indicate that there is no specific "memory center," but well-consolidated information is stored in a distributed fashion. When a memory is established—presumably as long-term synaptic changes—the hippocampal formation no longer seems necessary for storage and recall. The time required to reach this stage is not known, but, again on the basis of observations of patients with damage to medial parts of the temporal lobe, it may perhaps take as long as a year.[7] During this period we imagine a gradual consolidation of the memory traces in the relevant parts of the cortex (and probably in subcortical structures). It seems unlikely that the information is first held in the hippocampus for a certain period and then transmitted in a finally processed form out to the permanent stores. Probably, the consolidation takes place by a continuous "dialogue" between the hippocampus and other parts of the cortex. The nature of such a dialogue is so far only a matter of speculation, however.

Amnesia Can Be Caused by Lesions Outside the Medial Temporal Lobe

Clinical observations suggest that amnesia can arise after lesions of the *medial thalamus*, the *mammillary body*, or the connections from the latter to the thalamus (the mammillothalamic tract). Whether isolated damage to any one of these structures causes amnesia is not finally settled, however. As to thalamic lesions, inclusion of the MD nucleus seems necessary to cause amnesia, although destruction of the anterior nucleus and the internal medullary lamina close to the MD may contribute (perhaps due to interruption of fibers to and from MD). Severe amnesia was described in a patient who, as judged from computer tomography of the brain, had a small lesion confined to the anterior and medial parts of the thalamus on the left side.[6]

The role of the *mammillary body* in amnesia has attracted much interest because its involvement in *Korsakoff's psychosis*, in which the patient suffers from severe anterograde and retrograde amnesia (among other cognitive impairments). The disease is usually due to chronic alcohol abuse. In Korsakoff's psychosis cell loss is found regularly in the medial thalamus, and whether a lesion of the mammillary bodies alone causes amnesia has been a matter of controversy. In monkeys, however, bilateral destruction of the mammillary bodies produces a moderate memory loss. Since both the MD and the mammillary body receive afferents from medial parts of the temporal lobe, it seems likely that the amnesia after their destruction is due to interruption of their cortical connections. In support of this assumption, amnesia has been reported after bilateral interruption of the *fornix* in epileptic patients (cutting the pathway from the hippocampal formation to the mammillary body). In any case, it seems unlikely that the memory traces are stored in the thalamus or the mammillary body.

The MD sends efferents to the prefrontal cortex, and accurate testing of patients with Korsakoff's psychosis shows that they have also symptoms suggestive of prefrontal dysfunction. As to the relation between the site of a lesion and the distribution of functional disturbances, PET studies of glucose uptake in a group of patients with severe amnesia are illuminating. Thus, these patients all showed altered glucose uptake in the hippocampus, thalamus, cingulate gyrus, and ventral parts of the prefrontal cortex, although their lesions as identified with MRI were differently placed. It seems reasonable to conclude that *declarative memory, as usually tested, depends on the integrity of several cell groups that are mutually interconnected.* When one part of the network is damaged, this also has consequences for the functioning of the other parts. This illustrates the problems inherent in assessing the functional role of a cell group or a tract only from the symptoms caused by their destruction.

Finally, loss of memory also has been reported after lesions restricted to *cholinergic cell groups in the basal forebrain*, as discussed above (*Cholinergic Cell Groups Projecting to the Cerebral Cortex*).

Memories in a wide sense represent our knowledge of the world and the actions that are necessary to relate successfully to it. Not all this knowledge is accessible for conscious "inspection" and analysis (nondeclarative or implicit memory described above). Nevertheless, all memories presumably have as their substrate synaptic changes in specific parts of the central nervous system. The American neuropsychologist Antonio Damasio uses the term *"knowledge systems of the brain"* about the widespread networks dedicated to specific tasks. Examples are knowledge systems dealing with social interactions, faces, objects, language, or ourselves. When parts of the temporal lobe cortex is particularly important for recognition of faces, this does not necessarily mean that all information about faces is stored there. More likely, this part is unique because it has access to face-related information stored in many other areas. Presumably, the memory of faces fails after a stroke in the temporal lobe because there is "no one" to retrieve and process all the relevant information—not because the storehouse is empty.

BEHAVIOR AND THE LIMBIC STRUCTURES

The phylogenetically old parts of the brain that we have discussed in this chapter influence complex functions closely related to various aspects of behavior. Even though some structures appear to be especially important for certain functions, there is no sound basis for localizing complex brain functions to smaller, well-defined cell groups or parts of the brain and to use terms such as "centers" for memory, sexual behavior, aggression, and so forth. In general, the more complex a function is, the more distributed the neural network subserving it. Our present knowledge tells us that all complex behavioral reactions engage the amygdala, the septal nuclei, the hippocampal region, the reticular formation, the hypothalamus, and large parts of the cerebral cortex. As witnessed by their numerous interconnections, all of these regions cooperate to exert an integrated influence on the peripheral somatic and autonomic effectors. What the American psychologist Grossman said about the septal nuclei probably holds for the rest of the limbic structures too: "Just about every behavior and/or psychological function which has been investigated to date has been shown to be affected in some way by septal lesions. . . ."

Further studies of the limbic structures are of great importance to improve our understanding of the interplay between conscious, cognitive processes and the emotional and more or less subconscious processes that together determine our behavior. Such knowledge is presumably also of importance for a better understanding of psychiatric diseases, in which emotional disturbances as a rule constitute an important aspect.

NOTES

1. Some authors use the term "limbic system" even more extensively and include the hypothalamus and parts of the basal ganglia (primarily the ventral striatum; see Chapter 13).

2. Only parts of the cingulate gyrus belong to the allocortex; most of it probably belongs to the oldest parts of the neocortex.

3. The region containing the *septal nuclei* is called the precommissural part of the septum. The postcommissural part is the *septum pellucidum*, which contains no neurons.

4. Not all neurons in the basal forebrain projecting to the cortex are cholinergic. Some neurons, mingled with the cholinergic ones, are *GABAergic*. Some contain the neuropeptide *galanin*, partly colocalized with acetylcholine. In humans the diagonal band of Broca has many *somatostatin-containing* neurons, although it is not known whether they project to the cortex. Thus, although apparently most of the neurons in the basal forebrain projecting to the cortex are cholinergic, it is not a transmitter-specific system. This is of relevance when trying to explain the symptoms of diseases with loss of neurons in the basal forebrain (notably Alzheimer's disease, discussed in Chapter 4).

5. The old view was based on experiments with anterograde degeneration techniques, which require that the neurons be damaged. To produce lesions of the hippocampus without at the same time affecting the subiculum is virtually impossible. Some fibers in the fornix nevertheless arise from hippocampal pyramidal cells. They end in parts of the septal nuclei, however, and not in the mammillary body. The fibers arise from CA3 pyramdal cells; that is, the same neurons that emit the Schaffer collaterals to CA1 (Fig. 19.7).

6. In this particular case the verbal memory was more severely affected than the visual. The patient could with some difficulty remember objects he had seen some time ago, whereas words heard were completely forgotten.

7. In Korsakoff's psychosis the retrograde amnesia may be very pronounced—for example, more than 25 years. This in itself suggests that the pathology in these patients does more than interrupting connections between the medial temporal lobe and other parts of the cerebral cortex.

CHAPTER 20

CEREBRAL CORTEX

The human cerebral cortex consists of between 10 and 20 billion neurons and constitutes more than half of all gray matter of the central nervous system. This gives a rough impression of its functional importance. In lower vertebrates there are only very modest primordia of the cerebral cortex (allocortex), and it is first in mammals, particularly anthropoid apes and humans, that the cerebral cortex comes to dominate the rest of the nervous system quantitatively. This enormous increase in the volume of the cortex has necessitated a marked folding of the surface of the hemisphere. The outer layer of the human cerebral cortex is around 0.2 m^2, but only one-third of this is exposed on the surface. The neocortex constitutes most of the cerebral cortex in higher mammals, and this chapter will deal only with the neocortex.

To understand the relation between the performance of the cerebral cortex and the underlying neural processes, we need to address two levels of organization. The first concerns information processing in a small volume of cortex. We may term this *intracortical synaptic organization*. The second level concerns the interconnection of functionally different cortical units with long association and commissural fibers, which we term *interareal synaptic organization*. How are signals arriving in a small bit of the cortex treated before "answers" are sent to other parts of the cortex or subcortical nuclei? How are the many different cortical areas linked to form networks designed for solving specific tasks? The enormous number of neurons and synaptic couplings in the human cerebral cortex explain why we do not have complete answers to such questions. Furthermore, the tasks of the cerebral cortex are the most complex of all. To understand the relationship between the "machinery" of the brain and mental functions like personality, memory, thought, and feelings is indeed the most formidable and exciting challenge of modern neuroscience.

In previous chapters we have treated the role of the cerebral cortex in sensory processes (Chapters 7–10), control of body and eye movements (Chapters 12 and 16), and autonomic functions (Chapter 19). The role of the cerebral cortex in relation to sleep and consciousness is briefly discussed in Chapter 15.

Figure 20.1 *The basic six-layered structure of the neocortex.* The three columns show sections perpendicular to the cortical surface subjected to different staining methods. The **left** column shows the appearance in Golgi-impregnated sections, in which the perikarya and some of the dendrites can be seen. The **middle** column shows a thionine-stained section, in which only the perikarya are visible. The **right** column shows the appearance after myelin staining—that is, the main pattern of the myelinated axons is evident, with perpendicular bundles of fibers entering the cortex, and horizontal bundles of fibers interconnecting nearby parts of the cortex. After Brodmann and Vogt.

1. MOLECULAR LAYER

2. EXTERNAL GRANULAR LAYER

3. EXTERNAL PYRAMIDAL LAYER

4. INTERNAL GRANULAR LAYER

5. INTERNAL PYRAMIDAL LAYER

6. MULTIFORM LAYER

STRUCTURE OF THE CEREBRAL CORTEX

The Neocortex Consists of Six Layers

All parts of the neocortex share a common basic structure, with the neurons arranged in six *layers* or *laminae* oriented parallel to the surface of the cortex (Figs. 20.1, 20.2, and 20.4). Another general feature is the arrangement of the neurons in rows or columns oriented perpendicular to the cortical surface (Fig. 20.2). Both kinds of cellular aggregation are related to functional specializations among the neurons, as we will discuss below. Figure 20.1 shows the main features of the layering. It can be seen that the laminar pattern arises because cells of similar shape and size are collected in more or less distinct layers. The density of cell bodies also differs among the layers.

About two-thirds of the neurons are cortical *pyramidal cells* (the name refers to the triangular shape of their cell bodies). A typical pyramidal cell has a long axon arising from the base of the pyramid and a long *apical dendrite* that extends toward the cortical surface—it thus extends through several layers superficial to the layer in which the perikaryon is located (Figs. 1.1 and 20.5). The fairly large pyramidal cells are found in layers 3 and 5, but many of the smaller cells in the other layers are also pyramidal. The pyramidal cells are also characterized by their large number of *dendritic spines* (Figs. 1.1 and 20.5). The rest of the cortical neurons constitute a heterogenous group whose neurons have in common that their perikarya are not pyramidal; such neurons are therefore lumped to-

Figure 20.2 *Cytoarchitectonics of the cerebral cortex.* Photomicrograph of a thionine-stained section through the central region of the human brain. The section is perpendicular to the direction of the central sulcus. The six-layered structure is evident in area 4 (MI) and in area 3b (SI). Note, however, the difference in development and appearance of the various layers in the two areas, especially with regard to layers 4 and 5. The cortex of the MI in the precentral gyrus is much thicker than that of the SI. This is not because there are more neurons but because of more extensive dendritic trees, more axonal branches and boutons, and perhaps more glial cells. Note also the tendency for the cells to be arranged in vertically oriented rows or columns. See also Figure 12.3 with a corresponding section from the monkey. Magnification, ×170.

gether as *nonpyramidal cells*. Their shape and size vary considerably, but all of them are most likely interneurons.[1]

The most superficial cortical layer, *layer 1*, the *molecular layer*, is fiber-rich with few neurons (Figs. 20.1 and 20.2). Apart from axons, it contains the apical dendrites of pyramidal cells in the deeper layers. *Layer 2*, the *external granular layer*, contains densely packed, small perikarya.[2] *Layer 4*, the *internal granular layer*, is similarly built. In primary sensory cortical areas, layer 4 is especially well developed, and shows even a further laminar subdivision in the striate area (layer 4A, B, and C; Fig. 20.4). *Layer 3*, the *external pyramidal layer*, can be recognized by its content of medium-sized pyramidal cells, whereas *layer 5*, the *internal pyramidal layer*, also contains many large pyramidal cells. *Layer 6*, the *multiform layer*, contains many cells with spindle-shaped perikarya.

Considering only certain salient features, we can say that *layers 2 and 4 are mainly receiving*—being most developed in the primary sensory areas—whereas *layers 3 and 5 are mainly efferent* and send their axons out of the part of the cortex in which they are located. The pyramidal cells of layer 5 send their axons primarily to subcortical nuclei, and this layer is particularly well developed in MI (Figs. 12.3 and 20.2). The layer 3 pyramidal cells send their axons primarily to other areas of the cortex (association and commissural fibers). Layer 6 is also largely efferent and sends many axons to the thalamus.

Afferents from Different Sources End in Different Cortical Layers

The cortical layers differ with regard to the origin of their extrinsic afferents. Thus, there is some degree of specialization among the laminae with regard to what kind of information they process. As we will discuss below, however, connections between the lamina ensure integration of their outputs. Schematically, pathways conveying *precise sensory information* end primarily in layer 4. This concerns thalamocortical fibers from the somatosensory relay nucleus, VPL, and from the relay nuclei of the visual and auditory pathways, the lateral and medial geniculate bodies. *Association fibers* (that is, from other cortical areas) end preferentially in layers 2–4. *Subcortical afferents with modulatory effects* end in several layers, notably layer 1. Such fibers arise in the intralaminar thalamic nuclei, in several brain stem nuclei (the raphe nuclei, nucleus locus coeruleus, and dopaminergic cell groups in the mesencephalon), and in the basal nucleus.

The Cerebral Cortex Can Be Divided into Cytoarchitectonic Areas

Even though all parts of the neocortex consist of six cell layers, the thickness and structure of the various layers vary from one area to another. This is observed most easily in sections stained to visualize the cell bodies alone (Figs. 1.2, 1.3, 20.2, and 20.4). Such *cytoarchitectonic* differences form the basis of the subdivision of the entire cortex into cytoarchitectonic areas (Fig. 20.3), as done around the turn of the century by

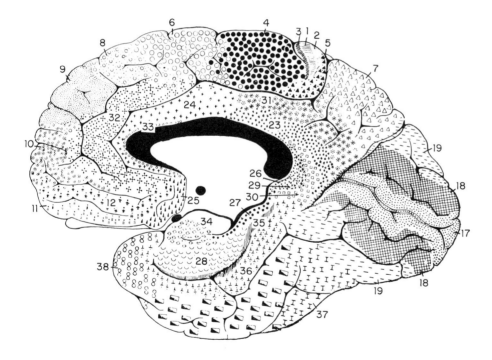

Brodmann and others (Fig. 20.3). This is described briefly in Chapter 3, and several of the cytoarchitectonic areas are mentioned in previous chapters.

The main importance of the division of the cortex into cytoarchitectonic areas is that these areas have proved in many instances to differ functionally, even though they were initially defined solely on the basis of the size,

Figure 20.3 *Brodmann's cytoarchitectonic map of the human brain.* The various areas are labeled with different symbols and numbers.

Figure 20.4 *The transition between area 17 (the striate area) and area 18.* Thionine-stained section from the human visual cortex. Note how the various layers change in cell size, cell density, and thickness at the transition between the two cytoarchitectonic areas. Most areal borders are less clearcut than this.

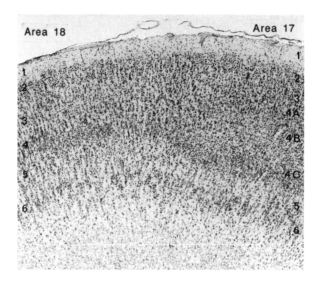

shape, and arrangement of the neuronal cell bodies. In many cases a cytoarchitectonically defined area is unique also with regard to its afferent and efferent connections and the physiological properties of its cells.

Although the borders between different cytoarchitectonic areas are sometimes easy to identify, as exemplified in Figure 20.4, more often the differences are rather subtle. Thus, it should not come as a surprise that authors often disagree with regard to the parcellation of the cortex into areas, as a comparison of their published maps will show. Today we try to *define a cortical area* not only on the basis of cytoarchitectonics but also by additional criteria, such as fiber connections, cellular markers, recordings of single-cell activity, and the behavioral effects of stimulation or ablation of the area in question. We will return to connections and functions of different cortical areas later in this chapter.

With regard to the *size of cortical areas*, there are surprisingly large individual variations. The volume of the striate area (the most easily identified one) varies by a factor of three among adult humans. Because the volume of the hemispheres does not show similar variations, this implies that in a brain with a large striate area, other areas are relatively smaller. Whether such anatomic differences also have functional significance is unknown, but conceivably they may contribute to the large differences between humans in mental and other capacities.

Intracortical Connectivity: Interneurons and Pyramidal Cell Collaterals

The pyramidal cells send their axon toward the white matter to reach other parts of the cortex or subcortical cell groups. Thus, they are the *projection neurons* of the cortex (Fig. 20.5), which most likely constitute more than two-thirds of all cortical neurons. The projection neurons send *recurrent collaterals* before the axon leaves the cortex and can thus influence the level of activity among the cortical neurons in their vicinity. The recurrent collaterals may, for example, excite inhibitory interneurons and thereby limit the activity of the parent cell and other pyramidal cells.

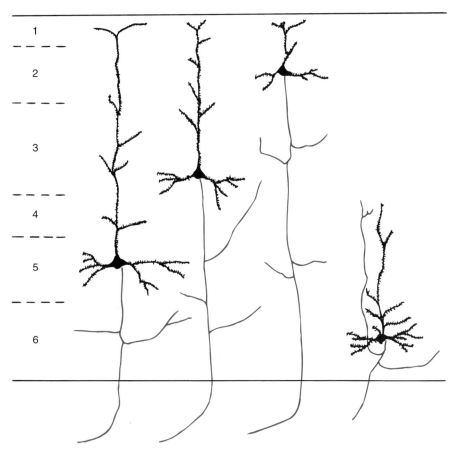

All cells belonging to the other main type of cortical neurons, the *non-pyramidal cells*, have locally branching axons that do not reach the white matter—that is, they are the cortical *interneurons* (Fig. 20.6). Such interneurons may be classified into three main types on the basis of the course and branching pattern of their axons. One type has an axon that forms numerous terminal branches close to the perikaryon. It mediates influence mainly to neighboring neurons within the lamina in which the cell body is located. A second type has an axon coursing perpendicularly or *vertically* toward either the cortical surface or the white matter, giving off collaterals on its way. This enables the interneuron to influence neurons in several layers. Finally, the third main type of interneuron sends its axon in a *horizontal* direction (parallel to the cortical surface).

Even though this division into three kinds of cortical interneurons is an oversimplification, it shows the main features of the *intracortical connections*, which permits interactions among neighboring neurons, among neurons within different layers, and among neurons located at some distance within the same layer. *Vertically oriented axons* (from either interneurons or pyramidal cell recurrent collaterals) ensures the communication among neurons within a narrow cortical cylinder or column. The *horizontal axonal branches* mediate communication among neurons in different columns. Such horizontal influences can be inhibitory or excitatory. In sensory cortical areas, the horizontal intracortical connections mediate *lateral inhibition*, which increases the spatial resolution of the

Figure 20.5 *Cortical projection neurons.* Schematic drawing. The axons, shown in red, give off several recurrent collaterals on their way to the white matter. The dendrites have numerous spines. The larges neurons, with the largest perikarya and the thickest axons, are located in layer 5. Schematic drawing based on studies by Jones (1988) of the central region of the monkey with the Golgi method.

1

2

3

4

5

6

Figure 20.6 *Main kinds of cortical interneurons.* Note three patterns of axonal distribution (in red): in the immediate vicinity of the perikaryon, horizontally in the layer of the perikaryon, and vertically spanning several layers. Based on Jones (1988).

sensory information (lateral inhibition is present at several levels of the sensory pathways, see Chapter 7). The may also contribute to *cortical plasticity* by modulating the size of the receptive fields of cortical neurons.

The majority of horizontal intracortical axons appear to be collaterals of pyramidal cells rather than of interneurons. They are generally longer in association areas than in primary sensory areas—measured up to 9 mm in monkey posterior parietal cortex, although the majority are probably less than 1–2 mm. Thus, cortical columns that are farther apart than this must communicate by means of projection neurons with an axon coursing in the white matter—that is, association fibers. Such connections are discussed later in this chapter.

Intracortical Impulse Traffic and Information Processing

Afferent fibers ending in a small volume of the cortex make excitatory synapses with a large number of projection neurons and interneurons. Thus, *one* afferent fiber from the thalamus has been estimated to contact about 5000 cortical neurons. The synaptic contacts are established in certain layers only, but the excitation is propagated to other layers by the pyramidal cell recurrent collaterals and excitatory interneurons (spiny stellate cells). At the same time, numerous inhibitory interneurons are activated. The inhibitory interneurons serve to focus the efferent cortical signals and to terminate the activity of the projection neurons. In addition, the inhibitory interneurons inhibit other inhibitory interneurons, with resulting disinhibition.

Horizontal axonal collaterals propagate both inhibition and excitation laterally from the focus of cortical excitation. This does not occur at random but so that functionally related neurons are interconnected. Finally, the integrated signals are issued—especially from layers 3 and 5 pyramids—to other parts of the cortex and subcortical cell groups (among them motoneurons).

As we see, the activity (that is, the frequency and pattern of action potentials) of each cortical neuron depends on the activity of the numerous other neurons with which it is synaptically connected. This is true of fibers reaching the cortex from other regions (subcortical nuclei and other parts of the cortex) and intracortical connections from cells in the immediate vicinity (within a radius of a few millimeters in the horizontal direction). *One cortical neuron, such as a pyramidal cell of the MI, integrates information from perhaps 600 nearby cortical cells and has been estimated to receive about 60,000 synapses* (monkey).

The enormous number of neurons and their complex interconnections within even a small volume of cortical tissue explain why we still do not understand the basic rules underlying intracortical information processing. Promising advances have been made, however, especially in the visual cortex (see below).

More About Intracortical Organization

Intracortical Impulse Traffic in the Visual Cortex

Regarding intracortical impulse traffic, detailed studies have been performed in the visual cortex with the use of methods enabling the recording of single-cell activity in relation to specific stimuli and subsequent intracellular injection of HRP. Thus, the dendritic and axonal patterns of individual, functionally characterized neurons can be determined. Successful attempts have also been made to abolish the activity of neurons in specific layers and then study how the properties of neurons in other layers are changed. As expected from the known terminal pattern of axons from the lateral geniculate body, neurons are first activated in layer 4 after visual stimuli (in addition, neurons in other layers with dendrites extending into layer 4 can be influenced). From layer 4, the excitation is propagated to layers 2 and 3, and from there to layers 5 and 6. Some cells in layer 6 send axons upward to layer 4. Presumably, at every step in such a pathway through the cortex some processing of the sensory information takes place, such as integration by one cell of the signals from other functionally different cells. In accordance with this assumption, the functional properties of cells in different layers vary, as shown with microelectrode recordings after natural stimulation of receptors. A projection neuron in layer 5 has quite different properties than a cell in layer 4; for example, the receptive fields of the layer 5 cells are larger (as a sign of convergence of signals from several neurons in layer 4). Other properties of layer 5 cells also suggest that signals from functionally different layer 4 cells converge on layer 5 cells (via processing in layers 2 and 3).

Horizontal Integration and Cortical Plasticity

The extensive horizontal intracortical connections appear to be crucial for the working of the cortex. They ensure, as mentioned above, that the receptive fields of cortical neurons are not static but subject to modification by inputs from their neighbors. For example, single cells in the visual cortex have smaller receptive fields and react more strongly when the *attention* of the animal is directed to the visual stimulus. Horizontal connections most likely also contribute to well-known psychophysical phenomena, such as the filling in of missing lines in otherwise meaningful visual images. When blocking GABA receptors (and thus inhibitory horizontal connections) the receptive fields of cortical neurons enlarge immediately. Stimulation of a small peripheral spot activates a much larger area in the SI after blocking GABA transmission than before. After amputation of a finger in monkeys, the area in SI activated from the neighboring fingers enlarges immediately. These examples show that excitatory connections must exist in the cortex (and at lower levels) that are suppressed under ordinary conditions. Furthermore, due to such modifiable connections there is a dynamic balance between the cortical representations of various body parts. Training of a sensory task can alter the cortical representation of the trained part (for example, training roughness discrimination with the index finger). It seems likely that such examples of cortical plasticity are due, at least partly, to changes in the synaptic efficacy of horizontal connections. The same mechanism probably operates during the recovery after brain damage affecting the cerebral cortex or its connections.

The horizontal connections may also help explain why the responses of cortical neurons as a rule are *context dependant*—that is, not only the stimulus hitting its receptive field determines the response of a cortical neuron but also stimuli in other locations.

Cortical Microstructure: Columns and Modules

We have mentioned previously that the cortical cells appear to be organized into small units formed by cylinders or *columns* of tissue extending perpendicular to the surface of the cortex. A tendency for cortical neurons to be arranged in perpendicular rows is evident from thionine-stained sections (Figs. 20.2 and 20.4). That neurons within a column share functional properties that differ from those within adjacent columns was first observed by Mountcastle in the monkey SI. He found that when a microelectrode was inserted perpendicular to the cortical surface, the cells encountered as the electrode traversed the thickness of the cortex had very similar receptive fields. They were furthermore similar with regard to their adequate stimulus, as if they were activated by the same kind of receptor. When, in contrast, the microelectrode was inserted obliquely, the receptive fields of the neurons moved with the advancement of the electrode. On the basis of such experiments, it was proposed that SI neurons with similar receptive fields and modalities are grouped together in columns with a diameter of some hundred micrometers. A similar columnar arrangement has been observed in the MI, but with relation to muscles rather than to receptors (neurons within one column act on one or a few synergistic muscles). Interestingly, a pyramidal cell with all its dendrites and recurrent collaterals is contained within a cortical tissue cylinder with a diameter of about 350 μm (of course, hundreds of other neurons are present within the same cylinder).

Module is a more general term for columns and other groups of neurons sharing important properties (in the cortex and elsewhere; see Chapter 8, *Modular Organization of the Visual Cortex*). Different criteria are used to define modules in the cortex, and depending on the criteria used, their shape and size vary greatly. Furthermore, the relation between the tendency for cortical neurons to be arranged in columns and the physiologically defined functional columns is not always clear. Also, the distribution in the cortex of neurons with different properties is less schematic than the modular concept might imply. In the visual cortex, in which the segregation of functionally different neurons has been most thoroughly investigated, cells sharing functional properties are arranged in bands rather than in cylinders (Fig. 8.20). Another more serious problem with the columnar concept is that neurons in different layers—for example, of the striate area—are not functionally identical (for example, cells that are color-specific and cells that are movement-specific are located in different layers). Thus, the modules may not always extend through the depth of the cortex but may be limited to one or a few layers. To apply the columnar concept to such examples of segregation of functionally different cortical neurons is rather confusing.

It may not be feasible to define *the* cortical module, that is, one found in all parts of the cortex. Nevertheless, it is striking how connections and cytochemical markers show a patchy distribution all over the cortex. For example, afferent projections—from the thalamus or from other parts of the cortex—end in many, regularly spaced patches in the cortex. This means that inputs from different sources may converge systematically on cortical neurons. Also, projection neurons with a common target tend to be lumped together similarly. There is, furthermore, a striking correspondence between the diameters of cortical dendritic trees and of the terminal patches formed by afferent fibers.

The *biologic significance* of modular organization in the cortex and elsewhere (for example, in the striatum and the cerebellum) is not fully understood. The modular pattern gives each cortical neuron a varied afferent input—each neuron receiving samples of information from several sources (several patches contact each neuron). In the motor cortex, for example, a neuron might need to integrate information from the thalamus (perhaps from different subgroups in the VL nucleus), from SI, and from the premotor cortex. Another advantage of modular organization may be that it permits shorter intracortical connections and thus saves nervous tissue. Modules may, furthermore, be advantageous during development by making it easier for growing axons to find their target. Some claim, however, that modular organization is merely a byproduct of how the nervous system develops, lacking an intrinsic functional meaning.

Fast Excitation and Inhibition in the Cortex: Glutamate and GABA

Most or perhaps all *projection neurons*—those sending their axons to subcortical nuclei and those forming association or commissural connections—use *glutamate* as a neurotransmitter. Accordingly, physiological studies show that they have fast, excitatory synaptic actions (however, there are also metabotropic, modulatory glutamate receptors in the cortex). Glutamate released from pyramidal cell intracortical collaterals can also bind to *NMDA receptors*, which are thought to be involved in plastic changes related to learning and restitution after brain damage.

A subgroup of cortical *interneurons* is most likely also excitatory, as judged from, among other things, the kind of synapse they form (asymmetrical synaptic thickening, in contrast to the symmetrical thickening found at most inhibitory cortical synapses). This kind of interneuron has numerous dendritic spines, in this respect resembling the (excitatory) pyramidal cells. Apart from such so-called *spiny stellate cells*, the rest of the interneurons (the "aspiny" ones) are probably inhibitory, with GABA as the predominant neurotransmitter. GABA-containing neurons constitute 20%–25% of all cortical neurons. Physiological studies also indicate that the *majority of cortical interneurons are inhibitory*. Most of the GABAergic interneurons also contain one or several neuropeptides (such as substance P, somatostatin, VIP, cholecystokinin, and neuropeptide Y).

There is some evidence that *epilepsy* may be related to selective loss of GABAergic cortical interneurons (even though this is just one of several possible mechanisms).

Modulatory Synaptic Effects in the Cerebral Cortex

Most cortical neurons receive inputs from the thalamus and other parts of the cortex with fast, excitatory synaptic actions (glutamate acting on AMPA receptors), and fast inhibition from interneurons (GABA acting on $GABA_A$ receptors). Such synapses are responsible for precise and specific information transfer in topographically organized connections. In addition, however, cortical neurons are influenced by slow, modulatory synaptic actions. This is partly due to glutamate acting on metabotropic receptors and GABA acting on $GABA_B$ receptors. In addition, neuropeptides colocalized with GABA exert modulatory effects, although we do not know their functional roles.

Most studied, however, are modulatory actions mediated by diffusely organized fiber systems from several brain-stem and basal forebrain cell groups. We have mentioned such connections in Chapter 2 (under *Modulatory Transmitter Systems*) and in Chapter 15 (under *Impulse Pathways and Transmitters for the Activation of the Cerebral Cortex*). The following neurotransmitters are involved: acetylcholine, norepinephrine, serotonin, dopamine, and histamine. In general, they act to improve the precision of cortical signal transfer, for example by *improving the signal-to-noise ratio*. Such effects are probably important in relation to arousal, focussed attention, and motivation. Acetylcholine, for example brings layer 5 pyramids in the motor cortex from a state with low-frequency burst firing to single-spike firing. In the latter state, the frequency of single spikes depends on the degree of depolarization, that is, the intensity of synaptic excitatory inputs to the neuron from, for example, the premotor cortex and the thalamus.

Cortical Neurons Are Coincidence Detectors

Many cortical neurons react primarily when information about two events reaches them simultaneously, like cells in the visual cortex that respond poorly to signals from one eye only but vigorously to simultaneous signals from both eyes (binocular cells). Like a good detective who has a special eye for *coincidences* (events occurring simultaneously) and disregards numerous trivial bits of information, the cortical neurons respond preferentially to certain coincidences of stimuli that have a survival value. This characteristic property of cortical cells is probably built into the inborn wiring pattern ("hardware") of the brain, but it also needs proper use to be further developed and maintained (see *The Parietal Lobe and the Development of the Ability to Integrate Somatosensory and Visual Information*, later in this chapter).

Glutamatergic thalamocortical fibers appear to act via AMPA receptors on cortical neurons but not via NMDA receptors (the latter being related to induction of LTP). The recurrent pyramidal cell collaterals, however, act also on NMDA receptors. There is experimental evidence that simultaneous activation of a cortical neuron from the thalamus (AMPA) and from other cortical neurons (NMDA) can induce LTP. In the monkey motor cortex LTP has been established during the learning of new motor skills. Thus, not only are the cortical neurons especially sensitive to coincident inputs, this may also be the cellular basis of associative learning in the cortex.

CONNECTIONS OF THE CEREBRAL CORTEX

The connections of the cerebral cortex with subcortical structures have been described in several of the previous chapters. We have dealt with the terminal regions of the major sensory pathways and the areas giving origin to the descending pathways involved in motor control. *Here we describe general aspects of connections between the thalamus and the cerebral cortex* and of the *corticocortical connections* (association and commissural connections). Such knowledge is a necessary basis for the following treatment of the cortical association areas and their functional roles.

A Brief Survey of Cortical Connections

We can classify the *afferent* connections of the cerebral cortex as follows:

1. Precisely, topographically organized connections from the *"specific" thalamic nuclei*; each thalamic nucleus supplies one particular part of the cortex;
2. Diffusely organized connections from the *intralaminar thalamic nuclei and several other subcortical nuclei* (the raphe nuclei, the nucleus coeruleus, dopaminergic cell groups in the mesencephalon, and cholinergic cell groups in the basal forebrain); such connections do not respect the cytoarchitectonic borders in contrast to the connections from the specific thalamic nuclei;
3. *Association fibers*—that is, precisely organized connections linking cortical areas within the same hemisphere;
4. *Commissural fibers*—that is, precisely organized connections between areas in the two hemispheres.

The *efferent* connections of the cerebral cortex can also be divided into subcortical and corticocortical ones (association and commissural connections). The *subcortical* fibers are destined for the thalamus, the striatum, various brain stem nuclei (among them the pontine nuclei projecting to the cerebellum), and the spinal cord. The *corticocortical* connections are for the most part reciprocal—that is, an area receives fibers from the same areas to which it sends fibers.

Thalamocortical Connections

The thalamus has been mentioned in several contexts (see Chapters 3 and 7 for descriptions of its gross anatomy and main subdivisions). *The thalamus supplies all parts of the neocortex with afferents.* Each part of the cortex receives fibers primarily from one of the specific thalamic nuclei. The main features of this topographic arrangement of the thalamocortical projection are shown in Figure 20.7 (as we believe it is organized in humans). Figures 7.20 and 14.14 show the projection from the ventral thalamic nucleus in more detail, based on experimental studies in monkeys with retrograde degeneration techniques and retrograde and anterograde axonal transport methods.

Conditions are more complex than shown in the diagrams, however. In the first place, the topographic arrangement is much more fine-grained. Thus, the projection from one thalamic nucleus is precisely arranged, with subdivisions of the nucleus supplying minor parts only of the large fields shown in Figure 20.7. As described in Chapters 7 and 8, the thalamocortical connections from the VPL and the lateral geniculate body are so-

Figure 20.7 *The thalamocortical projection*. Highly simplified scheme showing the main features of its topographic organization.

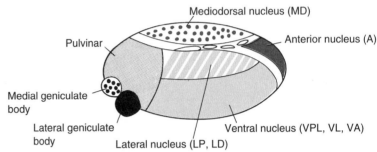

matotopically and retinotopically organized, respectively, with a precision that enables the cortex to extract information about minute spatial details. Furthermore, each thalamic nucleus sends fibers to more than one cortical area. We can take the MD as an example. In the scheme, it is depicted as sending fibers to the prefrontal cortex (without any topographic arrangement). In reality, the MD sends fibers to other parts of the cortex, too, such as parts of the cingulate gyrus. The MD furthermore consists of several subdivisions, each supplying a different part of the prefrontal cortex. The main point emerging from such knowledge is that the MD is not a functional unit. A small lesion, for example, must be expected to produce quite different effects depending on its exact location within the MD.

Some of the specific thalamic nuclei are relay stations in the *pathways for impulses from sensory receptors* (vision, hearing, cutaneous sensation, proprioception) to specific cortical areas. The *VPL* receives afferents from the somatosensory pathways and projects to the SI, areas 3, 1, and 2 (Figs. 7.14 and 7.15); the *lateral geniculate body* receives afferents from the retina and projects to the striate area (Fig. 8.14); the *medial geniculate body* is the last subcortical station in the auditory pathways and sends efferents to AI (Figs. 9.10 and 9.11). Other specific thalamic nuclei, the *VL* and *VA*, are relay stations in the pathways from the cerebellum and the basal ganglia to the motor and premotor cortical areas (Fig. 14.14). Other thalamic nuclei relay signals from limbic structures: The *anterior thalamic nucleus* receives afferents from the mammillary nucleus (which receives its main input from the subiculum of the hippocampal formation) and projects to the cingulate gyrus; and the *MD* (Fig. 20.8) can relay signals from the amygdala to the frontal lobes (Chapter

19). The posterior parietal cortex (areas 5 and 7) receives fibers from the posterior part of the thalamus, the *lateral posterior nucleus (LP)*, and parts of the *pulvinar* (Figs. 3.20, 3.28, and 20.7). Other parts of the pulvinar projects to the temporal lobe. The LP and the pulvinar receive afferents from nuclei related to vision and eye movements, such as the *superior colliculus* and the *pretectal nuclei*, and may relay such information to the posterior parietal cortex (see also Chapter 16, *Cortical Centers for Control of Eye Movements.*).

Figure 20.8 *The thalamus.* Frontal section through the middle part of the human thalamus. Myelin stain. (See also Figs. 3.23 and 3.26.)

The Corticothalamic Connections

All of the thalamic nuclei receive massive connections from the cerebral cortex. In general, the nuclei receive afferents from the cortical areas to which they send their efferents—that is, the thalamocortical and the corticothalamic connections are *reciprocal*. The corticothalamic projections are also precisely, topographically organized. As mentioned, corticothalamic neurons have their perikarya mainly in layer 6, whereas projections to other subcortical nuclei arise mainly in layer 5. This indicates that the information received by the thalamus is not merely a copy of information sent from the cortex to other regions.

In view of the massive corticothalamic connections, the function of the thalamus is probably not limited to mediating information from subcortical cell groups to the cortex. In addition, the thalamus receives and presumably processes vast amounts of information from the cortex and is therefore intimately involved in processes taking place in the cortex itself. That the corticothalamic fibers really influence the information processing in the thalamus is witnessed by observations of the lateral geniculate body; the properties of the relay cells (thalamocortical) of the nucleus are in part determined by signals from the striate area.

Inhibition in the Thalamus: Interneurons and The Reticular Thalamic Nucleus

Inhibitory interneurons (the majority GABAergic) probably constitute one-fourth or more of all neurons in some of the thalamic nuclei. In the thalamic sensory relay nuclei, the inhibitory interneurons may contribute to the enhancement of stimulus contrasts (by *lateral inhibition*) and to selection of certain kinds of stimuli by suppressing other kinds (for example, in relation to transmission of signals from nociceptors). *Opioid and other peptides* (such as SP) are present in several of the thalamic nuclei, including those relaying nociceptive signals.

The *reticular thalamic nucleus* is unique among the thalamic nuclei because virtually all neurons are GABAergic. The nucleus, which forms a thin shell at the lateral aspect of the thalamus (Fig. 20.8), sends its *efferent* fibers in the medial direction to end in the other thalamic nuclei (and not to the cortex, differing also in this respect from the other thalamic nuclei). Both the corticothalamic and thalamocortical fibers pass through the reticular nucleus on their way to and from the thalamus and give off numerous collaterals that end in the nucleus. Furthermore, the reticular nucleus receives *afferents* from the mesencephalic reticular formation and has reciprocal connections with the *PAG* (the latter nucleus is related to, among other things, the control of transmission of signals from nociceptors).

The function of the reticular thalamic nucleus is not fully understood, but its connections indicate that it can influence the activity of thalamocortical neurons and thus indirectly the activity of the cerebral cortex. Indeed, electrophysiological studies show that the reticular nucleus can synchronize the activity of neurons throughout the thalamus. Furthermore, its activity is closely correlated with changes of the EEG during sleep and wakefulness. Its relation to attention and control of sensory information transfer to the cortex may explain why lesions of the reticular nucleus reduce learning and memory (shown for spatial tasks).

The Intralaminar Thalamic Nuclei

Modern tracer studies have shown that the cortical projections from each of the intralaminar nuclei end in certain parts of the cortex only; for example, the CL nucleus sends fibers predominantly to the parietal cortex. Nevertheless, the projections are considerably more widespread and diffuse than those from the specific thalamic nuclei and do not respect areal borders (the intralaminar nuclei were formerly termed the unspecific thalamic nuclei). Physiological studies indicate that the intralaminar nuclei exert *general effects on the excitability of cortical neurons*. Thus, electrical stimulation produces a so-called *recruiting response* in extensive parts of the cortex, which resembles the EEG changes associated with arousal (desynchronization; see Chapter 15).

The tasks of the intralaminar nuclei are not only related to the cerebral cortex, since they have even stronger connections with the *striatum*. Such connections are precisely organized (another fact speaking against the use of the term unspecific thalamic nuclei). We do not know the role of these thalamostriatal connections for the functioning of the basal ganglia.

Extrathalamic, Modulatory Connections to the Cerebral Cortex

Apart from the massive afferent connections to the cerebral cortex from the thalamus, several other subcortical cell groups provide sparser cortical inputs. This concerns the *raphe nuclei* (serotonin), the *locus coeruleus* (norepinephrine), *dopaminergic cell groups in the mesencephalon* (apart from the substantia nigra), the *basal nucleus* (acetylcholine), and the *tuberomammillary nucleus* in the hypothalamus (histamine).

As mentioned above, all of these groups project to large parts of the cortex with no distinct topographic pattern. Nevertheless, recent studies in monkeys show that each nucleus (and thus fibers with a particular transmitter) projects with a higher density to some than to other parts of the cortex. For example, dopaminergic fibers end with highest density in the prefrontal and temporal neocortex, whereas noradrenergic fibers innervate especially the central region (MI, SI). Furthermore, fibers from the various nuclei end in somewhat different cortical layers. A striking feature of the fibers is that, after having entered the cortex, they run horizontally for a considerable distance (in contrast to the vertical organization of the afferents from the specific thalamic nuclei).

Fibers from the above-mentioned nuclei exert a *modulatory control over the excitability level of cortical neurons*, with relation to *wakefulness and phases of sleep*. In addition, they probably *control more specifically selected neuronal groups in connection with our attention being directed to relevant, novel stimuli* (see Chapter 2, *Modulatory Transmitter Systems*, and Chapter 15, *Impulse Pathways and Transmitters for the Activation of the Cerebral Cortex*).

Association Connections of the Cerebral Cortex

Vast numbers of association fibers ensure the cooperation of various parts of the cortex. The shortest association fibers connect minor parts within one area (so-called *U fibers*), whereas somewhat longer fibers link together neighboring areas. There are, for example, ample connections between the SI and area 5 posteriorly (Fig. 20.9) and the MI anteriorly. MI furthermore receives association fibers from the PMA and SMA (premotor areas). The longest association fibers interconnect functionally related areas in different lobes. There are, for example, connections from the extrastriatal visual areas and the posterior parietal cortex to the premotor and prefrontal areas (Figs. 20.9 and 20.13).

When we follow the *association connections "outward" from the primary sensory areas (SI, VI, and AI), they progress toward areas that integrate sensory information of different modalities*—somatosensory and visual information converge in one area, visual and auditory in another, and so forth. The areas outside the primary sensory areas (like the areas of the posterior parietal cortex and the extrastriate areas) send their efferent projections not only to their immediate neighbors but also to distant areas in the frontal lobe (premotor and prefrontal areas) and to "limbic" cortical areas (the cingulate gyrus and the hippocampal gyrus) (Figs. 20.9, 20.10, and 20.12).

The discussion so far may give the impression that the flow of information between various cortical areas goes only in one direction, but this is not the case. As a general rule the association connections are *reciprocal*, enabling areas to exert mutual influences. For example, there is not a one-way traffic outwards from the striate area through successive stages of extrastriate areas, since at all levels areas send fibers back to each other and to the striate area. Certain differences exist, however, between the connections going in opposite directions between two areas. For example, fibers going outward—also called *feedforward* connections—from

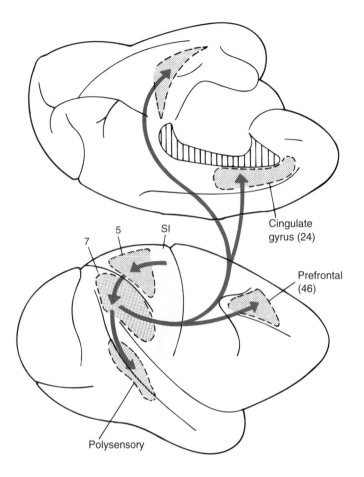

Figure 20.9 *Association connections of the SI* (monkey). Only some fiber connections are shown, to illustrate the flow of information progressing from SI to the posterior parietal cortical areas, and from there to polysensory areas in the temporal lobe, to the prefrontal cortex, and to limbic cortical regions. Based on Jones and Powell (1970).

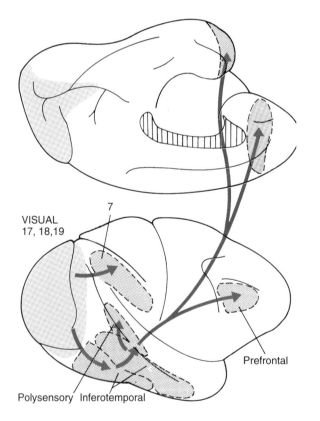

Figure 20.10 *Association connections of the visual cortex.* Compare with Figure 20.9 and note similarities with regard to the progression of information outward from the striate area. Only some connections are shown. Based on Jones and Powell (1970).

Figure 20.11 *The total distribution of commissural connections* (monkey). Note the absence of commissural fibers to the striate area and the SI hand region. The MI hand region likewise lacks commissural connections but is not seen in the figure because it is largely buried in the central sulcus. From Myers (1965).

the striate area to the extrastriate areas end primarily in layer 4, whereas the projections in the opposite direction end in layers 1, 5, and 6. Possibly, the connections that are efferent from the sensory areas are involved in increasing integration and higher-level processing of sensory information, whereas the "backward" connections are of a *feedback* nature (the term feedback in this connection lacks precise meaning, however).

As a rule, each cortical area establishes association connections with many other areas (Fig. 20.10); that is, there is a considerable *divergence* of information. At the same time, there is also considerable *convergence*, since each area receives afferents from several other areas. Together, the many areas of the cortex are extensively interconnected, forming complex networks specialized for specific tasks. More complex functions—such as control of attention and speech—are carried out by many areas in conjunction by way of their association connections. At the cellular level, the extensive association connections enable neurons to integrate many, specific pieces of information and act as coincidence detectors, as discussed above.

Commissural Connections of the Cerebral Cortex

Most commissural fibers are found in the *corpus callosum* (Figs. 3.25 and 3.26). A small fraction (in humans, 1%–2%) course in the *anterior commissure*. The latter fibers are believed to belong primarily to the olfactory pathways.[3] As a general rule, *commissural fibers interconnect corresponding areas in the two hemispheres*. The density of such fibers varies considerably among regions, however. Some regions are almost or totally devoid of commissural fibers (Fig. 20.11). This concerns primarily the striate area and parts of the MI and SI representing distal parts of the extremities (the regions representing the hands and feet). Thus, regions of the cortex dealing with parts of the body that usually work in a symmetrical fashion (such as the two halves of the back) are amply interconnected, whereas parts that usually work independently (such as the hands) have few commissural fibers. A corresponding organization is present in the somatosensory and the motor pathways; connections related to distal body parts are entirely crossed, whereas connections related to proximal parts are to a greater extent bilateral. It seems possible that commissural connections between, for example, the hand areas, would disturb the independent control of the hands. It should be emphasized, however, that via commissural connections of other cortical areas, information about movement commands and sensory signals pertaining to the distal body parts reach both hemispheres.

We will return to the corpus callosum and the commissural connections later in this chapter when dealing with the sharing of tasks by the two hemispheres.

FUNCTIONS OF THE CEREBRAL CORTEX

Association Areas

For some of the cortical areas, functional aspects have been discussed in previous chapters. This concerns areas related to movement control such as the MI, PMA, and SMA. We have also dealt with the primary sensory areas, SI, VI, and AI, and discussed further processing of sensory information in neighboring areas. Parts of the cortex of importance for control of autonomic functions have been discussed in Chapter 19.

Here we will address primarily functions that can be ascribed to the so-called *association areas* of the cerebral cortex. This term is not precisely defined but is traditionally used for parts of the cortex that neither receive direct sensory information via the major sensory pathways nor send direct fibers to motoneuronal groups. All of the cerebral lobes contain association areas for which such a definition is used.

The connections of the association areas indicate that they are able to integrate information from sensory and "limbic" parts of the cortex and thereafter issue commands to motor cortical areas and (indirectly) to the hypothalamus.

Comparison of the cerebral hemispheres of humans and monkeys (Figs. 20.3, 20.9, 20.10, and 20.13) shows that the association areas occupy a much larger fraction of the total in humans than in monkeys. Comparison of monkeys with other mammals, such as cats and dogs, shows again that the main difference between them with regard to the cerebral cortex is the relative size of the association areas. These parts of the cortex are of importance for what we may loosely call *higher mental functions*, as we will discuss below. One should realize, however, that the individual association areas cannot be regarded as "centers" for specific mental faculties. First, several areas—often located in quite different parts of the hemisphere—participate in one task or function, and, furthermore, one area participates in more than one function. This is witnessed by the high degree of divergence and convergence of the connections of the association areas, as discussed above. Second, the operations of the association areas cannot be understood if considered in isolation; the intimate connections between the association areas and subcortical cell groups, like the thalamus, the basal ganglia, the amygdala, and the hippocampus, are essential for normal functioning.

Measurements of regional cerebral blood flow and metabolism during the performance of various cognitive tasks indicate that *large parts of the cortex participate in all higher mental functions*. When a person is asked to imagine that she is walking from one place to another in a city she knows, the activity increases in the extrastriate visual areas, in the posterior parietal cortex, in parts of the temporal lobe, and in several prefrontal areas. Solving a mathematical problem activates many of the same cortical areas but with certain differences, and a verbal task activates multiple areas that partly coincide with and partly differ from those activated in the spatial and the mathematical tasks.

In Chapter 8 we discussed the cortical substrate of visual imagery (*Consciousness and Visual Experience*).

Agnosia and Apraxia

Lesions of association areas typically disturb higher-level aspects of sensory and motor functions. *Agnosia* is usually defined as the lack of ability to recognize objects (when not due to reduced sensation or dementia). *Apraxia* is used similarly about the loss of the ability to do certain, formerly well-known actions (such as dressing, using household tools, copy a drawing, and so forth). There is no clear-cut distinction between these two categories of symptoms, however. Loss of the ability to copy a drawing—called *constructional apraxia*—may, for example, be due to the patient not being able to perceive more than a small piece of the drawing at a time. Thus, she is not able mentally to put several pieces together, (this is called *simultanagnosia*). Cortical lesions, depending on their site and size, can produce a wide specter of difficulties with perception. This concerns not only objects (strictly defined) but all aspects of higher processing of sensory information. The word agnosia is therefore used more widely than the definition may suggest. For example, we use the term *visual agnosia* for loss of the ability to recognize objects and persons by sight, whereas *tactile agnosia* means loss of the ability to recognize objects by touch.

Visual agnosia is the most common kind, and has been studied the most. It may appear in several subvarieties, each with a specific name. For example, *prosopagnosia* means inability to recognize familiar *faces; autotopagnosia* is inability to recognize ones own *body parts; simultanagnosia* is the inability to perceive more than one object at a time, and so forth. Inability to recognize letters, *alexia*, is regarded by some as a special kind of agnosia. To some extent, the different kinds of agnosia can be attributed to lesions of specific parts of the cortex. For example, several kinds of visual agnosia are associated with lesions of specific parts of occipito-temporal extrastriate areas (see Chapter 8, *Further Processing of Sensory Information Outside the Striate Area*). Tactile agnosia has been described after lesions at the parieto-temporal junction (see Chapter 7, *Lesions of the Somatosensory Areas*). Disturbances of the body image are typical of lesions in the posterior parietal cortex (see below).

Agnosia as the only symptom occurs seldom, however, and even rarer are cases with isolated subcategories, such as prosopagnosia. Such cases are nevertheless of great theoretical interest since they shed light on how the brain works to solve specific tasks.

If we in the term agnosia include the inability to recognize complex sounds (like music, spoken words, laughter, and so forth), the distinction with speech disturbances after brain damage (*aphasia*) becomes blurred. Furthermore, there are elements of apraxia in aphasia when it includes (as often happens) the inability to write (*agraphia*). Patients with lesions of the association areas often have symptoms belonging to several categories mentioned above—that is, elements of aphasia, agnosia, and apraxia. This can only partly be explained by the fact that many lesions are large and affect several specialized regions. It also reflects that such regions—although often anatomically widely separated—are extensively interconnected, and that their normal functioning requires that they cooperate.

Figure 20.12 *The association connections of the posterior parietal cortex* (monkey). Connections with the limbic cortical areas are not shown (see Fig. 20.9). Note the convergence of visual and somatosensory information in area 7.

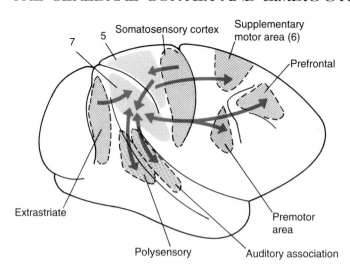

Parietal Association Areas

Usually areas 5 and 7—located in the upper and lower parietal lobules, respectively—are considered to constitute the parietal association cortex (Figs. 7.20, 20.3, and 20.12).[4] The term *posterior parietal cortex* is also used of this region. Both areas 5 and 7 can be further subdivided into parts differing in connections and functional properties. These areas are intercalated between the visual cortical areas in the occipital lobe and the somatosensory cortex in the anterior parietal cortex. Functionally, as one might expect from this location, areas 5 and 7 process and integrate somatosensory and visual information. From these areas, signals are conveyed to premotor and motor areas (Fig. 20.12), explaining why lesions of the posterior parietal cortex can produce disturbances of voluntary movements. The posterior parietal cortical areas also have ample connections (both ways) with the *cingulate gyrus* (Fig. 19.3) and the *prefrontal cortex*. These connections are assumed to mediate the influence of emotions, attention, and motivation on behavior produced by somatosensory and visual stimuli.

Experiments with recording of *single-cell activity* in *area 5* of the monkey indicate that this area is essential for the *proper use of somatosensory information, for goal-directed voluntary movements, and for the manipulation of objects*, as expressed by the Finnish neurophysiologist Hyvärinen. This fits well with the symptoms occurring in humans after damage to the posterior parietal cortex, as will be discussed below.

Single-cell recordings indicate that *area 7* has an important role in the *integration of visual and somatosensory stimuli, which is essential for the coordination of the eye and the hand*—that is, for visual guidance of movements. Area 7 is also involved in the control of eye movements, as discussed in Chapter 16.

Lesions of the posterior parietal cortex in humans can cause different symptoms, depending on which parts are most affected. Some of the symptoms can be summarized as *difficulties with the transformation of sensory stimuli into adequate motor actions*. This can probably be explained by lack of parietal influence on the premotor areas. The understanding of the meaning of sensory stimuli is seriously impaired (but usually not the mere recognition of a stimulus). This *agnosia* concerns especially the recognition of the form and spatial position of objects. A typical symptom after right-sided lesions is a tendency to *neglect* visual stimuli from the opposite side, and often from the opposite body half. The patient is also unable to use well-known tools and objects (*apraxia*). They furthermore have problems with *visually guided movements* (such as stretching out the arm to obtain an object). Similar symptoms may occur also after lesions of other parts of the hemisphere, for example apraxia caused by a frontal lobe lesion. The reciprocal connections between the posterior parietal cortex and the prefrontal cortex probably explain such phenomena.

Properties of Single Cells in the Posterior Parietal Cortex

Studies of monkeys with permanently implanted electrodes have demonstrated a wide repertoire of properties among neurons in areas 5 and 7. Common to many is that a task-related increase in firing frequency occurs only when a stimulus is relevant and the attention of the animal is directed toward the stimulus. Thus, it is virtually impossible to activate many neurons when the animal is drowsy and inattentive. Some cells respond to stimulation of proprioceptors, but their response is much more vigorous when a movement (stimulating the proprioceptors) is self-initiated by the monkey than when the joint is passively manipulated by the examiner. In area 5, many neurons change their firing frequency in relation to manipulatory hand movements. Other neurons increase their firing in relation to reaching movements, but only when the hand is moved toward an object the monkey wants to obtain (such as an orange). The increase of firing in such neurons starts at the time the animal discovers the object—that is, before the arm movement starts—and is therefore not a result of proprioceptive stimulation. Mountcastle, who first described such neurons, suggested that they may function as *command neurons* for the target-directed exploration of our immediate surrounding extrapersonal space. Such neurons appear to respond to the coincidence of two events: a sensory stimulus (for example, the sight of an orange) and a signal that depends on motivation (whether the monkey is hungry and wants the orange).

The Parietal Lobe and the Development of the Ability to Integrate Somatosensory and Visual Information

The ability to integrate somatosensory and visual information and to use visual information to guide voluntary movements is not inborn but learned in infancy and early childhood. Persons who were born blind but get back the visual sense as young adults do not manage to coordinate the visual information with the other senses and therefore cannot utilize the "new" sense. They usually continue to use tactile sensation to "see" objects, and the visual information can in fact be more confusing than helpful (this is vividly described by Oliver Sacks in *An Anthropologist on Mars*).

Studies by Hyvärinen and co-workers show that the properties of single cells in the parietal cortex change during the phase in which an infant monkey learns to coordinate visual and somatosensory information. Monkeys were prevented from seeing from birth (by suturing the eyelids) until they were between 6 months and 1 year old. At that time few cells in area 7 responded to visual stimuli, in contrast to the normal situation at that age. An abnormally large fraction of the cells were activated by passive somatosensory stimuli and by active movements. Most striking was the almost total absence of cells that could be activated by both so-

More About Symptoms after Lesions of the Posterior Parietal Cortex

The most marked symptom produced by *bilateral parietal lesions* is the *inability to grasp and to manipulate objects*. Thus, the patient may be unable to move the hand toward an object that is clearly seen, even though there are no pareses and no visual defects. Movements that do not require visual guidance, such as buttoning, bringing an object to the mouth, and so forth, are performed normally. When the patient is asked to pour water from a bottle into a glass, he pours the water outside the glass over and over again, even though he can see clearly both the bottle and the glass. Such patients also have severe difficulties with the *appraisal of distances and the size of objects*. Furthermore, to *fix the gaze* becomes difficult, especially to direct the gaze toward a point in the periphery of the visual field. The *identification of objects is difficult*, because of the inability to attend to more than one detail at a time (such as seeing a cigarette but not the person who smokes it). This may be a fundamental defect after parietal lobe lesions, perhaps also explaining the difficulties mentioned above with pouring water into a glass (the patient is unable to locate in space the bottle and the glass at the same time).

Patients with parietal lobe lesions typically have difficulties with *drawing* an object or a scene; again the inability to perceive more than one feature at a time is the probable basic defect. The parts of an object are drawn separately, without the proper spatial relations, or the drawing gives an extremely simplified representation. This symptom occurs most often after damage to the right parietal cortex, in cases of unilateral lesions. The *use of tools* is also difficult or impossible: For example, the patient no longer knows how to use a hammer (apraxia).

Unilateral lesions of the right parietal lobe typically produce *negligence of the opposite body half and visual space*. Such a patient behaves as if the left part of his body does not exist. He dresses only the right side, shaves only the right half of the face, and so forth. He may, for example, deny that the left leg belongs to him and claim that it belongs to the person in the adjacent bed. A similar symptom is denial of the disease and the functional loss (*anosognosia*). The patient may deny that the limb is paralytic, or that he is blind. Thus, certain aspects of body knowledge no longer exist in the mind of the patient, but the loss is not consciously perceived. When drawing a face, for example, the right side is drawn normally, whereas the left side is vague or not included in the drawing.

Even though the symptoms mentioned above are most often seen after damage of the posterior parietal cortex, most of them have been described after lesions in other parts of the brain too, especially of the prefrontal cortex, the thalamus, and the basal ganglia (all of these have connections with the parietal cortex).

A peculiar constellation of symptoms, the *Gerstmann syndrome*, can occur after lesions of the parietal lobe at the transition to the temporal lobe (usually of the left hemisphere). The symptoms are as follows: *finger agnosia* (the patient cannot recognize and distinguish the various fingers on her own or other people's hands), *agraphia* (inability to write), sometimes *alexia* (inability to read), *right–left confusion*, and, finally, *dyscalculia* (reduced ability to perform simple calculations, especially to distinguish categories of numbers such as tens, hundreds, and so forth). The most distinctive feature of the syndrome is the finger agnosia, which can occur in isolation. That finger agnosia can be the only symptom of a parietal lobe lesion indicates that a disproportionally large part of the human parietal cortex is devoted to the hand. Thus, the hand has a unique role as an exploratory sense organ and as a tool, and, furthermore, it has a special place in our inner, mental, body image. The British neurologist Critchley expressed it as follows: "The hand is largely an organ of the parietal lobe."

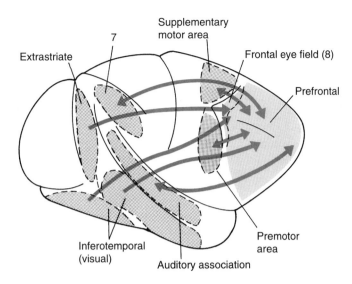

Figure 20.13 *The association connections of the prefrontal cortex* (monkey). Note the convergence of all kinds of processed sensory information and the connections with PMA and SMA. Connections with limbic cortical areas are not shown (see Figs. 19.3 and 19.5).

matosensory and visual stimuli. Even 2 years after reestablishment of normal vision, the single-cell properties of area 7 remained virtually unaltered, with very few cells responding to visual stimuli. Properties of cells of the extrastriate cortex (area 19) were also altered in the visually deprived monkeys; some cells were, for example, activated by somatosensory stimuli (which never occurred in normal monkeys), and there were fewer than normal visually driven cells.

Behaviorally, the monkeys were blind after opening of the eyes, and no improvement occurred during the next month. They bumped into obstacles, fell off tables, and were unable to retrieve food by sight alone. They were not frightened by threatening faces, in contrast to normal monkeys at the same age. One monkey that was observed for 3 years improved to some extent, but it never regained the full use of the visual sense.

The above data indicate that the *functional properties of neurons in the association areas, and thus the capacity of the areas to contribute to certain tasks, are determined to a large extent in early childhood.* Furthermore, there is only a limited possibility of regaining the proper function of these regions at a later stage.

The experiments also show that when one kind of sensory information is lacking during an early stage of development, other sensory modalities take over parts of the cortex not normally used for processing that kind of sensory information. This has been shown also after early lesions of the auditory system.

Frontal Association Areas

In this context we use the term association cortex only about the *prefrontal cortex*—that is, the parts of the frontal lobe in front of areas 6 (PMA, SMA) and 8 (the frontal eye field) (Fig. 20.3). The prefrontal cortex consists of several different cytoarchitectonic areas, each with a specific set of connections. Together, the areas receive strong connections from areas in the occipital, parietal, and temporal lobes and, in addition, from the cingulate gyrus (Fig. 20.13). Thalamic afferents come from the

MD (Fig. 20.7), which in turn receives afferents from the amygdala and the ventral pallidum (among other places). Together, the prefrontal cortex appears to receive *information about all sensory modalities and also about the motivational and emotional state of the individual*. The prefrontal cortex sends fibers back to most of the areas from which it receives afferents, among them the SMA and the PMA. In addition, many prefrontal efferents reach the caudate nucleus of the striatum (Fig. 13.6). Finally, some efferents reach the hypothalamus.

The symptoms that occur in humans and monkeys with *lesions of the prefrontal cortex* are at least partially different from those occurring after lesions of other parts of the hemispheres. For example, there are usually changes of mood and personality. Commonly, large lesions produce apathy, indifference, and emotional leveling-off. The patient appears to be uncritical compared with before the damage. He may, for example, behave in a complacent and boastful manner, which he would never have done before. The ability to alter the behavior on the basis of experience from previous actions appears to be reduced. Clear-cut symptoms occur usually only after bilateral damage to the prefrontal cortex. Occassionaly, however, the first signs of a frontal-lobe tumor are changes of behavior and personality.

More About the Human Prefrontal Cortex

Symptoms After Lesions

A striking defect after bilateral lesions of the dorsolateral prefrontal cortex is the lack of the so-called *delayed response*. A monkey sees that food is put into one of two bowls. Then the sight of the bowls is blocked for up to 10 minutes before the monkey is allowed to choose one of the two. In contrast to normal monkeys, the lesioned ones do not remember which bowl contained the food (even though they do not show reduced performance in other more complicated memory tests). The dorsolateral parts of the prefrontal cortex thus appear to be necessary for the *ability to form and retain an inner conception of the existence of an object in time and space when the object is no longer seen*. Interestingly, humans manage a similar test first at the age of about 1 year. Before that age, everything that is not seen or felt is presumably nonexistent for the infant.

A characteristic symptom in humans with prefrontal lesions is the *inability to alter the response when the stimulus changes*—they continue to make the same response even though it is no longer adequate. This phenomenon is called *perseveration*. The so-called *Wisconsin card sort test* is often used to reveal such a defect. The person is asked to sort cards in accordance with certain general rules, such as color, number, shape, and so forth. The correct rule to be applied is indicated by the response given by the examiner to the first attempts at sorting the cards. The rules can be changed without warning. Normal persons understand fairly quickly that the rule has been changed and alter their responses accordingly, whereas patients with prefrontal lesions continue sorting in accordance with the first rule, in spite of repeated warnings that they are making mistakes.

Emotional and personality changes after frontal lobe lesions are difficult to evaluate, and the premorbid personality of the patients appears to play a decisive role. Nevertheless, a general tendency is for the patients to become less emotional and to show reduced emotional reactions to events. They also have difficulties in extracting the salient features from a complex situation, making their responses unpredictable and often inadequate. A test designed for such symptoms utilizes drawings of complex situations, in part with a dramatic content, such as a man who has fallen through the ice on a lake and is in danger of drowning. Patients with frontal lesions usually attend only to details, saying, for example, "Since there is a sign saying 'Careful!' on the beach, there may be a high-voltage cable nearby." This kind of reduction results in inability to foresee the consequences of one's own actions, and poor insight into other people's circumstances. This leads to poor social adaptation, with isolation as the final result.

The reduced capacity to retain inner conceptions is most likely the reason why such patients have increased *distractibility*, with reduced ability to perform tasks that require continuous activity and attention. Motor hyperactivity, which can be a symptom, may perhaps result from the increased distractibility. Thus, in monkeys with prefrontal lesions, the hyperactivity disappears when they are placed in an environment with few stimuli.

In humans with frontal lobe tumors (for example, a glioma or a metastasis from a malignant tumor elsewhere), a depressive disorder has been observed. This may rather be a condition of de-emotionalization and social isolation.

The Prefrontal Cortex and Psychiatric Disease

In Chapter 19 we discuss the role of the amygdala in certain kinds of serious (endogenous) *depression*. Changes are also found, however, in other limbic structures (such as the hippocampus, the hypothalamus, and the prefrontal cortex). These parts have intimate connections with the amygdala. It is to be expected that diseases affecting complex functions like emotions, personality, sense of reality, and thought would involve both limbic structures and the neocortex, and also many neurotransmitters. In endogenous depression a typical finding is a disturbance of monoamine metabolism in the brain, especially of serotonin and norepinephrine (also other transmitters may show changes, however). Alteration of adrenergic β receptors has been shown in the hippocampus in a rat model of learned helplessness. It is likely that in humans corresponding alterations would occur in the prefrontal cortex . Such findings are important because they show that *purely psychological processes can alter transmitter receptors, and that these alterations are associated with altered behavior*. Thus, the finding of altered neurotransmitters or receptors in a psychiatric disease does not prove that the disease is caused by a defect in the brain rather than by psychological factors.

Ever since the first accurate description of psychiatric diseases such as *schizophrenia*, it has been postulated that the disease is caused by alteration of the frontal lobes. This assumption was partly based on similarities between the symptoms in schizophrenia and in cases of frontal lobe damage. This question is still not clarified, and parts of the brain other than the frontal lobes have been implicated, such as certain limbic structures. In Chapter 13 (*The Ventral Striatum, Psychosis, and Drug Addiction*) we discussed the role of the ventral striatum (especially the nucleus accumbens) as a target for antipsychotic drugs. The fact that the drugs commonly used for the treatment of psychotic disorders are antidopaminergic gave rise to the *hypothesis that schizophrenia is caused by disturbances of dopamine actions pre- or postsynaptically*. Recent studies have strenghtened this theory; for example, by showing an increased level of a subgroup of D_2 receptors (D_4) in the brains of schizophrenic patients. Other monoamines may be involved in schizophrenia as well, and PET studies suggest that untreated patients have reduced glutamate concentrations in the prefrontal cortex.

The problem with examining the brains of schizophrenic patients after their death is that they almost always have been treated with antidopaminergic drugs for a long time. Thus, observed changes of, for example, dopamine receptor density and dopamine content can therefore be a result of the treatment and not of the disease. The same reservations hold for the interpretation of postmortal structural changes.

Various *morphological changes* have been observed in the brains of schizophrenic patients, including cell loss in the frontal lobes and in limbic structures (the hippocampal formation and the amygdala), but often such findings are not confirmed by later studies. Measurements of *regional blood flow* lend some support to the theory that the frontal lobes may be involved in some manner. Thus, many schizophrenics have been reported to have abnormally low blood flow in the prefrontal cortex, and various tasks that give increased flow in normal people failed to do so in these patients. Even these results are controversial, however.

We should also bear in mind that altered neuronal activity in the prefrontal cortex (or any other structure) does not tell us that the primary pathology is there. Thus, the alterations in one area may be secondary to changed activity in other areas with which it is connected. Considering the many connections between the prefrontal cortex and the amygdala, ventral striatum, and hippocampal formation (among others) it seems likely that even if the primary pathology should arise in one of these structures only, the symptoms would be due to malfunctioning of the whole network. These parts of the brain are intimately involved in normal emotions and cognitive processes in response to interactions with our environment. Therefore, the final symptomatology in a disease like schizophrenia would reflect both the dysfunction caused by neuronal pathology and the attempts by the rest of the brain to cope with the disturbed functions. This would be so, regardless of whether schizophrenia turns out to be due to a defect receptor gene, a prenatal disturbance of neuronal migration, or (most likely) a combination of many factors.

The Temporal Association Cortex

A unitary functional role is even less evident for the temporal association areas than for those in the parietal and frontal lobes. Apart from the auditory cortex (areas 41 and 42) (Fig. 9.11) and the phylogenetically old parts at the medial aspect (Fig. 19.1), the temporal lobe consists largely of areas 20, 21, and 22, which here are considered the association areas (Fig. 20.3).

The cortex of the *superior temporal gyrus* is characterized by its connections with the *auditory cortex*, whereas the inferior parts of the temporal lobe—the *inferotemporal cortex*—are dominated by processed visual information from the extrastriate visual areas. In addition, there are strong connections with *limbic structures* such as the hippocampal formation (via the entorhinal area) and the amygdala (Figs. 19.5 and 19.9). Finally, long association fibers interconnect the temporal association areas with the *prefrontal cortex* (Fig. 20.13).

Bilateral damage of the temporal lobes produces the so-called *Klüver-Bucy syndrome*[5] with pronounced *amnesia*, among other symptoms. The amnesia can be ascribed largely to the destruction of the hippocampal formation and neighboring areas in the hippocampal gyrus. There are also emotional changes caused by the concomitant destruction of the amygdala located in the tip of the temporal lobe. These aspects are discussed in Chapter 19. In addition, the patients become very *distractible*—they have difficulties in maintaining their attention on a certain stimulus or task. Finally, psychic blindness or *visual agnosia* is a typical symptom of temporal lobe lesions affecting the inferotemporal parts. The patient is unable to recognize objects and persons she sees, even though her vision is normal. As for other association areas, it is the interpretation of sensory information that is deficient, not the sensory experience as such. In-

Experimental Studies of the Temporal Association Cortex

Electrical stimulation of the temporal association cortex in awake humans can recall memories of past events or produce dreamlike sequences of imagined events. Such data come largely from pioneer studies made by the Canadian neurosurgeon Penfield, in which he stimulated the temporal lobe and other parts of the cortex in awake patients (in whom the cortex was exposed under local anesthesia for therapeutic reasons). In monkeys, some single neurons of the temporal cortex respond only when the monkey sees, for example, a *face* or a *hand*. Some neurons respond preferentially to one particular face, whereas other neurons respond to any face. A neuron that responds briskly when the monkey is shown a drawing of a face may stop firing when important features are removed, such as the mouth or the eyes.

The inferotemporal cortex is of importance especially for the interpretation of complex visual stimuli, as judged from experiments in monkeys. Thus bilateral removal of these regions makes the monkeys unable to recognize and distinguish complex visual patterns. These and other observations lead to the conclusion that the inferotemporal cortex is of special importance for the *categorization of complex visual stimuli*.

Stimulation of the *insula*, which is hidden at the bottom lateral fissure (Fig. 3.28), produces mostly chewing movements, changed respiratory pattern, abdominal sensations, altered peristaltic movements of the gut, and other vegetative phenomena. As discussed in Chapter 7 (*Further Processing of Sensory Information Outside SI*), single units in parts of the insula have large somatosensoy receptive fields, and lesions of the SII and adjoining parts of the insula can produce *tactile agnosia*.

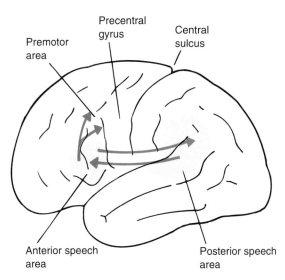

Premotor
area

Precentral
gyrus

Central
sulcus

Anterior speech
area

Posterior speech
area

Figure 20.14 *Speech areas of the human brain.* Lesions of the anterior speech area (of Broca) produce predominantly motor aphasia, whereas lesions of the posterior speech area produce mainly sensory aphasia. The posterior speech area as shown here comprises parts of the inferior parietal lobulus that were not included in the area described by Wernicke. Note the long association fibers interconnecting the two areas. These connections explain why a lesion in between the two speech areas can produce aphasia (so-called conductance aphasia).

formation about size and shape of objects may nevertheless be available to the posterior parietal cortex to be used in movement control, as discussed in Chapter 8 (*Consciousness and Visual Experience*).

Language Functions and "Speech Areas" of the Cerebral Cortex

Clinical observations in the past century led to the identification of two so-called *speech areas* in the left hemisphere (Fig. 20.14). The frontal area is named after the French physician Paul Broca who in 1861 described loss of speech—*aphasia*—caused by a lesion in the left frontal lobe just in front of the motor face area. The posterior speech area is named after the German neurologist Carl Wernicke. He discovered in 1874 that one of the clinically observed kinds of aphasia was associated with a lesion in the posterior part of the superior temporal gyrus. *Aphasia* is defined as loss (or disturbance) of speech due to a brain lesion. That speech depends almost entirely on only one hemisphere—in most people, the left—is the most marked and best-known example of laterlization (of function) or hemispheric dominance. We will return to the topic of lateralization below.

What are termed speech areas should, more correctly, be termed "areas of aphasia," since we know that their destruction produces various disturbances of language functions (aphasia), but we know little of how these areas contribute to the normal production of language and speech. Furthermore, the speech areas are not the only parts of the brain participating. Language depends on several different processes, such as storage of words in short-term memory, phonologic (sound), and semantic (meaning) processing in relation to the "lexicon" in long-term memory, arranging words into sentences, and the issuing of commands to motor areas about sound production. Functional MRI and PET show that various tests of language functions activate regions corresponding approximately to the areas of Broca and Wernicke. Silent reading or repetition of words activates primarily Broca's area. Specific tests for semantic analysis activate extensive areas in the temporal, prefrontal, and inferior parietal cortices—including Broca's and Wernicke's areas (primarily in the left hemisphere). Tests of phonologic analysis (like choosing matching words by sound similarity) activate partly the same, partly different areas than semantic tests. The main tendency is—as for other complex mental functions—that extensive regions of the hemisphere participate in language and speech, and that different tasks activate overlapping regions. Although the many studies with neuroimaging techniques do not agree on all points, they confirm the relation of Broca's and Wernicke's areas to normal language functions, but show that they are not alone in this respect. So far, this kind of study gives little information about *how* the various cortical areas contribute.

Aphasia

There is an enormous literature dealing with the disturbances of speech and language, and there are numerous classifications of aphasias. Also, there is no lack of hypotheses, whereas understanding of the basic mechanisms underlying language and speech is still limited. This should come as no surprise, however, considering the complexity of the function in question.

Very schematically, there are *two main types of aphasia*. The simplest type is the so-called *motor aphasia*. This occurs most often after destruction of *Broca's area* (the anterior speech area). The patient more or less completely loses the ability to speak, and typically produces only single words in a sort of telegraphic style. The few words used may also be applied wrongly. Other names used for this type are *nonfluent aphasia* (because the speech becomes stuttering) and *expressive aphasia*. The understanding of language is usually preserved, whereas the production of speech is deficient. Nevertheless, there are no signs of pareses of the muscles involved in speech production. Often, motor aphasia is combined with *agraphia*—the inability to express language in writing.

In patients with *sensory* or *receptive aphasia*, the lesion usually affects more posterior parts of the hemisphere at the junction between the parietal, temporal, and occipital lobes, that is in or close to the *Wernicke's* or the *posterior speech area* (Fig. 20.14). Typically, the comprehension of language is most severely affected. The various elementary sounds are not properly put together to form meaningful words and sentences. Words that are heard cannot be repeated. In contrast to motor aphasia, spontaneous speech is fluent, but sounds are often put together into meaningless words, and proper words lack relation to each other ("word–salad"). Usually, sensory aphasia is combined with *alexia*—the inability to read.

In reality, *pure forms of aphasia as described above are very seldom encountered*; in most patients there is a mixture of motor and sensory symptoms, with one or the other dominating. Often there are other symptoms as well, since lesions of the hemispheres are very seldom confined to the speech areas. There are, furthermore, similarities between *word blindness* (*alexia, dyslexia*) and visual agnosia, which may be caused by lesions of the parietal lobe and the inferotemporal cortex. On the other hand, elementary symptoms of aphasia—such as agraphia or alexia—may sometimes occur in isolation or in combination with other kinds of symptoms (cf. Gerstmann's syndrome, described above).

It should also be emphasized that the relationship between specific aphasic symptoms and the anatomic location of a brain lesion is not absolute. Virtually all forms of aphasia have been described after lesions in unexpected parts of the brain. Thus, we can only say that the probability of speech disturbances is highest when the lesion affects one or both of the areas depicted in Figure 20.14 (or the association fibers interconnecting the anterior and posterior speech areas).

The Function of the Commissural Connections: The Corpus Callosum

The fact that the two hemispheres are connected by afferent and efferent fiber tracts with the opposite body half is proof that there is a division of tasks between the hemispheres. This does not mean, of course, that the two hemispheres are independent units—the *commissural connections* ensure that information reaching one hemisphere also reaches the other and that commands issued to lower parts of the brain also are known to both hemispheres. Complex functions are often carried out by cooperation of the two hemispheres, and we have mentioned in examples above that lesions of the association areas often have to be bilateral to produce clear-cut functional deficits.

We will mention a few examples of the significance of the commissural connections. When the optic nerve fibers that cross in the chiasma are cut (Figs. 8.14 and 8.22), impulses from one eye reach only the hemisphere of the same side. After such an operation, monkeys are trained in a *visual discrimination* task (to distinguish a triangle and a circle to obtain a fruit reward) with a patch occluding vision in the left eye. The learning must depend on processes taking place in the right hemisphere, which receives visual information from the right eye. When the monkey has learned the task with the right eye, the occlusion is reversed. Nevertheless, even when using the left eye, the monkey solves the task as well as when using the right eye. Thus, the left hemisphere also has learned the task. This must be dependent on an effective transmission of visual information from one hemisphere to the other, as can be demonstrated by cutting also the corpus callosum (and the anterior commissure) before the discrimination training starts. Then the animal learns the task only with the right hemisphere when the left eye is occluded. The transmission of visual information from one hemisphere to the other in this experiment must depend on commissural connections between the extrastriate and probably the inferotemporal areas, since the striate area lacks commissural fibers (Fig. 20.11).

Corresponding experiments have shown that *tactile* and *kinesthetic sensations* are also transferred through the corpus callosum. A monkey with transection of the corpus callosum (and the anterior commissure) is trained to open a box with the right hand only (without being allowed to see the box). After some training, the opening is performed swiftly. If, however, the monkey then is prevented from using the right hand, the task has to be learned over again with the left hand—no learning had taken place in the right hemisphere (which controls the left hand). A monkey with an intact corpus callosum uses both hands with identical dexterity to solve this task, even though only one hand was used during the training period.

There is a certain topographic arrangement of the commissural fibers within the corpus callosum. As one might expect, the posterior parts are necessary for the transfer of visual information, whereas the anterior and middle parts are necessary for transfer of somatosensory signals. (see Chapter 15, *Can Consciousness Be Explained in Neurobiological Terms?"* with a description of a patient with damage of the middle part of the corpus callosum and abolished transfer of tactile information.)

The ample commissural connections make it possible for the two hemispheres to specialize and to share tasks between them. Both are not required to be equally good at all tasks. Nevertheless, they keep each other constantly informed (just as one would expect of hospital specialists sharing the responsibility for one patient). The brain, even though in a sense consisting of two anatomic parts, functions as a unit for the whole body and our extrapersonal space. The degree of hemispheric specialization or lateralization of functions can be studied only after eliminating the callosal transfer of information.

Cerebral Lateralization and Dominance

Data showing that the two hemispheres are different have received much attention since the early 1970s, and many simplistic statements about the functions of the right and the left hemispheres have been put forward. Recent studies provide a much more complex picture, however. A specialist in the field of cerebral lateralization wrote a few years ago: "... the time has come to put the brain back together again." Another scientist launched the expression "dichotomania" about the urge to equate the many examples of duality in human nature with the two halves of the brain (left–right): scientist–artist, conscious–subconscious, rational–mysticist, masculine–feminine, and so forth. The truth is that both hemispheres take part in most functions—the differences concern mainly how efficient they carry out individual processes, like elements of language functions, emotional behavior, and visual object recognition, and so forth. We will discuss a few examples below.

A wealth of information on the topic of hemispheric specializations (lateralization) has been provided by the study of patients in whom the corpus callosum has been transected (this is done in severe cases of epilepsy, to prevent spread of the abnormal discharges from one hemisphere to the other). The American Roger Sperry was awarded the Nobel Prize in 1981 for his pioneering studies of so-called *split brain* patients. Even though lateralization is probably most marked in humans, there is much evidence that it occurs also in animals (for example, the ability to sing depends on cell groups in the left side of the brain in birds).

Split-brain patients manage well in everyday life, mainly because visual information reaches both hemispheres (because we move the gaze constantly) and there are some bilateral sensory and motor pathways. They get into trouble, however, if, for example, somatosensory information is not supplemented with visual information. The above example of the commissurotomized monkey and tactile learning is relevant for split-brain patients, too. In some situations conflicts may arise between commands issued from the two hemispheres; the left hemisphere may, for example, command the right hand to start dressing, whereas the left hand is ordered to undress.

When one hemisphere is most important for a certain function, we say that it is *dominant* for that function, whereas the other hemisphere is *recessive*. The most clear-cut example of such cerebral dominance—or, in other words, lateralization of function—is *speech*, as mentioned above. Thus, for most people, even for most left-handed persons, the left hemisphere is responsible for language functions.[6] Various investigations have confirmed the lateralization of language. Studies of *split-brain* patients are especially instructive in this respect. They confirm, among other things, that the right hemisphere is mute in most people (even though it may express single words when strong emotions are aroused). When a split-brain patient is asked to identify with the right hand an object that is not seen, he can easily tell the name of the object, what it is used for, and so forth. This is because the tactile information comes to the left, speech-dominant hemisphere. When the left hand is used for the same test, however, the patient is unable to name the object, because the information reaches only the "mute" right hemisphere. The patient nevertheless shows signs of adequate emotional reactions to the object. That the right hemisphere "understands" the nature of the object is further supported by other experiments in which the right hemisphere is presented with a picture of, for example, a key. Even though the patient cannot say anything about the object, he nevertheless picks out with the left hand a key among several objects (which are not seen). Such data show that the *right hemisphere can understand concrete language.* It understands both speech and writing of this kind but cannot express understanding through language—only through action. The right hemisphere can utter a few words, however, especially when they are emotionally loaded. It cannot manage however, abstract or rare words, or grammatical analysis.

Not all aspects of language function are necessarily localized to the dominant hemisphere. The modulation and melody of the sounds of speech, *prosody,* may be localized to the right hemisphere, as witnessed by several clinical reports (some aspects of prosody may neveretheless depend on the left hemisphere). Thus, in some patients who have had a stroke without aphasia, prosody has been reported to be changed or reduced. Patients with loss of prosody may also be unable to judge the emotional aspects of the speech of other persons—for example, they cannot decide whether the person is sad or happy. Such an "intonational agnosia" may have serious effects on the social life of the patient. The importance of the prosody illustrates that much of what we regard as verbal communication is in fact non-verbal.

With regard to lateralization of *hand functions*, the hemispheric differences are less clear-cut than for language. It is of course not a question of the ability to use the hand, but a matter of preference of one hand for most or all tasks. Even though hand preference is inheritable, there are also strong social factors that contribute to the final outcome of hand preference, for example, in writing. There is most likely a gradual transition with regard to the strength of hand preference, from those with a strong tendency to use the right hand for all tasks if possible (writing, drawing, use of tools, eating, and so forth) to those with an equally strong tendency to use the left hand. The latter group probably constitutes 2%–3% of the total population. Hand preference starts to become expressed from the second year of life and is usually finally established at the age of 5 to 6.

There is not a strong correlation between the *lateralization of speech and hand preference.* Thus, for about 95% of the population, the left hemisphere is dominant for speech, whereas the corresponding number for left-handedness is 70%. Thus, only about 30% of left-handed people have right-hemisphere speech dominance.

Whereas many studies show that the *left hemisphere* usually is superior with regard to *analytical and logical thinking* as expressed verbally and in numbers, the *right hemisphere* is superior with regard to *spatial abilities*, the comprehension of complicated patterns, and drawing.

Studies of split-brain patients raise interesting questions, such as whether the two hemispheres have independent consciousness and what the relation is between consciousness and language and between intelligence and language. No simple answers are available to such questions addressing phenomena in the transition zone between neuroscience, philosophy, and religion. To argue that man consists of two personalities, one in each of the hemispheres, is of course a gross oversimplification. The normal cooperation and interaction between the hemispheres is so intimate that our mental life and behavior are caused by their collective activities.

Are the Two Hemispheres Anatomically Different?

Certain *anatomic differences* between the two hemispheres appear to exist in most humans. Thus, the upper face of the temporal lobe (the *temporal plane*) in the vicinity of the auditory cortex is more extensive on the left than on the right side in about 70% (in more than 90% of persons the language function depends on the left hemisphere; thus, the relationship between speech lateralization and anatomic asymmetry is not absolute). The difference appears to be present before birth, and recent studies indicate that the lateralization of language functions is determined prenatally. It is well known that early brain damage (in infancy, before language has been acquired) has less severe effects on language functions than lesions occurring later. Since, obviously, in such early cases of brain damage the right hemisphere takes over the language functions, it was concluded that language function is not initially lateralized. However, a more likely interpretation is that even though there is an inborn tendency for lateralization of speech, at an early stage the right hemisphere has not been fully occupied by other tasks and therefore can substitute for the left hemisphere. At later stages, both hemispheres are fully used and specialized for specific tasks and therefore unable to take over new complex functions.

More About Lateralization

Emotions

Early observations of split-brain patients suggest that the right hemisphere is dominant for the expression of emotions. Further studies show, however, that the *right hemisphere does not dominate all aspects of emotional behavior*. Thus, the two hemispheres appear both to be specialized for specific aspects of emotions. We mentioned prosody as an example of right hemisphere dominance. Overall, the *right hemisphere* appears to be the best at *perceiving* emotional expressions, whereas *both hemispheres are involved in the experience and expression of emotions*. The left hemisphere may, however, be the best judge of certain kinds of emotional expressions. Some data have been interpreted to show that the right hemisphere is dominant as to the experience of strongly negative feelings (and the left as to positive feelings). Even this division may be too general, however (apart from the fact that the terms negative and positive feelings lack precision).

Patients with *strokes* affecting the left hemisphere tend to have more depressive reactions than patients with corresponding right-sided lesions (the right hemisphere understands the agony of the left?). Right hemisphere lesions, especially when they affect the frontal lobe, appear to have a stronger tendency to produce a somewhat inadequate elevation of mood.

Music

It has proved difficult to localize the ability to appreciate and express *music* to one of the two hemispheres. It has been customary to say that the right hemisphere is dominant with regard to, for example, the perception of a melody and that with high-level musical training (professional musicians), the left hemisphere becomes increasingly important. Studies of musicians after brain strokes have not confirmed such assumptions, however. *Amusia* most often occurs together with aphasia, but it has also been reported to occur in isolation. This strongly suggests that language and music use largely separate parts of the cortex, although they appear to lie close together. This is supported by PET studies of musicians practicing sight-reading (that is, at the same time reading and playing an unfamiliar score).

Ear and Visual Field Dominance

A certain degree of "*ear dominance*" exists in most people, which correlates well with the speech lateralization—that is, the right ear is dominant for most people. This phenomenon can be studied by use of so-called *dichotic listening*. Two words are presented at the same time, one to each ear. Afterwards, most people say that they heard the word presented to the right ear.

Visual field dominance has been described in studies in which different visual stimuli are presented to the two hemispheres simultaneously. With regard to written words and letters, there is a tendency to prefer those presented in the right visual field (that is, those transferred to the left hemisphere). For the recognition of faces, the reverse situation appears to exist for most people, as can be demonstrated by the presentation of so-called chimeric portraits composed of two left halves and two right halves, respectively. The person is asked which of the chimeric portraits most resembles the original (authentic) portrait. Most persons claim that the *chimeric portrait* consisting of two right facial halves most resembles the original. This is taken to suggest that the right hemisphere dominates in the analysis of faces and other complex visual patterns. Another indication of this is that when the shape of letters is made sufficiently ornate, the right hemisphere appears to become necessary for their interpretation.

Results That Do Not Fit the Usual Right–Left Dichotomy

Studies with detailed analyses of specific aspects of broader categories of cerebral functions, reveal that the division of labor between right and left is more complicated than apparent from the first split-brain observations.

Sophisticated studies of visual perception show that the *right hemisphere* is superior to perceive and remember *specific* characteristics of objects (for example, the face of a person), whereas the left is better at categories (a face versus other kinds of objects). A different picture emerged in a study comparing patients with lesions in the superior temporal gyrus as to their ability to identify letters. Those with right-hemisphere lesions had difficulties with identification of a letter when it was composed of many small ones—but perceived easily the small letters. Those with a left-hemisphere lesion had difficulties with identification of the small letters but identified easily the big one. Thus, the right hemisphere is good at identifying the overall shape, whereas the left is good at seeing the details. It may seem paradoxical that the left hemisphere is specialized both for identification of broad categories *and* details (and that the right hemisphere is specialized for identification of specific properties *and* the overall shape). Most likely, however, this reflects that different principles govern lateralization of visual and semantic analysis and memory.

Another lateralization of a specific function does not fit with the usual right–left dichotomy of functions. Thus, the right hemisphere is best at measuring distance (for example, the distance between a dot and a line), whereas the left hemisphere excels at judging mutual positions (whether the dot is above or below the line).

Lateralization and Sex Differences

Many studies show that men, on the average, perform better than women on certain spatial tasks (shown most convincingly for the ability to imaginally rotate a figure), mathematical reasoning, and targetting ability (for example, throwing a dart). Women, on the other hand, excel on tasks requiring verbal fluency, perceptual speed, and some fine motor skills. Many speculative explanations have been offered. From an evolutionary point of view, it is now common to explain the arise of such sex differences by the living conditions during early human history, and the different roles played by men and women. Although cognitive sex differences thus may have a genetic basis, environmental influences interact with genetic predispositions to produce the final cognitive make-up of the individual. It should be emphasized, however, that the cognitive sex differences are on the average small, and very much smaller than the variability among individuals of the same sex. As said by the Canadian psychologist Doreen Kimura: ". . . in the larger comparative context, the similarities between human males and females far outweigh the differences."

Cognitive sex differences have been speculatively linked with more or less convincingly demonstrated sex differences in lateralization and brain structure. Some observations suggest for example that men have stronger lateralization of, for example, visuospatial abilities, whereas women to a higher degree use both hemispheres (it is not obvious, however, that a strong lateralization gives a higher visuospatial ability—the reverse might just as well be the case). It was then studied whether there might be sex differences in the cross-sectional area of the corpus callosum, which would correlate with differences in lateralization; that is, a corpus callosum with relatively few fibers was expected to correlate with a high degree of lateralization. Indeed, some studies reported that the corpus callosum is relatively larger in cross section in women than in men. The above speculations have not been confirmed by further and more comprehensive studies, however. Firstly, the reported differences as for visuospatial abilities constitute merely a few percent of the individual variations among members of the same sex. Furthermore, the notion that men have more marked lateralization than women cannot be accepted as generally valid. Finally, several studies have not been able to confirm the sex differences in the size of the corpus callosum. They are at best small, whereas the individual variations again are surprisingly large. In monkeys the number of axons in the corpus callosum varies with a factor of two among individuals. One report claimed in fact that the corpus callosum is about 10% larger in left-handers (and persons using both hands equally) than in right-handers. This does not support a correlation between superior visuospatial abilities, strong lateralization, and a small corpus callosum. Thus, left-handedness is most common among boys, and it is usually considered that left-handers have better visuospatial (and mathematical) abilities than right-handers.

Regarding *mathematical abilities*, a small sex difference in favor of men seems well documented. A large American study found that the sex difference was related to a greater variability among men, with more men than women performing at a very high level. They furthermore concluded that the sex difference was due to both biologic and environmental factors. A causal relationship between mathematical sex differences and differences in lateralization seems unlikely, however.

In conclusion, the available data do not support that sex differences in cognitive and other abilites can be explained by differences in lateralization.

Psychological Differences and Biology

Men and women differ perhaps more obviously in other aspects of their psychology than cognition (such as aggression, emotional reactions, and so forth). Some differences are expressed very early, for example regarding preferred activities. Most researchers today would ascribe such differences to both biologic and environmental factors, as discussed above.

In which respects are the brains of men and women different? We discussed above that sex differences in the corpus callosum are very small at best, and can hardly explain the observed cognitive differences. The most obvious anatomic differences between the brains of men and women are found in the *hypothalamus* (see Chapter 18, *The Hypothalamus, Sexual Functions, and Sex Differences*). Although the structural sex differences in the hypothalamus presumably are mainly related to differences in sexuall functions, we cannot exclude sex differences also in hypothalamic influences on other cell groups, such as the amygdala and the cerebral cortex. We furthermore know that receptors for *sex hormones* are found in many parts of the brain outside the hypothalamus (for example, the amygdala and the prefrontal cortex, just to mention two regions related to emotions and emotional reactions). Experiments in rats and monkeys clearly show that exposure to male sex hormones during early critical phases of development leads to certain behavioral characteristics in later life. Indirect evidence suggests that this may be so also in humans, for example, regarding spatial abilities. Furthermore, some cognitive functions have been shown to vary in the same individual with variations in the level of sex hormones (both in men and women). Thus, sex differences in distribution and densities of hormone receptors, in conjunction with different hormonal makeup, may form the basis for psychological sex differences. The excitability of specific neuronal populations would then be modulated by the blood level of hormones. In addition, although we are not yet able to prove them, subtle differences in the cerebral wiring patterns and synaptic organizations might contribute to the sex differences (as they would contribute to differences among persons of the same sex).

The final performance of the brain is a product of genetic *and* environmental influences, as is discussed in Chapter 4. Environmental challenges induce structural and neurochemical adaptations in the nervous system expressed through altered behavior. A crucial point is that all development—either genetically determined or not—involves synaptic changes. Thus, from the time of birth there is a dynamic interplay between the biology and the environment. A certain genetically determined disposition—for example, regarding temperament—evokes a certain kind of response from other people. The response induces synaptic and neurochemical changes in the brain as a basis for behavior adaptations. To sort out the mutual roles of nature and nurture in the formation of a person's psychology and behavior becomes then virtually impossible.

NOTES

1. Some of the nonpyramidal cells are multipolar and are called stellate cells. Others are called basket cells because their axonal branches form a wickerwork around the perikarya of pyramidal cells. There are in addition several other varieties, given names that as a rule reflect the shape of the neuron.

2. Formerly, the term granule cells was used of the small cortical neurons, explaining the names of layers 2 and 4, which contain mainly small perikarya. Many of the so-called granule cells are in fact small pyramidal cells, and the term granule cell should therefore not be used of cortical neurons.

3. In the monkey the anterior commissure contains about 5% of all commissural fibers, many of which link corresponding parts of the temporal lobes.

4. There is some disagreement in the literature with regard to the parcellation of the posterior parietal cortex in humans. Brodmann (Fig. 20.3) placed areas 5 and 7 in the superior parietal lobule, whereas the inferior lobule contained areas 39 and 40. Vogt (and others), however, describe area 5 as located in the superior parietal lobule and area 7 in the inferior—that is, corresponding to the situation in monkeys.

5. The constellation of symptoms occurring after bilateral destruction of the temporal lobes is named after the two American neurosurgeons Klüver and Bucy who first described it in monkeys. Besides *amnesia*, the animals *lack emotional responses and aggressive behavior (increases tameness)* and they *withdraw from social contact*, presumably due to damage of the amygdala. Furthermore, the syndrome includes *visual agnosia*, a tendency to *examine all objects by mouth*, a tendency to *pay attention to all visual stimuli*, and an irresistible urge to *touch everything*, and *hypersexuality*.

6. It was formerly often assumed that one hemisphere, usually the left, was dominant for all functions and that the right hemisphere was recessive in all respects. It was also assumed that dominance for speech and for hand functions was closely linked.

LITERATURE

Textbooks and Reference Works

Adams, J. H., and Duchen, L. W. *Greenfield's neuropathology*, 5th ed. Edward Arnold, 1992.

Adams, R. D., and Victor, M. *Principles of neurology*, 5th ed. McGraw-Hill, Inc., 1993.

Adelman, G. *Encyclopedia of neuroscience*. Birkhauser, 1987.

Brodal, A. *Neurological anatomy in relation to clinical medicine*. Oxford University Press, 1981.

Finger, S. *Origins of neuroscience. A history of explorations into brain function.* Oxford University Press, 1994.

Heimer, L. *The human brain and spinal cord. Functional neuroanatomy and dissection guide*, 2nd ed. Springer-Verlag, 1995.

Gazzaniga, M. *The cognitive neurosciences*. The MIT Press, 1995.

Kandel, E., et. al. *Principles of neural science*, 3rd ed. Elsevier, 1991.

Levitan, I.B., and Kaczmarek, L.K. *The neuron. Cell and molecular biology*, 2nd ed. Oxford University Press, 1997.

Lockard, I. *Desk reference for neuroanatomy. A guide to essential terms.* Springer-Verlag, 1977.

Martin, J. H. *Neuroanatomy. Text and atlas*. Elsevier, 1989.

Matthews, G. *Cellular physiology of nerve and muscle*. Blackwell, 1985.

Nichols J.G., et al. *From neuron to brain*, 3rd ed. Sinauer Associates, 1992.

Parent, A. *Carpenter's human neuroanatomy*, 9th ed. Williams and Wilkins, 1996.

Paxinos, G. *The human nervous system*. Academic Press, 1990.

Rauber/Kopsch. *Anatomie des Menschen*. Band III. Nervensystem. Sinnesorgane. Georg Thieme Verlag, 1987.

Schmidt, R. F. *Fundamentals of neurophysiology*, 3rd ed. Springer-Verlag, 1985.

Schmidt, R. F. *Fundamentals of sensory physiology*, 3rd ed. Springer-Verlag, 1986.

Shepherd, G. M. *Neurobiology*, 3rd ed. Oxford University Press, 1994.

Smith, C. U. M. *Elements of molecular neurobiology*. John Wiley & Sons, 1989.

Atlases

DeArmond, S. J., et al. *Structure of the human brain. A photographic atlas*, 3rd ed. Oxford University Press, 1989.

Gouaze, A., and Salomon, G. *Brain anatomy and magnetic resonance imaging*. Springer-Verlag, 1988.

Haines, D. E. *Correlative neuroanatomy. The anatomical basis for some common neurological deficits*. Urban & Schwarzenberg, 1985.

Haines, D. E. *Neuroanatomy. An atlas of structures, sections, and systems*, 2nd ed. Urban & Schwarzenberg, 1987.

Miller, R. A., and Burack, E. *Atlas of the central nervous system in man*, 3rd ed. Williams & Wilkins, 1983.

Nieuwenhuys, R. *Chemoarchitecture of the brain.* Springer-Verlag, 1985.

Nieuwenhuys, R., Voogd, J., and van Huijzen, C. *The human central nervous system. A synopsis and atlas*, 3rd ed. Springer-Verlag, 1988.

Olszewski, J. *Cytoarchitecture of the human brain stem.* Karger, 1954.

Paxinos, G., and Huang, X.-F. *Atlas of the human brainstem.* Academic Press, 1995.

Roberts, M. P. *Atlas of the human brain in section.* Lea & Febiger, 1987.

Review Journals

ANNUAL REVIEW OF NEUROSCIENCE, ANNUAL REVIEWS INC.

Contains about twenty reviews by leading neuroscientists. Covers a wide range of topics. Requires background knowledge.

CLINICAL NEUROSCIENCE. WILEY-LISS, INC.

Quarterly. Issues focused on themes with a clinical origin, such as "Alzheimer's disease," "Neuroscience of Depression," and "Pain: Mechanisms and therapy." Aims at integrating basic neuroscience with clinical neurology, neurosurgery, and psychiatry.

CURRENT OPINION IN NEUROBIOLOGY. CURRENT BIOLOGY LTD.

Six issues anually. Concise reviews of the development the last few years within a special subfield of. High scientific standard. Contains comprehensive reference lists. Some key references are supplied with brief, focused abstracts.

NEURON. CELL PRESS.

Monthly. Each issue features one reveiw article (basic neuroscience) of high standard (in addition to many research articles).

SCIENTIFIC AMERICAN. SCIENTIFIC AMERICAN INC.

Monthly. Regularly one or more articles on various aspects of neuroscience. Requires less prior knowledge than the specialized neuroscince review journals. Well-written, easy-to-follow articles with often superb illustrations.

SEMINARS IN THE NEUROSCIENCES. SAUNDERS/ACADEMIC PRESS LTD.

Six issues yearly. Thematic focus with reviews by leading scientists ("The neurobiology of pain," "Imaging the brain," "Circadian rhythms," and so forth).

THE NEUROSCIENTIST. WILLIAMS & WILKINS.

Bi-monthly. Multi-disciplinary reviews, aiming at bridging the gap between basic and clinical neuroscience.

TRENDS IN NEUROSCIENCES, ELSEVIER.

Monthly. Brief reviews of neurobiological topics in rapid development. Written by leading scientists. Requires fairly broad prior knowledge of neuroscience.

Chapter 1

Neuronal Structure

Abbott, N. J. The neuronal microenvironment. Trends Neurosci. 9:3–6, 1986.

Atwood, H. L., Lnenicka, G.A. Structure and function in synapses: Emerging correlations. Trends Neurosci. 9:248–250, 1986.

Cajal, R. Y. *Histologie du systeme nerveux*, Vol. I–II. Instituto Ramon Y Cajal, 1952.

Harris, K. M., and Kater, S. B. Dendritic spines: Cellular specializations imparting both stability and flexibility to synaptic function. Annu. Rev. Neurosci. 17:341–371, 1994.

Dermietzel, R., Spray, D. C. Gap junctions in the brain: Where, what type, how many and why? Trends Neurosci. 16:186–192, 1993.

Emson, P. C. *Chemical neuroanatomy.* Raven Press, 1983.

Jones, E. G. The nervous tissue. In: *Cell and tissue biology.* Weiss, L., ed. Urban & Schwarzenberg, 1988, pp 279–350.

Matus, A. Microtubule-associated proteins: Their potential role in determining neuronal morphology. Annu. Rev. Neurosci. 11:29–44, 1988.

Peters, A., et al. *The fine structure of the nervous system: Neurons and their supporting cells.* 3rd ed. W. B. Saunders, 1991.

Segev, I. Single neurone models: Oversimple, complex and reduced. Trends Neurosci. 15:414–421, 1992.

Vallee, R. Molecular analysis of the microtubule motor dynein. Proc. Natl. Acad. Sci. USA 90:8769–8772, 1993.

Vallee, R. B., and Bloom, G. S. Mechanisms of fast and slow axonal transport. Annu. Rev. Neurosci. 14:59–92, 1991.

Glia

Altman, J. Microglia emerge from the fog. Trends Neurosci. 17:47–49, 1994.

Barron, K.D. The microglial cell. A historical review. J. Neurol. Sci. 134 Suppl:57–68, 1995.

Kimelberg, H. K., and Norenberg, M.D. Astrocytes. Sci. Am. 260:44–55, 1989.

Glass, J. D. Human immunodeficiency virus and the brain. Annu. Rev. Neurosci. 19:1–26, 1996.

Hart, M. N., and Fabry, Z. CNS antigen presentation. Trends Neurosci. 18:475–481, 1995.

Lassmann, H. Bone marrow derived elements and resident microglia in brain inflammation. Glia 7:19–24, 1993.

Perry, V. H., et al. Macrophages and inflammation in the central nervous system. Trends Neurosci. 16:268–273, 1993.

Silver, R., et al. Mast cells in the brain: evidence and functional significance. Trends Neurosci. 19:25–31, 1996.

Stevens, A., Bähr, M. Origin of macrophages in central nervous tissue. J. Neurol. Sci. 118:117–122, 1993.

Tolbert, L. P., and Oland, L. A. A role for glia in the development of organized neuropilar structures. Trends Neurosci. 12:70–75, 1989.

Walz, W. Role of glial cells in the regulation of the brain ion microenvironment. Prog. Neurobiol. 33:309–333, 1989.

Chapter 2

Electrophysiology and Synaptic Function

Armstrong, R. C., and Montminy, M. R. Transsynaptic control of gene expression. Annu. Rev. Neurosci. 16:17–29, 1993.

Artola, A., and Singer, W. Long.term depression of excitatory synaptic transmission and its relationship to long-term potentiation. Trends Neurosci. 16:480–487, 1993.

Bear, M. F., and Malenka, R. C. Synaptic plasticity: LTP and LTD. Curr. Opin. Neurobiol. 4:389–399, 1994.

Bialek, W., and Rieke, F. Reliability and information transmission in spiking neurons. Trends Neurosci. 15:428–434, 1992.

Catteral, W. A. Structure and function of voltage-gated ion channels. Trends Neurosci. 16:500–506, 1993.

Changeux, J-P. Chemical signaling in the brain. Sci. Am. 269:30–37, 1993.

Clapham, D. E. Direct G protein activation of ion channels? Annu. Rev. Neurosci. 17:441–464, 1994.

Clarke, K. A. *Neurophysiology. Applications in the behavioral and biomedical sciences.* Ellis Horwood, 1990.

Eccles, J. C. *The physiology of synapses.* Springer-Verlag, 1964.

Hall, Z. W., and Sanes, J. R. Synaptic structure and development: The neuromuscular junction. Neuron 10 Suppl:99–121, 1993.

Jessel, T. M., andKandel, E. R. Synaptic transmission: A bidirectional and self-modifiable form of cell-cell communication. Neuron 10 Suppl:77–98, 1993.

Johnston, D., et al. Active properties of neuronal dendrites. Annu. Rev. Neurosci. 19:165–186, 1996.

Kaczmarek, L. Molecular biology of vertebrate learning: is *c-fos* a new beginning. J. Neurosci. Res. 34:377–381, 1993.

Kostyuk, P. G., and Verkhratsky, A.N. *Calcium signalling in the nervous system.* John Wiley & Sons, 1995.

Kuno, M. *The synapse.* Oxford University Press, 1994.

Linden, D. J. Long-term synaptic depression in the mammalian brain. Neuron 12:457–472, 1994.

Matthews, G. Neurotransmitter release. Annu. Rev. Neurosci. 19:219–233, 1996.

McCormick, D. A. Cellular mechanisms underlying cholinergic and noradrenergic modulation of neuronal firing mode in the cat and guinea pig dorsal lateral geniculate nucleus. J. Neurosci. 12:278–289, 1992.

Meyer, F. B. Calcium, neuronal hyperexcitability and ischemic injury. Brain Res. Brain Res. Rev. 14:227–243, 1989.

Riederer, P., et al. *An introduction to neurotransmission in health and disease.* Oxford University Press, 1990.

Sather, W. A., et al. Structural basis of ion channel permeation and selectivity. Curr. Opin. Neurobiol. 4:313–323, 1994.

Schmidt, R. F. Fundamentals of neurophysiology, 3rd ed. Springer-Verlag, 1985.

Searle, J. R. Is the brain's mind a computer program? Sci. Am. 262:20–25, 1990.

Segal, M. Dendritic spines for neuroprotection: A hypothesis. Trends Neurosci. 18:468–471, 1995.

Shepherd, G. M. *The synaptic organization of the brain.* 3rd. ed. Oxford University Press, 1990.

Unwin, N. Neurotransmitter action: Opening of ligand-gated ion channels. Neuron 72 Suppl. 10:31–41, 1993.

Vizi, E. S. *Non-Synaptic interactions between neurons. Modulation of neurochemical transmission, pharmacological and clinical aspects.* John Wiley & Sons, 1984.

Zucker, R. S. Short-term synaptic plasticity. Annu. Rev. Neurosci. 12:13–31, 1989.

Neurotransmitters and Receptors

Amara, S. G., and Kuhar, M. J. Neurotransmitter transporters: Recent progress. Annu. Rev. Neurosci. 16:73–93, 1993.

Descartes, L., and Umbriaco, D. Ultrastructural basis of monoamine and acetylcholine function in CNS. Semin. Neurosci. 7:309–318, 1995.

Edwards, F. A. ATP receptors. Curr. Opin. Neurobiol. 4:313–323, 1994.

Hökfelt, T. Neuropeptides in perspective: The last ten years. Neuron 7:867–879, 1991.

Finley, P. R. Selective serotonin reuptake inhibitors. Ann. Pharmacother. 28:1359–1369, 1994.

Kelly, R. B. Storage and release of neurotransmitters. Neuron 10 Suppl:43–53, 1993.

Lipton, S.A. Prospects for clinically tolerated NMDA antagonists: Open-channel blockers and alternative redox states of nitric oxide. Trends Neurosci. 16:527–532, 1993.

Lodge, D. *Excitatory amino acids in health and disease.* John Wiley & Sons, 1988.

Malenka, R. C., and Nicoll, R. A. NMDA-receptor-dependent synaptic plasticity: Multiple forms and mechanisms. Trends Neurosci. 16:521–527, 1993.

Mansour, A., et al. Anatomy of CNS opioid receptors. Trends Neurosci. 11:308–314, 1988.

Mason, T. Noradrenaline in the brain: Progress in theories of behavioural function. Prog. Neurobiol. 16:263–303, 1981.

Matsumoto, R. R. GABA receptors: Are cellular differences reflected in function? Brain Res. Brain Res. Rev. 14:203–225, 1989.

Mesulam, M.-M. The cholinergic contribution to neuromudulation in the cerebral cortex. Semin. Neurosci. 7:297–307, 1995.

Monck, J. R., and Fernandez, J. M. The exocytotic fusion pore and neurotransmitter release. Neuron 12:707–716, 1994.

Ottersen, O. P., et al. Amino acid transmitters. In: *The rat nervous system,* 2nd ed. Paxinos, G, ed. Academic Press, 1995, pp 1017–1037.

Peroutka, S. J. 5–hydroxytryptamine receptor subtypes: Molecular, biochemical and physiological characterization. Trends. Neurosci. 11:496–500, 1988.

Pin, J.-P., and Duvoisin, R. Neurotransmitter receptors I. The metabotropic glutamate receptors: structure and function. Neuropharmacology 34:1–21, 1995.

Salter, M. W., et al. Physiological roles for adenosine and ATP in synaptic transmission in the spinal dorsal horn. Prog. Neurobiol. 41:125–156, 1993.

Seeburg, P. H. The molecular biology of mammalian glutamate receptor channels. Trends Neurosci. 16:359–365, 1993.

Schofield, P. R. et al. The role of receptor subtype diversity in the CNS. Trends Neurosci. 13:8–11, 1990.

Schumann, E. M., and, Madison, D. V. Nitric oxide and synaptic function. Annu. Rev. Neurosci. 17:153–183, 1994.

Tecott, L. H., and Julius, D. A new wave of serotonin receptors. Curr. Opin. Neurobiol. 3:310–315, 1994.

Tracey, D. J., et al. *Neurotransmitters in the human brain*. Plenum Press, 1995.

Westbrook, G. L.. Glutamate receptor update. Curr. Opin. Neurobiol. 4:337–346, 1994

Zimmermann, H. Signalling via ATP in the nervous system. Trends Neurosci. 17:420–426, 1994.

Chapter 3

Abbott, N. J. The neuronal microenvironment. Trends Neurosci. 9:3–6, 1986.

Bargman, W. A., et al. Meninges, choroid plexuses, ependyma, and their relations. In: *Histology and histopathology of the nervous system*. Haymaker, W., and Adams, R. D., eds. Thomas, 1982.

Brown, A. G. *Organization in the spinal cord. The anatomy and physiology of identified neurones*. Springer-Verlag, 1981.

Cassone, V. M. Effects of melatonin on vertebrate circadian systems. Trends Neurosci. 13:457–464, 1990.

Davson, H., and Segal, M. B. *Physiology of the CSF and blood-brain barriers*. CRC Press, 1996.

Dudley, A. W. Cerebrospinal blood vessels: Normal and diseased. In: *Histology and histopathology of the nervous system*. Haymaker, W., and Adams, R. D., eds. Thomas, 1982.

Erlich, S. S., and Apuzzo, M. L. J. The pineal gland: Anatomy, physiology, and clinical significance. J. Neurosurg. 63:321–341, 1985.

Landon, D. N. *The peripheral nerve*. Chapman and Hall, 1976.

Olesen, J., and Edvinsson, L. Migraine: A research field matured for the basic sciences. Trends Neurosci. 14:3–5, 1991.

Rechthand, E., and Rapoport, S. I. Regulation of the microenvironment of peripheral nerve: Role of the blood–nerve barrier. Prog. Neurobiol. 28:303–343, 1987.

Rexed, B. The cytoarchitectonic organization of the spinal cord in the cat. J. Comp. Neurol. 96:415–495, 1952.

Sasaki, T., and Kassell, N. F. Cerebrovascular system. In: *The human nervous system*. Paxinos, G., ed. Academic Press, Inc., 1990, pp 1135–1149.

Scheibel, M. E., and Scheibel, A. Terminal axonal patterns in cat spinal cord. I. The lateral corticospinal tract. Brain Res. 2:333–350, 1966.

Risau, W., and Wolburg, H. Development of the blood–brain barrier. Trends Neurosci. 13:174–184, 1990.

Walz, W. Role of glial cells in the regulation of the brain ion microenvironment. Prog. Neurobiol. 33:309–333, 1989.

Wood, J. H. *Neurobiology of cerebrospinal fluid* (2 vols.). Plenum Press, 1983.

Chapter 4

Development and Plasticity

Brody, B. A., et al. Sequence of central nervous system myelination in human infancy. J. Neuropathol. Exp. Neurol. 46:283–301, 1987.

Conel, J. L. *The postnatal development of the human cerebral cortex*, Vol.1–6 Harvard University Press, 1939–1959.

Cragg, B. G. The development of synapses in the cat visual cortex. Invest. Ophthalmol Vis Sci, 11:377–389, 1972.

Bonhoeffer, T. Neurotrophins and activity-dependent development of the neocortex. Curr. Opin. Neurobiol. 6:119–126, 1996.

Bourgeois, J.-P., and Rakic, P. Changes of synaptic density in the primary visual cortex of the macaque monkey from fetal to adult stage. J. Neurosci. 13:2801–2820, 1993.

Davies, A. M. Intrinsic programmes of growth abd survival in developing vertebrate neurons. Trends Neurosci. 17:195–199, 1994.

Dekaban, A. S., and Sadowsky, D. Changes in brain weights during the span of human life: Relation of brain weights to body heights and body weights. Ann. Neurol. 4:345–356, 1978.

Duman, R. S., et al. Stress, antidepressant treatments, and neurotrophic factors: molecular and cellular mechanisms. The Neuroscientist 1:351–360, 1995.

Finlay, B. L. Cell death and the creation of regional differences in neuronal numbers. J. Neurobiol. 23:1159–1171, 1992.

Fox, K. The critical period for long-term potentiation in primary sensory cortex. Neuron 15:485–488, 1995.

Goodman, C. S., and Shatz C. J. Developmental mechanisms that generate precise patterns of neuronal connectivity. Neuron 10 Suppl:77–98, 1993.

Guthrie, S. The status of the neural segment. Trends Neurosci. 18:74–79, 1995.

Hamilton, W. J., et al. *Human embryology. Prenatal development of form and function*, 4th ed. Williams & Wilkins, 1972.

Harris, W. A., and Holt, C. E. From Tags to RAGS: Chemoaffinity finally has receptors and ligands. Neuron 15:241–244, 1995.

Herschman, H. R. Polypeptide growth factors and the CNS. Trends Neurosci. 9:53–57, 1986.

Jacobson, M. *Developmental neurobiology*, 2nd ed. Plenum Press, 1978.

Kalil, R. E. Synapse formation in the developing brain. Sci. Am. 261:38–45, 1989.

Keynes, R., and Krumlauf, R. Hox genes and regionalization of the nervous system. Annu. Rev. Neurosci. 17:109–132, 1994.

Korsching, S. The neurotrophic factor concept: A reexamination. J. Neurosci. 13:2739–2748, 1993.

Kuang, R. Z., and Kalil, K. Development of specificity in corticospinal connections by axon collaterals branching selectively into appropriate spinal targets. J. Comp. Neurol. 334:270–282, 1994.

Larsen, W. J. *Human embryology*. Churchill Livingston, 1993.

Le Douarin, E., and Dupin, E.Cell lineage analysis in neural crest ontogeny. J. Neurobiol. 24:146–161, 1993.

Lewin, G. L. Physiology of the neurotrophins. Annu. Rev. Neurosci. 19:289–317, 1996.

Liestøl, K., et al. Selective synaptic connections: Significance of recognition and competition in mature sympathetic ganglia. Trends Neurosci. 9:21–24, 1986.

Norman, M. G. Malformations of the brain. J. Neuropathol. Exp. Neurol. 55:133–143, 1996.

O'Leary, D. M., et al. Specification of neocortical areas and thalamocortical connections. Annu. Rev. Neurosci. 17:419–439, 1994.

Patterson, P.H., and Nawa, H. Neuronal differentiation factors/cytokines and synaptic plasticity. Neuron10 Suppl:123–137, 1993.

Purves, D., and Lichtman, J. W. *Principles of neural development*. Blackwell, 1985.

Ruiz i Altaba, A. Pattern formation in the vertebrate neural plate. Trends Neurosci. 17:233–242, 1994.

Shatz, C. J. Impulse activity and the patterning of connections during CNS development. Neuron 5:745–756, 1990.

Sanes, J. R. Extracellular matrix molecules that influence neural development. Annu. Rev. Neurosci. 12:491–516, 1989.

Wall, J. T. Variable organization in cortical maps of the skin as an indication of the life-long adaptive capacities of the circuits in the mammalian brain. Trends Neurosci. 11:549–558, 1988.

Williams, R. W., and Herrup, K. The control of neuron number. Annu. Rev. Neurosci. 11:423–453, 1988.

Aging and Alzheimer's Disease
Arnsten, A. T. Catecholamine mechanisms in age-related cognitive decline. Neurobiol. Aging 14:639–641, 1993.

Aubert, I., et al. Cholinergic markers in aged cognitively impaired Long-Evans rats. Neuroscience 67:277–292, 1995.

Barnes, C. A. Normal aging: regionally specific changes in hippocampal synaptic transmission. Trends Neurosci. 17:13–18, 1994.

Baloh, R. W., et al. The effect of aging on visual-vestibuloocular responses. Exp. Brain Res. 95:509–516, 1993.

Birren, J. E. and Fisher, L. M. Aging and speed of behavior: Possible consequences for psychological functioning. Annu. Rev. Psychol. 46:329–353, 1995.

Giaquinto, S. *Aging and the nervous system.* Wiley, 1988.

Kaplan, F. S., et al. Age-related changes in proprioception and sensation of joint position. Acta Orthop. Scand. 56:72–74, 1985.

Katzman, R. Clinical and epidemiological aspects of Alzheimer's disease. Clin. Neurosci. 1:165–170, 1993.

Lishman, W. A. *Organic psychiatry: the psychological consequences of cerebral disorder.* 2nd ed. Blackwell, 1987.

Masliah, E., and Terry, R. D. Role of synaptic pathology in the mechanisms of dementia in Alzheimer's disease. Clin. Neurosci. 1:192–198, 1993.

Mullan, M., and Crawford, F. Genetic and molecular advances in Alzheimer's disease. Trends Neurosci. 16:398–403, 1993.

Peters, A. The absence of significant neuronal loss from cerebral cortex with age. Neurobiol. Aging 14:657–658, 1993.

Rapp, P.R., and Amaral, D.G. Individual differences in the cognitive and neurobiological consequences of normal aging. Trends Neurosci. 15:340–345, 1992.

Richardson, R. T., and DeLong, M. R. A reappraisal of the functions of the nucleus basalis of Meynert. Trends Neurosci. 11:264–267, 1988.

Shimamura, A. P. Neuropsychological perspectives on memory and cognitive decline in normal human aging. Semin. Neurosci. 6:387–394, 1994.

Strittmatter, W. J., and Roses, A. D. Apolipoprotein E and Alzheimier's disease. Annu. Rev. Neurosci. 19:53–77, 1996.

Terry, R.D. et al. Neocortical cell counts in normal human adult aging. Ann. Neurol. 21:530–539, 1987.

Wallace, W., et al. Amyloid precursor protein in the cerebral cortex is rapidly and persistently induced by loss of subcortical innervation. Proc. Natl. Acad. Sci. USA 90:8712–8716, 1993.

West, M. J. Advances in the study of age-related neuron loss. Semin. Neurosci. 6:403–411, 1994.

Yankner, B. A. Mechanisms of neuronal degeneration in Alzheimer's disease. Neuron 16(5):921–932, 1996.

Restitution

Aguayo, A. J., et al. Degenerative and regenerative responses of injured neurons in the central nervous sytem of adult mammals. Phil. Trans. R. Soc. Lond. B. 331:337–343, 1991.

Bähr, M., and Bonhoeffer, F. Perspectives on axonal regeneration in the mammalian CNS. Trends Neurosci. 17:473–479, 1994.

Bignami, A., et al. *Central nervous system plasticity and repair.* Raven Press, 1985.

Fisher, C. M. Concerning the mechanism of recovery in stroke hemiplegia. Can. J. Neurol. Sci. 19:57–63, 1992.

Fries, W., et al. Motor recovery following capsular stroke. Role of descending pathways from multiple motor areas. Brain 116:369–382, 1993.

Goldberger, M. E., and Murray, M. Recovery of movement and axonal sprouting may obey some of the same laws. In: *Neuronal plasticity.* Cotman, C.W. ed. Raven Press, 1978, pp 73–96.

Keller, A., et al. Formation of new synapses in the cat motor cortex following lesions of the deep cerebellar nuclei. Exp. Brain Res. 80:23–33, 1990.

Lindsay, R. M., et al. Neurotrophic factors: From molecule to man. Trends Neurosci. 17:182–190, 1994.

Lindvall, O., et al. Neurotrophins and brain insults. Trends Neurosci. 17:490–496, 1994.

Mackel, R. The role of the monkey sensory cortex in the recovery from cerebellar injury. Exp. Brain Res. 66:638–652, 1987.

Nicholls, J. G. Repair and regeneration of the central nervous system. Springer-Verlag, 1982.

Schallert, T., and Jones, T. A. "Exuberant" neuronal growth after brain damage in adult rats: The essential role of behavioral experience. J. Neural Transplant. Plast. 4:193–198, 1993.

Schnell, L., and Schwab, M.E. Sprouting and regeneration of lesioned corticospinal tract fibres in the adult rat spinal cord. Eur. J. Neurosci. 5:1156–1171, 1993.

Weiller, C., et al. Individual patterns of functional reorganization in the human cerebral cortex after capsular infarction. Ann. Neurol. 33:181–189, 1993.

Weiller, C., et al. Functional reorganization of the brain in recovery from striatocapsular infarction in man. Ann. Neurol. 31:463–472, 1992.

Wictorin, K., et al. Reformation of long axon pathways in adult rat central nervous system by human forebrain neuroblasts. Nature 347:556–558, 1990.

Chapter 5

Bolz, J., et al. Pharmacological analysis of cortical circuitry. Trends Neurosci. 12:292–296, 1989.

Cohen, M. S., Bookheimer, S. Y. Localization of brain function using magnetic resonance imaging. Trends Neurosci. 17:268–276, 1994.

Damasio, H., and Damasio, A. R. *Anatomical correlates of neuropsychological disorders. A neuroimaging approach.* Oxford University Press, 1989.

Heimer, L., and Zaborsky, L. *Neuroanatomical tract-tracing methods. 2. Recent progress.* Plenum Press, 1989.

Kristeva-Feige, R. et al. A neuromagnetic study of the functional organization of the sensorimotor cortex. Eur. J. Neurosci. 6:632–639, 1994.

Kuhar, M. J., et al. Neurotransmitter receptor mapping by autoradiography and other methods. Annu. Rev. Neurosci. 9:27–59, 1986.

Magistretti, P. J. Cellular bases of brain energy metabolism and their relevance to functional brain imaging: Evidence for a prominent role of Astrocytes. Cereb. Cortex 6:50–61, 1996.

Martin, J. B. Molecular genetic studies in the neuropsychiatric disorders. Trends Neurosci. 12:130–137, 1989.

Mesulam, M. M. Tracing neural connections with horseradish peroxidase. John Wiley & Sons, 1982.

Mills, K. R. Magnetic brain stimulation: A tool to explore the action of the motor cortex on single human spinal motoneurons. Trends Neurosci. 14:401–405, 1991.

Mora, B. M., et al. In vivo functional localization of the human cortex using positron emission tomography and magnetic resonance imaging. Trends Neurosci. 12:282–284, 1989.

Mountcastle, V. B. The neural mechanisms of cognitive functions can now be studied directly. Trends Neurosci. 9:505–508, 1986.

Newberg, A. B. The study of neurological disorders using positron emission tomography and single photon emission computed tomography. J. Neurol. Sci. 135:91–108, 1996.

Olesen, J. Migraine and cerebral blood flow. Trends Neurosci. 8:318–321, 1985.

Ottersen, O. P. Quantitative electron microscopic immunocytochemistry of neuroactive amino acids. Anat. Embryol. 180:1–15, 1989.

Raichle, M. E. Visualizing the mind. Sci. Am. 270:36–42, 1994.

Sawle, G. V. and Myers, R. The role of positron emission tomography in the assessment of human neurotransplantation. Trends Neurosci. 16:172–176, 1993.

Sergent, J. Brain-imaging studies of cognitive function. Trends Neurosci. 17:221–227, 1994.

Shallice, T. *From neuropsychology to mental structure.* Cambridge University Press, 1988.

Sharif, N. A., and Lewis, M. E. *Brain imaging. Techniques and applications.* John Wiley & Sons, 1989.

Stahl, S. M., et al. Imaging neurotransmitters and their receptors in living human brain by positron emission tomography. Trends Neurosci. 9:241–245, 1986.

Swash, M., and Kennard, C. *Scientific basis of clinical neurology.* Churchill Livingstone, 1985.

Valentino, K. L., et al. Applications of monoclonal antibodies to neuroscience research. Annu. Rev. Neurosci. 8:199–223, 1985.

Young, S. W. In situ hybridization histochemistry and the study of the nervous system. Trends Neurosci. 9:549–551, 1986.

Chapter 6

Darian-Smith, I. Sensory processes. In: *Handbook of physiology*, Section 1: The nervous system. American Physiological Society, 1984.

Hamill, O. P., and McBride, D. W. Jr. The cloning of a mechano-gated membrane ion channel. Trends Neurosci. 17:439–443, 1994.

Koutalos, Y., and Yau, K.-W. A rich complexity emerges in phototransduction. Curr. Opin. Neurobiol. 3:513–519, 1993.

Schmidt, R. F. Fundamentals of sensory physiology. Springer Verlag, 1986.

Stock, J., et al. Chemosensing and signal transduction in bacteria. Curr. Opin. Neurobiol. 4:474–480, 1994.

Chapter 7

Somatosensory Receptors

Bjurholm, A. et al. Noradrenergic and peptidergic nerves in the synovial membrane of the Sprague-Dawley rat. Arthritis Rheum. 33:859–865, 1990.

Gandevia, S.C., et al. Kinaesthetic signals and muscle contraction. Trends Neurosci. 15:62–65, 1992.

Giles, L. G. F., and Harvey, A. R. Immunohistochemical demonstration of nociceptors in the capsule and synovial folds of human zygoapophyseal joints. Br. J. Rheumatol. 26:362–364, 1987.

Hasan, Z., and Stuart, D. G. Animal solutions to problems of movement control: The role of proprioceptors. Annu. Rev. Neurosci. 11:199–223, 1988.

Kellgren, J. H., and Samuel, E. P. The sensitivity and innervation of the articular capsule. J. Bone Joint Surg. 32B:84–92, 1950.

Macefield, G., et al. Perceptual responses to microstimulation of single afferents innervating joints, muscle and skin of the human hand. J. Physiol. 429:113–129, 1990.

Matthews, P. B. C. Evolving views on the internal operation and functional role of the muscle spindle. J. Physiol. 320:1–30, 1981.

McCloskey, I., et al. Sensory effects of pulling or vibrating tendons in man. Brain 106:21–37, 1983.

Proske, U., et al. Joint receptors and kinaesthesia. Exp. Brain Res. 72:219–224, 1988.

Rothwell, J. C., et al. Manual motor performance in a deafferented man. Brain 105:515–542, 1982.

Sacks, O. *The man who mistook his wife for a hat*. Pan Books Ltd. 1986.

Simone, D. A., et al. Identification of muscle afferents subserving sensation of deep pain in humans. J. Neurphysiol. 72:883–889, 1994.

Torebjörk, H. E., et al. Intraneural microstimulation in man. Its relation to specificity of tactile sensations. Brain 110:1509–1529, 1987.

Vallbo, B., et al. Somatosensory, proprioceptive and autonomic activity in human peripheral nerves. Physiol. Rev. 59:919–957, 1979.

The Spinal Cord and Somatosensory Pathways

Albe-Fessard, D., et al. Diencephalic mechanisms of pain sensation. Brain Res. Brain Res. Rev. 9:217–296, 1985.

Brown, A. G. *Organization in the spinal cord. The anatomy and physiology of identified neurones*. Springer-Verlag, 1981.

Cooper, B. Y., et al. Finger movement deficits in the stumptail macaque following lesions if the fasciculus cuenatus. Somatosens. Motor. Res. 10:17–29, 1993.

Foerster, O. The dermatomes in man. Brain 56:1–40, 1933.

Giesler, G. J., et al. Direct spinal pathways to the limbic system for nociceptive information. Trends Neurosci. 17:244–250, 1994.

Glendenning, D. S., and Vierck, Jr., C. J. Lack of proprioceptive deficit after dorsal column lesions in monkeys. Neurology 43:363–366, 1993.

Gordon, G. *Active Touch. The mechanism of recognition of objects by manipulation. A multi-disciplinary approach.* Pergamon Press, 1978.

Groenewegen, H. J., and Berendse, H. W. The specificity of the "nonspecific" midline and intralaminar thalamic nuclei. Trends Neurosci. 17:52–57, 1994.

Keegan, J. J., and Garret, F. D. The segmental distribution of cutaneous nerves in the limbs of man. Anat. Rec. 102:409–437, 1948.

Laidlaw, R. W., et al. The occurrence of dissociated disturbances of pallesthesia and kinesthesia. Bull. Neurol. Inst. N.Y. 7:303–320, 1938.

Liguori, R., et al. Determination of the segmental sensory and motor innervation of the lumbosacral spinal nerves. An electrophysiological study. Brain 115:915–934, 1992.

Levine, J. D. et al. Peptides and the primary afferent nociceptor. J. Neurosci. 13:2273–2286, 1993.

Macchi, G. et al. *Somatosensory integration in the thalamus.* Elsevier, 1990.

Maxwell, D. J., and.Rethelyi, M. Ultrastructure and synaptic connections of cutaneous afferent fibres in the spinal cord. Trends Neurosci. 10:117–123, 1987.

Nathan, P. W., et al. Sensory effects in man of lesions of the posterior columns and of some other afferent pathways. Brain 109:1003–1041, 1986.

Ralston, H. J., and Ralston, D. D. Medial lemniscal and spinal projections to the macaque thalamus: An electron microscopic study of differing GABAergic circuitry serving thalamic somatosensory mechanisms. J. Neurosci. 14:2485–2502, 1994.

Stevens, R. T., et al. Spinothalamocortical projections to the secondary somatosensory cortex (SII) in squirrel monkey. Brain Res. 631:241–246, 1993.

Todd, A. J., and Spike, R. C. The localization of classical transmitters and neuropeptides within neurons in laminae I-III of the mammalian spinal dorsal horn. Prog. Neurobiol. 41:609–645, 1993.

Urban, L., et al. Modulation of spinal excitability: Co-operation between neurokinin and excitatory amino acid neurotransmitters. Trends Neurosci. 17:432–438, 1994.

Somatosensory Cortical Areas

Caselli, R. Ventrolateral and dorsomedial somatosensory association cortex damage produces distinct soemsthetic syndromes in humans. Neurology 43:762–771, 1993.

DiPiero, V., et al. cerebral blood flow study in tonic pain activation in man. Pain 56:167–173, 1994.

Cohen, L. G., and Starr, A. Localization, timing and specificity of gating of somatosensory evoked potentials during active movement in man. Brain 110:451–467.

Darian-Smith, D., et al. Ipsilateral cortical projections to area 3a, 3b, and 4 in the macaque monkey. J. Comp. Neurol. 335:200–213, 1993.

Hari, R., et al. Functional organization of the human first and second somatosensory cortices: A neuromagnetic study. Eur. J. Neurosci. 5:724–734, 1993.

Pavlides, C., et al. Projection from the sensory to the motor cortex is important in learning motor skills in the monkey. J. Neurophysiol. 70:733–741, 1993.

Schneider, R. J. A modality-specific somatosensory area within the insula of the rhesus monkey. Brain Res. 621:116–120, 1993.

Van Buren, J. M. Sensory responses from stimulation of the inferior Rolandic and Sylvian regions in man. J. Neurosurg. 59:119–130, 1983.

Woolsey, C. N. Organization of somatic sensory and motor areas of the cerebral cortex. In: *Biological and biochemical bases of behavior.* Harlow, H. F. and Woolsey, C. N., eds. University of Wisconsin Press, 1958, pp 63–81.

Pain

Beric, A. Central pain: "New" syndromes and their evaluation. Muscle & Nerve 16:1017–1024, 1993.

Besson, J.-M., et al. *Thalamus and pain.* Excerpta Medica, 1987.

Brownstein, M.J. A brief history of opiates, opioid peptides, and opioid receptors. Proc. Natl. Acad. Sci. USA 90:5391–5393, 1993.

Carrive, P. The periaqueductal gray and defensive behavior: functional representation and neuronal organization. Behav. Brain Res. 58:27–47, 1993.

Devor, M. Pain mechanisms. The Neuroscientist 2:233–244, 1996.

Dougherty, P.M., et al. Combined application of excitatory amino acids and substance P produces long-lasting changes in responses of primate spinothalamic tract neurons. Brain Res. Rev. 18:227–246, 1993.

Fitzgerald, M. Monoamines and descending control of nociception. Trends Neurosci. 9:51–52, 1986.

Gamsa, A. The role of psychological factors in chronic pain. II. A critical appraisal. Pain 57:17–29, 1994.

Gybels, J.M., and Sweet, W.H. *Neurosurgical treatment of persistent pain. Physiological and pathological mechanisms of human pain.* Karger, 1989.

Koltzenburg, M., and McMahon, S. B. The enigmatic role of the sympathetic nervous system in chronic pain. Trends Pharm. Sci. 12:399–402, 1991.

Mansour, A., et al. Anatomy of CNS opioid receptors. Trends Neurosci. 11:308–314, 1988.

Mense, S. Nociception from skeletal muscle in relation to clinical muscle pain. Pain 54:241–289, 1993.

Marchettini, P. Muscle pain: animal and human experimental and clinical studies. Muscle Nerve 16:1033–1039, 1993.

Padawer, W. J., and Levine, F. M. Exercise-induced analgesia: Fact or artifact? Pain 48:131–135, 1992.

Reynolds, D. V. Surgery in the rat during electrical analgesia induced by focal brain stimulation. Science 164:444–445, 1969.

Roberts, W. J., and Foglesong, M. E. Spinal recordings suggest that wide-dynamic-range neurons mediate sympathetically maintained pain. Pain 34:298–304, 1988.

Schaible, H.-G., and Grubb, B. D. Afferent and spinal mechanisms of joint pain. Pain 55:5–54, 1993.

Turner, J. A., et al. The importance of placebo effects in pain treatment and research. JAMA 271:1609–1614, 1994.

Wall, P.D. Pain and the placebo response. In: *Experimental and theoretical studies of consciousness*, (Ciba Found. Symp. 174) Wiley, 1993, pp 187–216.

Wall, P. D., and McMahon, S. B. The relationship of perceived pain to afferent nerve impulses. Trends Neurosci. 9:254–255, 1986.

Wall, P.D., and Melzack, R. *Textbook of pain.* 2nd ed. Churchill Livingstone, 1988.

Woolf, J., and Doubell, T. P. The pathophysiology of chronic pain—increased sensitivity to low threshold Aβ-fibre inputs. Curr. Opin. Neurobiol. 4:525–534, 1994.

Chapter 8

Albright, T. D. Why do things look as they do? Trends Neurosci. 17:175–177, 1994.

Allison, T., et al. Face recognition in human extrastriate cortex. J. Neurophysiol. 71:821–825, 1994.

Daw, N. W., et al. Rod pathways in mammalian retina. Trends Neurosci. 13:110–115, 1990.

Desimone, R., and Duncan, J. Neural mechanisms of selective visual attention. Annu. Rev. Neurosci. 18:193–222, 1995.

Dowling, J. *The retina: An approachable part of the brain.* Harvard University Press, 1987.

Goodale, M. A., and Milner, A. D. Separate visual pathways for perception and action. Trends Neurosci. 15:20–25, 1992.

Holmes, G. Disturbancies of vision by cerebral lesions. In: *Selected papers of Gordon Holmes*, Phillips, C. G., ed. Chap. 6. Oxford University Press, 1979, pp 337–367.

Hubel, D., and Wiesel, T. Receptive fields, binocular interaction and functional architecture in the cat's visual cortex. J. Physiol. 160:106–154, 1962.

Kaas, J. H. Why does the brain have so many visual areas? J. Cogn. Neurosci. 1:121–135, 1989.

Livingston, M. S., and Hubel, D. H. Psychophysical evidence for separate channels for the perception of form, color, movement, and depth. J. Neurosci. 7:3416–3468, 1987.

Logothetis, N. K., and Sheinberg, D. L. Visual object recognition. Annu. Rev. Neurosci. 19:577–621, 1996.

Malach, R. et al. Relationship between intrinsic connections and functional architecture revealed by optical imaging and *in vivo* targeted biocytin injections in primate striate cortex. Proc. Natl. Acad. Sci. USA 90:10469–10473, 1993.

Martin, K. A. C. From enzymes to visual perception: A bridge too far? Trends Neurosci. 11:280–387, 1988.

Merigan, W. H., and Maunsell, J. H. R. How parallell are the primate visual pathways? Annu. Rev. Neurosci. 16:369–402, 1993.

Mora, B. M., et al. In vivo functional localization of the human visual cortex using positron emission tomography and magnetic resonance imaging. Trends Neurosci. 12:282–284, 1989.

Nealey,T. A., and Maunsell, J. H. R. Magnocellular and parvocellular contributions to the responses of neurons in macaque striate cortex. J. Neurosci 14:2069–2079, 1994.

Peterhans, E., and von der Heydt, R. Subjective contours—bridging the gap between psychophysics and physiology. Trends Neurosci. 14:112–119, 1991.

Roland, P. E., and Gulyás, B. Visual imagery and visual representation. Trends Neurosci. 17:281–287, 1994.

Schiller, P. H. The ON and OFF channels of the visual system. Trends Neurosci. 15:86–92, 1992.

Shapley, R., and Perry, V. H. Cat and monkey retinal ganglion cells and their visual functional roles. Trends Neurosci. 9:229–235, 1986.

van Essen, D. C. Functional organization of primate visual cortex. In: *Cerebral Cortex*, Vol. 3. Peters, A., and Jones, E. G., Eds. Plenum Press, 1985.

Van Essen, D. C., and Gallant, J. L. Neural mechanisms of form and motion processing in the primate visual system. Neuron 13:1–10, 1994.

Wilson, F. A. W., et al. Dissociation of object and spatial domains in primate prefrontal cortex. Science 260:1055–1958, 1993.

Zeki, S. *A vision of the brain*. Backwell Scientific Publications, 1993.

Chapter 9

Ashmore, J. F., and Kolston, P. J. Hair cell based amplification in the cochlea. Curr. Opin. Neurobiol. 4:503–508, 1994.

Bisiach, E., et al. Disorders of perceived auditory lateralization after lesions of the right hemisphere. Brain 107:37–52, 1984.

Brainard, M. S. Neural substrates of sound localization. Curr. Opin. Neurobiol. 4:557–562, 1994.

Corwin, J. T., and Warchol, M. E. Auditory hair cells: Structure, function, development and regeneration. Annu. Rev. Neurosci. 14:301–333, 1991.

Creutzfeldt, O., et al. *Hearing mechanisms and speech*. Springer-Verlag, 1979.

Edelman, G. M., et al. *Auditory function. Neurobiological bases of hearing*. John Wiley & Sons, 1988.

Ehret, G., and Romand, R. *The central auditory system*. Oxford University Press, 1997.

Hirsh, I. J., and Watson, C. S. Auditory psychophysics and perception. Annu. Rev. Psychol. 47:461–484, 1996.

Loeb, G. E. Cochlear prosthesics. Annu. Rev. Neurosci. 13:357–371, 1990.

Masterton, R.B. Role of the central auditory system in hearing: the new direction. Trends Neurosci. 15:280–285, 1992.

Miller, S. L., et al. Speech and other central auditory processes: Insights from cognitive neuroscience. Curr. Opin. Neurobiol. 5:198–204, 1995.

Penfield, W., and Perot, P. The brain's record of auditory and visual experience. Brain 86:596–696, 1963.

Pickles, J. O. *An introduction to the physiology of hearing*, 2nd ed. Academic Press, 1988.

Tanaka, Y., et al. "So-called" cortical deafness. Brain 114:2385–2401, 1991.

Chapter 10

Arnholt, R. R. H. Molecular neurobiology of olfaction. Crit. Rev. Neurobiol. 7:1–22, 1993.

Barbas, H. Organization of cortical afferent input to orbitofrontal areas in the rhesus monkey. Neuroscience 56:841–864, 1993.

Carr, W. E. S., et al. The role of perireceptor events in chemosensory processes. Trends Neurosci. 13:212–215, 1990.

DeVries, S. H., Baylor, D. A. Synaptic circuitry of the retina and olfactory bulb. Neuron 10 Suppl:139–149, 1993.

Dionne, V. E. How do you smell? Principle in question. Trends Neurosci. 11:188–199, 1988.

Finger, T. E., and Silver, W. L. *Neurobiology of taste and smell.* John Wiley & Sons, 1987.

Gilbertson, T.A. The physiology of vertebrate taste reception. Curr. Opin. Neurobiol. 3:532–539, 1993

Haberly, L. B., and Bower, J. M. Olfactory cortex: Model circuit for study of associative memory. Trends Neurosci. 12:258–264, 1989.

Hudson, R. Olfactory imprinting. Curr. Opin. Neurobiol. 3:548–552, 1993

Kauer, J. S. Contributions of topography and parallel processing to odor coding in the vertebrate olfactory pathway. Trends Neurosci. 14:79–85, 1991.

Kinnamon, S. C. Taste transduction: A diversity of mechanisms. Trends Neurosci. 11: 491–496, 1988.

Margolis, F. L., and Getchel, T. V. *Molecular neurobiology of the olfactory system: Molecular, membranous, and cytological studies.* Plenum Press, 1988.

Margolskee, R.F. The biochemistry and molecular biology of taste transduction. Curr. Opin. Neurobiol. 3:526–531, 1993.

Price, J. L. Olfactory system. In Paxinos, G.: *The human nervous system*, Chapter 29. Academic Press, 1990, pp 979–998.

Richardson, J. T. E., and Zucco, G. M. Cognition and olfaction: A review. Psychol. Bull. 105:352–360, 1989.

Ressler, K. J., et al. A molecular dissection of spatial patterning in the olfactory system. Curr. Opin. Neurobiol. 4:588–596, 1994.

Ronnett, G.V., and Payne, R. A tale of two senses. Neuron 15:11–16, 1995.

Roper, S. D. The cell biology of vertebrate taste receptors. Annu. Rev. Neurosci. 12:329–354, 1989.

Travers, J. B., et al. Gustatory neural processing in the hindbrain. Annu. Rev. Neurosci. 10;595–632, 1987.

Trombley, P. Q., and Shepherd, G. M. Synaptic transmission and modulation in the olfactory bulb. Curr. Opin. Neurobiol. 3:540–547, 1993.

Chapter 11

Basmajian, J. V. *Muscles alive. Their functions revealed by electromyography*, 5th ed. Williams & Wilkins, 1985.

Bennett, D.J. Stretch reflex responses in the human elbow joint during a voluntary movement. J. Physiol. 474:339–351, 1994.

Brushart, T.M.E. Motor axons preferentially reinnervate motor pathways. J. Neurosci. 13:2730–2738, 1993.

Cody, F. J. W., et al. Observations on the genesis of the stretch reflex in Parkinsons' disease. Brain 109:229–249, 1986.

Cody, F. J. W., et al. Stretch and vibration reflexes of wrist flexor muscles in spasticity. Brain 110:433–450, 1987.

Corcos, D. M., et al. Movement deficits caused by hyperexcitable stretch reflexes in spastic humans. Brain 109:1043–1058, 1986.

Fawcett, J. W., and Keynes, R. J. Peripheral nerve regeneration. Annu. Rev. Neurosci. 13:43–60, 1990.

Fellows, S. J., et al. Changes in the short- and long-latency stretch reflex components of the triceps surae muscle during ischaemia in man. J. Physiol. 472:737–748, 1993.

Fitzpatrick, R. C., et al. Ankle stiffness of standing humans in response to imperceptible perturbation: reflex and task-dependent components. J. Physiol. 454:533–547, 1992.

Futagi, Y., et al. Primitive reflex profiles in infants: differences based on categories of neurological abnormality. Brain Dev. 14:294–298, 1992.

Granit, R. *The basis of motor control. Integrating the activity of muscles, alpha and gamma motoneurons and their leading control system.* Academic Press, 1970.

Hammond, P. H. The influence of prior instruction to the subject on an apparently involuntary neuromuscular response. J. Physiol. (Lond.) 132:17–18P, 1956.

Henneman, E., et al. Rank order of motoneurons within a pool: Law of combination. J. Neurophysiol. 37:1338–1349, 1974.

Horowits, R. Passive force generation and titin isoforms in mammalian skeletal muscle. Biophys. J. 61:392–398, 1992.

Jenny, A. B., and Inukai, J. Principles of motor organization of the monkey cervical spinal cord. J. Neurosci. 3:567–575, 1983.

Lacquaniti, F., et al. Transient reversal of the stretch reflex in human arm muscles. J. Neurophysiol. 66:939–954, 1991.

Liddell, E. G. T. *The discovery of reflexes.* Oxford University Press, 1960.

Macefield, V. G., et al. The contribution of transcortical pathways to long-latency stretch and tactile reflexes in human hand muscles. Exp. Brain Res. 108:147–154, 1996.

Marsden, C. D., et al. Stretch reflex and servo action in a variety of human muscles. J. Physiol. (Lond.) 259:531–560, 1976.

Matthews, P. B. C. Muscle spindles and their motor control. Physiol. Rev. 44:219–288, 1964. Matthews, P. B. C. The human stretch reflex and the motor cortex. Trends Neurosci. 14:87–91, 1991.

Navarrete, R., and Vrbová, G. Activity-dependent interactions between motoneurones and muscles: their role in the development of the motor unit. Prog. Neurobiol. 41:93–124, 1993.

Piehl, F., et al. Calcitonin gene-related petide-like immunoreactivity in motoneuron pools innervating different hind limb muscles in the rat. Exp. Brain Res. 96:291–303, 1993.

Rafuse, V. F., et al. Proportional enlargement of motor units after partial denervation of cat triceps surae muscles. J. Neurophysiol. 68:1261–1276, 1992.

Sherrington, C. S. *The integrative action of the brain.* Cambridge University Press, 1947.

Stein, R. B., et al. Analysis of short-latency reflexes in human elbow flexor muscles. J. Neurophysiol. 73:1900–1911, 1995.

Swash, M., et al. Focal loss of anterior horn cells in the cervical cord in motor neuron disease. Brain 109:939–952, 1986.

Van der Meché, F. G. A., and Van Gijn, J. Hypotonia: An erronous clinical concept? Brain 109:1169–1178, 1986.

Chapter 12

Amblard, B. Visuo-vestibular integration in the development of posture and gait. Arch. Ital. Biol. 134:249–276, 1996.

Armstrong, D. M. The supraspinal control of mammalian locomotion. J. Physiol. 405:1–37, 1988.

Asanuma, H. *The motor cortex.* Raven Press, 1989.

Bennett, K. M. B., and Lemon, R. N. Corticomotoneuronal contribution to the fractionation of muscle activity during precision grip in the monkey. J. Neurophysiol. 75:1826–1842, 1996.

Brooks, V. B. *The neural basis of motor control.* Oxford University Press, 1986.

Danek, A., et al. Tracing of neuronal connections in the human brain by magnetic resonance imaging *in vivo.* Eur. J. Neurosci. 2:112–115, 1990.

Deiber, M. P., et al. Cerebral structures participating in motor preparation in humans: A positron emission tomography study. J. Neurophysiol. 75:233–247, 1996.

Englander, R.N. et al. The location of human pyramidal tract in the internal capsule: Anatomic evidence. Neurology 25:823–826, 1975.

Foerster, O. Motorische Felder und Bahnen. Hdb. d. Neurol. 6:1–448, 1936.

Goodwin, A. W., and Darian-Smith, I. *Hand function and the neocortex.* Springer Verlag, 1985.

Georgopoulos, A. P. New concepts in generation of movement. Neuron 13:257–268, 1994.

Glendenning, D. S. The effect of fasciculus cuneatus lesions on finger positioning and long-latencey reflexes in monkeys. Exp. Brain Res. 93:104–116, 1993.

Grillner, S. Neural networks for vertebrate locomotion. Sci. Am. 274:64–69, 1996.

Halsband, U. et al. The role of the premotor cortex and the supplementary motor area in the temporal control of movement in man. Brain 116:243–266, 1993.

He, S.-Q., et al. Topographic organization of corticospinal projections from the frontal lobe: Motor areas on the lateral surface of the hemisphere. J. Neurosci. 13:952–980, 1993.

Ibrahim, I. K., et al. Stretch-induced electromyographic activity and torque in spastic elbow muscles. Brain 116:971–989, 1993.

Jacobs, B. L., and Fornal, C. A. 5–HT and motor control: A hypothesis. Trends Neurosci. 16:346–352, 1993.

Jeannerod, M. *The neural and behavioural organization of goal-directed movements*. Oxford University Press, 1988.

Keller, A. Intrinsic synaptic organization of the motor cortex. Cereb. Cortex 3:430–441, 1993.

Kennedy, P. R. Corticospinal, rubrospinal and rubro-olivary projections: A unifying hypothesis. Trends Neurosci. 13:474–478, 1990.

Monrad-Krohn, G. H. *The clinical examination of the nervous system*, 10th ed. H. K. Lewis & Co., 1954.

Nathan, P.W. et al. The corticospinal tracts in man. Course and location of fibres at different segmental levels. Brain 113:303–324, 1990.

Paus, T. et al. Role of the human anterior cingulate cortex in the control of oculomotor, manual, and speech responses: A positron emission tomography study. J. Neurophysiol. 70:453–469, 1993.

Phillips, C. G. *Movements of the hand*. Liverpool University Press, 1986.

Phillips, C. G., and Porter, R. *Corticospinal neurones*. Their role in movement. Academic Press, 1977.

Picard, N., and Strick, P. L. Motor areas of the medial wall: A review of their location and functional activation. Cereb. Cortex 6:342–253, 1996.

Prochazka, A. Sensorimotor gain control: A basic strategy of motor systems? Prog. Neurobiol. 33:281–307, 1989.

Quinn, N., and Jenner, P. *Disorders of movement. Clinical, pharmacological and physiological aspects*. Academic Press, 1989.

Ralston, D. D., and Ralston, H. J. III. The terminations of corticospinal tract axons in the macaque monkey. J. Comp. Neurol. 242:325–337, 1985.

Ropper, A. H., et al. Pyramidal infarction in the medulla: A cause of pure motor hemiplegia sparing the face. Neurology 29:91–95, 1979.

Schieber, M. H. How might the motor cortex individuate movements? Trends Neurosci. 13:440–445, 1990.

Sinkjær, T., et al. Non-reflex and reflex mediated ankle joint stiffness in multiple sclerosis patients with spasticity. Muscle Nerve 16:69–76, 1993.

Sherrington, C. S. *The integrative action of the brain*. Cambridge University Press, 1947.

Sjölund, B., and Björklund, A. *Brain stem control of spinal mechanisms*. Elsevier, 1982.

Tanji, J. The supplementary motor area in the cerebral cortex. Neurosci. Res. 19:251–268, 1994.

Wilson, S. A., et al. Transcranial magnetic stimulation mapping of the motor cortex in normal subjects. The representation of two intrinsic hand muscles. J. Neurol. Sci. 118:134–144, 1993.

Woolsey, C. N. Organization of somatic sensory and motor areas of the cerebral cortex. In: *Biological and biochemical bases of behavior*. Harlow, H. F., and Woolsey, C. N., eds. University of Wisconsin Press, 1958.

Chapter 13

Albin, R. L., et al. The functional anatomy of basal ganglia disorders. Trends Neurosci. 12:366–375, 1989.

Alexander, G. E., et al. Parallel organization of functionally segregated circuits linking basal ganglia and cortex. Annu. Rev. Neurosci. 9:357–381, 1986.

Alheid, G.F., et al. Basal ganglia. In: *The human nervous system*. Paxinos, G., ed. Academic Press, Inc. 1990, pp 483–582.

Brandt, J., and Butters, N. The neuropsychology of Huntington's disease. Trends Neurosci. 9:118–120, 1986.

Brown, R. G., and Marsden, C. D. Cognitive function in Parkinson's disease: From description to theory. Trends Neurosci. 13:21–29, 1990.

Chevalier, G., and Deniau, J. M. Disinhibition as a basic process in the expression of striatal functions. Trends Neurosci. 13:277–280, 1990.

Di Chiara, G., et al. Modulatory functions of neurotransmitters in the striatum: Ach/dopamine/NMDA interactions. Trends Neurosci. 17:228–233, 1994.

Defer, G.L., et al. Long-term outcome of unilaterally transplanted Parkinsonian patients. 1. Clinical approach. Brain 119(1):41–50, 1996.

Ellison, G. Stimulant-indiced psychosis, the dopamine theory of schizophrenia, and the habenula. Brain Res. Brain Res. Rev. 19:223–239, 1994.

Flaherty, A. W., and Graybiel, A. M. Input-output organization of the sensorimotor striatum in the squirrel monkey. J. Neurosci. 14:599–610, 1994.

Gerfen, C. R. The neostriatal mosaic: multiple levels of compartmental organization. Trends Neurosci. 15:133–138, 1992.

Groenewegen, H. J., et al. Organization of the output of the ventral striatopallidal system in the rat: Ventral pallidal afferents. Neuroscience 57:113–142, 1993.

Hallett, M. Physiology of basal ganglia disorders: An overview. Can. J. Neurol. Sci. 20:177–183, 1993.

Hattori, T. Conceptual history of the nigrostriatal dopamine system. Neurosci. Res. 16:239–262, 1993.

Holloway, M. Rx for addiction. Sci. Am. 264:70–79, 1991.

Jellinger, K. A. Pathology of Parkinson's disease. Changes other than the nigrostriatal pathway. Mol. Chem. Neuropathol. 14:153–197, 1991.

Nestler, E. J., et al. Drug addiction: A model for the molecular basis of neural plasticity. Neuron 11:995–1006, 1993.

Parent, A., Hazrati, L.-N. Anatomical aspects of information processing in primate basal ganglia. Trends Neurosci. 16:111–116, 1993.

Paulson, H.L., and Fischbeck, K.H. Trinucleotide repeats in neurogenetic disorders. Annu. Rev. Neurosci. 19:79–107, 1996.

Sacks, O. *Awakenings.* Picador, 1990.

Sacks, O. *The man who mistook his wife for a hat.* Chapter 10: Witty Ticcy Ray. Pan Books Ltd., 1986.

Sawle, G. V., Myers, R. The role of positron tomography in the asessment of human transplantation. Trends Neurosci. 16:172–176, 1993.

Selemon, L. D., et al. Islands an striosomes in the neostriatum of the rhesus monkey: Nonequivalent compartments. Neuroscience 58:183–192, 1994.

Surmeier, D. J., et al. Are neostriatal dopamine receptors co-localized? Trends Neurosci. 16:299–305, 1993.

White, F. J. Synaptic regulation of mesocorticolimbic dopamine neurons. Annu. Rev. Neurosci. 19:405–436, 1996.

Wichmann, T., et al. The primate subthalamic nucleus. I. Functional properties in intact animals. J. Neurophysiol. 72:494–506, 1994.

Wise, R. A. Neurobiology of addiction. Curr. Opin. Neurobiol. 6:243–251, 1996.

Chapter 14

Akshoomoff, N. A., and Courchesne, E. A new role for the cerebellum in cognitive operations. Behav. Neurosci. 106:731–738, 1992.

Brodal, P., and Bjaalie, J. G. Organization of the pontine nuclei. Neurosci. Res. 13:83–118, 1992.

Brooks, V.B. *The neural basis of motor control.* Oxford University Press, 1986.

Deuschl, G., et al. Adaptation motor learning of arm movements in patients with cerebellar disease. J. Neurol. Neurosurg. Psychiatry 60:515–519, 1996.

Dow, R. S., and Moruzzi, G. *The physiology and pathology of the cerebellum.* The University of Minnesota Press, 1958.

Eccles, J. C., et al. *The cerebellum as a neuronal machine.* Springer-Verlag, 1967.

Fiez, J.A. Cerebellar contributions to cognition. Neuron 16:13–15, 1996.

Holmes, G. The cerebellum. In: *Selected papers of Gordon Holmes.* Phillips, C.G.. ed. Chapter 5. Oxford University Press, 1979, pp 186–247.

Gorassani, M., et al. Cerebellar ataxia and muscle spindle sensitivity. J. Neurophysiol. 70:1853–1862, 1993.

Ito, M. *The cerebellum and neural control.* Raven Press, New York, 1984.

Ito, M. The cellular basis of cerebellar plasticity. Curr. Opin. Neurobiol. 1:616–620, 1991.

Jahnsen, H. Electrophysiological characteristics of neurones in the guinea-pig deep cerebellar nuclei *in vitro*. J. Physiol. 372:129–147, 1986.

Jueptner, M., et al. Localization of a cerebellar timing process using PET. Neurology 45:1540–1545, 1995.

Keele, S. W., and Ivry, R. Does the cerebellum provide a common computation for diverse tasks? Ann. N. Y. Acad. Sci. 608:179–207, 1990.

Kim, S.-G., et al. Activation of a cerebellar output nucleus during cognitive processing. Science 265:949–951, 1994.

King, J. S. *New concepts in cerebellar neurobiology*. Alan R. Liss Inc., 1987.

Leiner, H. C., et al. The human cerebro-cerebellar system: its computing, cognitive, and language skills. Behav. Brain Res. 44:113–128, 1991.

Lisberger, S. G. Neural basis for motor learning in the vestibuloocular reflex of primates. J. Neurophysiol. 72:974–998, 1994.

Llinás, R., and Welsh, J. P. On the cerebellum and motor learning. Curr. Opin. Neurobiol. 3:958–965, 1993.

Llinás, R., and Sugimori, M. The electrophysiology of the cerebellar purkinje cell revisited. In: *The cerebellum revisited*: Llinás, R., and Sotelo, C., eds. Springer 1992, pp 167–181.

Müller, F., and Dichgans, J. Dyscoordination of pinch and lift forces during grasp in patients with cerebellar lesions. Exp. Brain Res. 101:485–492, 1994.

Optican, L. M., and Robinson, D. A. Cerebellar-dependent adaptive control of primate saccadic system. J. Neurophysiol. 44:1058–1076, 1980.

Osborn, C. E., and Poppele, R. E. Sensory integration by the dorsal spinocerebellar tract circuitry. Neuroscience 54:945–956,1993.

Pascual-Leone, A., et al. Procedural learning in Parkinson's disease and cerebellar degeneration. Ann. Neurol. 34:594–602, 1993.

Paulin, M. G. The role of the cerebellum in motor control and perception. Brain Behav. Evol. 41:39–50, 1993.

Raymond, J. L., et al. The cerebellum: a neuronal learning machine? Science 272:1126–1131, 1996.

Thatch, T. The cerebellum and the adaptive coordination of movement. Annu. Rev. Neurosci. 15:403–442, 1992.

Thach, T., et al. Cerebellar output: multiple maps and modes of control in movement coordination. In: *The cerebellum revisited*. Llinas, R., and Sotelo, C., eds. Springer, 1992, pp 283–300.

Welsh, J. P., and Harvey, J. A. The role of the cerebellum in voluntary and reflexive movements: history and current status. In: *The cerebellum revisited*. Llinás, R., and Sotelo, C., eds. Springer, 1992, pp. 301–334.

Wiesendanger, R., and Wiesendanger, M. Cerebello-cortical linkage in the monkey as revealed by transcellular labeling with the lectin wheat germ agglutinin conjugated to the marker horseradish peroxidase. Exp. Brain Res. 59:105–117, 1985.

Chapter 15

Aldrich, M. S. Narcolepsy. Neurology 42 Suppl 6:34–43, 1992.

Barlow, J. S. The electroencephalogram: its patterns and origins. MIT Press, 1993.

Berridge, C. W., Foote, S. L. Effects of locus coeruleus activation on electroencephalographic activity in neocortex and hippocampus. J. Neurosci. 11:3135–3145, 1991.

Brodal, A. *The reticular formation of the brain stem. Anatomical aspects and functional correlations.* Oliver and Boyd, 1957.

Driver, J., and Mattingley, J. B. Selective attention in humans: Normality and pathology. Curr. Opin. Neurobiol. 5:191–197, 1995.

Fields, H. L. Neural mechanisms of opiate analgesia. In: *Advances in pain research and therapy*, Vol. 9. Fields, H. L., et al., eds. Raven Press, 1985, pp 479–486.

Foote, S. L., and Morrison, J. H. Extrathalamic modulation of cortical function. Annu. Rev. Neurosci. 10:67–95, 1987.

Gazzaniga, M. S. Brain mechanisms and conscious experience. In: *Experimental and theoretical studies of consciousness*. John Wiley & Sons (Ciba Foundation Symposium 174), 1993, pp 247–262.

Grantyn, A., et al.Tracing premotor brain stem networks of orienting movements. Curr. Opin. Neurobiol. 3:973–981, 1993.

Hobson, J. A. Sleep and dreaming: Induction and mediation of REM sleep by cholinergic mechanisms. Curr. Opin. Neurobiol. 2:759–763, 1992.

Jordan, L. M., et al. Control of functional systems in the brainstem and spinal cord. Curr. Opin. Neurobiol. 2:794–801, 1992.

Lagercrantz, H. Neuromodulators and respiratory control during development. Trends Neurosci. 10:368–372, 1987.

Mancia, M. One possible function of sleep: To produce dreams. Behav. Brain Res. 69:203–206, 1995.

Martin, G. F. et al. Reticular formation of the pons and medulla. In: *The human nervous system*. Paxinos, G., ed. Academic Press, Inc.1990, pp 203–220.

McGinty, D., and Szymusiak, R. Keeping cool: A hypothesis about the mechanisms and fucntions of slow-wave sleep. Trends Neurosci. 13:480–487, 1990.

Miller, K. W. Are lipids or proteins the target of general anaesthetic action? Trends Neurosci. 9:49–51, 1986.

Moruzzi, G., and Magoun, H. W. Brain stem reticular formation and activation of the EEG. Electroenceph. Clin. Neurophysiol. 1:455–473, 1949.

Müller, C. M., et al. Structures mediating cholinergic reticular facilitation of cortical structures in the cat: Effects of lesions in immunocytochemically characterized projections. Exp. Brain Res. 96:8–18, 1993.

Plazzi, G., et al. Pontine lesions in idiopathic narcolepsy. Neurology 46:1250–1254, 1996.

Richter, D. W. et al. Mechanisms of respiratory rhythm generation. Curr. Opin. Neurobiol. 2:788–793, 1992.

Saper, C. B. Function of the locus coeruleus. Trends Neurosci. 10:343–344, 1987.

Scheibel, M. E., and Scheibel, A. B. structural substrates for integrative patterns in the brain stem reticular core. In: *Reticular formation of the brain*, Jasper, H. H., et al., eds. Little Brown, 1958, pp 31–55.

Siegel, J. M., and Rogawski, M. A. A function of REM sleep: Regulation of noradrenergic receptor sensitivity. Brain Res. Rev. 13:213–233, 1988.

Sjölund, B., and Björklund, A. *Brain stem control of spinal mechanisms*. Elsevier, 1982.

Steriade, M. Thalamocortical oscillations in the sleeping and aroused brain. Science 262:679–685, 1993.

Steriade, M. Central core modulation of spontaneous oscillations and sensory transmission in thalamocortical systems. Curr. Opin. Neurobiol. 3:619–625, 1993.

Searle, J. R. The problem of consciousness. In: *Experimental and theoretical studies of consciousness*. John Wiley & Sons (Ciba Found. Symp. 174), 1993, pp. 61–80.

Winson, J. The meaning of dreams. Sci. Am. 263:42–48, 1990.

Chapter 16

Amarenco, P., and Hauw, J.-J. Cerebellar infarction in the territory of the anterior and inferior cerebellar artery. Brain 113:139–155, 1990.

Andersen, R. A., et al. Evidence for the lateral intraparietal area as the parietal eye field. Curr. Opin. Neurobiol. 2:840–846, 1992.

Brodal, A. *The cranial nerves. Anatomy and anatomico-clinical correlations*, 2nd ed. Munksgaard, 1967.

Büttner-Ennever, J. A. *Neuroanatomy of the oculomotor system*. Elsevier, 1988.

Carpenter, R. H. S. *Movements of the eyes*, 2nd ed. Pion Limited, 1988.

Dean, P., Redgrave, P., and Westby, G. V. M. Event or emergency? Two systems in the mammalian superior colliculus. Trends Neurosci. 12:137–147, 1989.

Gaymard, B., et al. Smooth pursuit eye movement deficits after pontine nuclei lesions in humans. J. Neurol. Neurosurg. Psychiatry 56:799–807, 1993.

Grüsser, O.-J., et al. Cortical representation of head-in-space movement and same psychophysical experiments on head movement. In: *The head-neck sensory motor system*, Berthoz, A., et al., eds. Oxford University Press, 1992, pp. 497–509.

Keller, E. L., and Heinen, S. J. Generation of smooth-pursuit eye movements: Neuronal mechanisms and pathways. Neurosci. Res. 11:79–107, 1991.

Kennard, C., and Clifford Rose, F. *Physiological aspects of clinical neuro-ophthalmology*. Chapman and Hall Medical, 1988.

Knox, A. P., et al. The central connections of the vagus nerve in the ferret. Brain Res. Bull. 33:49–63, 1994.

Latto, R. The role of the inferior parietal cortex and the frontal eye-fields in visuospatial discriminations in the macaque monkey. Behav. Brain Res. 22:41–52, 1986.

Lee, B. H., et al. Calcitonin gene-related peptide in nucleus ambiguus motoneurons in rat: Viscerotopic organization. J. Comp. Neurol. 320:531–543, 1992.

Lewis, R. F., et al. Extraocular muscle proprioception functions in control of ocular alignment and eye movement conjugacy. J. Neurophysiol. 72:1028–1031, 1994.

Lindeman, H. H. Anatomy of the Otolith organs. Adv. Oto-Rhino-Laryng. 20:405–433, 1973.

Lisberger, S. G., et al. Visual motion processing and sensory-motor integration of smooth pursuit eye movements. Annu. Rev. Neurosci. 10:97–129, 1987.

Monrad-Krohn, G. H. *The clinical examination of the nervous system*, 10th ed. H. K. Lewis & Co., 1954.

Moschovakis, A. K., and Highstein, S. M. The anatomy and physiology of primate neurons that control rapid eye movements. Annu. Rev. Neurosci. 17:465–488, 1994.

Mumenthaler, M. *Neurologie*, 6th ed. Thieme Verlag, 1979.

Petit, L., et al. Functional neuroanatomy of the human visual fixation system. Eur. J. Neurosci. 7:169–174, 1995.

Pickles, J. O., and Corey, D. P. Mechanoelectrical transduction by hair cells. Trends Neurosci. 15:254–259, 1992.

Samii, M., and Janetta, P. J. *The cranial nerves. Anatomy, pathology, pathophysiology, diagnosis, treatment.* Springer-Verlag, 1981.

Sparks, D. L., and Mays, L. Signal transformations required for the generation of saccadic eye movements. Annu. Rev. Neurosci. 13:309–336, 1990.

Stanton, G. B., et al. Topography of projections to posterior cortical areas from the macaque frontal eye fields. J. Comp. Neurol. 353:291–305, 1995.

Strominger, N. L., et al. The connectivity of the area postrema in the ferret. Brain Res. Bull. 33:33–47, 1994.

Waterston, J. A., et al. A quantitative study of eye and head movements during smooth pursuit in patients with cerebellar disease. Brain 115:1343–1358, 1992.

Wilson, V. J., and Melvill Jones, G. *Mammalian vesitbular physiology*. Plenum Press, 1979.

Chapter 17

Andersson, K.-E., and Sjögren, C. Aspects of the physiology and pharmacology of the bladder and urethra. Prog. Neurobiol. 19:71–89, 1982.

Appel, N. M., and Elde, R. P. The intermediolateral cell column of the thoracic spinal cord is comprised of target-specific subnuclei: Evidence from retrograde transport studies and immunohistochemistry. J. Neurosci. 8:1767–1775, 1988.

Appenzeller, O. *The autonomic nervous system. An introduction to basic and clinical concepts.* Elsevier, 1990.

Bell, C. *Novel peripheral neurotransmitters.* International encyclopedia of pharmacology and therapeutics. Section 135. Pergamon Press, 1991.

Berkley, K. J., et al. Responses of neurons in and near the thalamic ventrobasal complex of the rat to stimulation of uterus, cervix, vagina, colon, and skin. J. Neurophysiol. 69:557–568, 1993.

Bernard, J. F., et al. The parabrachial area: electrophysiological evidence for an involvement in visceral nociceptive processes. J. Neurophysiol. 71:1660–1664, 1994.

Berntson, G. G., et al. Autonomic space and psychophysical response. Psychophysiology 31:44–61, 1994.

Burnstock, G. The changing face of autonomic neurotransmission. Acta Physiol. Scand. 126:67–91, 1986.

Cervero, F. Visceral pain: mechanisms of peripheral and central sensitization. Ann. Med. 27:235–239, 1995.

Cervero, F., and Sharkey, K. A. More than just gut feelings about visceral sensation. Trends Neurosci. 8:188–190, 1985.

Creazzo, T., et al. Neural regulation of the heart. A model for modulation of voltage-sensitive channels and regulation of cellular metabolism by neurotransmitters. Trends Neurosci. 6:430–433, 1983.

Elfvin, L.-G., et al. The chemical neuroanatomy of sympathetic ganglia. Annu. Rev. Neurosci. 16:471–504, 1993.

Fugère, F., and Lewis, G. Coeliac plexus block for chronic pain syndromes. Can. J. Anaesth. 40:954–963, 1993.

Furness, J. B., et al. Roles of peptides in transmission in the enteric nervous system. Trends Neurosci. 15:66–71, 1992.

Hakusui, S., et al. Postprandial hypotension: Microneurographic analysis and treatment with vasopressin. Neurology 41:712–715, 1991.

Hirst, G. D. S., and Edwards, F. R. Sympathetic neuroeffector transmission in arteries and arterioles. Physiol. Rev. 69:546–604, 1989.

Jänig, W. Spinal visceal afferents, sympathetic nervous system and referred pain. In: *New trends in referred pain and hyperalgesia*. Vecchiet, L., et al., eds. Elsevier 1993, pp. 83–98.

Jänig, W., and McLachlan, E. M. Characteristics of function-specific pathways in the sympathetic nervous system. Trends Neurosci. 15:475–481, 1992.

Gabella, G. *Structure of the autonomic nervous system*. Chapman and Hall, 1976.

Goyal, R. J., and Hirano, I. The enteric nervous system. N. Engl. J. Med. 334:1106–1115, 1996.

Gybels, J. M., and Sweet, W. H. Neurosurgical treatment of persistent pain. Physiological and pathological mechanisms of human pain. Karger, 1989.

Haymaker, W., and Woodhall, B. *Peripheral nerve injuries. Principles of diagnosis*. W. B. Saunders, 1945.

Laskey, W., and Polosa, C. Characteristics of the sympathetic preganglionic neuron and its synaptic input. Prog. Neurobiol. 31:47–84, 1988.

Loewy, A. D., and Spyer, K. M. *Central regulation of autonomic functions*. Oxford University Press, 1990.

Mathias, C. J. Orthostatic hypotension: Causes, mechanisms, and influencing factors. Neurology 45 Suppl. 5:S6–S11, 1995.

Miolan, J. P., and Niel, J. P. The mammalian sympathetic prevertebral ganglia: Integrative properties and role in the nervous control of digestive tract motility. J. Auton. Nerv. Syst. 58:125–138, 1996.

Pick, J. *The autonomic nervous system. Morphological, comparative, clinical and surgical aspects*. Lippincott, 1970.

Pyner, S., and Coote, J. H. Evidence that sympathetic preganglionic neurones are arranged in target-specific columns in the thoracic spinal cord of the rat. J. Comp. Neurol. 342:15–22, 1994.

Schott, G. D. Visceral afferents: Their contribution to "sympathetic dependent" pain. Brain 117:397–413, 1994.

Simmons, M. A. The complexity and diversity of synaptic transmission in the prevertebral sympathetic ganglia. Prog. Neurobiol. 24:43–93, 1985.

Treede, R.-D., et al. The plasticity of cutaneous hyperalgesia during sympathetic ganglion blockade in patients with neuropathic pain. Brain 115:607–621, 1992.

Wallin, B. G., et al. Coherence between the sympathetic drives to relaxed and contracting muscles of different limbs of human subjects. J. Physiol. 455:219–233, 1992.

Wood, J. D. Application of classification schemes to the enteric nervous system. J. Auton. Nerv. Syst. 48:17–19, 1994.

Wallin, B. G., and Fagius, J. The sympathetic nervous system in man—aspects derived from microelectrode recordings. Trends Neurosci. 9:63–67, 1986.

Chapter 18

Arnold, A. P., and Gorski, R. A. Gonadal steroid induction of structural sex differences in the central nervous system. Annu. Rev. Neurosci. 7:413–442, 1984.

Bloom, F. E. Intrinsic regulatory systems of the brain. In: *Handbook of Physiology*. Section 1: The nervous system. American Physiological Society, 1986.

Breedlove, M. Regional sex differences in steroid accumulation in the nervous system. Trends Neurosci. 6:403–406, 1983.

Cassone, V. M. Effects of melatonin on vertebrate circadian systems. Trends Neurosci. 13:457–464, 1990.

Ciriello, J., et al. *Organization of the autonomic nervous system: Central and peripheral mechanisms.* Alan R. Liss, 1987.

Clark, Le Gros W. E., et al. *The hypothalamus. Morphological, functional, clinical, and surgical aspects.* Oliver and Boyd, 1936.

Cohen, S., and Herbert, T. B. Health psychology: Psychological factors and physical disease from the perspective of human psychoneuroimmunology. Annu. Rev. Psychol. 47:113–142, 1996.

Cooper, K. E. *Fever and antipyresis. The role of the nervous system.* Cambridge University Press, 1995.

Cross, B. A., and Leng, G. *The neurohypophysis: structure, function and control.* Progress in Brain Research, Vol. 60. Elsevier, 1983.

Bandler, R., and Shipley, M. T. Columnar organization in the midbrain periaqueductal gray: Modules for emotional expression? Trends Neurosci. 17:379–389, 1994.

DeVoogd, T. J. Androgens can affect the morphology of mammalian CNS neurons in adulthood. Trends Neurosci. 10:341–342, 1987.

Ericsson, A., et al. A functional anatomical analysis of central pathways subserving effects of interleukin-1 on stress-related neuroendocrine neurons. J. Neurosci. 14:897–913, 1994.

Felten, D. L. Direct innervation of lymphoid organs: substrate for neurotransmitter signaling of cells of the immune system. Neuropsychobiology 28:110–112, 1993.

Ganten, D., and Pfaff, D. *Central cardiovascular control. Basic and clinical aspects.* Curr Top Neuroendocrinol, Vol. 3. Springer-Verlag, 1985.

Ganten, D., and Pfaff, D. *Actions of progesterone on the brain.* Curr Top Neuroendocrinol, Vol. 4. Springer-Verlag, 1985.

Ganten, D., and Pfaff, D. *Morphology of Hypothalamus and its connections.* Curr Top Neuroendocrinol, Vol. 7. Springer-Verlag, 1986.

Giesler,G.J ., et al. Direct spinal pathways to the limbic system for nociceptive information. Trends Neurosci. 17:244–250, 1994.

Hori, T., et al. The autonomic nervous system as a communication channel between the brain and the immune system. Neuroimmunomodulation 2:203–215, 1995.

Kellner, R. Psychosomatic syndromes, somatization and somatoform disorders. Psychother. Psychosom. 61:4–24, 1994.

Kluger, M. J., et al. Cytokines and fever. Neuroimmunomodulation 2:216–223, 1995.

Lagercrantz, H. Neuromodulators and respiratory control during development. Trends Neurosci. 10:368–372, 1987.

LeVay, S. *The sexual brain.* The MIT Press, 1993.

Madden, K. S., et al. Sympathetic nervous system modulation of the immune system. J. Neuroimmunol. 49:77–87, 1994.

Morin, L. P. The circadian visual system. Brain Res. Brain Res. Rev. 67:102–127, 1994.

Marazziti, D., et al. Immune cell imbalance in major depressive and panic disorders. Neuropsychobiology 26:23–26, 1992.

Miller, M. J., and Bell, G. I. JAK/STAT eats the fat. Trends Neurosci. 19:159–161, 1996.

Mtui, E. P., et al. Medullary visceral reflex circuits: Local afferents to nucleus tractus solitarii synthesize catecholamines and project to thoracic spinal cord. J. Comp. Neurol. 351:5–26, 1995.

Plata-Salamán, C.R. Immunoregulators in the nervous system. Neurosci. Behav. Rev. 15:185–215, 1991.

Raine, C. S. *Advances in Neuroimmunology.* New York Academy of Sciences, 1988.

Toates, F. *Stress. Conceptual and biological aspects.* John Wiley & Sons, 1995.

Rinner, I., and Schauenstein, K. The parasympathetic nervous system takes part in the immunoneuroendocrine dialogue. J. Neuroimmunol 34:165–172, 1991.

Rusak, B., and Bina, K. G. Neurotransmitters in the mammalian circadian system. Annu. Rev. Neurosci. 13:397–401, 1990.

Schwaab, D. F., et al. Functional neuroanatomy and neuropathology of the human hypothalamus. Anat. Embryol. 187:317–330, 1993.

Smith, O., and DeVito, J. L. Central neural integration for the control of autonomic responses associated with emotion. Annu. Rev. Neurosci. 7:43–65, 1984.

Swanson, L. W. The neural basis of motivated behavior. Acta Morphol. Neerl.-Scand. 26:165–176, 1989.

Ursin, H., and Olff, M. Psychobiology of coping and defence strategies. Neuropsychobiology 28:66–71, 1993.

Zeisberger, E., and Roth, J. Neurobiological concepts of fever generation and suppression. Neuropsychobiology 28:106–109, 1993.

Yoshimura, F., andGorbman, A. *Pars distalis of the pituitary gland. Structure, function and regulation.* International congress series 673. Elsevier, 1986.

Chapter 19

Adolphs, R., et al.. Impaired recognition of emotion in facial expression following bilateral damage to the human amygdala. Nature 372:669–672, 1994.

Aggleton, J. The contribution of the amygdala to normal and abnormal emotional states. Trends Neurosci. 16:328–333, 1993.

Alheid, G. F., and Heimer, L. New perspectives in basal forebrain organization of special relevance for neuropsychiatric disorders: The striatopallidal, amygdaloid, and corticopetal components of substantia innominata. Neuroscience 27:1–39, 1988.

Amaral, D. G. Emerging principles of intrinsic hippocampal organization. Curr. Opin. Neurobiol. 3:225–229, 1993.

Andersen, P., et al. Lamellar organization of excitatory hippocampal pathways. Exp. Brain Res. 13:222–238, 1971.

Bancaud, J., et al. Anatomical origin of *déjà vu* and vivid 'memories' in human temporal lobe epilepsy. Brain 117:71–90, 1994.

Bernard, J. F., et al. Nucleus centralis of the amygdala and the globus pallidus ventralis: electrophysiological evidence for an involvement in pain processes. J. Neurophysiol. 68:551–569, 1992.

Chan-Palay, V., and Köhler, C. *The hippocampus. New vistas.* Alan R. Liss Inc., 1989.

Changeux, J.-P. *The neural and molecular bases of learning.* John Wiley & Sons, 1987.

Cohen, N. J., and Eichenbaum, H. *Memory, amnesia, and the hippocampal system.* The MIT Press, 1993.

Courtney, S.M., et al. Object and spatial visual working memory activate separate neural systems in human cortex. Cereb Cortex 6:39–49, 1996.

Damasio, A. R., and Tranel, D. Knowledge systems. Curr. Opin. Neurobiol. 2:186–190, 1992.

Davis, M., et al. Neurotransmission in the rat amygdala related to fear and anxiety. Trends Neurosci. 17:208–214, 1994.

Doane, B.K., and Livingston, K.E. *The limbic system. Functional organization and clinical disorders.* Raven Press, 1985.

Drevet, W.C., et al. A functional anatomical study of unipolar depression. J. Neurosci. 12:3628–3641, 1992.

Dudai, Y. *The neurobiology of memory. Concepts, findings, trends.* Oxford University Press, 1989.

Eichenbaum, H., Otto,T. LTP and memory: Can we enhance the connection? Trends Neurosci. 16:163–164, 1993.

Ekman, P. Expression and the nature of emotion. In: *Approaches to emotion.* Scherer, K.R., and Ekman, P., L., eds. Erlbaum 1984.

Everitt, B. J., et al. The basolateral amygdala-ventral striatal system and conditioned place preference: Further evidence of limbic-striatal interactions underlying reward-related processes. Neuroscience 42:1–18, 1991.

Fisher, R. S. Animal models of the epilepsies. Brain Res. Brain Res. Rev. 14:245–278, 1989.

Gaffan, D., and Gaffan, E. A. Amnesia in man following transection of the fornix. Brain 114:2611–2618, 1991.

Grossman, S. P. Behavioral functions of the septum: A re-analysis. In: *The septal nuclei,* Plenum Press, 1976, pp 361–422.

Heilig, M., et al. Corticotropin-releasing factor and neuropeptide Y: Role in emotional integration. Trends Neurosci. 17:80–85, 1994.

Heimburger, R. F., et al. Stereotactic amygdalotomy for convulsive and behavioral disorders. Appl. Neurophysiol. 41:43–51, 1978.

Isaacson, R. L. *The limbic system.* 2nd ed. Plenum Press, 1982.

Jacobson, R. Disorders of facial recognition, social behaviour and affect after combined bilateral amygdalotomy and subcaudate tractotomy—a clinical and experimental study. Psychol. Med. 16:439–450, 1986.

Kuhar, M. J. Neuroanatomical substrates of anxiety: a brief survey. Trends Neurosci. 9:307–310, 1986.

Laitinen, L. V., and Livingston, K. E. *Surgical approaches in psychiatry.* University Park Press, 1973.

Morris, M. K., et al. Amnesia following a discrete basal forebrain lesion. Brain 115:1827–1847, 1992.

Murray, E. A. What have ablation studies told us about the neural substrates of stimulus memory? Sem. Neurosci. 8:13–22, 1996.

Narabayashi, H., et al. Stereotactic amygdalectomy for behavior disorders. Arch. Neurol. 9:11–26, 1963.

O'Keefe, J., and Nadel, L. *The hippocampus as a cognitive map.* Clarendon Press 1978.

Perani, D., et al. Evidence of multiple memory systems in the human brain. Brain 116:903–919, 1993.

Rosenzweig, M.R. Aspects of the search for neural mechanisms of memory. Annu. Rev. Psychol. 47:1–32, 1996.

Scoville, W. B., and Milner, B. Loss of recent memory after bilateral hippocampal lesions. J. Neurol. Neurosurg. Psychiatry 20:11–21, 1957.

Shaikh, M. B., et al. Basal amygdaloid facilitation of midbrain periaqueductal gray elicited defensive rage behavior in the cat mediated trough NMDA receptors. Brain Res. 635:187–195, 1994.

LeDoux, J. E. Brain mechanisms of emotion and emotional learning. Curr. Opin. Neurobiol. 2:191–197, 1992.

LeDoux, J. E. The amygdala: Contributions to fear and stress. Semin. Neurosci. 6:231–237, 1994.

Sakai,K., and Miyashita, Y. Memory and imagery in the temporal lobe. Curr. Opin. Neurobiol. 3:166–170, 1993.

Shallice, T. *From neuropsychology to mental structure.* Cambridge University Press, 1988.

Squire, L. R. *Memory and brain.* Oxford University Press, 1987.

Suzuki, W. Neuroanatomy of the monkey entorhinal, perirhinal and parahippocampal cortices: Organization of cortical inputs and interconnections with amygdala and striatum. Semin. Neurosci. 8:3–12, 1996.

Wilson, F.A.W. The relationship between learning, memory and neuronal responses in the primate basal forebrain. In: *The basal forebrain: Anatomy to function.* Napier,T. C. et al. eds. Plenum Press, 1992, pp. 1–13.

Zola-Morgan, S., et al. Human amnesia and the medial temporal region: Enduring memory impairment following a bilateral lesion limited to field CA1 of the hippocampus. J. Neurosci. 6:2950–2967, 1986.

Zola-Morgan, S., and Squire, L. R. Neuroanatomy of memory. Annu. Rev. Neurosci. 16:547–563, 1993.

Chapter 20

Structure and Function

Barlow, H. The mechanical mind. Annu. Rev. Neurosci. 13:15–24, 1990.

Bear,M. F., and Kirkwood, A. Neocortical long-term potentiation. Curr. Opin. Neurobiol. 3:197–202, 1993.

Bentivoglio, M., and Sperafico, R. *Cellular thalamic mechanisms.* Excepta Medica, 1988.

Bolz, J., et al. Pharmacological analysis of cortical circuitry. Trends Neurosci. 12:292–296, 1989.

Bressler, S. L. The gamma wave: A cortical information carrier? Trends Neurosci. 13:161–162, 1990.

Brodmann, K. Vergleichende *Lokalisationslehre der Grosshirnrinde.* J. A. Barth, 1909.

Connor, B. W., and Gutnik, M. J. Intrinsic firing patterns of diverse neocortical neurons. Trends Neurosci. 13:99–104, 1990.

Creutzfeldt, O. D. *Cortex Cerebri.* Oxford Science Publications, 1995.

Foote, S. L., and Morrison, J. H. Extrathalamic modulation of cortical function. Annu. Rev. Neurosci. 10:67–95, 1987.

Gilbert, C. D. Horizontal integration and cortical dynamics. Neuron 9:1–13, 1992.

Hornung, J.-P., and De Tribolet, N. Distribution of GABA-containing neurons in human frontal cortex: A quantitative immunocytochemical study. Anat. Embryol. 189:139–145, 1994.

Groenewegen, H. J., and Berendse, H. W. The specificity of the 'nonspecific' midline and intralaminar thalamic nuclei. Trends Neurosci. 17:52–57, 1994.

Gutnick, M. J. The *cortical neuron.* Oxford University Press, 1995.

Jones, E. G. The *thalamus.* Plenum Press, 1985.

Jones, E. G., and Peters, A. Functional properties of cortical cells. In: *Cerebral cortex,* Vol. 2. Plenum Press, 1984.

Lee Robinson, D., and Petersen, S.E. The pulvinar and visual salience. Trends Neurosci. 15:127–132, 1992.

Macchi, G., Rustioni, A., and Spreafico, R. *Somatosensory integration of the thalamus.* Elsevier, 1990.

McCormick, D. A., et al. Neurotransmitter control of neocortical neuronal activity and excitability. Cereb. Cortex 3:387–398, 1993.

Myers, R. E. Phylogenetic studies of commissural connexions. In: *Functions of the corpus callosum.* Ciba Foundation Study Group, No. 20, Churchill, 1965, pp 138–142.

Olesen, J., and Edvinsson, L. Migraine: A research field matured for the basic sciences. Trends Neurosci. 14:3–5, 1991.

Parnavelas, J. G., and Papadopolous, G. C. The monoaminergic innervation of the cerebral cortex is not diffuse and nonspecific. Trends Neurosci. 12:315–319, 1989.

Penfield, W., and Rasmussen, T. *The cerebral cortex of man.* Macmillan, 1950.

Peters, A. Morphological correlates of epilepsy: Cells in the cerebral cortex. In: *Antiepileptic drugs: Mechanisms of action.* Glaser, G. H., et al., eds. Raven Press, 1980, pp. 21–48.

Peters, A., and Jones, E. G. Cellular components of the cerebral cortex. In: *Cerebral cortex,* Vol. 1. Plenum Press, 1984.

Peters, A., and Jones, E. G. Development and maturation of cerebral cortex. In: *Cerebral cortex,* Vol. 7. Plenum Press, 1988.

Rakic, P., and Singer, W. *Neurobiology of neocortex.* John Wiley & Sons, 1988.

Searle, J. R. Is the brain's mind a computer program? Sci. Am. 262:20–25, 1990.

Swindale, N. V. Is the cerebral cortex modular? Trends Neurosci. 13:487–492, 1990.

Wall, J. T. Variable organization in cortical maps of the skin as an indication of the lifelong adaptive capacities of the circuits in the mammalian brain. Trends Neurosci. 11:549–558, 1988.

Association Areas

Critchley, M. *The parietal lobes.* Edward Arnold, 1953.

Damasio, A. R., et al. Face agnosia and the neural substrates of memory. Annu. Rev. Neurosci. 13:89–109, 1990.

Farah, M.J. Agnosia. Curr. Opin. Neurobiol. 2:162–164, 1992.

Fuster, J.M. Frontal lobes. Curr. Opin. Neurobiol. 3:160–165, 1993.

Fuster, J. *The prefrontal cortex. Anatomy, physiology, and neuropsychology of the frontal lobe,* 2nd ed. Raven Press, 1989.

Goldman-Rakic, P. S. Topography of cognition: Parallel and distributed networks in primate association cortex. Annu. Rev. Neurosci. 11:137–156, 1988.

Gross, C.G., et al. Inferior temporal cortex as a pattern recognition device. In: *Computational learning and cognition.* Baum, E., ed. 1993, pp. 44–73.

Hyvärinen, J. *The parietal cortex of monkey and man.* Springer-Verlag, 1982.

Jones,E. G., and Powell, T. P. S. An anatomical study of converging sensory pathways within the cerebral cortex of the monkey. Brain 93:793–820, 1970.

Linsker, R. Perceptual neural organization: Some approaches based on network models and information theory. Annu. Rev. Neurosci. 13:257–281, 1990.

Molchan, S. E., et al. A functional anatomical study of associative learning in humans. Proc. Natl. Acad. Sci. USA 91:8122–8126, 1994.

Pandya, D. N., and Selzer, B. Association areas of the cerebral cortex. Trends Neurosci. 5:386–390, 1982.

Petrides, M. Frontal lobes and behaviour. Curr. Opin. Neurobiol. 4:207–211, 1994.

Posner, M.I., and Dehaene, S. Attentional networks. Trends Neurosci. 17:75–79, 1994.

Rafal, R. D. Neglect. Curr. Opin. Neurobiol. 4:231–236, 1994.

Rauschecker, J. P., and Korte, M. Auditory compensation for early blindness in cat cerebral cortex. J. Neurosci. 13:4538–4548, 1993.

Sacks, O. *An anthropologist on Mars*. Picador, 1995.

Van Hoesen, G. The modern concept of association cortex. Curr. Opin. Neurobiol. 3:150–154, 1993.

Lateralization, Sex Differences, and Language

Aboitiz, F., et al. Morphometry of the sylvian fissure and the corpus callosum, with emphasis on sex differences. Brain 115:1521–1541, 1992.

Bates, E. Language development. Curr. Opin. Neurobiol. 2:180–185, 1992.

Benbow, C.P. Sex differences in mathematical reasoning ability in intellectually talented preadolescents: their nature, effects, and possible causes. Behav. Brain Sci. 11:169–232, 1988.

Biver, F., et al. Sex difference in $5HT_2$ receptor in the living human brain. Neurosci. Lett. 204:25–28, 1996.

Bleier, R., et al. Can the corpus callosum predict gender, handedness, or cognitive differences? Trends Neurosci. 9:391–394, 1986.

Brown, H. D., and Kosslyn, S. M. Cerebral lateralization. Curr. Opin. Neurobiol. 3:183–186, 1993.

Brust, J. C. M. Music and language. Musical alexia and agraphia. Brain 103:367–392, 1980.

Bryden, M. P., et al. Handedness is not related to self-reported disease incidence. Cortex 27:605–611, 1991.

Caramazza, A. Some aspects of language processing revealed through the analysis of acquired aphasia: The lexical system. Annu. Rev. Neurosci. 11:395–421, 1988.

Davidson, R. J., and Hugdahl, K. *Brain Asymmetry*. The MIT Press, 1995.

Damasio, A. R. Category-related recognition defects as a clue to the neural substrates of knowledge. Trends Neurosci. 13:95–98, 1990.

Démont, J.-F. et al. The anatomy of phonological and semantic processing in normal subjects. Brain 115:1753–1768, 1992.

Frackowiak, R. S. J. Functional mapping of verbal memory and language. Trends Neurosci. 17:109–114, 1994.

Galaburda, A.M.: Neurology of developmental dyslexia. Curr. Opin. Neurobiol. 3:237–242, 1993.

Geschwind, N., and Galaburda, A. M. *Cerebral lateralization. Biological mechanisms, associations and pathology*. MIT Press, 1986.

Glass, A. Individual differences in hemispheric specialization. Plenum Press, 1987.

Greenfield, P.M. Language, tools and brain: the ontogeny and phylogeny of hierarchially organized sequential behavior. Behav. Brain Sci. 14:531–595, 1991.

Hellige, J.B. *Hemispheric asymmetry: what's right and what's left*. Harvard University Press 1993.

Hinke, R.M., et al. Functional magnetic resonance imaging of Broca's area during internal speech. NeuroReport 4:675–678, 1993.

Howard, D., et al. The cortical localization of the lexicons. Positron emission tomography evidence. Brain 115:1769–1782, 1992.

Kim, S.-G., et al. Functional magnetic resonance imagin of motor cortex: Hemispheric asymmetry and handedness. Science 261:615–617, 1993.

Kimura, D. Sex, sexual orientation and sex hormones influence human cognitive function. Curr. Opin. Neurobiol. 6:259–263, 1996.

Lecours, A. R., et al. *Aphasiology*. Bailliere Tindall, 1983.

Lent, R., and Schmidt, S. L.The ontogenesis of the forebrain commissures and the determination of brain asymmetries. Progr. Neurobiol. 40:249–276, 1993.

Mehler, J., et al. Cross-linguistic approaches to speech processing. Curr. Opin. Neurobiol. 4:171–176, 1994.

Ottoson, D. *Duality and unity of the brain. Unified functioning and specialization of the hemispheres*. Plenum Press, 1987.

Penfield, W., and Roberts, L. *Speech and brain mechanisms.* Princeton University Press, 1959.

Petersen, S. E., and Fiez, J. A. The processing of single words studied with positron emission tomography. Annu. Rev. Neurosci. 16:509–530, 1993.

Poizner, H., et al. Biological foundations of language: Clues from sign language. Annu. Rev. Neurosci. 13:283–307, 1990.

Ross, E. D. Right hemisphere's role in language, affective behavior and emotion. Trends Neurosci. 7:342–346, 1984.

Sergent, J. Music, the brain and Ravel. Trends Neurosci. 16:168–172, 1993.

Sergent, J., et al. Distributed neural network underlying musical sight-reading and keyboard performance. Science 257:106–109, 1992.

Sperry, R. W. Lateral specialization in the surgically separated hemispheres. In: *The Neurosciences. Third study program*, Schmidt, F. O. and Worden, F. G., eds. MIT Press, 1974, pp 5–19.

Springer, S. P., and Deutsch, G. *Left brain, right brain.* Freeman, 1989.

Weiskrantz, L. *Thought without language.* Oxford University Press, 1988.

Woods, B. T. Is the left hemisphere specialized for language at birth? Trends Neurosci. 6:115–117, 1983.

The Cerebral Cortex and Mental Disease

Andreasen, N. C. Pieces of the schizophrenia puzzle fall into place. Neuron 16:697–700, 1996.

Goodwin, F. K. Neurobiology of manic-depressive illness. Clin. Neurosci. 1:157–162, 1993.

Henn, F. A. Animal models of depression. Clin. Neurosci. 1:152–156, 1993.

McEntee, W. J., and Mair, R. G. The Korsakoff syndrome: A neurochemical perspective. Trends Neurosci. 13:340–344, 1990.

Miller, R. Schizophrenia as a progressive disorder: Relation to EEG, CT, neuropathological and other evidence. Prog. Neurobiol. 33:17–44, 1989.

Reynolds, E. H., and Trimble, M. R. *The bridge between neurology and psychiatry.* Churchill Livingstone, 1989.

Roberts, G. W. Schizophrenia: The cellular biology of a functional psychosis. Trends Neurosci. 13:207–211, 1990.

Seeman, P., et al. Dopamine D4 receptors elevated in schizophrenia. Nature, 365:441–445, 1993.

van Ree, J. M., and Matthysse, S. Psychiatric disorders: Neurotransmitters and neuropepetides. Prog. Brain Res. 65:1–228, 1986.

Winn, P. Schizophrenia research moves to the prefrontal cortex. Trends Neurosci. 17:265–268, 1994.

Index

Italic numbers indicate figures; "n" following page numbers refers to "Note."